DATE DUE

MAY 0 9 2012

d

ꓶ

DSM-IV-TR **Casebook** and **Treatment Guide** for

Child
Mental Health

EDITED BY

CATHRYN A. GALANTER, M.D.

PETER S. JENSEN, M.D.

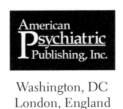

Washington, DC
London, England

If you would like to buy between 25 and 99 copies of this or any other APPI title, you are eligible for a 20% discount; please contact APPI Customer Service at appi@psych.org or 800-368-5777. If you wish to buy 100 or more copies of the same title, please e-mail us at bulksales@psych.org for a price quote.

Copyright © 2009 American Psychiatric Publishing, Inc.
ALL RIGHTS RESERVED

Manufactured in the United States of America on acid-free paper
13   12   11   10   09   5   4   3   2   1
First Edition

Typeset in Adobe Electra and ITC Highlander.

American Psychiatric Publishing, Inc.
1000 Wilson Boulevard
Arlington, VA 22209-3901
www.appi.org

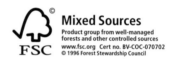

Mixed Sources
Product group from well-managed forests and other controlled sources
www.fsc.org Cert no. BV-COC-070702
© 1996 Forest Stewardship Council

Library of Congress Cataloging-in-Publication Data
DSM-IV-TR casebook and treatment guide for child mental health / edited by Cathryn A. Galanter, Peter S. Jensen. — 1st ed.
  p. ; cm.
  Includes bibliographical references and index.
  ISBN 978-1-58562-310-5 (alk. paper)
  1. Child psychiatry—Case studies. I. Galanter, Cathryn A., 1968– II. Jensen, Peter S. III. Diagnostic and statistical manual of mental disorders.
  [DNLM: 1. Diagnostic and statistical manual of mental disorders. 4th ed., text revision. 2. Mental Disorders—diagnosis—Case Reports. 3. Adolescent.
4. Child. 5. Diagnosis, Differential—Case Reports. 6. Mental Disorders—therapy—Case Reports. WS 350 D811 2009]
  RJ499.D758 2009
  618.92'89—dc22

                                                              2008044429

British Library Cataloguing in Publication Data
A CIP record is available from the British Library.

Contents

Cathryn A. Galanter, M.D.
Peter S. Jensen, M.D.

Peter S. Jensen, M.D.
Cathryn A. Galanter, M.D.

Part I: Classic Cases

Peter S. Jensen, M.D.
Cathryn A. Galanter, M.D.

■ 1
Stephen P. Hinshaw, Ph.D.

William E. Pelham, Jr., Ph.D., A.B.P.P.
James Waxmonsky, M.D.

Laurence L. Greenhill, M.D.

Stephen P. Hinshaw, Ph.D.

Part II: Comorbid Complexity

Part III: Toughest Cases: Diagnostic and Treatment Dilemmas

Part IV: Kids in Crisis
Psychopathology in the Context
of Social Stressors

Part V: Diagnostic and Treatment Decision Making

■ **Contributors** ■

J. Stuart Ablon, Ph.D.
Associate Clinical Professor of Psychiatry, Harvard Medical School; Associate Director and Cofounder, Collaborative Problem Solving Institute, Department of Psychiatry, Massachusetts General Hospital, Boston, Massachusetts

Jean Addington, Ph.D.
Professor of Psychiatry, University of Toronto; Research Scientist, Director of Psychosocial Treatments, First Episode Psychosis Program, and Director or the PRIME Research Clinic, Centre for Addiction and Mental Health, Toronto, Ontario, Canada

Anne Marie Albano, Ph.D, A.B.P.P.
Associate Professor of Clinical Psychology, Division of Child and Adolescent Psychiatry, and Director, Columbia University Clinic for Anxiety and Related Disorders, Columbia University, New York, New York

L. Eugene Arnold, M.D., M.Ed.
Professor Emeritus of Psychiatry; Former Director, Division of Child and Adolescent Psychiatry; Former Vice Chair of Psychiatry; Interim Director, Nisonger Center of Excellence in Developmental Disabilities, The Ohio State University, Columbus, Ohio

Andrea Auther, Ph.D.
Assistant Director, Recognition and Prevention (RAP) Program, The Zucker Hillside Hospital, Glen Oaks, New York

Susan Bacalman, M.S.W.
The M.I.N.D. Institute (Medical Investigation of Neurodevelopmental Disorders Institute), University of California, Davis Medical Center, Sacramento, California

Gail A. Bernstein, M.D.
Head, Program in Child and Adolescent Anxiety and Mood Disorders; Endowed Professor in Child and Adolescent Anxiety Disorders, Division of Child and Adolescent Psychiatry, University of Minnesota Medical School, Minneapolis

Boris Birmaher, M.D.
Endowed Chair in Early-Onset Bipolar Disease and Professor of Psychiatry, University of Pittsburgh School of Medicine, Pittsburgh, Pennsylvania

Bruce Black, M.D.
Founder and Director, Comprehensive Psychiatric Associates, Wellesley, Massachusetts. Assistant Professor of Psychiatry, Tufts University School of Medicine, Boston, Massachusetts

Caroline Lewczyk Boxmeyer, Ph.D.
Research Scientist, Center for the Prevention of Youth Behavior Problems; Supervising Psychologist, Psychology Clinic, University of Alabama.University of Alabama, Tuscaloosa

David A. Brent, M.D.
Academic Chief of Child and Adolescent Psychiatry, Western Psychiatric Institute and Clinic; Professor of Child Psychiatry, Pediatrics, and Epidemiology; Endowed Chair of Suicide Studies, University of Pittsburgh School of Medicine, Pittsburgh, Pennsylvania

Oscar G. Bukstein, M.D., M.P.H.
Associate Professor of Psychiatry, University of Pittsburgh School of Medicine, Pittsburgh, Pennsylvania

John V. Campo, M.D.
Chief, Division of Child and Adolescent Psychiatry; Medical Director, Pediatric Behavioral Health; Professor of Clinical Psychiatry, The Ohio State University and Nationwide Children's Hospital, Columbus, Ohio

Gabrielle A. Carlson, M.D.
Professor of Psychiatry and Pediatrics and Director, Division of Child and Adolescent Psychiatry, State University of New York at Stony Brook

Bruce F. Chorpita, Ph.D.
Professor of Psychology, University of California, Los Angeles

Greg Clarke, Ph.D.
Kaiser Permanente Center for Health Research, Portland, Oregon

Barbara J. Coffey, M.D., M.S.
Director, Institute for Tourette and Tic Disorders, New York University Child Study Center; Associate Professor, Department of Child and Adolescent Psychiatry, New York University School of Medicine, New York, New York

Judith A. Cohen, M.D.
Medical Director, Center for Traumatic Stress in Children and Adolescents, Allegheny General Hospital, Pittsburgh, Pennsylvania

Christine A. Conelea, M.S.
Graduate Student, Clinical Psychology Doctoral Program, University of Wisconsin–Milwaukee

Cheryl M. Corcoran, M.D.
Florence Irving Assistant Professor of Clinical Psychiatry and Director of the Center of Prevention and Evaluation, Columbia University/New York State Psychiatric Institute, New York, New York

Barbara A. Cornblatt, Ph.D., M.B.A.
Professor of Psychiatry, Albert Einstein College of Medicine, Bronx, New York; Investigator, Feinstein Institute for Medical Research; Director, Recognition and Prevention Program, The Zucker Hillside Hospital, Glen Oaks, New York

Christoph U. Correll, M.D.
Medical Director, Recognition and Prevention Program, The Zucker Hillside Hospital, Glen Oaks, New York; Assistant Professor of Psychiatry and Behavioral Sciences, Albert Einstein College of Medicine, Bronx, New York

Sarah A. Crawley, M.A.
Doctoral Student in Clinical Psychology, Temple University, Philadelphia, Pennsylvania

Kathryn R. Cullen, M.D.
Assistant Professor, Child Psychiatry Division, Department of Psychiatry, University of Minnesota Medical School, Minneapolis, Minnesota

Lisa M. Cullins, M.D.
Corporate Medical Director, EMQ Children and Family Services, Campbell, California; Adjunct Assistant Clinical Professor of Psychiatry, University of California, San Francisco

Ronald E. Dahl, M.D.
Staunton Professor of Psychiatry and Pediatrics and Professor of Psychology, University of Pittsburgh, Pittsburgh, Pennsylvania

Tara L. Deliberto, B.S.
Laboratory Manager, Laboratory for Clinical and Developmental Research, Department of Psychology, Harvard University, Cambridge, Massachusetts

David R. DeMaso, M.D.
Professor of Psychiatry and Pediatrics, Harvard Medical School; Psychiatrist-in-Chief, Children's Hospital Boston, Boston, Massachusetts

Thomas A. Dixon, B.S.
Research Assistant, Children's Hospital of Philadelphia Mood and Anxiety Disorders Center, Philadelphia, Pennsylvania

Stacy S. Drury, M.D., Ph.D.
Assistant Professor, Department of Psychiatry and Neurology, Section of Child and Adolescent Psychiatry, Tulane University Medical Center, New Orleans, Louisiana

Helen Egger, M.D.
Assistant Professor, Center for Developmental Epidemiology, Department of Psychiatry and Behavioral Sciences, Duke University Medical Center; Clinical Director, Duke Preschool Psychiatric Clinic, Durham, North Carolina

Graham J. Emslie, M.D.
Professor, Charles E. and Sarah M. Seay Chair in Child Psychiatry, and Chief, Child and Adolescent Psychiatry Division, University of Texas Southwestern Medical Center at Dallas and Children's Medical Center of Dallas, Dallas, Texas

Jeffery N. Epstein, Ph.D.
Associate Professor of Pediatrics, Division of Behavioral Medicine and Clinical Psychology, Cincinnati Children's Hospital Medical Center; Department of Psychology, University of Cincinnati; Director, Cincinnati Children's Center for Attention Deficit Hyperactivity Disorder Cincinnati, Ohio

Christianne Esposito-Smythers, Ph.D.
Assistant Professor (Research), Department of Psychiatry and Human Behavior, Brown University; Training Faculty, Brown University Center for Alcohol and Addiction Studies, Providence, Rhode Island

Sheila M. Eyberg, Ph.D., A.B.P.P.
Distinguished Professor, Department of Clinical and Health Psychology, University of Florida, Gainesville, Florida

Robert L. Findling, M.D.
Rocco L. Motto, M.D. Chair of Child and Adolescent Psychiatry, Case Western Reserve University School of Medicine; Director, Division of Child and Adolescent Psychiatry, University Hospitals Case Medical Center, Cleveland, Ohio

E. Blake Finkelson, B.A.
Doctoral Student in Clinical Psychology, and Graduate Research Assistant, Children, Families and Cultures (CFC) Laboratory, Catholic University of America, Washington, D.C.

Mary A. Fristad, Ph.D., A.B.P.P.
Professor of Psychiatry and Psychology and Director of Research and Psychological Services, Division of Child and Adolescent Psychiatry, The Ohio State University, Columbus, Ohio

Jami M. Furr, M.A.
Doctoral Student in Clinical Psychology and Student Research Assistant, Child and Adolescent Anxiety Disorders Clinic, Temple University, Philadelphia, Pennsylvania

Cathryn A. Galanter, M.D.
Assistant Professor of Clinical Psychiatry, Division of Child and Adolescent Psychiatry, Columbia University/New York State Psychiatric Institute, New York, New York

Mary Kay Gill, R.N., M.S.N., J.D.
Program Coordinator of Course and Outcome for Bipolar Youth and Longitudinal Assessment of Manic Symptoms, Western Psychiatric Institute and Clinic, University of Pittsburgh Medical Center, Pittsburgh, Pennsylvania

Mary Margaret Gleason, M.D.
Assistant Professor, Department of Psychiatry and Human Behavior, Warren Alpert Medical School; Acting Associate Training Director for Child Psychiatry and Triple Board (Pediatrics, Psychiatry, Child Psychiatry) Training, Brown University, Providence, Rhode Island

Daniel A. Gorman, M.D., F.R.C.P.C.
Staff Psychiatrist, Neuropsychiatry Program, The Hospital for Sick Children; Assistant Professor, Department of Psychiatry, University of Toronto, Ontario, Canada

Ross W. Greene, Ph.D.
Associate Clinical Professor, Department of Psychiatry, Harvard Medical School; Founding Director, Collaborative Problem Solving Institute, Department of Psychiatry, Massachusetts General Hospital, Boston

Laurence L. Greenhill, M.D.
Ruane Professor of Psychiatry and Pediatric Psychopharmacology, Columbia University; Director, New York State Research Unit of Pediatric Psychopharmacology, New York State Psychiatric Institute; Attending and Consultant Physician, Disruptive Behavior Disorders Clinic, Columbia Presbyterian Medical Center, New York, New York

Angela S. Guarda, M.D.
Associate Professor of Psychiatry and Behavioral Sciences, Johns Hopkins School of Medicine, Baltimore, Maryland

Allison G. Harvey, Ph.D.
Associate Professor of Clinical Psychology and Director, Sleep and Psychological Disorders Laboratory, University of California, Berkeley

Robert L. Hendren, D.O.
Professor of Psychiatry, Executive Director, and Tsakopoulos-Vismara Chair of the M.I.N.D. Institute (Medical Investigation of Neurodevelopmental Disorders Institute); Chief of Child and Adolescent Psychiatry, University of California, Davis; President, American Academy of Child and Adolescent Psychiatry, 2007–2009

Scott W. Henggeler, Ph.D.
Professor of Psychiatry and Behavioral Sciences and Director, Family Services Research Center, Medical University of South Carolina, Charleston

Stephen P. Hinshaw, Ph.D.
Professor of Psychology and Chair, Department of Psychology, University of California, Berkeley

Brian L. Isakson, Ph.D.
Clinical Child Psychology Intern, Department of Psychiatry, University of New Mexico Health Science Center, Albuquerque

Peter S. Jensen, M.D.
President and Chief Executive Officer, REACH Institute (Resource for Advancing Children's Health), New York, New York

Paramjit T. Joshi, M.D.
Endowed Professor and Chair, Department of Psychiatry and Behavioral Sciences, Children's National Medical Center; Professor of Psychiatry, Department of Behavioral Sciences and Pediatrics, George Washington University School of Medicine, Washington, D.C.

Yifrah Kaminer, M.D., M.B.A.
Professor of Psychiatry, Department of Psychiatry and Alcohol Research Center; Codirector of Research, Division of Child and Adolescent Psychiatry, University of Connecticut Health Center, Farmington, Connecticut

Sandra J. Kaplan, M.D.
Director, Division of Trauma Psychiatry, North Shore University Hospital–The Zucker Hillside Hospital, Long Island Jewish Medical Center, Manhasset, New York; Professor of Psychiatry, New York University School of Medicine; Director, Adolescent Trauma Treatment Development Center, National Child Traumatic Stress Network, and of the Florence and Robert A. Rosen Center for Law Enforcement and Military Personnel and Their Families

Niranjan S. Karnik, M.D., Ph.D.
Assistant Adjunct Professor, Department of Psychiatry and Department of Anthropology, History and Social Medicine, University of California School of Medicine, San Francisco; Staff Psychiatrist, Palo Alto Medical Foundation, Fremont, California

Courtney Pierce Keeton, Ph.D.
Instructor of Psychiatry and Behavioral Sciences, Division of Child and Adolescent Psychiatry, Johns Hopkins Medical Institutions, Baltimore, Maryland

Philip C. Kendall, Ph.D., A.B.P.P.
Laura H. Carnell Professor of Psychology and Director, Child and Adolescent Anxiety Disorders Clinic, Temple University, Philadelphia, Pennsylvania

Clarice J. Kestenbaum, M.D.
Professor of Clinical Psychiatry and Director of Training Emerita, Division of Child and Adolescent Psychiatry, Columbia University College of Physicians and Surgeons, New York, New York

Dena A. Klein, Ph.D.
Staff Psychologist and Director, Child and Adolescent Psychological Assessment Service, Child Outpatinet Psychiatry Department and Adolescent Depression and Suicide Program, Montefiore Medical Center, Bronx, New York

Rachel G. Klein, Ph.D.
Fascitelli Family Professor of Child and Adolescent Psychiatry and Director, Institute for Anxiety and Mood Disorders, Child Study Center, New York University Langone Medical Center, New York, New York

Penelope Knapp, M.D.
Professor Emeritus of Psychiatry and Pediatrics, University of California Davis; Medical Director, California Department of Mental Health, Sacramento, California

Robert A. Kowatch, M.D., Ph.D.
Professor of Psychiatry and Pediatrics and Director of Psychiatry Research, Cincinnati Children's Hospital Medical Center, Cincinnati, Ohio

Harvey N. Kranzler, M.D.
Professor of Clinical Psychiatry and Director, Division of Child and Adolescent Psychiatry, Albert Einstein College of Medicine; Clinical Director, Bronx Children's Psychiatric Center, Bronx, New York

Christopher J. Kratochvil, M.D.
Professor, Department of Psychiatry; Graduate Faculty Member and Assistant Director, Psychopharmacology Research Consortium, University of Nebraska Medical Center, Omaha, Nebraska

Sanjiv Kumra, M.D., M.S.
Associate Professor of Psychiatry and Division Chief, Department of Child and Adolescent Psychiatry, University of Minnesota, Minneapolis, Minnesota

Joshua M. Langberg, Ph.D.
Assistant Professor, Center for ADHD, Cincinnati Children's Hospital Medical Center, Cincinnati, Ohio

Christopher M. Layne, Ph.D.
Director of Treatment and Intervention Development, University of California, Los Angeles/Duke National Center for Child Traumatic Stress, Los Angeles, California

Patricia K. Leebens, M.D.
Consulting Child and Adolescent Psychiatrist, Family and Children's Aid, Danbury, Connecticut; Assistant Clinical Professor of Child Psychiatry, Yale Child Study Center, New Haven and the University of Connecticut School of Medicine, Farmington, Connecticut

Daniel le Grange, Ph.D.
Associate Professor of Psychiatry, Department of Psychiatry, Section for Child and Adolescent Psychiatry; Director, Eating Disorders Program, The University of Chicago, Chicago, Illinois

Alicia F. Lieberman, Ph.D.
Irving B. Harris Endowed Chair of Infant Mental Health, Professor in Psychiatry, and Vice Chair for Academic Affairs, University of California, San Francisco; Director, Child Trauma Research Project, San Francisco General Hospital; Director, Early Trauma Treatment Network; and President (2008), Board of Zero to Three: The National Center for Infants, Toddlers and Families

John E. Lochman, Ph.D., A.B.P.P.
Professor and Doddridge Saxon Chairholder in Clinical Psychology, and Director, Center for Prevention of Youth Behavior Problems, The University of Alabama, Tuscaloosa, Alabama

Joan L. Luby, M.D.
Associate Professor of Psychiatry (Child) and Founder and Director, Early Emotional Development Program, Washington University School of Medicine, St. Louis, Missouri

Richard P. Malone, M.D.
Professor of Psychiatry, Drexel University College of Medicine, Philadelphia. Pennsylvania

Anthony P. Mannarino, Ph.D.
Director, Center for Traumatic Stress in Children and Adolescents; Vice President, Department of Psychiatry, Allegheny General Hospital, Pittsburgh, Pennsylvania; Professor of Psychiatry, Drexel University College of Medicine, Philadelphia, Pennsylvania

John S. March, M.D., M.P.H.
Professor of Psychiatry and Chief, Child and Adolescent Psychiatry, Duke University Medical Center, Durham, North Carolina

Carla E. Marin, M.S.
Doctoral Candidate in Life Span Developmental Science, Florida International University, Miami, Florida

Jon McClellan, M.D.
Professor, Department of Psychiatry and Behavioral Sciences, University of Washington, Seattle; Medical Director, Child Study and Treatment Center, Division of Mental Health, Washington State

Alec L. Miller, Psy.D.
Professor of Clinical Psychiatry and Behavioral Sciences, Chief of Child and Adolescent Psychology, Director of the Adolescent Depression and Suicide Program; and Associate Director of the Psychology Internship Training Program, Montefiore Medical Center/Albert Einstein College of Medicine, Bronx, New York

Jodi A. Mindell, Ph.D., C.B.S.M.
Professor of Psychology, Saint Joseph's University; Professor of Pediatrics, University of Pennsylvania School of Medicine, Philadelphia, Pennsylvania; Associate Director, Sleep Center at The Children's Hospital of Philadelphia

Robert Miranda, Jr., Ph.D.
Assistant Professor (Research), Department of Psychiatry and Human Behavior, Brown University, Providence, Rhode Island

David A. Mrazek, M.D., F.R.C.Psych.
Chair, Department of Psychiatry and Psychology, Mayo Clinic; Professor of Psychiatry and of Pediatrics, Mayo Clinic College of Medicine, Rochester, Minnesota

Matthew K. Nock, Ph.D.
John L. Loeb Associate Professor of the Social Sciences and Director, Laboratory for Clinical and Developmental Research, Department of Psychology, Harvard University, Cambridge, Massachusetts

Judith A. Owens, M.D., M.P.H., D'A.B.S.M.
Associate Professor of Pediatrics, Brown Medical School; Director, Pediatric Sleep Disorders Clinic, Hasbro Children's Hospital and the Learning, Attention, and Behavior Program, Rhode Island Hospital, Providence, Rhode Island

Mani Pavuluri, M.D., Ph.D.
Founding Director, Pediatric Mood Program, Center for Cognitive Medicine, University of Illinois, Chicago

William E. Pelham, Jr., Ph.D., A.B.P.P.
Distinguished Professor of Psychology, Pediatrics, and Psychiatry and Director, Center for Children and Families, State University of New York at Buffalo

Bradley S. Peterson, M.D.
Suzanne Crosby Murphy Professor in Pediatric Neuropsychiatry and Director of Magnetic Resonance Imaging Research, Department of Psychiatry, Columbia University/New York State Psychiatric Institute, New York, New York

Cynthia R. Pfeffer, M.D.
Professor of Psychiatry and Director, Childhood Bereavement Program, Weill Cornell Medical College, New York Presbyterian Hospital, White Plains, New York

John Piacentini, Ph.D., A.B.P.P.
Professor of Psychiatry and Biobehavioral Sciences, David Geffen School of Medicine; Director, Child OCD, Anxiety, and Tic Disorders Program, Semel Institute for Neuroscience and Human Behavior, University of California, Los Angeles

Daniel Pine, M.D.
Chief, Section on Development and Affective Neuroscience; Chief, Emotion and Development Branch; and Chief, Child and Adolescent Research, Mood and Anxiety Disorders Program, National Institute of Mental Health Intramural Research Program, Bethesda, Maryland

Nicole Powell, Ph.D, M.P.H.
Research Psychologist, Center for the Prevention of Youth Behavior Problems, The University of Alabama, Tuscaloosa

Frank W. Putnam, M.D.
Professor of Pediatrics and Psychiatry and Director, Mayerson Center for Safe and Healthy Children, Cincinnati Children's Hospital Medical Center, Cincinnati, Ohio

Judith L. Rapoport, M.D.
Chief, Child Psychiatry Branch, National Institute of Mental Health, Bethesda, Maryland

M. Jamila Reid, Ph.D.
Staff, Parenting Clinic and Affiliate Assistant Professor, Department of Psychology, University of Washington, Seattle

Mark A. Riddle, M.D.
Professor of Psychiatry and Pediatrics and Director, Division of Child and Adolescent Psychiatry, Johns Hopkins University School of Medicine; Vice President for Psychiatric Sciences, Kennedy Krieger Institute, Baltimore, Maryland

Paula Riggs, M.D.
Associate Professor of Psychiatry, University of Colorado School of Medicine, Denver, Colorado

Irwin N. Sandler, Ph.D.
Regents' Professor, Department of Psychology, and Director, Prevention Research Center for Families in Stress, Arizona State University, Tempe, Arizona

Lawrence Scahill, M.S.N., Ph.D.
Professor of Nursing and Child Psychiatry and Director, Research Unit on Pediatric Psychopharmacology, Child Study Center, Yale University School of Nursing, New Haven, Connecticut

Laura Schreibman, Ph.D.
Distinguished Professor of Psychology, University of California, San Diego, La Jolla, California

Wendy K. Silverman, Ph.D., A.B.P.P.
Professor of Psychology, Florida International University, Miami, Florida

Lacramioara Spetie, M.D.
Assistant Professor of Psychiatry, The Ohio State University, Columbus, Ohio

Kevin D. Stark, Ph.D.
Professor of Educational Psychology, University of Texas, Austin

Hans Steiner, Dr. med. univ., F.A.P.A., F.A.A.C.A.P., F.A.P.M.
Professor in Psychiatry and Behavioral Sciences, Child and Adolescent Psychiatry, and Human Development, Stanford University School of Medicine, Palo Alto, California

Susan E. Swedo, M.D.
Tenured Investigator, National Institute of Mental Health Intramural Research Program; Chief, Pediatrics and Developmental Neuropsychiatry Branch, National Institute of Mental Health, Bethesda, Maryland

Eva M. Szigethy, M.D., Ph.D.
Assistant Professor of Psychiatry and Pediatrics, University of Pittsburgh School of Medicine; Director, Medical Coping Clinic, Department of Gastroenterology, Children's Hospital of Pittsburgh, Pittsburgh, Pennsylvania

Julia W. Tossell, M.D.
Staff Clinician, Child Psychiatry Branch, National Institute of Mental Health, Bethesda, Maryland

Andrea M. Victor, Ph.D.
Assistant Professor, Child and Adolescent Anxiety and Mood Disorders Clinic, University of Minnesota Medical School, Minneapolis, Minnesota

Karen Dineen Wagner, M.D., Ph.D.
Marie B. Gale Professor and Vice Chair, Department of Psychiatry and Behavioral Sciences, and Director, Division of Child and Adolescent Psychiatry, University of Texas Medical Branch in Galveston

John T. Walkup, M.D.
Associate Professor of Psychiatry and Behavioral Sciences and Deputy Director, Division of Child and Adolescent Psychiatry, Johns Hopkins Medical Institutions, Baltimore, Maryland; Medical Director, Research Unit of Pediatric Psychopharmacology

B. Timothy Walsh, M.D.
Ruane Professor of Pediatric Psychopharmacology, Department of Psychiatry, College of Physicians and Surgeons, Columbia University, and Director, Division of Clinical Therapeutics, New York State Psychiatric Institute, New York, New York

Bruce Waslick, M.D.
Staff Child Psychiatrist, Division of Child Behavioral Health, Baystate Medical Center, Springfield, Massachusetts; Associate Professor of Psychiatry, Tufts University School of Medicine, Boston, Massachusetts

James Waxmonsky, M.D.
Faculty, Department of Psychiatry, State University of New York at Buffalo; Staff, Women and Children's Hospital of Buffalo, Buffalo, New York

Carolyn Webster-Stratton, Ph.D.
Professor and Director, Parenting Clinic, University of Washington, Seattle, Washington

Lynn M. Wegner, M.D., F.A.A.P.
Associate Clinical Professor and Director, Developmental/Behavioral Pediatrics Division, Department of Pediatrics, University of North Carolina at Chapel Hill School of Medicine, Chapel Hill, North Carolina

Elizabeth B. Weller, M.D.
Professor of Psychiatry and Pediatrics, University of Pennsylvania, Philadelphia, Pennsylvania

Ronald A. Weller, M.D.
Faculty, Departments of Psychiatry and of Neuroscience, University of Pennsylvania, Philadelphia

Karen C. Wells, Ph.D.
Associate Professor of Medical Psychology; Director, Family Studies Program and Clinic; and Director of Psychology Internship, Department of Psychiatry, Duke University Medical Center, Durham, North Carolina

Helen Nelson Willard, M.Ed., CCC-SLP
Private Practice, Cary, North Carolina

Jeffrey J. Wilson, M.D.
Assistant Professor of Clinical Psychiatry, Columbia University/New York State Psychiatric Institute, New York, New York

Nancy C. Winters, M.D.
Associate Professor, Department of Psychiatry, Division of Public Psychiatry, Oregon Health and Science University, Portland, Oregon; Chief Psychiatrist, Children's Mental Health and Addictions, State of Oregon

Sharlene A. Wolchik, Ph.D.
Professor, Department of Psychology, Arizona State University, Tempe, Arizona

Douglas W. Woods, Ph.D.
Associate Professor and Director of Clinical Training, University of Wisconsin–Milwaukee

Charles H. Zeanah, M.D.
Sellars Polchow Professor of Psychiatry and Vice Chair and Chief of Child and Adolescent Psychiatry, Tulane University School of Medicine, New Orleans, Louisiana

Alison Zisser, M.S.
Graduate Student, Department of Clinical and Health Psychology, University of Florida, Gainesville

■ Acknowledgments ■

We gratefully acknowledge the children, adolescents, and families that we have treated over the years. Their challenges and successes have inspired us; we hope that aspects of their experiences documented in this book will contribute to the improvement in assessment and treatment of others. We would like to thank Leigh Garrett Lyndon, Stephanie Hundt, and Lucine Petite for their administrative and editorial assistance. We would also like to thank Jim Rosenfeld for his careful reading of several of the chapters.

Cathryn would like to thank Marc Galanter, M.D., and Wynne Galanter, Ph.D., for their years of encouragement and very early exposure to the emotional and intellectual rewards of clinical care of children, adults, and families and research about mental health.

■ Preface ■

When we were approached by American Psychiatric Publishing, Inc., about writing *DSM-IV-TR Casebook and Treatment Guide for Child Mental Health*, we were very excited. Given our shared passion for working with other clinicians to improve mental health care provided to children, we saw this book as one tool that could help in that mission. In the United States, approximately 20% of children and adolescents have diagnosable mental health problems, and 11% of the population is significantly impaired (U.S. Department of Health and Human Services 1999). Of these children in need, 75%–80% do not receive specialty services, with a majority failing to receive any services at all. For example, young people who are in treatment for attention-deficit/hyperactivity disorder (ADHD), one of the best-studied conditions, may have received an inaccurate diagnosis (and likely are receiving inappropriate treatment; Jensen 2000), and among children correctly diagnosed with ADHD, most do not receive optimal treatment ("Moderators and Mediators of Treatment Response" 1999; MTA Cooperative Group 1999). The Institute of Medicine has estimated that across all of medicine, a 17-year lag exists from the time that researchers develop a new effective treatment to the point of its implementation in the community (Committee on Quality of Health Care in America 2001). In child mental health, these health care gaps appear to be even greater and are getting worse: in the 2001 Surgeon General's Conference on Children's Mental Health, David Satcher noted that unmet needs for child mental health services remain as high as they were 20 years ago and that child neuropsychiatric disorders will rise proportionately by half, to become one of the five most common causes of childhood morbidity and mortality across the world by 2020 (U.S. Department of Health and Human Services 2001).

We set out to write a book that would begin to address some of the challenges that clinicians face in diagnosing and treating children. In this book, we present 30 cases written by experts in the field to provide readers with realistic examples of the types of children and adolescents that may be encountered in practice; each case is accompanied by, in most cases, three commentaries from field-leading clinicians (including child and adolescent psychiatrists, psychologists, social workers, and nurses) who draw from the combination of evidence-based interventions, biopsychosocial approaches, a systems perspective, and commonsense thinking. In addition to providing a diagnostic formulation, the commentaries purposely address different treatment approaches—psychotherapeutic, psychopharmacologic, and integrative—and how each of these approaches may be "called for" in specific situations.

We have grouped the cases into four parts in the book. The cases in Part I, "Classic Cases," have fairly clear diagnoses. Various experts explain their conceptualizations of a case and their recommendations for treatment. In Part II, "Comorbid Complexity," authors describe cases in which the youth have several diagnoses or the actual diagnosis is unclear. Readers will have the opportunity to read how experts in the field conceptualize diagnoses and recommend treatment for these complex situations. Part III, "Toughest Cases: Diagnostic and Treatment Dilemmas," includes examples in which the diagnosis is unclear, the patient has not responded to previous treatment, and/or only limited evidence is available on the correct means of treatment. Part IV, "Kids in Crisis," concerns youth who have psychopathology in the context of extreme psychosocial stressors.

The closing section, Part V, "Diagnostic and Treatment Decision Making," includes two chapters on clinical and research issues in the diagnosis and treatment of child psychopathology. Chapter 31, "Diagnostic Decision Making," focuses on diagnosis, including the importance of maintaining a developmental perspective, weighing information from different informants and considering culture, context, impairment, comorbidity, and subthreshold disorders. Chapter 32, "Research and Clinical Perspectives on Diagnostic and Treatment Decision Making: Whence the Future?" considers how a better understanding of the role of clinical decision making can lead to improvements in diagnosis, treatment, and implementation of evidence-based approaches. In the appendix, we have compiled an extensive table of screening tools and rating scales (i.e., "decision-making tools"); we provide information about how to acquire these tools.

We hope that this book can serve as an invaluable tool for trainees, trainers, and clinicians who work in child and adolescent psychiatry. Because it provides points of view from different disciplinary approaches, the book is appropriate for all clinicians of all disciplines—social workers, child and adolescent psychiatrists, psychologists, nurse-clinicians, and others—who are involved in treating children and adolescents with mental health problems.

The book can be used as a teaching tool for clinicians at all levels of training. For the preclinical student, it provides an opportunity to read about a case that pops out of the page. More experienced students, interns, or residents have an opportunity to read how experts in the field conceptualize diagnosis and treatment. Reading each case and the associated commentaries will have the value of meeting with three expert supervisors. For more experienced clinicians, the cases and commentaries can serve as a proxy for a consultation, or second opinion, with three experts in the field. The book may be useful for child and adolescent psychiatrists studying for their board exams because it offers concise, research-based, and clinically applicable perspectives on diagnosing and treating childhood psychopathology. We trust that readers will find the book to be an interesting and educational experience, much as we found in preparing it.

Cathryn A. Galanter, M.D.
Peter S. Jensen, M.D.

REFERENCES

Committee on Quality of Health Care in America, Institute of Medicine: Crossing the Quality Chasm: A New Health System for the 21st Century. Washington, DC, National Academy Press, 2001

Jensen PS: Stimulant treatment for children: a community perspective: commentary. J Am Acad Child Adolesc Psychiatry 39:984–987, 2000

Moderators and mediators of treatment response for children with attention-deficit/hyperactivity disorder: the Multimodal Treatment Study of children with attention-deficit/hyperactivity disorder. Arch Gen Psychiatry 56:1088–1096, 1999

MTA Cooperative Group: A 14-month randomized clinical trial of treatment strategies for attention-deficit/hyperactivity disorder. Multimodal Treatment Study of Children with ADHD. Arch Gen Psychiatry 56:1073–1086, 1999

U.S. Department of Health and Human Services: Children and mental health, in Mental Health: A Report of the Surgeon General. Rockville, MD, Department of Health and Human Services, Substance Abuse and Mental Health Services Administration, Center for Mental Health Services, National Institutes of Health, National Institute of Mental Health, 1999

U.S. Department of Health and Human Services: Report of the Surgeon General's Conference on Children's Mental Health: a national action agenda. 2001. Available at: http://www.surgeongeneral.gov/topics/cmh/childreport.html. Accessed May 19, 2008.

Introduction

Our Conceptualization of the Cases

Peter S. Jensen, M.D.
Cathryn A. Galanter, M.D.

For each case and the respective commentaries presented in *DSM-IV-TR Casebook and Treatment Guide for Child Mental Health*, we asked different experts to prepare their diagnostic formulation and treatment recommendations for a specific case. At the outset, experts were asked to prepare each case and then write an "integrative commentary," drawing freely from the range of etiologic and therapeutic perspectives—whether psychotherapeutic, psychopharmacologic, or ecological/environmental—in terms of their preferred and optimal approach to understanding the specific case and its overall management.

In addition to the case writers (who also provide integrative commentaries), additional experts, usually one each from child psychiatry and child psychology, were asked to review each vignette and approach the case from a psychopharmacologic treatment perspective and from a psychosocial treatment perspective, respectively. These commentators read only the case vignette, not the case writer's integrative commentary. Through this means, we deliberately attempted to "tie the hands" of two of each of the three commentators, thereby highlighting to our readers how different training backgrounds and experiences might lead one expert to one set of conclusions and another expert to quite different recommendations.

This was a difficult, perhaps even unfair, task for our experts, all of whom tended to be quite integrative. As is evident from their commentaries, our experts usually wished to draw upon multiple treatment perspectives in approaching the cases—as most experts are wont to do, in our opinion. Nonetheless, the differences among commentaries often illustrate the self-evident fact of what happens in the real world: clinicians' conceptualizations of a patient's presenting problem, making one or more diagnoses, and formulations of treatment plans vary.

Because the cases presented here are only snippets of real cases, these variations among commentators may reflect the lack of complete information that is otherwise obtained from face-to-face interviews. But incomplete information is part and parcel of real cases as well, and as clinicians, we are all prone to filling in such gaps with our own assumptions and inferences, based on our past experiences and theoretical biases. We believe that in the real world, such differences in diagnostic formulations and treatment recommendations are often a function of the lack of specific targeted research evidence, and can signal the need for more research.

It is in that spirit—to highlight where we need more data, either from patients themselves or from additional studies of patients represented by the vignettes—that we hope readers will review the differences and similarities across experts' commentaries. In some instances, despite tied hands, psychopharmacologic experts indicated that their preferred approach was psychotherapeutic. In other instances, psychotherapeutic experts indicated preferences for a psychopharmacologic approach to case management. When our experts agreed on overall diagnostic and treatment approaches, despite tied hands, we were either impressed with the robustness and maturity of the research in that area or led to conclude that a single dominant theoretical persuasion underpinned the field's approach to the disorder, with or without much research. Our assigning a given expert or team of experts to prepare one perspective or another is not a statement about their expertise per se and is more a statement of our intention to illustrate these different perspectives toward diagnosis and treatment.

Despite the difficulty encountered by our experts in restricting themselves to one viewpoint or another, we hope that the message throughout this casebook is clear: depending on which clinical discipline and door the patient happens to enter, he or she may hear different perspectives on diagnosis and treatment—sometimes subtle from the clinician's perspective, but rarely subtle from the patient's and family's perspective. In fact, families tend to reify these diagnoses and may shop from one clinician to the next, wondering what the patient's real "diagnosis" is.

Much more problematic is when the clinician diagnostician reifies the diagnosis: "Which disorder does the patient *really* have?" The *Diagnostic and Statistical Manual of Mental Disorders*, 4th Edition, Text Revision (DSM-IV-TR; American Psychiatric Association 2000), is meant to be a communication system for purposes of scientific study, clinical decision making, and even billing practices. As such, it is important that we understand that it is a system in evolution. As more research is conducted, some new diagnostic categories might be defined, and others might be subsumed and collapsed.

To illustrate our perspective as editors: rather than only the three types of attention-deficit/hyperactivity disorder (ADHD) currently described in DSM-

IV-TR (i.e., combined type, predominantly hyperactive-impulsive type, and predominantly inattentive type), future research and more distant DSMs will reveal that there are in fact many different kinds of ADHD, each with different sets of gene combinations and etiological factors, pathways to disorder development, and potential points for prevention or early intervention. By analogy, many different types of cough exist—coughs that are seasonal with a nonpurulent sputum; winter coughs that are associated with high fever; rare coughs that are associated with high fever, bloody sputum, difficulties breathing, and positive smears for pneumococcal bacteria; coughs that are associated with weight loss, decreased appetite, sometimes bloody sputum, and metastasizing masses into other parts of the body; and coughs that seem associated with no known biological factors but appear with other associated habits such as nose wrinkling, grimacing, shoulder shrugging, and so forth. Medical research has demonstrated that all of these coughs appear to have different origins and prognoses, and therefore often require different treatments and treatment combinations. Therefore, as neuropsychiatric and behavioral research advance, so too should our understanding of different psychiatric symptom profiles and correlated factors, yielding new knowledge about etiology, clinical presentation, associated factors, prognosis, prevention, and treatment—the eventual goal of DSM and progress in scientific research.

In preparing this volume, we wished to illustrate the range of different kinds of cases, including fairly classic cases illustrating DSM-IV-TR criteria (Part I); cases with comorbid complexity in which it would be unclear whether a child had one or more conditions and, if so, which came first (Part II); tough cases that reflect the current difficulties in establishing diagnoses and treatment plans (Part III); and cases that illustrate the impact of environmental factors on children's outcomes, thereby raising the question of whether the disorder was internal to the child or should instead (or also) be conceptualized as a problem in the environment (Part IV). In considering the last-mentioned cases—that is, those involving psychopathology in the context of social stressors—depending on one's theoretical persuasions in such instances, one might take a preventive approach, seeking to address environmental factors, much like the public health scientist might approach the prevention of dental disease through water fluoridation rather than ensuring that there is a dentist on every block to fill cavities as they arise—an impractical and imperfect solution. In our view, the need for a biopsychosocial perspective for case understanding and management is most easily seen in Part IV but applies to earlier sections of the book as well.

In reviewing all of the cases presented in this book, we realize that some cases might seem to fit better under another section heading. Thus, some of our intended "classic" cases illustrate comorbid complexity, and even seemingly "easy" cases can constitute diagnostic dilemmas. This realization also illustrates the key point that classic cases are often complex and may be approached quite differently by different experts. Moreover, most cases are comorbid; impairment can be difficult to judge even among experts, and quite different treatments are recommended for the same child. We suggest that in instances where differences are prominent among commentators, the need for further research is especially acute.

We admit that our experts were given a difficult task. They did not have a patient to interview and were unable to reconcile discrepant information from multiple informants. Although checklists and rating scales were summarized in some instances, our expert commentators could not review single response items from these scales or determine through interview whether information was valid or invalid. Obviously, a vignette necessarily collapses an enormous quantity of details from a rich human history. By definition, the case writers presented details most salient to themselves and their own conceptualization of the case, despite a common framework for taking a history and conducting a mental status exam that is commonly taught in psychiatry and psychology. The two commentator-only experts were subject to the clinical judgments and filters imposed by the case writer and, therefore, saw the case only through the case writer's eyes. But so it is in actual practice: We as clinicians all tend to view clinical phenomena within patients and families as a function of how we are trained to see and what we have seen before.

What we expect to see we all see easily, but what we do not expect to see is difficult to ascertain. Hence the need for continually broadening our vision, not just in obtaining clinical data from multiple informants about the child's presentation, but also in eliciting the child's developmental history, as well as all potentially contributing factors that may have given rise to the child's current condition—too often limited to what the field knows now and the models that we have been taught.

From this perspective, clinicians need to consider DSM-IV-TR as a temporary stepping-stone. On the one hand, it temporarily limits the background noise and the field of observations about a complex set of behaviors within a child that may in fact have to do with a vast combination of inborn/genetic, biological/constitutional, developmental/psychological, and environmental/societal forces. In view of our current understanding that etiologic factors exert differing degrees of influence within the same disorder across multiple persons with that condition, our use of DSM-IV-TR needs to be treated with both respect and "gentle bemusement"; we must respect its role as a necessary communication system. We must understand that when appropriately used, the diagnostic system can serve as a communication tool among clinicians, researchers, and policy makers, and that all research done using any particular definition is more likely to be applicable to patients for whom the same description applies. In addition, policy decisions about reimbursement and medical necessity have some coherence within that diagnostic system, as do scientific statements about prognosis, outcomes, and impairment—as long as we use the system carefully, consistently, and coherently.

On the other hand, the system is imperfect and a work in progress (Jensen et al. 2006). As new research is done, we learn that some disorders that have previously been lumped together might better be split, in terms of their etiologic, associated, and prognostic factors, as is currently much discussed concerning the predominantly inattentive type of ADHD versus other forms of ADHD (Diamond 2005). Robins and Guze (1970) provided a much needed standard for the field that has changed only modestly (see Cantwell 1995) since they outlined the core criteria for validating a disorder: an onset of clustering symptoms that frequently co-occur more than other sets of symptoms; a coherent set of associated psychosocial factors; biological and laboratory findings consistent with that system profile; a particular natural course and set of outcomes; family history and/or genetic factors; and response to treatment. The coherence of these factors or lack thereof enables physicians to separate different types of cough, such as those resulting from seasonal allergies, lung cancer, pneumococcal pneumonia, and nervous tics. The same type of research has been well under way for some time in many areas of child and adolescent psychopathology (Cantwell 1995) and is illustrated in the cases described in this book. As seen in some cases, however, the differences among commentators suggest that much more research is needed.

In preparing this volume, we have been left with a twofold sense: a combination of incremental progress and a humbling perspective. Significant strides have been made through the careful application of DSM-III, DSM-III-R, and DSM-IV nosologies (American Psychiatric Association 1980, 1987, 1994, 2000). For some conditions, we now know a great deal about etiology, diagnosis, prognosis, and treatment, and we have much to offer our patients and families. Yet we find other areas—rare or rarely studied conditions, comorbid cases, and such—where research is urgently needed and where we are left with the unavoidable conclusion that our patients have a lot to teach us still. Thus, in the course of our clinical activities with patients and our clinical and basic science research on the difficulties from which patients suffer, it is important that we not take ourselves or our current diagnostic systems too seriously—yet our patients' suffering *must* be taken seriously. We hope and trust that our readers will learn as much from this volume as we have in working with an outstanding group of colleagues in preparing it.

REFERENCES

American Psychiatric Association: Diagnostic and Statistical Manual of Mental Disorders, 3rd Edition. Washington, DC, American Psychiatric Association, 1980

American Psychiatric Association: Diagnostic and Statistical Manual of Mental Disorders, 3rd Edition, Revised. Washington, DC, American Psychiatric Association, 1987

American Psychiatric Association: Diagnostic and Statistical Manual of Mental Disorders, 4th Edition. Washington, DC, American Psychiatric Association, 1994

American Psychiatric Association: Diagnostic and Statistical Manual of Mental Disorders, 4th Edition, Text Revision. Washington, DC, American Psychiatric Association, 2000

Cantwell DP: Child psychiatry: introduction and overview, in Comprehensive Textbook of Psychiatry, 6th Edition. Edited by Kaplan HI, Sadock BJ. Baltimore, MD, Williams & Wilkins, 1995, pp 2151–2154

Diamond A: Attention-deficit disorder (attention-deficit/ hyperactivity disorder without hyperactivity): a neurobiologically and behaviorally distinct disorder from attention-deficit/hyperactivity disorder (with hyperactivity). Dev Psychopathol 17:807–825, 2005

Jensen PS, Knapp P, Mrazek DA (eds): Toward a New Diagnostic System for Child Psychopathology: Moving Beyond the DSM. New York, Guilford, 2006

Robins E, Guze SB: Establishment of diagnostic validity in psychiatric illness: its application to schizophrenia. Am J Psychiatry 126:983–987, 1970

• Part 1 •

CLASSIC CASES

Introduction to Classic Cases

Peter S. Jensen, M.D.
Cathryn A. Galanter, M.D.

Our intention in Part I was to illustrate "classic" or "easy" cases, yet as we reviewed the experts' commentaries, we realized that even these so-called easy cases illustrate the complexity of patient presentations in typical real-world conditions. Associated conditions are common with classic cases, whether they be attention-deficit/hyperactivity disorder (ADHD), autism, bipolar disorder, or schizophrenia. Even a vignette of our best-studied disorder, ADHD, may render different opinions about diagnostic subtypes as well as different treatment recommendations. As demonstrated in the first two cases—"Trouble Paying Attention: Attention-Deficit/Hyperactivity Disorder" (Chapter 1) and "Trouble With Transitions: Does My Child Have Autism?" (Chapter 2)—subtleties in the wording of the clinical presentation and history may lead to differences in diagnosis. Although among clinicians "in the know" about diagnosis, the distinctions between ADHD, inattentive type, and ADHD, combined type, may be subtle, as may be the differences among autism, Asperger's disorder, and pervasive developmental disorder, and we as clinicians and researchers may view such disorders as "differences without a distinction," possibly because we view some of these disorders as a spectrum of disorders along several continua. However, our clinical appreciation of these subtleties is often lost on parents and caregivers, and sometimes leads to confusion, anger, disappointment, and doctor shopping.

For example, whether one chooses to employ or not to employ the hierarchical exclusionary criteria of DSM-IV-TR (American Psychiatric Association 2000) in the diagnosis of an autism spectrum disorder (vis-à-vis the diagnosis of ADHD) may not only confuse a parent but also lead to clinical differences in whether one identifies and chooses to treat the attentional and hyperactive symptoms in a child with an autism spectrum disorder. Yet, imagine how these differences are perceived by the parent. Without careful education and guidance of the parent of what the diagnoses "mean," and whether one chooses to employ hierarchical criteria or not, and whether one chooses to treat or not to treat inattention symptoms regardless of the primary diagnosis, these so-called subtleties can be very confusing to parents looking for firm and fast answers, even introducing them to perplexing treatment decisions (e.g., whether to treat the inattentive symptoms) that they may find hard to fathom.

Thus, we feel it is incumbent upon the diagnostician, regardless of disciplinary roots—child psychiatry, pediatrics, psychology, neurology, or social work—to educate the parent about the sometimes subtle differences among categories and the manner in which the diagnoses are used and can be used by other diagnosticians. This simple, often overlooked step is necessary to avoid the confusion experienced by families when different labels are applied to the same child by various diagnosticians over time. Families must also be helped to understand what has been shown to work for the primary condition, as well as evidence about effective interventions for associated problems, such as various medications for inattention, hyperactivity, anxiety, or aggression that often accompanies many disorders.

In discussing the case of "Living in Her Parents' Shadow: Separation Anxiety Disorder" (Chapter 3), all of the commentators generally recommend the same treatments, even though they demonstrate subtle differences in how etiological factors are invoked. It is important to note that although behavioral therapies tend to be recommended in all of the commentaries, the extent to which child psychiatrists and even many psychologists and social workers have actually been fully trained and supervised in using cognitive-behavioral therapy and exposure therapies is unclear.

The case of "Chatterbox at Home: Selective Mutism" (Chapter 4) epitomizes the lack of treatment studies for some disorders and demonstrates that diagnosticians often must rely on inferred evidence from related fields. Thus, because we know that anxiety disorders are treated with a combination of methods, including psychotherapy and cognitive-behavioral therapies, the commentators draw upon this research in discussing the optimal treatments for the patient. Notice also that the patient had seen three therapists before obtaining appropriate treatment.

In the case of "Everything Bothers Her: Major Depressive Disorder" (Chapter 5), the experts use a wide range of questionnaires in the evaluation of this youth's depression. The rating scales even span disruptive behaviors and obsessive-compulsive symptoms, and in one instance the commentator suggests a questionnaire concerning the youth's readiness for treatment based on the stages of change model, an elegant and often neglected approach to understanding the patient's readiness for treatment.

This case also nicely illustrates the overlap of inattentive symptoms common to both depression and ADHD, leaving commentators in some cases to make the diagnosis of ADHD, predominantly inattentive type. Note also that the commentators astutely speculate whether her ADHD symptoms predisposed the patient to depression, and if so, which should be treated first, the ADHD or the depression. Available treatment algorithms, such as the Texas medication algorithms for depression and ADHD, do offer guidance (Hughes et al. 2007; Pliszka et al. 2006), yet the ultimate decision in most instances comes down to the clinician's determination of what he or she feels is the etiology of the child's depression. Is the ADHD etiological or incidental? Is the depression severe and the most impairing problem that must be currently treated, or is it the ADHD?

Also of interest in Chapter 5 is March's commentary on the traditional narrative approach to a case history versus his application of an evidence-based medicine approach. Here we find much to agree with and a model that needs to be taught and to permeate training programs.

"Excessively Silly: Bipolar Disorder" (Chapter 6) presents the case of a 9-year-old girl with bipolar disorder who, not surprisingly, presented with other comorbid conditions. It is interesting to note that in this classic presentation of bipolar disorder, the commentators have very similar diagnostic impressions and treatment recommendations. Also of interest is that the use of rating scales with well-established thresholds for mania may be of help in such cases.

Also worth noting in this case is the important role of psychoeducation and family support over and above the formal treatments employed by the clinician. Although it may be easy for us to take parental psychoeducation and support as a "given" and for granted, it is not clear that we always do this as intensively or intelligently as we might. Systematic parent education and support programs, such as Pavuluri's Rainbow Program (Pavuluri et al. 2004), are important components and ought to be more systematically studied as well as provided to parents as part of an overall intervention approach. Such programs seem likely to lead also to better medication adherence and long-term family adjustment and accommodation to a child's chronic disabilities.

In "Life of the Party: Chronic Marijuana Use" (Chapter 7), the case of a marijuana-abusing teen is presented. In their commentaries, the experts tend to disagree on the question of marijuana abuse versus dependence, and subtle distinctions are drawn between the psychological factors that might underpin this discrimination. Also of note is the fact that although research evidence tends to support the likelihood of a marijuana withdrawal syndrome, such a syndrome is not present in DSM-IV-TR and represents another research area in need of further study.

In "My Mind Is Breaking: Psychosis" (Chapter 8), the experts note that childhood-onset schizophrenia is difficult to study. It also is difficult to diagnose; a lapse of 2 years between symptom onset and accurate diagnosis is commonplace. Also of note is the range of determinations regarding the child's level of impairment, with Global Assessment of Functioning (GAF) scores ranging from 25 to 40. Although all commentators agree that the child is severely impaired, readers should note that many putative symptoms of childhood and adolescent schizophrenia, such as odd behaviors and even hallucinations, can occur on a continuum with normality and as a function of cultural context, making such symptoms difficult to identify as true "symptoms" without the use of multiple informants and abundant contextual and developmental information. For this case, we relied on only two commentaries because we could find no credible expert in the field who was willing to discuss the use of psychosocial treatments alone—a marked advance from 30 years ago, when the proposed psychological approaches for schizophrenia invoked commonplace but misguided concepts such as the double bind hypothesis.

In "She Just Won't Eat a Thing: Anorexia Nervosa" (Chapter 9), the experts demonstrate differences of opinion regarding the diagnostic subtype (anorexia nervosa, restricting type, vs. anorexia nervosa, binge-eating/purging type). Although the commentators operated on the assumption that anorexia has important biological determinants, their recommended treatments tended to be therapeutically agnostic—that is, the use of behavioral approaches to restore the child to a metabolically safe state. Notice also the lack of evidence for any effective psychopharmacologic treatments. Also of interest is the range of GAF scores from 40 to 70.

In considering treatment options, the commentators cite evidence from the large multisite Treatment for Adolescents with Depression Study (TADS) (March et al. 2004). Across the field of child and adolescent psychiatry, large multisite clinical trials have become commonplace—not only TADS but also the National Institute of Mental Health Multimodal Treatment Study of Children With Attention Deficit Hyperactivity Disorder (MTA) study ("Moderators and Mediators of Treatment Response" 1999; MTA Cooperative Group 1999) and the Research Units on Pediatric Psychopharmacology studies of anxiety disorders (Research Unit on Pediatric Psychopharmacology Anxiety Study Group 2001) and autism (Research Units on Pediatric Psychopharmacology [RUPP] Autism Network 2005). Because many of these studies contrasted psychological and psychopharmacologic treatments alone and in combination (MTA and TADS, in particular), they appear to have narrowed the differences of opinion between psychiatric versus psychological clinicians as well as pointed the way for the benefits of treatments combining both psychopharmacologic and psychotherapeutic approaches in treatment-resistant or difficult cases.

In "The Blinker: Tourette's Disorder" (Chapter 10), the case presenters and the commentators alike make clear that psychiatric syndromes sometimes are misdiagnosed as medical conditions (in this case, blepharitis). When the disorder is appropriately diagnosed, however, both psychopharmacologic and psychotherapeutic (habit reversal training) interventions can be effective.

In "She Never Falls Asleep: Disordered Sleep in an Adolescent" (Chapter 11), subtle diagnostic discriminations are made by the commentators. Sleep disorders have been increasingly researched over the last decade. Their diagnosis becomes increasingly important as effective approaches can be applied; in addition to environmental strategies, medications can now be employed with these disorders. Of note also is the use of daily diaries as a means to track symptoms. Such approaches increasingly have a role in better understanding a particular symptom and in monitoring the onset, frequency, and determinants of and factors associated with these types of symptoms.

Other areas in which diaries may be especially helpful include tracking aggressive symptoms and bipolar symptoms. The case commentators emphasize the recommendation and need for motivational methods in working with patients and parents. Increasingly, intervention approaches must rely not only on medications and formal psychotherapies but also on psychoeducational and motivational methods to ensure compliance and adherence. Patients' willingness and readiness to change is an important area that clinicians must assess, particularly when motivation is low or when interventions are complex and arduous.

In the last case in Part I, "The World Is a Very Dirty Place: Obsessive-Compulsive Disorder" (Chapter 12), again findings from one of the major multisite studies are considered regarding the use of medication, therapy, or both. Just because "evidence-based treatments" exist does not mean that they are effectively deployed. As the chapter's contributors note, in the multisite Pediatric OCD [obsessive-compulsive disorder] Treatment Study, therapists employing cognitive-behavioral therapy at one site were three times more effective than at another site (Pediatric OCD Treatment Study [POTS] Team 2004). This case also illustrates—despite the editors' expressed wish for "classic" (i.e., noncomorbid cases)—that "typical" cases are often complicated by comorbidity.

REFERENCES

American Psychiatric Association: Diagnostic and Statistical Manual of Mental Disorders, 4th Edition, Text Revision. Washington, DC, American Psychiatric Association, 2000

Hughes CW, Emslie FH, Crismon ML, et al; Texas Consensus Conference Panel on Medication Treatment of Childhood Major Depressive Disorder: Texas Children's Medication Algorithm Project: update from Texas Consensus Conference Panel on Medication Treatment of Childhood Major Depressive Disorder. J Am Acad Child Adolesc Psychiatry 46:667–686, 2007

March J, Silva S, Petrycki S, et al; Treatment for Adolescents with Depression Study (TADS) Team: Fluoxetine, cognitive-behavioral therapy, and their combination for adolescents with depression: Treatment for Adolescents with Depression Study (TADS) randomized controlled trial. JAMA 292:807–820, 2004

Moderators and mediators of treatment response for children with attention-deficit/
    hyperactivity disorder: the Multimodal Treatment Study of children with attention-
    deficit/hyperactivity disorder. Arch Gen Psychiatry 56:1088–1096, 1999
MTA Cooperative Group: A 14-month randomized clinical trial of treatment strategies
    for attention deficit hyperactivity disorder. Multimodal Treatment Study of Chil-
    dren With ADHD. Arch Gen Psychiatry 56:1073–1086, 1999
Pavuluri MN, Graczyk PA, Henry DB, et al: Child- and family-focused cognitive-
    behavioral therapy for pediatric bipolar disorder: development and preliminary re-
    sults. J Am Acad Child Adolesc Psychiatry 43:528–537, 2004
Pediatric OCD Treatment Study (POTS) Team: Cognitive-behavior therapy, sertra-
    line, and their combination for children and adolescents with obsessive-compulsive
    disorder: the Pediatric OCD Treatment Study (POTS) randomized controlled trial.
    JAMA 292:1969–1976, 2004
Pliszka SR, Crismon ML, Hughes CW, et al; Texas Consensus Conference Panel on
    Pharmacotherapy of Childhood Attention Deficit Hyperactivity Disorder: The
    Texas Children's Medication Algorithm Project: a revision of the algorithm for medi-
    cation treatment of childhood attention deficit/hyperactivity disorder (ADHD). J Am
    Acad Child Adolesc Psychiatry 45:520–526, 2006
Research Unit on Pediatric Psychopharmacology Anxiety Study Group: Fluvoxamine
    for the treatment of anxiety disorders in children and adolescents. N Engl J Med
    344:1279–1285, 2001
Research Units on Pediatric Psychopharmacology (RUPP) Autism Network: Random-
    ized, controlled, crossover trial of methylphenidate in pervasive developmental dis-
    order with hyperactivity. Arch Gen Psychiatry 62:1266–1274, 2005

■ CHAPTER 1 ■

Trouble Paying Attention

Attention-Deficit/ Hyperactivity Disorder

Stephen P. Hinshaw, Ph.D.

CASE PRESENTATION

IDENTIFYING INFORMATION

Alicia is an 8½-year-old, second-generation Mexican American girl who lives with her parents and 11-year-old brother. She attends her local public school and is in third grade in a regular education classroom. Her father is a small business owner, her mother works half-time in a day care center, and the family lives in a middle-class neighborhood of a moderate-sized city.

CHIEF COMPLAINT

Alicia's parents saw a newspaper advertisement for a study of children "who may be having trouble paying attention." This ad caught their eye because at the most recent parent-teacher conference, Alicia's teacher stated that Alicia might have attention-deficit/hyperactivity disorder (ADHD) and recommended that the parents get her evaluated.

HISTORY OF PRESENT ILLNESS

Alicia's parents are drained from the nightly battles with Alicia over homework and discouraged by her passivity, lack of focus, and "spaciness." She seems not to care about doing well academically. Her parents complain that the more they cajole,

Stephen P. Hinshaw, Ph.D., is Professor of Psychology and Chair of the Department of Psychology at the University of California, Berkeley (for complete biographical information, see "About the Contributors," p. 613).

beg, and threaten punishments, the less responsive Alicia seems to be. Now in third grade, she is showing marked variability in her school performance, ranging from grades of B down to D. Her performance in reading is noted to be particularly poor.

Since kindergarten, teachers have complained of a pattern of Alicia's "not seeming to listen," "poor concentration," and "wandering about." Her teachers also have commented on Alicia's undirected and unfocused activity in the classroom, plus a style characterized as "daydreamy." During second grade, when expectations for homework increased substantially, Alicia's parents began to get into nightly battles with her about completing such work; they continue to be exasperated by her struggles with attention, focus, and motivation.

Alicia has never had close friends. Other children do not openly dislike her but rather seem to avoid her because she will not stay with a game or activity for long. She tends to tune out when others are talking. In group activities, the leaders must constantly prompt her to give eye contact and stay on task, which bothers the other children in the group. On the girls' soccer team, her teammates sometimes tease her for not following the coach's directions and for occasionally "spacing out" during matches.

PAST PSYCHIATRIC HISTORY

As noted earlier, since kindergarten, Alicia has had difficulty with daydreaming and wandering about. She has persisted with typical preschool anxieties for several years longer than most of her peers. For example, she still worries about nightmares, storms, and whether she will be safe when her parents go out for the evening and leave her with a babysitter.

MEDICAL HISTORY

Alicia had several ear infections at age 2, some of which were quite protracted, requiring several rounds of antibiotics. Tubes for her ears were considered but never inserted.

DEVELOPMENTAL HISTORY

Alicia was born at 36 weeks through assisted vaginal delivery and weighed 6 lbs 1 oz. She reached nearly all major milestones within normal time frames, although her speech was mildly delayed in that she was still using two- to three-word phrases by almost age 2½ years. By age 3½, when she was evaluated for preschool, her expressive language had improved and was considered to be within normal limits. She also had difficulties with following multipart directions, although it was never clear whether this problem related to her not having really heard the request or to an underlying language processing problem. Her pediatrician and preschool teachers noted some awkwardness of gait; this issue has shown improvement over time.

Social History

Alicia lives with both parents. Her father is age 38. His family immigrated to the United States when he was age 4. He has an associate's degree; his current employment is running a car repair shop. His family describes him as a "people person." Alicia's mother, age 37, comes from a large extended family that emigrated from Mexico several generations ago. She received a high school diploma and has obtained certification, through part-time attendance at a community college, in preschool education.

Family History

Alicia's father had difficulty learning to read as a child, but it was not clear whether this problem was related to a learning disability or to the fact that English was not his native language. He has no evident psychiatric disorders at present. The paternal grandmother was reported to have suffered from depression back in Mexico. Alicia's mother has multiple phobias; for example, she does not drive a car and is afraid of elevators. She appears mildly dysphoric but does not meet criteria for dysthymia or major depression. Alicia's maternal aunt was recently diagnosed as having "adult ADHD," following a long history of school failure and multiple, transitory jobs throughout her adult life. Alicia's great-grandfather died of suicide after several mental hospitalizations.

Mental Status Examination

Alicia was reluctant to maintain eye contact or to discuss school or homework situations. No gross neurological signs were present. Her sensory, perceptual, and cognitive functions were intact. She brightened when the examiner got her to discuss her pets at home and her eventual desire to be an animal trainer. Still, there were often marked delays in her making verbal responses to the clinician's questions; she seemed preoccupied with internal thoughts or anxieties, and she often needed the question repeated several times before emerging with an answer.

The initial evaluation included the obtaining of parent and teacher rating scales, a developmental history from the parents (which yielded the information presented above), a structured interview with them, and an examination of Alicia, which included a brief office neurological exam as well as cognitive and attention testing.

Rating Scales and Additional Information

Alicia's parents and her second- and third-grade teachers completed the SNAP Rating Scale (Swanson 1992). Results were consistent across raters: Alicia was scored as positive for either seven, eight, or nine symptoms (out of the nine listed in DSM-IV-TR [American Psychiatric Association 2000]) of inattention-disorganization, depending on the informant, but she was scored as positive for only zero, one, or two symptoms of hyperactivity/impulsivity (out of the nine from the DSM-IV-TR list) across informants. The Child Behavior Checklist and Teacher Report Form (Achenbach 1991a, 1991b) each revealed T-scores above 65 for the narrow-band Attention Problems scale and at or above 70 for the Anxious-Depressed scale.

Alicia's performance on the Conners' Continuous Performance Test (Conners 1995) showed clinically significant elevations on omission errors and reaction time variability. Self-report on the Children's Depression Inventory (Kovacs 1992) showed a mild level of depressive symptomatology. The parental structured interview revealed evidence for several specific phobias (dogs, dark), but Alicia did not meet criteria for any other anxiety disorders.

During a classroom observation, the clinician noted that Alicia was a loner in the class: Alicia initially engaged in the assignments or group projects directed by the teacher but quickly became disengaged when the teacher was reading instructions or giving directions, often staring out the window or occasionally talking with peers. Finally, during a videotaped parent-child interaction in the clinic, the initial free play portion was marked by positive interchange. Once, however, the instructions called for the parents to ask her to perform academic tasks; Alicia became sullen and resistant, and the parents began to cajole and beg her to perform, their exasperation at her lack of responsiveness readily apparent.

COMMENTARIES

Psychotherapeutic Perspective

William E. Pelham, Jr., Ph.D., A.B.P.P.
James Waxmonsky, M.D.

DIAGNOSTIC FORMULATION

To diagnose ADHD, information should be gathered from parents and teachers, and this is most efficiently done through the use of rating scales (Pelham et al. 2005b). For Alicia, both parents and teachers reported seven or more symp-

---

William E. Pelham, Jr., Ph.D., A.B.P.P, is Distinguished Professor of Psychology, Pediatrics, and Psychiatry and Director of the Center for Children and Families at the State University of New York at Buffalo.

James Waxmonsky, M.D., is on the faculty in the Department of Psychiatry at the State University of New York at Buffalo, and a staff member at Women and Children's Hospital of Buffalo in Buffalo, New York.

For complete biographical information, see "About the Contributors," p. 613.

toms of inattention and two or fewer symptoms of hyperactivity/impulsivity. Therefore, Alicia meets DSM-IV-TR Criterion A for the inattentive type of ADHD. It is also important to obtain an estimate of the child's function at home, at school, and with peers, because functioning in these domains predicts impairment better than symptom counts do (Pelham et al. 2005b). The Children's Impairment Rating Scale, an eight-item visual analogue scale on which parents and teachers rate a child's functioning in key domains, can be used to quickly measure functional impairments (Fabiano et al. 2006). For Alicia, her teacher and parents reported impairment related to inattention (finishing classwork, completing homework, and attending during soccer). These problems date back to kindergarten and are consistently impairing across domains, fulfilling the DSM-IV-TR B, C, and D criteria for ADHD. The parent and teacher rating scales are the key to diagnosis. Neither neuropsychological tests (e.g., a continuous performance test) nor child self-reports are necessary in cases like Alicia's in which ADHD-related impairment is clearly present in multiple domains (Pelham et al. 2005b).

A brief screen (e.g., Child Behavior Checklist) for anxiety and mood disorders is useful when parents also report possible problems in this domain. Alicia's Child Behavior Checklist profile and the parental report suggest some evidence of internalizing symptoms, but direct interview of the parents and child did not confirm that Alicia's worries impair her daily functioning. Although Alicia's worries may be contributing to her inattention or vice versa, there is not sufficient evidence of anxiety-related impairment to make a separate diagnosis of an anxiety disorder.

Whenever evidence (e.g., a parent or teacher report) indicates academic struggles, the child should be evaluated for learning disabilities and/or other developmental delays. Given Alicia's academic struggles and increased behavior problems during academic tasks at school and home, standardized achievement and intelligence tests should be given. Further, it is important to know whether Alicia is receiving any classroom-based behavioral or academic interventions or other special education services and what impact they have had, if any.

Because up to half of children with ADHD will meet criteria for oppositional defiant disorder or conduct disorder (MTA Cooperative Group 1999), any child with ADHD should be screened for these disorders. Alicia argues with her parents during homework, likely due to the repeated prompts she needs to stay on task. However, she does not demonstrate other symptoms of oppositional defiant disorder or conduct disorder.

No clear evidence exists that comorbidities influence treatment development or response in children with ADHD (Pelham and Fabiano 2008). The emphasis of diagnosis and assessment, therefore, should be on functional impairments and functional analyses.

DSM-IV-TR DIAGNOSIS

Axis I   314.00 ADHD, predominantly inattentive type

            Rule out a reading disorder

Axis II   History of recurrent ear infections

Axis III   None

Axis IV   Moderate impairment with peers, primary supports, and education

Axis V   Global Assessment of Functioning=55

            Moderate impairment in multiple realms

TREATMENT RECOMMENDATIONS

Behavioral modification (BMOD) therapies are the only evidence-based psychosocial approach for ADHD, as supported by more than 175 studies (Pelham and Fabiano 2008). BMOD is as effective as medication for achieving functional improvements (academic achievement, peer relations, aggression) (MTA Cooperative Group 1999, 2004), improves the chances of a successful treatment response with medication (Pelham et al. 2005a), allows reduced medication dosages (MTA Cooperative Group 1999; Pelham et al. 2005a), and is preferred by families over medication alone (Pelham and Fabiano 2008). After 36 months in the Multimodal Treatment Study of Children With ADHD (MTA study), children treated with BMOD improved as much as those treated with medication in all domains (Jensen et al. 2007). Because children with comorbid anxiety symptoms exhibited an enhanced response to BMOD in the MTA study (Pelham and Fabiano 2008), Alicia is an excellent candidate for BMOD.

By focusing on functional impairments during the diagnostic assessment, the clinician will have compiled a list of target behaviors to be used as treatment goals. For Alicia, this list would include needing instructions repeated during class and staying on task/completing assignments. The antecedent and consequent conditions that influence these behaviors should be identified. For example, does Alicia have greater difficulty attending when she sits close to the window? The list of target behaviors can be converted into a daily report card (DRC) to create a set of daily and weekly goals. For example, classroom DRC goals might include "needs three or fewer reminders per day to complete seatwork" and "completes assignments accurately within designated time." Alicia's access to free-time classroom activities might be made contingent on completion of her daily goals, with extra rewards for exemplary behavior. The initial DRC goals should be achievable so that Alicia can experience the benefits of good behavior, with goals increased in difficulty as she improves. The DRC provides parents with daily school feedback while simplifying the level of detail that teachers provide to parents. Instead of discussing recurrent negative feedback about school, her parents can now praise and reward Alicia when she achieves her DRC goals. A standardized packet for developing a DRC can be downloaded (http://ccf.buffalo.edu/resources.php).

To address Alicia's functional impairments at home (e.g., arguing during homework), the clinician might recommend that Alicia's parents participate in a group parent training course using any one of the evidence-based programs (e.g., Barkley 1987; Cunningham et al. 1998; McMahon and Forehand 2003). These courses emphasize praising good behavior and developing structured behavioral plans for recurrent negative behaviors. Periodic group booster sessions are necessary to facilitate maintenance.

Alicia's problems with peers appear to be relatively minor and secondary to her inattentiveness. Thus, the prescribed interventions at home and school may be sufficient to improve her peer relationships.

After these initial interventions, the clinician can assess the need for additional and/or more intensive treatments. If a learning disability is found, Alicia may need specialized educational supports at school. If BMOD does not improve Alicia's anxieties, an evidence-based program for anxiety should be implemented. If peer problems worsen, Alicia may need a more intensive social skills program, such as a therapeutic summer camp (Pelham and Fabiano 2008). Concurrent stimulant medication is another consideration. The choice between medication and more intensive behavioral interventions and/or special education is the parent's responsibility and will depend on parental preferences and resources and the severity of the child's problems. The ideal sequencing of medication and behavioral treatments has not been well studied and remains a point of debate (Pelham 2007).

Psychopharmacologic Perspective

Laurence L. Greenhill, M.D.

DIAGNOSTIC FORMULATION

In summary, Alicia is an 8½-year-old Mexican American girl with a 4-year history of lack of focus, variability in school performance, poor reading performance, daydreaming in school, battles over homework, lack of friends, and

Laurence L. Greenhill, M.D., is Ruane Professor of Psychiatry and Pediatric Psychopharmacology at Columbia University; Director of the New York State Research Unit of Pediatric Psychopharmacology at New York State Psychiatric Institute; and Attending and Consultant Physician in the Disruptive Behavior Disorders Clinic at Columbia Presbyterian Medical Center in New York, New York (for complete biographical information, see "About the Contributors," p. 613).

spaciness during team sports. These behaviors are consistent with a diagnosis of ADHD, inattentive type (ADHD-I). In addition, she has a history of persistent preschool anxieties, including worries over storms, and difficulty separating from parents. Other symptoms of concern include a history of delayed language milestones, difficulties in following multipart directions, problems with reading, poor social skills, and rejection by peers. She has a history of chronic ear infections, requiring several rounds of antibiotics. The father had difficulty learning to read as a child, and the mother is afflicted with multiple phobias, unwilling to drive a car or to take elevators. Alicia's maternal aunt has adult ADHD, based on chronic school failure and multiple transitory jobs.

Alicia's lengthy history meets the DSM-IV-TR duration criterion (more than 6 months). She also meets the DSM-IV-TR criteria for impairment in more than one setting (classroom, at home, and on the sports field), onset before age 7 (problems first appeared in kindergarten), required number of ADHD symptoms endorsed by multiple observers, differential diagnosis, and a set of problems not better explained by another Axis I disorder.

Rating scales completed by the parents and two teachers were confirmatory of ADHD-I. All raters endorsed a minimum of seven inattention symptoms and two or fewer symptoms of overactivity-impulsivity, consistent with a diagnosis of ADHD-I. Confirmatory were the Child Behavior Checklist and Teacher Report Form (Achenbach 1991a, 1991b), which revealed T-scores in the clinical range for attention problems and for anxious-depressed behavior. Alicia demonstrated significantly elevated omission error rates on the Conners' Continuous Performance Test (Conners 1995) and clinically significant reaction time variability, also supportive of a serious impairment in attention. Her classroom behavior, characterized by distractibility, staring out of the window, and daydreaming when the teacher is reading instructions or giving directions, is also consistent with ADHD-I. Similarly, Alicia was sullen and resistant toward her parents when they asked her to perform academic tasks during the videotaped parent-child interaction in the clinic.

DSM-IV-TR DIAGNOSIS

Axis I   314.00 ADHD, predominantly inattentive type
          Rule out generalized anxiety disorder
          Rule out adjustment disorder with depressed or mixed anxiety and depressed mood
          Rule out reading disorder
Axis II   None present
Axis III Chronic ear infections, past, in remission
Axis IV   Level of psychosocial stressors: mild-moderate
          Social issues (i.e., peer rejection)
Axis V   Global Assessment of Functioning=55

SUGGESTED DIAGNOSTIC ASSESSMENT TOOLS

Instruments that can facilitate assessment of level of severity of the primary symptoms:

1. *ADHD:* SNAP-IV is a rating scale for ADHD based on DSM-IV-TR symptoms rated by a parent or teacher (Swanson 1992).
2. *Anxiety:* the Multidimensional Anxiety Scale for Children (March et al. 1997) is a validated self-report on anxiety symptoms.
3. *Depressed mood:* the Children's Depression Rating Scale—Revised (Poznanski et al. 1985) is a clinician-rated scale used as a screening and diagnostic tool and a measure of severity of depression in children.

TREATMENT RECOMMENDATIONS

ADHD is a disorder that begins in childhood and shows a worldwide prevalence of 5.4% of the school-age population (Polanczyk and Rhode 2007). It also causes disability and impairment in adults (Kessler et al. 2006). ADHD-I and associated comorbid disorders are optimally treated with a multimodal treatment approach that uses a combination of psychoeducation, parent guidance and support, consultation to the teacher(s), and pharmacologic and psychotherapeutic interventions (MTA Cooperative Group 1999).

Alicia and her parents will need psychoeducation regarding the nature, phenomenology, comorbidity (particularly with ADHD-I and anxiety disorder), and expected course and outcome of ADHD-I. As for all newly diagnosed children and families, Alicia's family should be referred to an organization such as Children and Adults with Attention Deficit Disorders (CHADD), a national advocacy and support group.

Because evidence indicates that Alicia may be suffering from a reading disability, she is a candidate for a neuropsychological screen to rule out a reading disorder or other processing disorder (Pliszka 2007). Neuropsychological testing could also provide information on whether there is evidence of impairment in executive functioning, given her problems with following instructions, daydreaming in class, and withdrawal when the teacher is giving directions.

Alicia's teacher may be contacted about implementing an individualized education program (IEP) tailored to improve Alicia's classroom attentiveness to directions. The teacher can move Alicia's seat next to the teacher's desk to be able to refocus Alicia with a physical touch or gesture.

From the pharmacologic perspective, stimulant medications, such as methylphenidate and mixed salts of amphetamine, have been approved to treat the symptoms of ADHD in preschoolers (Greenhill et al. 2001), school-age children (Pliszka 2007), and adolescents (Wilens et al. 2006). Although used in the basic short-acting formulation in the MTA study (Greenhill et al. 2001), dopamine reuptake blocking agents are available in long-duration preparations, such as osmotic-release (OROS) methylphenidate (Concerta) or mixed salts of amphetamine, extended release (Adderall XR). These preparations can be given once daily, in the morning by the parent, so the child will not require dosing at school. These medications have robust efficacy for extending attention span, increasing seatwork productivity, improving completion of academic tasks, and increasing cooperativeness during academic tasks. The primary adverse effects are reduction of appetite, associated weight loss or lack of weight gain, and delay in sleep onset if the medication is taken too late during the day (Greenhill et al. 2006). If the stimulants are not effective or have too many adverse events, another pharmacologic option to consider for treatment of ADHD, inattentive type, is the noradrenergic reuptake blocker atomoxetine (Pliszka 2007).

Psychotherapeutic interventions to be considered include behavioral intervention techniques found useful during the MTA study, such as the DRC, whereby the teacher sends home a daily positive note, for parental reinforcement, for each day that the child reaches a behavioral target (MTA Cooperative Group 1999). Alicia's parents should also be referred for parent training to strengthen their understanding of behavioral treatment principles in establishing a contingency management plan at home to reinforce homework behavior.

Integrative Perspective

Stephen P. Hinshaw, Ph.D.

DIAGNOSTIC FORMULATION

Alicia's parents, along with her second- and third-grade teachers, completed the SNAP (Swanson 1992). Results were consistent across raters: Alicia scored as positive for seven to nine symptoms (of the nine listed in DSM-IV-TR) of inattention-disorganization, depending on informant, but she was positive for only two or fewer symptoms of hyperactivity-impulsivity (out of the nine from the DSM-IV-TR list) across informants. The Child Behavior Checklist and Teacher Report Form (Achenbach 1991a, 1991b) each revealed T-scores >65 for the narrow-band Attention Problems scale and ≥70 for Anxious-Depressed behavior.

On the basis of a structured interview held with the parents (Diagnostic Interview Schedule for Children; Shaffer et al. 2000), the clinician determined that Alicia met full DSM-IV-TR criteria for ADHD-I. Specifically, she met criteria for eight of nine inattentive-disorganized symptoms but only one hyper-active-impulsive symptom. The symptoms of inattention were exhibited in school and at home; they were clearly yielding impairment, in the form of underachievement at school, considerable friction at home, and impairments in peer relationships.

Her performance on the Conners' Continuous Performance Test (Conners 1995) showed clinically significant elevations on omission errors and reaction time variability. Self-report on the Children's Depression Inventory (Kovacs 1992) showed a mild level of depressive symptomatology. The parental structured interview also revealed evidence that Alicia has several specific phobias (dogs, dark), but Alicia did not meet criteria for any other anxiety disorders.

During a classroom observation, the clinician noted that Alicia was a loner in the class and that although she was initially engaged in the assignments or group projects directed by the teacher, she quickly became disengaged when the teacher was reading instructions or giving directions, often staring out the window or occasionally talking with peers. Finally, during a videotaped parent-child interaction in the clinic, the initial free play portion was marked by positive interchange. However, when the instructions called for the parents to ask her to perform academic tasks, Alicia became sullen and resistant, and the parents began to cajole and beg her to perform, their exasperation at her lack of responsiveness readily apparent.

Overall, the pattern of assessment data clearly reveals a diagnosis of ADHD-I. This may well be the most common form of ADHD in the community, although the bulk of clinical referrals are for the combined type (American Psychiatric Association 2000). As with other childhood-onset conditions, boys with ADHD outnumber girls with the disorder at a ratio of approximately 3:1, yet there is some evidence that for the predominantly inattentive type, the male-predominant sex ratio may be reduced (closer to 2:1; see Lahey et al. 1994).

Alicia's clinical presentation suggests the presence of "sluggish cognitive tempo," which characterizes a subset of individuals with ADHD. Here, the presenting problems pertain to a slow cognitive style, with the descriptors of "spacy" and "daydreamy" commonly applied (McBurnett et al. 2001). Whether this variant of ADHD-I comprises a distinct form of the condition—and, indeed, whether ADHD-I differs from the other types of ADHD in a qualitative way—is the subject of active debate (Milich et al. 2001).

In terms of comorbid diagnoses, Alicia met criteria for specific phobias. Despite the presence of symptoms of mild depression and signs of anxiety, however, she did not cross the threshold for mood disorders or other anxiety disorders. Importantly, additional evaluation will be needed to ascertain the presence of formal learning disorders. Although ADHD is frequently associated with academic impairment (Hinshaw 2002), in perhaps 25% of cases an independent reading or mathematics disorder is also apparent. The recommendation was made for full IQ testing as well as a series of achievement tests, particularly in reading.

DSM-IV-TR DIAGNOSIS

Axis I   314.00 ADHD, predominantly inattentive type

300.29 Specific phobia

Rule out reading disorder

Rule out mathematics disorder

Axis II   None

Axis III   Chronic ear infections, past, in remission

Axis IV   Educational problems

Axis V   Global Assessment of Functioning, highest in past year=58

TREATMENT RECOMMENDATIONS

Alicia's parents were referred to a psychologist who conducts behaviorally oriented parent training. They were also provided a referral to a developmental-behavioral pediatrician who specializes in evaluations of stimulant medication for children and adolescents with ADHD. In addition, they were encouraged to obtain a full workup of her educational and learning issues. Along this line, the possibility of an IEP was raised with Alicia's teacher.

Considerable evidence exists regarding the efficacy of stimulant medication for ADHD, combined type (MTA Cooperative Group 1999), but far less is known about medication or psychosocial treatments for ADHD-I. Thus, whether medication or behavioral intervention is the treatment of choice for this condition remains under active debate.

Alicia's parents met with the psychologist and decided to join the parent training group (for a model of such training, see Anastopoulos and Farley 2003). The group, which included five other sets of caregivers, was quite active. The leader provided education about ADHD, instructions in using a structured reward program, role-plays and rehearsals of the kinds of situations that "push the buttons" of the parents, and guided practice in de-escalating angry, emotionally explosive discipline procedures and using time-out and other consequences instead. Through the group, Alicia's parents realized that they were not alone in their situation. They also came to learn that although they could take the blame off themselves for having caused their daughter's ADHD, they were still clearly responsible for helping Alicia to realize her potential. Through engagement in treatment, they received social support, practical strategies for home management and school consultation, and a sense that openly discussing their daughter's condition with professionals and other families—and with Alicia herself—was far preferable to silence and denial.

Some of the initial work was quite frustrating. Alicia responded to initial limit setting with anger and defiance. At other times, she was tearful, wondering why she was so different from other girls and why other kids in her class teased her for being behind in her schoolwork. Essential to the process was learning how to work with the school system more productively. The family did obtain an IEP. Indeed, the school psychologist's testing revealed the presence of normal-range IQ but markedly depressed reading scores and uncovered the presence of significant deficits in phonemic awareness and phonological processing. The school and parents are currently working out accommodations, such as modifications of homework and some small-group supplements for Alicia's reading skills.

Through their efforts, the parents have noticed some improvements in Alicia's behavior, particularly the amount of time she can stay on task during homework and school lessons. They are encouraged to have been able to manage her issues (and their own frustration) more consistently at home. The parents are still wary of setbacks, however, as well as their own tendencies to stop the rewards when Alicia shows some improvement.

At this point, they still want to try to manage without any medication for their daughter, even though other families in the group have indicated that medication has been useful in their situations. Although Alicia's parents have not accepted the referral to the developmental-behavioral pediatrician, they are increasingly tempted to do so. If they do, one piece of guidance from the extremely limited evidence regarding medication effectiveness for ADHD-I is that efficacious dosages tend to be lower than those for ADHD, combined type. It will therefore be crucial that the physician be aware to perform an initial titration, with the inclusion of several dosage levels.

In the future, if Alicia's internalizing symptoms crystallize into more serious anxiety or mood disorders, cognitive-behavioral therapy could be a viable treatment option (Kendall et al 2003).

REFERENCES

Achenbach TM: Manual for the Child Behavior Checklist, 4-18 and 1991 Profile. Burlington, VT, University Associates in Psychiatry, 1991a

Achenbach TM: Manual for the Teacher Report Form and 1991 Profile. Burlington, VT, University Associates in Psychiatry, 1991b

American Psychiatric Association: Diagnostic and Statistical Manual of Mental Disorders, 4th Edition, Text Revision. Washington, DC, American Psychiatric Association, 2000

Anastopoulos AD, Farley SE: A cognitive-behavioral training program for parents of children with attention-deficit/hyperactivity disorder, in Evidence-Based Psychotherapies for Children and Adolescents. Edited by Kazdin AE, Weisz JR. New York, Guilford, 2003, pp 187–203

Barkley RA: Defiant Children: A Clinician's Manual for Parent Training. New York, Guilford, 1987

Conners CK: Conners' Continuous Performance Test and Computer Program User's Manual. Toronto, Ontario, Canada, Multi-Health Systems, 1995

Cunningham CE, Bremner R, Secord-Gilbert M: The Community Parent Education (COPE) program: a school-based family systems oriented course for parents of children with behavior disorders. Hamilton, ON, Chedoke-McMaster Hospitals and McMaster University, 1998

Fabiano G, Pelham W Jr, Gnagy E, et al: A practical measure of impairment: psychometric properties of the impairment rating scale in samples of children with attention deficit hyperactivity disorder and two school-based samples. J Clin Child Adolesc Psychol 35:369–385, 2006

Greenhill LL, Swanson JM, Vitiello B, et al: Impairment and deportment responses to different methylphenidate doses in children with ADHD: the MTA titration trial. J Am Acad Child Adolesc Psychiatry 40:180–187, 2001

Greenhill LL, Kollins S, Abikoff H, et al: Efficacy of immediate-release methylphenidate treatment for preschoolers with ADHD. J Am Acad Child Adolesc Psychiatry 45:1284–1294, 2006

Hinshaw SP: Is ADHD an impairing condition in childhood and adolescence? in Attention-Deficit Hyperactivity Disorder: State of the Science, Best Practices. Edited by Jensen PS, Cooper JR. Kingston, NJ, Civic Research Institute, 2002, pp 5-1–5-21

Jensen PS, Arnold LE, Swanson JM, et al: 3-year follow-up of the NIMH MTA study. J Am Acad Child Adolesc Psychiatry 46:989–1002, 2007

Kendall PD, Aschenbrand SG, Hudson JL: Child-focused treatment of anxiety, in Evidence-Based Psychotherapies for Children and Adolescents. Edited by Kazdin AE, Weisz JR. New York, Guilford, 2003, pp 81–100

Kessler R, Adler L, Barkley R, et al: The prevalence and correlates of adult ADHD in the United States: results from the National Comorbidity Survey Replication. Am J Psychiatry 163:716–723, 2006

Kovacs M: Children's Depression Inventory (CDI) Manual. Toronto, Ontario, Canada, Multi-Health Systems, 1992

Lahey BB, Applegate B, McBurnett K, et al: DSM-IV field trials for attention deficit hyperactivity disorder. Am J Psychiatry 151:1673–1685, 1994

March J, Parker J, Sullivan K: The Multidimensional Anxiety Scale for Children (MASC): factor structure, reliability, and validity. J Am Acad Child Adolesc Psychiatry 36:554–565, 1997

McBurnett K, Pfiffner LJ, Frick PJ: Symptom properties as a function of ADHD type: an argument for continued study of sluggish cognitive tempo. J Abnorm Child Psychol 29:207–213, 2001

McMahon R, Forehand R: Helping the Noncompliant Child: Family Based Treatment for Oppositional Behavior, 2nd Edition. New York, Guilford, 2003

Milich R, Balentine AC, Lynam DR: ADHD combined type and ADHD predominantly inattentive type are distinct and unrelated disorders. Clin Psychol 8:463–488, 2001

MTA Cooperative Group: A 14-month randomized clinical trial of treatment strategies for attention-deficit/hyperactivity disorder. Multimodal Treatment Study of Children with ADHD. Arch Gen Psychiatry 56:1073–1086, 1999

MTA Cooperative Group: National Institute of Mental Health Multimodal Treatment Study of ADHD follow-up: changes in effectiveness and growth after the end of treatment. Pediatrics 113:762–769, 2004

Pelham WE Jr: Against the grain: a proposal for a psychosocial-first approach to treating ADHD—the Buffalo Treatment Algorithm, in Attention Deficit Hyperactivity Disorder: A 21st Century Perspective. Edited by McBurnett K, Elliott R, Elliott G, et al. London, CRC Press, 2007, pp 301–316

Pelham WE Jr, Fabiano G: Evidence-based psychosocial treatments for attention-deficit/hyperactivity disorder: an update. J Clin Child Adolesc Psychol 37:185–214, 2008

Pelham WE Jr, Burrows-MacLean L, Gnagy EM, et al: Transdermal methylphenidate, behavioral, and combined treatment for children with ADHD. Exp Clin Psychopharmacol 13:111–126, 2005a

Pelham WE Jr, Fabiano G, Massetti G: Evidence-based assessment of attention deficit hyperactivity disorder in children and adolescents. J Clin Child Adolesc Psychol 34:449–476, 2005b

Pliszka S; AACAP Work Group on Quality Issues: Practice parameter for the assessment and treatment of attention-deficit/hyperactivity disorder. J Am Acad Child Adolesc Psychiatry 46:894–921, 2007

Polanczyk G, Rhode L: Prevalance of ADHD: a meta analysis. Am J Psychiatry 164:942–948, 2007

Poznanski E, Freeman L, Mokros H: Children's Depression Rating Scale—Revised. Psychopharmacol Bull 21:979–989, 1985

Shaffer D, Fisher P, Lucas C, et al: NIMH Diagnostic Interview Schedule for Children, Version IV (NIMH DISC-IV): description, differences from previous versions, and reliability of some common diagnoses. J Am Acad Child Adolesc Psychiatry 39:28–38, 2000

Swanson JM: School-Based Assessments and Interventions for ADD students. Irvine, CA, KC Press, 1992

Wilens TE, McBurnett K, Bukstein O, et al: Multisite controlled study of OROS methylphenidate in the treatment of adolescents with attention-deficit/hyperactivity disorder. Arch Pediatr Adolesc Med 160:82–90, 2006

■ CHAPTER 2 ■

Trouble With Transitions

Does My Child Have Autism?

Susan Bacalman, M.S.W.
Robert L. Hendren, D.O.

CASE PRESENTATION

IDENTIFYING INFORMATION

Sebastian, who is 10 years old, lives with both parents and an older sister and younger brother.

CHIEF COMPLAINT

Sebastian was referred by his parents, who were seeking a second opinion. They think that his current diagnoses, attention-deficit/hyperactivity disorder (ADHD) and obsessive-compulsive disorder (OCD), do not adequately explain his behavior problems. They recently read an article describing autism spectrum disorders and feel that they finally know what is wrong with their son.

Susan Bacalman, M.S.W., is with The M.I.N.D. Institute (Medical Investigation of Neurodevelopmental Disorders Institute) at the University of California, Davis Medical Center in Sacramento, California.

Robert L. Hendren, D.O., is Professor of Psychiatry, Executive Director, and Tsakopoulos-Vismara Chair of the M.I.N.D. Institute, and Chief of Child and Adolescent Psychiatry at the University of California, Davis. As of this writing, he is also President of the American Academy of Child and Adolescent Psychiatry (2007–2009).

For complete biographical information, see "About the Contributors," p. 613.

History of Present Illness

Many of the behaviors that concern Sebastian's parents have been present since he was much younger. Currently, he is easily distracted, fidgety, always out of his seat, overly talkative, and unable to wait his turn. The compulsive and rigid behaviors that he has exhibited since early childhood have become more pronounced. For example, he becomes upset if his mother does not always drive the same route, and he is preoccupied with searching for railroad crossing gates. Changes in routine are difficult for Sebastian. He flies into a rage if his mother changes their afternoon schedule. He has difficulty following directions, and although school staff view this behavior as oppositional, his parents suspect he has difficulty processing their requests.

Sebastian's parents feel that his play behavior has always been unusual. He is more interested in taking things apart than engaging in pretend play. He does not play with children in the neighborhood and is disinterested in other children at the park or playground.

Past Psychiatric History

Sebastian's parents had vague concerns about Sebastian when, at 12 months of age, he preferred to spin the wheels of his pull toy rather than pull it around. Their concerns intensified when Sebastian was age 4 as he became more irritable and argumentative. When he entered kindergarten at age 5, Sebastian was aggressive with classmates when they invaded his physical space. He did not understand how to engage with other children in conversation or in play. He did not join in group games such as hide-and-seek and seemed unaware of how to share or take turns. As Sebastian progressed through the early elementary grades, his behavior problems worsened. He was frequently suspended from school because of his aggressive outbursts and refusal to comply with teacher directions. He had difficulty in unstructured settings, particularly those that were overstimulating, such as the playground at recess.

Over the years, his parents obtained several evaluations for Sebastian, including psychoeducational testing and a comprehensive pediatric neurology workup, but the diagnoses of ADHD and OCD remained unchanged.

In an effort to treat his problems with attention and difficulties making transitions, doctors prescribed trials of several medications for Sebastian, including clonidine, stimulants, and a selective serotonin reuptake inhibitor (SSRI). Clonidine was discontinued because it was too sedating. Osmotic-release (OROS) methylphenidate (Concerta) was modestly effective in treating Sebastian's inattention and distractibility and was continued at a low dose. The SSRI, paroxetine (Paxil), was stopped because Sebastian complained of a dry mouth.

MEDICAL HISTORY

A neurologist evaluated Sebastian at age 6 because he periodically "spaced out." The results of the electroencephalogram and hearing and vision tests were normal. The neurologist noted motor clumsiness, difficulty holding a pencil correctly, and poor handwriting.

DEVELOPMENTAL HISTORY

Sebastian was the product of a normal, full-term pregnancy and uncomplicated delivery. No problems were noted during his early infancy. He walked at age 12 months and began using single words between 24 and 28 months. He rapidly progressed from using single words to using complex sentences. Although Sebastian used grammatically correct sentences, his parents felt that they were always prompting him to communicate appropriately. For example, he typically greeted other people by asking them what type of vacuum cleaner they own.

It has been difficult to obtain adequate educational services for Sebastian. On numerous psychoeducational assessments, his IQ has been in the average range with superior to gifted abilities in information and block design. Despite Sebastian's high cognitive abilities, he was withdrawn from a regular classroom due to his behavior problems and placed in an alternative program for children with severe behavior disturbances. He was lost in this program and easily targeted for teasing by his more socially competent classmates.

SOCIAL HISTORY

Sebastian's parents are both professionals who work outside the home. There are no significant economic or health stressors and no history of abuse or neglect.

FAMILY HISTORY

A second-degree relative on the paternal side has ADHD. No other psychiatric or learning problems are present in either parent or the extended family.

MENTAL STATUS EXAMINATION

Sebastian was an appropriately dressed, attractive 10-year-old boy. He appeared restless, fidgeting in his seat. He was not interested in answering questions and instead asked the interviewer what type of car she drove. Once she responded, he immediately listed all of her vehicle's design features and commended her on her choice. When Sebastian talked about the technicalities of cars, his eye contact improved and his tone of voice became more expressive. Otherwise, it was difficult to engage Sebastian in conversation. He could not describe how he was feeling or elaborate on why he was experiencing problems at school. He acknowledged that he did not have many friends but could not explain why this was so. Given his limited range of facial expressions and inability to describe his feelings, it was difficult to assess the quality of Sebastian's mood. He denied ever wanting to hurt himself, and his mother never observed him losing interest in favorite activities or becoming lethargic. Sleep and appetite were normal. Sebastian denied hearing voices or seeing things that were not present, and his mother never observed him responding to internal stimuli.

Diagnostic Measures

In addition to taking a comprehensive history and observing Sebastian, we administered the Social Communication Questionnaire (SCQ; Rutter et al. 2003) to his parents and conducted the Autism Diagnostic Observation Schedule — Generic (ADOS-G; Lord et al. 1999) with Sebastian. These instruments were developed in recent years and are widely used to facilitate the detection of autism or pervasive developmental disorder (PDD) in children and adolescents.

The SCQ, a screening tool that can be completed by a parent or caregiver, is used to examine behaviors associated with autism based on criteria from the *Diagnostic and Statistical Manual of Mental Disorders*, 4th Edition (DSM-IV; American Psychiatric Association 1994). Persons who receive a score of 15 or higher on the SCQ are considered at increased risk for autism and should be referred for further assessment (Eaves et al. 2006). Sebastian's score on this measure was 22. The ADOS-G is a semistructured play interaction (with children) or interview (with adolescents) administered to elicit and observe the quality of an individual's social and communication behaviors. It has four modules, each geared to a different developmental level and verbal ability. Sebastian received a total score of 12 on this measure, which was above the autism cutoff of 10.

Children presenting with significant social and communication difficulties should be screened for autism, because early identification and intervention can positively affect their prognosis.

COMMENTARIES

Psychotherapeutic Perspective

Laura Schreibman, Ph.D.

DIAGNOSTIC FORMULATION

Sebastian meets criteria for an autistic disorder, specifically Asperger's disorder. He meets criteria for an autistic disorder based on evidence of autistic behaviors prior to age 36 months. His parents became concerned and noted odd behavior when he was age 12 months. He subsequently exhibited behaviors consistent with autism, including compulsive, ritualistic behaviors; lack of interest in pretend play with toys; difficulties with transitions and changes in routine; lack of interest in other children; failure to participate in social group games; absence of sharing or turn-taking; and insensitivity to or lack of awareness of needs of social/communicative partners. In addition, both the SCQ and the ADOS-G confirmed an autism diagnosis. The administration of the Autism Diagnostic Interview—Revised (Lord et al. 1994), as an adjunct to the ADOS-G, could be helpful in confirming the diagnosis by indicating specific behaviors and deficits that have been present since a very early age.

Sebastian meets the diagnostic criteria for Asperger's disorder because of his failure to develop peer relationships appropriate to his developmental level, lack of social or emotional reciprocity, an encompassing preoccupation with one or more stereotyped and restricted patterns of interest that is abnormal either in intensity or focus (his obsession with cars, burned-out city lights), and an inflexible adherence to specific, nonfunctional routines or rituals (he does not tolerate changes in schedule or his mother's changes in driving speed). In addition, the disturbance causes clinically significant impairment in social functioning, as is evidenced by Sebastian's difficulty in social interaction, dislike of children standing too close, aggression, and inappropriate social initiations. The description of his approaching an examiner by asking her the make of car she drives and pursuing that topic with far more detail and persistence than is socially appropriate is an excellent example of the egocentric, hyperverbose, and insensitive social interactions typical of individuals with

Laura Schreibman, Ph.D., is Distinguished Professor of Psychology at the University of California, San Diego, in La Jolla, California (for complete biographical information, see "About the Contributors," p. 613).

Asperger's disorder. The fact that Sebastian is the subject of teasing by peers is a common consequence of disordered social functioning in children with this disorder. He also does not have a history of clinically significant delay in language development, cognitive development, or acquisition of other (nonsocial) adaptive behaviors. Although his language is not delayed, he does show deficits in the ability to describe his emotions. Motor clumsiness is also mentioned in Sebastian's evaluation, and this characteristic is often noted in individuals with Asperger's disorder.

Differential diagnosis from autistic disorder is possible primarily because Sebastian was not significantly delayed in language acquisition or cognitive development. He does show a pronounced difficulty with change (routine and transitions) but lacks the motor mannerisms often apparent in individuals with autistic disorder. Rett's disorder and childhood disintegrative disorder can be ruled out because Sebastian lacks the behavioral deterioration, mental retardation, and language impairment characterizing these disorders. Schizophrenia in childhood is ruled out because of the absence of delusions, hallucinations, and disorganized speech. Also, schizophrenia in childhood is preceded by years of normal development, whereas Sebastian exhibited symptoms in very early childhood.

The additional diagnosis of ADHD is made, although with the caveat that according to the framework of DSM-IV-TR, ADHD cannot be applied in addition to an autistic spectrum disorder. However, given the significant clinical impact of the ADHD symptoms on Sebastian's functioning, it is included here.

DSM-IV-TR DIAGNOSIS

Axis I   299.80 Asperger's disorder
            314.01 ADHD, combined type
Axis II   None
Axis III   None
Axis IV   Possible inappropriate classroom placement
Axis V   Global Assessment of Functioning=55

TREATMENT RECOMMENDATIONS

Treatment should be preceded by a thorough evaluation of Sebastian's current needs to determine treatment targets. Several areas of his functioning need to be addressed. Sebastian needs direct intervention for social deficits, inappropriate social initiations, behavioral control (outbursts, aggression, and oppositional behavior), compulsive and ritualistic behaviors, and self-control.

One area of concern is the parents' difficulty in dealing with their child's behavioral outbursts, behavioral rigidity, compulsiveness, and oppositional behavior. Parent behavioral training would likely be beneficial in assisting the parents to improve Sebastian's behavior in the home and community settings. Thus, instruction in behavioral management for the parents with the assistance of an in-home behavior specialist is recommended.

Intervention in the classroom setting is also recommended. Ideally, Sebastian would be transitioned from his current highly structured classroom to a less structured classroom. A clear description of individualized education program (IEP) goals, including social goals, should be obtained and addressed first within a more highly structured and individual format; as Sebastian attains these goals, the transition to a less structured classroom should be possible. A shadow aide in the classroom should facilitate this transition, with the goal of fading the aide as soon as possible. Programmed consistency with the behavioral procedures being implemented by the parents in the home is very important to help generalize behavioral improvements across the environments.

Perhaps the most critical need for individuals with Asperger's disorder is training in elements of social interaction. These individuals often need training in basic social discourse skills, such as the proper distance to stand from someone, eye contact with a social partner when engaging in discourse, and of course the discourse itself. Instruction is needed in avoiding persistence on a specific (often compulsive) topic, changing topics, asking questions of the social partner, and attending to the answer. Instruction in how to read facial expressions of others is also important. Such instruction is highly recommended for Sebastian both on an individual level and as part of a group experience. His participation in a social group program would help him learn a variety of specific skills with a variety of social interaction partners. This program should facilitate acquisition and generalization of skills, reduce Sebastian's stigmatizing social eccentricities, and reduce teasing by peers.

Self-management techniques would likely help Sebastian with several behavioral issues. Self-management has been used effectively with a variety of populations, including individuals with developmental disabilities and those with ADHD (Apple et al. 2005; Gureasko-Moore et al. 2006; Hinshaw 2006; Newman and Ten Eyck 2005; Schreibman and Koegel 2005). Generally, the procedure involves choosing a target behavior (the choice is ideally that of the client but can be made by a caregiver, as might be expected in cases of developmental disability) and then teaching the patient to identify an occurrence of the behavior, record the behavior, evaluate performance, and then self-reinforce. For a child such as Sebastian, self-management would likely prove useful in addressing behaviors such as social approaches, initiations, and topic shifts, as well as controlling excess motor activity, following directions, reducing rituals, and other behavioral targets.

Psychopharmacologic Perspective

Lawrence Scahill, M.S.N., Ph.D.

DIAGNOSTIC FORMULATION

Sebastian's history and examination are consistent with a diagnosis of autism. Sebastian exhibits behaviors in all three domains that define autism. In clinical practice, many would use the term *high-functioning autism*. In the differential diagnosis would be ADHD, OCD, Asperger's disorder, and pervasive developmental disorder, not otherwise specified (PDD-NOS).

The primary cues for the diagnosis of high-functioning autism are Sebastian's long-standing social delay and isolation, which are central to the diagnosis of all PDDs. Although not described in detail, the history suggests delayed language development, which would argue against Asperger's disorder. Further support for the diagnosis of autism is provided by Sebastian's rigid adherence to routine, preoccupation with parts of objects (e.g., the wheels of his pull toy), and restricted interest in cars (American Psychiatric Association 2000; Scahill 2005).

Despite the historical diagnosis of OCD, the clinical picture is not consistent with that diagnosis. In its classic presentation, OCD in children is characterized by the intrusion of unwanted thoughts accompanied by anxiety and often punctuated by repetitive behaviors that reduce the anxiety (Scahill et al. 2003), although many children do not show this clear-cut presentation. However, Sebastian demonstrates rigid adherence to routines and restrictive interests. He enjoys thinking and talking about cars—he is not struggling against intrusive thoughts or unwanted repetitive behavior that he does not want to perform.

Given the history, the diagnosis of ADHD is not surprising. By convention, DSM-IV-TR advises against a diagnosis of ADHD in children with autism, Asperger's disorder, or PDD-NOS. Although inattention, hyperactivity, and impulsiveness are not core features of autism, these behaviors are relatively common in children with autism. This DSM-IV-TR convention suggests that a separate diagnosis of ADHD is not needed to explain these behaviors.

Lawrence Scahill, M.S.N., Ph.D., is Professor of Nursing and Child Psychiatry and Director of the Research Unit on Pediatric Psychopharmacology at the Child Study Center in the Yale University School of Nursing in New Haven, Connecticut (for complete biographical information, see "About the Contributors," p. 613).

In the past, many clinicians might have been reluctant to apply the diagnosis of autism to a child with normal intelligence. Indeed, early epidemiological studies indicated that a high percentage of children with autism were functioning in the mentally retarded range. Better sampling of the general population and improved precision of the diagnosis of autism and related PDDs suggest that children with autism and normal intelligence were systematically undercounted in the earlier surveys (Fombonne 2005).

DSM-IV-TR DIAGNOSIS

Axis I   299.00 Autistic disorder

Axis II   None

Axis III   None

Axis IV   Problems related to the social environment
            Educational problems

Axis V   Global Assessment of Functioning=50 (current)

TREATMENT RECOMMENDATIONS[1]

Currently, there are three primary approaches for the treatment of autism: education, behavioral interventions, and medication. Education is in many ways the place to begin with treatment planning. Sebastian has failed in school for several years because of his medical condition. The history suggests that the school has viewed him as a boy with ADHD and severe emotional disturbance. Thus, when he did not succeed in the mainstream classroom, he was placed in a special education environment for children with behavior problems. Federal law specifies that children with a medical condition that interferes with academic progress are entitled to special education services in a least restrictive and appropriate setting. Sebastian's placement does not appear to be consistent with this mandate. Sebastian's parents need information and coaching on how to call for a formal meeting with school personnel—often called the pupil placement team (PPT)—to plan his educational program based on the diagnosis and clinical characteristics of autism, not ADHD or OCD. The formal document that follows from the PPT is called an Individualized Education Plan (IEP). In Sebastian's case, the PPT should recognize his social disability, which is central to the diagnosis of autism. His school placement should promote his social skills not simply for his enrichment but because his social dis-

---

[1]A wide range of complementary and alternative treatments for autism have been proposed, such as megavitamin therapy, vitamin B_{12} injections, oral vitamin B_6, special diets, chelation, and hyperbaric oxygen, to name a few. Although there are anecdotal reports describing the benefits of these treatments, they have not been well studied, and the rationale for such treatments is often unclear.

ability is fundamentally interfering with his academic success. Thus, placement in a school where he is lost in the shuffle at best, but also is teased and bullied, is not dealing with an essential component of his medical condition. In some instances, the selection of placement may require visiting programs in the home school district or neighboring districts. In other cases, the undisputed diagnosis of *autism* prompts the school district to offer specific programs that are available and more appropriate. Because Sebastian's IQ is in the normal range, the parents will need to be vigilant about placements that are primarily for lower-functioning children.

Behavioral interventions are typically focused on specific maladaptive behavior (e.g., aggression) or specific skill building (e.g., everyday living skills). In Sebastian's case, the situations and circumstances that precede his aggression, explosive outbursts, and noncompliance at school and at home need to be determined. In addition, the frequency, duration, and intensity of these behaviors need to be better understood. Finally, the impact and consequences of his maladaptive behavior should be documented. For example, if his tantrums result in his escaping environmental demands, his tantrums are being inadvertently reinforced. This type of functional analysis should be repeated following Sebastian's placement in a more appropriate educational environment. The same approach may be useful at home.

Medication therapy for children with autism is an underdeveloped science. Until recently, precious few medications had been evaluated in large-scale trials. In the current state of the art, medications are directed at target behaviors rather than the diagnosis of autism. Common targets include tantrums, aggression and self-injury, hyperactivity, and repetitive behavior. In Sebastian's case, an important first step would be to have his parents and teacher complete a behavioral rating scale such as the Aberrant Behavior Checklist (ABC) to help identify the appropriate target symptoms. The ABC is a 58-item scale consisting of five subscales: Irritability (aggression, tantrums, and self-injury), Stereotypies, Social Withdrawal, Hyperactivity, and Inappropriate Speech (Aman et al. 1985). The ABC provides normative data for populations with developmental disabilities (Brown et al. 2002) and is sensitive to change (Research Units on Pediatric Psychopharmacology [RUPP] Autism Network 2005).

If Sebastian's PPT meeting resulted in a new and more appropriate placement in a timely manner, a prudent decision would be to hold off on medication until the classroom change has been made. His behavior may appear quite different in a more appropriate school setting. If the time lag for placement in a new school program is likely to be prolonged, considering medication in his current situation would make sense. The history suggests that hyperactivity was a prominent problem in the past. If it is a current problem, as evidenced by a high score (>27 for boys in this age group) on the Hyperactivity subscale on the ABC from a parent and his teacher, another stimulant trial may be worth considering. A large-scale study conducted by the federally funded RUPP Autism Network (2005) showed that methylphenidate was indeed superior to placebo for the target problem of hyperactivity in children with PDDs; however, the average improvement was only about 20% over placebo. This difference is considerably lower in magnitude than the level of improvement associated with methylphenidate in typically developing children with ADHD. Although less well studied, the α_2 agonist drug guanfacine may also be useful for reducing hyperactivity in children with PDD and is probably less sedating than clonidine (Scahill et al. 2006).

The case vignette also mentions a past trial of paroxetine (Paxil). The SSRIs are commonly used in children with PDD. To date, however, the SSRIs have been poorly studied. The rationale for their use in PDD is their perceived safety and their demonstrated efficacy for the treatment of OCD in adults and children. As already noted, there are fundamental differences between the repetitive behaviors of children with autism and those of children with OCD. In a study of 39 children and adolescents with PDD, Hollander et al. (2005) showed only modest improvement in repetitive behavior, hardly a ringing endorsement.

The frequency, duration, and intensity of Sebastian's emotional outbursts need to be understood better. In addition to the functional analysis mentioned above, the ABC Irritability subscale provides an index of severity for these behaviors. A score over 20 on the 15-item Irritability subscale is the threshold for considering a potent medication such as a risperidone (e.g., Risperdal). In a study of 101 children with autism, the RUPP Autism Network (2002) showed that risperidone was superior to placebo for reducing tantrums, aggression, and self-injury. Seventy percent of the children randomly assigned to risperidone improved, showing an average reduction of 50% in Irritability subscale score. This medication is now approved by the U.S. Food and Drug Administration for the treatment of tantrums, aggression, and self-injury in children with autism (Scahill et al. 2007). However, risperidone is a potent medication and should only be used for children with serious behavior problems.

In conclusion, several initial steps are needed to forge a treatment plan. First, the clinical team, family, and school personnel need to resolve Sebastian's school placement. In the meantime, a functional analysis of his explosive behaviors both at home and at school should be undertaken immediately. For the team to gain better insight into the severity of Sebastian's disruptive behavior and hyperactivity, a parent and a teacher should complete the ABC. Children with autism with an ABC Irritability score >20 are candidates for risperidone treatment (0.75–1.5 mg/day in two divided doses). Risperidone is also likely to reduce hyperactivity. However, if the ABC Hyperactivity subscale score is high (>27) and the Irritability scale score is not (<20), a trial of guanfacine or methylphenidate would be more appropriate. The results of the functional analysis could also point to specific behavioral interventions that could be implemented in combination with either medication. The impact of the medication and behavioral intervention could be reconsidered in 3–4 weeks via a review of target problems and readministration of the ABC.

Integrative Perspective

Susan Bacalman, M.S.W
Robert L. Hendren, D.O.

DIAGNOSTIC FORMULATION

Autism is the most common of the pervasive developmental disorders, a group of disorders characterized by severe impairments in social interaction and communication. Autism and the related PDDs are not rare, with current prevalence rates estimated to be 65 per 10,000 in the general population (Fombonne 2005).

According to DSM-IV-TR, an autism diagnosis is based on impairments in three domains: communication; reciprocal social interactions; and restricted, repetitive behaviors and interests. For an individual to meet diagnostic criteria, a minimum of six symptoms must be present, at least two symptoms from the social domain and at least one from each of the other two.

Many signs indicative of autism, which were apparent in Sebastian's early history, were missed. His language onset was slightly delayed; as his language development progressed, Sebastian developed superficially sophisticated sentences that had a scripted quality and that he did not use for social communication. He always had difficulty initiating and maintaining a conversation unless it centered on his interests. Only when asked about his early development did Sebastian's parents belatedly recognize that he did not look at them when babbling, did not point to share interests, and did not use language to communicate socially.

Sebastian's early social development was also consistent with autism. He showed little interest in other children of the same age. Although he could tolerate limited parallel play, he preferred to play by himself. The quality of Sebastian's play was also typical of children with autism. He disliked pretend play with dolls or action figures, and he did not role-play by himself or with peers. He was always drawn to the parts of toys or objects and would rather take toys apart than play with them as they were intended to be used.

Sebastian has always displayed restrictive interests, including an earlier pre-occupation with vacuum cleaners and a more recent preoccupation with the technical specifications of automobiles.

DSM-IV-TR DIAGNOSIS

Axis I   299.00 Autistic disorder

Axis II   799.9 Diagnosis deferred

Axis III   None

Axis IV   Educational problems

Axis V   Global Assessment of Functioning=48

DISCUSSION

Why did other clinicians miss the autism diagnosis? There are several likely explanations. First, Sebastian's IQ is in the normal range. Second, his advanced vocabulary and use of complex sentences masked his underlying communication deficits. Finally, his fidgetiness, inability to remain seated, and striking out at classmates were more prominent and caused acute management problems in school, leading to a diagnosis of ADHD and overshadowing his problems associated with autism.

A misdiagnosis of autism, particularly in high-functioning children, is not uncommon. In a well-documented article, Perry (1998) described five boys seen in his private practice, all initially diagnosed with ADHD and then subsequently rediagnosed with PDD. He proposed several possible reasons for the misdiagnoses. None of the boys presented with the more obvious signs of PDD such as echolalia and self-stimulating behaviors, and none of them had cognitive delay (mental retardation). Although the boys all struggled with friendships, their difficulties were considered less severe than those typically seen in children with autism (Perry 1998).

Restlessness, impulsivity, and difficulty in maintaining attention are common in children with autism (Ghaziuddin 2005); however, DSM-IV-TR discourages a diagnosis of ADHD in children meeting autism criteria. Ghaziuddin (2005) proposed that it is not helpful to disregard a diagnosis of ADHD in a child with autism, particularly if the child presents with unresolved symptoms of hyperactivity and impulsivity. To establish a co-occurring diagnosis of ADHD, a clinician should perform a comprehensive evaluation to determine whether other psychiatric or medical conditions may be contributing to the child's hyperactivity and impulsivity (Ghaziuddin 2005).

Another diagnostic dilemma in Sebastian's case is whether his presentation is more consistent with either high-functioning autism or Asperger's disorder. DSM-IV-TR distinguishes Asperger's disorder from autism based on IQ and the presence or absence of a language delay. To meet criteria for Asperger's disorder, a child must have at least a normal IQ and no history of language delay. Technically, Sebastian would meet criteria for high-functioning autism because he had a slight delay in onset of language. Much debate has occurred over whether these are distinct disorders or exist on a continuum of social and communication impairment (Miller and Ozonoff 2000). Kasari and Rotheram-Fuller (2005) reviewed a number of studies and found that the majority did not find empirical support for different disorders. Often, autism and Asperger's disorder are considered on a continuum or spectrum, thus the term *autism spectrum disorder.*

TREATMENT RECOMMENDATIONS

Our treatment plan for Sebastian included returning him to his regular elementary school with a one-to-one aide and providing additional interventions to address his behavior problems, social skills deficits, and language problems. We suggested that Sebastian have a comprehensive speech and language evaluation focusing on language pragmatics, processing, and comprehension.

Verbal children with autism often have problems with the pragmatics of language (Prizant and Wetherby 2005). Pragmatics involves the "how to" of language, the ability to master the socially relevant aspects of communication (Westby 1999). Sebastian was having significant problems in this area. He did not understand how to initiate a conversation or to build on another child's comments. He wanted to highjack the topic so that he could discuss his special interest in cars, and he was clueless when other children quickly became bored and disinterested.

We recommended that in addition to language pragmatics, the speech-language pathologist look at Sebastian's language processing abilities, including his ability to rapidly process incoming speech, hold information in short-term memory, and follow through with directions. Many autistic children tend to be visual learners and understand instructions better when presented with visual support (Prizant and Wetherby 2005). Pairing auditory information with pictures or written text often helps them process information more effectively.

To address Sebastian's outbursts and disruptions, we recommended that a behavioral specialist perform a functional analysis of his behavior. The results of this analysis would inform the treatment plan for teachers and other support staff. The one-to-one aide would be fully versed in how to identify and avoid triggers that would cause Sebastian to have an outburst or become unmanageable. The aide would also be given instruction on how to diffuse and redirect Sebastian when necessary.

We felt Sebastian would benefit from participation in a social skills group that would teach him prosocial behaviors. A well-run group can help children with autism learn social rules and better identify subtle social cues. Groups can foster a child's interactions with other members in a safe setting where the child can practice social interactions without fear of being teased or excluded.

Finally, we recommended a medication trial to target Sebastian's inattentiveness and his compulsive and rigid behaviors. Because Concerta had been mildly effective, we suggested increasing the dose to maximize its effect. Our other recommendation was to begin a trial of a different SSRI to decrease his compulsive behaviors and inflexibility.

Sebastian's parents were relieved to have a diagnosis that more fully explained his behaviors. Our team worked collaboratively with Sebastian's parents, school personnel, and therapists; with school staff we emphasized that Sebastian's oppositional behavior likely stemmed from autism. Sensitizing teachers and staff about Sebastian's pragmatic language deficits, processing problems, and poor adaptability to change enabled them to see him in a different light. We encouraged parents and school staff to cultivate Sebastian's many strengths, including his exquisite attention to detail, facility with facts, and excellent memory.

The family and school implemented our recommendations and reported improvement in Sebastian's school adjustment and overall functioning.

EDITORS' NOTE

Subtle differences in clinical presentation and history may lead to differences in diagnosis. Although those of us "in the know" about the subtleties of diagnosis recognize the likelihood that some diagnoses such as autism, Asperger's disorder, and PDD are best viewed as a spectrum of disorders along several continua, these subtleties may be lost on parents and caregivers, and sometimes lead to confusion, anger, disappointment, and doctor shopping. Interestingly, all of the commentators in this chapter noted Sebastian's language delay, but two interpreted it as significant and the third interpreted it as within the normal range. The presence of a delay would indicate autism, whereas the absence would indicate Asperger's disorder, thus highlighting a complex interplay of knowledge of symptom delay and placing them in a developmental context. Similarly, whether or not one applies hierarchical criteria in determining whether the diagnosis of an autism spectrum disorder (ASD) preempts the diagnosis of ADHD may not only confuse a parent but also lead to differences in whether one chooses to treat the attentional and hyperactive symptoms in a child with ASD. The current DSM framework precludes a diagnosis of ADHD in a child with autism. This hierarchical distinction is under review for DSM-V. These diagnostic distinctions may not make much of a difference in terms of one's recommended treatment approach but, when misunderstood by parents, may lead to dramatic differences in continued health care seeking in hopes of finding a cure and possibly even exposure of the patient to ineffective or dangerous treatments. Such is the case in the history of purported cures for autism.

Regardless of his or her disciplinary roots, such as psychiatry, pediatrics, psychology, or social work, the diagnostician is responsible for educating the parent about the differences across diagnostic categories. The goal is to avoid uncertainty for families when different labels are applied over time to the same child. Families must also be helped to understand what has been shown to work for the primary condition (e.g., intensive behavioral interventions), as well as effective interventions for any associated problems, such as various medications for inattention, hyperactivity, aggression, and irritability symptoms that often accompany ASD.

REFERENCES

Aman MG, Singh NN, Stewart AW, et al: The Aberrant Behavior Checklist: a behavior rating scale for the assessment of treatment effects. Am J Ment Defic 89:485–491, 1985

American Psychiatric Association: Diagnostic and Statistical Manual of Mental Disorders, 4th Edition. Washington, DC, American Psychiatric Association, 1994

American Psychiatric Association: Diagnostic and Statistical Manual of Mental Disorders, 4th Edition, Text Revision. Washington, DC, American Psychiatric Association, 2000

Apple AL, Billingsley F, Schwartz IS: Effects of video modeling alone and with self-management on complement-giving behaviors of children with high-functioning ASD. Journal of Positive Behavior Interventions 7:33–46, 2005

Brown EC, Aman MG, Havercamp SM: Factor analysis and norms for parent ratings on the Aberrant Behavior Checklist—Community for young people in special education. Research in Developmental Disabilities 23:45–60, 2002

Eaves LC, Wingert HD, Ho HH, et al: Screening for autism spectrum disorders with the Social Communication Questionnaire. J Dev Behav Pediatr 27 (2 suppl):S95–S103, 2006

Fombonne E: Epidemiology of autistic disorder and other pervasive developmental disorders. J Clin Psychiatry 66 (suppl 10):3–8, 2005

Ghaziuddin M: Mental Health Aspects of Autism and Asperger Syndrome. Philadelphia, PA, Jessica Kingsley, 2005

Gureasko-Moore S, DuPaul G, White GP: The effects of self-management in general education classrooms on the organizational skills of adolescents with ADHD. Behav Modif 30:159–183, 2006

Hinshaw SP: Treatment for children and adolescents with attention-deficit/hyperactivity disorder, in Child and Adolescent Therapy: Cognitive-Behavioral Procedures, 3rd Edition. Edited by Kendall PC. New York, Guilford, 2006, pp 82–113

Hollander E, Phillips A, Chaplin W, et al: A placebo controlled crossover trial of liquid fluoxetine on repetitive behaviors in childhood and adolescent autism. Neuropsychopharmacology 30:582–589, 2005

Kasari C, Rotheram-Fuller E: Current trends in psychological research on children with high-functioning autism and Asperger disorder. Curr Opin Psychiatry 18:497–501, 2005

Lord C, Rutter M, Le Couteur A: Autism Diagnostic Interview—Revised: a revised version of a diagnostic interview for caregivers of individuals with possible pervasive developmental disorders. J Autism Dev Disord 24:659–685, 1994

Lord C, Rutter M, DiLavore P, et al: Autism Diagnostic Observation Schedule. Los Angeles, CA, Western Psychological Services, 1999

Miller JN, Ozonoff S: The external validity of Asperger disorder: lack of evidence from the domain of neuropsychology. J Abnorm Psychol 109:227–238, 2000

Newman B, Ten Eyck P: Self-management of initiations by students diagnosed with autism. The Analysis of Verbal Behavior 21:177–122, 2005

Perry R: Misdiagnosed ADD/ADHD; rediagnosed PDD. J Am Acad Child Adolesc Psychiatry 37:113–114, 1998

Prizant BM, Wetherby AM: Critical issues in enhancing communication abilities for persons with autism spectrum disorders, in Handbook of Autism and Pervasive Developmental Disorders, 3rd Edition. Edited by Volkmar FR, Paul R, Klin A, et al. Hoboken, NJ, Wiley, 2005, pp 925–945

Research Units on Pediatric Psychopharmacology (RUPP) Autism Network: Randomized, controlled, crossover trial of methylphenidate in pervasive developmental disorder. Arch Gen Psychiatry 62:1266–1274, 2005

Rutter M, Bailey A, Berument S, et al: Social Communication Questionnaire. Los Angeles, CA, Western Psychological Services, 2003

Scahill L: Diagnosis and evaluation of pervasive developmental disorders. J Clin Psychiatry 66 (suppl 10):19–25, 2005

Scahill L, Kano Y, King RA, et al: Influence of age and tic disorders on obsessive-compulsive disorder in a pediatric sample. J Child Adolesc Psychopharmacol 13 (suppl 1):7–18, 2003

Scahill L, Aman MG, McDougle CJ, et al: A prospective open trial of guanfacine in children with pervasive developmental disorders. J Child Adolesc Psychopharmacol 16:589–598, 2006

Scahill L, Koenig K, Carroll DH, et al: Risperidone approved for the treatment of serious behavioral problems in children with autism. J Child Adolesc Psychiatr Nurs 20:188–190, 2007

Schreibman L, Koegel RL: Training for parents of children with autism: pivotal responses, generalization and individualization of interventions, in Psychosocial Treatments for Child and Adolescent Disorders: Empirically Based Strategies for Clinical Practice, 2nd Edition. Edited by Hibbs ED, Jensen PS. Washington, DC, American Psychological Association, 2005, pp 605–631

Westby C: Assessment of pragmatic competence in children with psychiatric disorders, in Communication Disorders and Children With Psychiatric and Behavioral Disorders (School-Age Children Series). Edited by Rogers-Adkinson DL, Griffith PL. San Diego, CA, Singular, 1999, pp 177–258

■ CHAPTER 3 ■

Living in Her Parents' Shadow
Separation Anxiety Disorder

Andrea M. Victor, Ph.D.
Gail A. Bernstein, M.D.

CASE PRESENTATION

IDENTIFYING INFORMATION

Susan, who is 7 years old, was referred for an evaluation by her pediatrician due to concerns regarding anxiety and school refusal.

CHIEF COMPLAINT

"Susan is afraid I will forget her at school," mother stated.

HISTORY OF PRESENT ILLNESS

For the past 3 months, Susan has had fears about separating from her parents to go to school, and these fears have become progressively worse. She has extreme distress on Sunday nights when thinking about going to school the next day. Susan has trouble falling asleep because she is plagued with worries about bad

Andrea M. Victor, Ph.D., is Assistant Professor at the Child and Adolescent Anxiety and Mood Disorders Clinic at the University of Minnesota Medical School in Minneapolis.

Gail A. Bernstein, M.D., is Head of the Program in Child and Adolescent Anxiety and Mood Disorders and Endowed Professor in Child and Adolescent Anxiety Disorders in the Division of Child and Adolescent Psychiatry at the University of Minnesota Medical School in Minneapolis.

For complete biographical information, see "About the Contributors," p. 613.

things happening to her parents while she is at school. Specifically, she worries that her mother will get into a car accident or that a burglar will break into their house and kill her mother. When it is time for school, Susan actively resists going by hiding under the bed, locking herself in the bathroom, or clinging to her mother as she begs to stay home because of a stomachache. Several times on the way to school, Susan has threatened to jump out of the car if forced to attend school and has tried to get out of the moving car on one occasion.

If Susan's parents are successful in getting her to school, she usually settles down within 30 minutes of arrival in the classroom. However, Susan intermittently appears sad and tearful. At those times, she tells her teacher that she needs to call home to make sure that her mother is safe. Susan frequently asks to go to the nurse's office because of stomach pain and feeling faint, in hopes that she will be sent home from school.

Susan's mother works in a retail store and cannot take Susan to work with her on days that Susan refuses to attend school. Therefore, her father, a construction worker, takes Susan with him to the construction site when she refuses to go to school, and she sits in his truck for up to 8 hours while he works. Her parents are considering the option of Susan's mother quitting her job so she can homeschool their daughter. Her parents have also stopped going out to dinner or the movies on Saturday nights because Susan has severe tantrums when a babysitter arrives.

While at home, Susan constantly shadows her parents. Sometimes she agrees to stay in her bedroom alone if her dog is with her. Most evenings, Susan starts out in her own bed. However, she invariably slips into the master bedroom and climbs into her parents' bed, stating that she is afraid she will fall asleep and never wake up. Susan reports scary dreams of monsters capturing her and locking her in a cave so she cannot escape and of her parents being swept up by a tornado and never returning.

Susan also worries that she is not as smart as her classmates, that the girls at school do not like her, and that her family does not have enough money to pay their taxes. However, these worries are not as severe as those related to separation from her parents, and Susan is able to control these worries. These worries do not interfere with Susan's sleep and concentration and are not associated with somatic complaints.

Past Psychiatric History

Susan has never participated in therapy or been given a prescription for psychotropic medication.

Medical History

Susan was small for gestational age, weighing 5 lbs at term. She was prone to illnesses as an infant.

DEVELOPMENTAL HISTORY

As an infant and toddler, Susan was slow to warm up to new people and approached novel or unfamiliar situations with distress or avoidance. She showed prolonged separation reactions for up to 90 minutes when left at day care during her preschool years.

SOCIAL HISTORY

Susan lives with her biological parents, 3-year-old sister, and 17-year-old brother. Her mother recently returned to work as a manager of a retail store, and her father is employed as a construction worker. There is no history of abuse or neglect. Susan is currently in second grade at a small parochial school that she has attended since kindergarten. She gets along well with peers but has limited contact with them outside of school.

FAMILY HISTORY

Susan's mother has a history of panic disorder. Her father has been diagnosed with recurrent major depression and is being treated with antidepressant medication. Susan's older brother has social phobia and dropped out of high school because of impairing fears and avoidance of social and performance situations.

MENTAL STATUS EXAMINATION

Susan was nicely dressed and well groomed, and appeared her stated age. She sat on her mother's lap during the evaluation and engaged in minimal eye contact with the interviewer. When asked direct questions, Susan provided limited responses and often looked to her mother to provide additional information. She refused to separate from her mother and would not allow her mother to leave the interview room without her. She expressed worries that her mother would not return if her mother went to the waiting room and left Susan to talk to the interviewer alone. Susan's mood was described by her mother as "nervous and irritable" at times of separation. Susan's affect was anxious. Her thinking was logical and coherent. There was no evidence of psychosis. Susan stated that she would jump out of her mother's moving car if required to go to school.

COMMENTARIES

Psychotherapeutic Perspective

Jami M. Furr, M.A.
Sarah A. Crawley, M.A.
Philip C. Kendall, Ph.D., A.B.P.P.

DIAGNOSTIC FORMULATION

Susan, a 7-year-old girl, presented with symptoms suggesting separation anxiety disorder (SAD) and problems with school refusal. She experiences distress upon separation from her parents, worries that harm will befall them, is afraid that she will be forgotten at school, refuses to go to school in response to her separation concerns, becomes distressed when she is home without her parents, will not sleep alone during the night, has nightmares with a separation theme, and reports stomach pain and faintness when away from her parents at school. It appears that her separation concerns have been present since preschool. Importantly, Susan's symptoms are reported to interfere meaningfully with her academic and social functioning (e.g., she has not been able to attend school and has limited contact with peers outside of school).

Susan is also experiencing generalized worrying and shyness, suggesting possible diagnoses of generalized anxiety disorder (GAD) and/or social phobia. Because anxiety disorders are highly comorbid with affective, conduct, and other anxiety disorders (Verduin and Kendall 2003), Susan's evaluation should include related assessments. A semistructured diagnostic interview would be appropriate. The Anxiety Disorders Interview Schedule for DSM-IV—Child Version (Silverman and Albano 1996), assesses a range of disorders and would rule out thought disorder or pervasive developmental disorder.

A multi-informant assessment would be helpful in this case, to obtain data from Susan, her parents, and her school teacher. Specifically, in Susan's case,

Jami M. Furr, M.A., is a doctoral student in clinical psychology and a student research assistant in the Child and Adolescent Anxiety Disorders Clinic at Temple University in Philadelphia, Pennsylvania.

Sarah A. Crawley, M.A., is a doctoral student in clinical psychology at Temple University in Philadelphia, Pennsylvania.

Philip C. Kendall, Ph.D., A.B.P.P., is Laura H. Carnell Professor of Psychology and Director in the Child and Adolescent Anxiety Disorders Clinic at Temple University in Philadelphia, Pennsylvania.

For complete biographical information, see "About the Contributors," p. 613.

the following assessments would be beneficial: self- and teacher-report measures of anxiety (see Furr et al. 2008) and related emotional concerns (e.g., depression), parent- and teacher-report measures of Susan's behavior, an index of academic achievement, and a physical exam to rule out medical factors that may contribute to her symptoms. Finally, given Susan's family history of maternal panic disorder and paternal depression, assessment of parental psychopathology may be beneficial. Child assessments should be administered before and after treatment, with some measures of anxiety being administered weekly to both Susan and her parents to track progress.

Both biological and psychosocial factors likely play a role in Susan's behavior. Susan may be predisposed to psychopathology given her family history of depression, panic disorder, and social phobia, as well as her likely behavioral inhibition as a young child. Susan may also have been exposed to her parents' anxious and depressed affects, and they possibly have modeled avoidance of anxiety-provoking situations as a result of their own psychopathology. Finally, Susan's parents behave in a manner that allows her to avoid school and other anxious situations (e.g., they pick her up when the nurse calls; they let her sleep in their bed; they allow her to go to work with Dad instead of working on classwork). This pattern of parental accommodation to Susan's avoidance contributes to and maintains her anxious avoidance, which may prevent her from mastering age-appropriate developmental challenges.

DSM-IV-TR DIAGNOSIS

Axis I   309.21 Separation anxiety disorder, accompanied by school refusal
             Rule out generalized anxiety disorder
             Rule out social phobia

Axis II   None

Axis III   Low gestational weight

Axis IV   Parents' psychopathology
             Brother's social phobia, brother's school refusal

Axis V   Global Assessment of Functioning=47 (current)

TREATMENT RECOMMENDATIONS

PSYCHOLOGICAL TREATMENT

A first-choice treatment for Susan is cognitive-behavioral therapy (CBT), such as the Coping Cat Program, a time-limited, manualized anxiety treatment with an accompanying child workbook (Kendall and Hedtke 2006a, 2006b). Numerous independent studies have supported the short-term (e.g., Kendall 1994; Kendall et al. 1997) and long-term (Kendall and Southam-Gerow 1996; Kendall et al. 2004) efficacy of CBT treatments.

The 16-session CBT program would include having Susan identify her somatic reactions to anxiety, identify and challenge her anxious thoughts, develop a plan to cope with the anxiety-provoking situation(s), practice her coping plan, engage in exposure tasks, evaluate her efforts at managing anxiety, and administer self-reward as appropriate. The therapist facilitates progress by "normalizing" anxiety, providing imaginal and in vivo exposure tasks (for a practical discussion of exposure tasks, see Kendall et al. 2005), orchestrating role-play opportunities, teaching relaxation skills, modeling coping behavior, and rewarding effort. Treatment gains are also facilitated by out-of-session activities, such as practicing skills learned in session, completing workbook tasks, and engaging in exposure tasks. Parents consult and collaborate with the therapist throughout treatment, and two sessions are devoted entirely to parents. Susan's parents would be oriented to the treatment components, educated about avoidance and how it can increase anxiety, and encouraged to model coping. Susan's parents may also be asked to participate in exposure tasks (e.g., appropriately responding to Susan's physical complaints and avoidance behavior). For example, the therapist would use in vivo exposure tasks and reward systems to help Susan return to school and would encourage her parents to set limits on Susan's avoidance to help her separate from them to go to school and other places.

Treatment Goals

Several treatment goals should be established for Susan. Susan will demonstrate improved coping skills by learning to use relaxation techniques, to identify anxious thoughts, to use appropriate coping thoughts and problem-solving strategies, and to self-reward for effort. As a result of applying these skills, Susan will show a reduction in avoidance and anxious arousal. Additionally, Susan will demonstrate a reduction in her avoidance of school, as evidenced by her return to school for partial and full days and by a reduction in phone calls made to her parents during the school day. Eventually, Susan's parents will require her to remain in school for the entire school day. Susan will also show an increase in self-confidence, as evidenced by a reduction in avoidance of and distress about separating from her parents. For example, Susan will be able to stay at home with a babysitter and play in a separate room from her parents without disproportionate distress. Lastly, Susan will have an increase in social and extracurricular activities. For instance, Susan will have a greater number of play dates with peers and will join an after-school activity (e.g., Girl Scouts). Susan will also demonstrate an increased tolerance for interaction with unfamiliar children and adults.

Additional Interventions

If academic difficulties are found in Susan's initial assessments, further neuropsychological and psychoeducational testing may be needed, because limitations in cognitive functioning could detract from her treatment outcome. Additionally, if Susan's parents are experiencing distressing psychological symptoms, they should be provided with appropriate referrals for focused evaluation and treatment. Susan's therapist should monitor the parents' emotional and behavioral responses throughout treatment. Similarly, appropriate referrals for evaluation and treatment may need to be provided for Susan's brother.

If the treatment is unsuccessful (partially or completely), the following recommendations may be useful. The number of treatment sessions can be extended, with a focus on furthering treatment gains beyond the accomplishments made to date. Augmenting CBT with medication, such as a selective serotonin reuptake inhibitor (SSRI), should also be considered. Additional treatment sessions for Susan's parents might provide a more optimal environment for Susan to show and maintain progress; if parent psychopathology is severe or interfering, the team can consider postponing Susan's treatment until after treatment for her mother or father. Similarly, if Susan's comorbid diagnoses (e.g., depression, learning difficulties) interfere, the team can consider postponing her anxiety treatment until after these difficulties are addressed. Finally, the team can consider providing Susan's parents with additional parent training, helping them with setting limits, providing rewards, granting developmentally appropriate autonomy, and being supportive of Susan's independence. This slant would be akin to the greater focus on the parents' role in CBT treatment that is designed for younger children (ages 4–8; Choate et al. 2005).

Psychopharmacologic Perspective

Rachel G. Klein, Ph.D.

DIAGNOSTIC FORMULATION

Anxiety about attending school, the main presenting problem in this case, can be a manifestation of various concerns, such as performance anxiety, social anxiety, or separation anxiety. In Susan's case, severe separation anxiety is salient, as evi-

Rachel G. Klein, Ph.D., is Fascitelli Family Professor of Child and Adolescent Psychiatry and Director of the Institute for Anxiety and Mood Disorders at the Child Study Center at the New York University Langone Medical Center in New York, New York (for complete biographical information, see "About the Contributors," p. 613).

denced by morbid thoughts about her parents' welfare, an overwhelming wish to contact her mother whenever school attendance has been forced, and somatic symptoms in school that have led to requests to return home. Unlike many children her age, Susan is able to articulate specific negative events that might befall her mother and that cause Susan anguish. School is not the only setting that has provoked separation concerns in Susan, as attested by her strong negative reaction when her parents have gone out in the evening, something which they have stopped doing. Moreover, her parents have capitulated with regard to school, allowing Susan to spend her days at the father's job. These are good examples of parents accommodating a child's anxiety by protecting her from provocative situations. This parental behavior is often interpreted as reflecting the parents' own anxiety about separating from the child and as serving the parents' needs for closeness to the child. However, such parental behavior can also, and often does, represent an expedient maneuver that relieves parents from making demands that inflict pain on the child and that cause familial disruption.

In addition, as is typical of children with separation anxiety, Susan has difficulty sleeping in her own bed and wanders into the parents' room, due to her fear of dying when alone at night. Concerns about death and dying are not unusual in separation anxiety. Thus, there is clear documentation for a diagnosis of SAD in this 7-year-old girl.

Many children with separation anxiety also have another anxiety disorder. The rate of comorbidity across anxiety disorders has been found to vary depending on the type of sample studied and assessments used (Pine and Klein 2008). In addition to having separation concerns, Susan is reported to worry about her school performance, family finances, and peer acceptance. If these worries reached clinical significance, one would consider a diagnosis of GAD. More detailed information about the frequency of these concerns and their exact impact on Susan's well-being would be helpful. The impression from the case description is that these worries do not affect her significantly. Consequently, a diagnosis of generalized anxiety is not judged as applicable.

Scales of anxiety for children are not likely to contribute meaningfully to Susan's diagnosis or management. A clinical evaluation with parent and child is the best tool for evaluating children's anxiety symptoms. The only purpose that scales might serve would be to indicate elevated anxiety not reported during the clinical evaluation. If high ratings were obtained for various items, the clinician would elicit further information to determine their clinical import. However, the scales would not contribute to a judgment regarding diagnosis or the severity of anxiety symptoms.

DIAGNOSIS

The only diagnosis that is appropriate for Susan is separation anxiety disorder. Susan's mother is reported to have suffered from panic disorder and her father from depression. Each disorder is significantly associated with SAD in off-spring, and a history of both further increases liability for separation anxiety in offspring (Pine et al. 2005).

DSM-IV-TR DIAGNOSIS

Axis I   309.21 Separation anxiety disorder

Axis II   None

Axis III   None

Axis IV   No psychosocial or environmental problems

Axis V   Global Assessment of Functioning=50

TREATMENT RECOMMENDATIONS

The treatment of childhood anxiety disorders is consistent with all other child psychopharmacology in that agents effective in adults are subsequently used in children. The well-documented efficacy of SSRIs in virtually all adult anxiety disorders has led to their application in children with anxiety disorders. Five placebo-controlled trials have been published describing the use of SSRIs in children with anxiety disorders: two were done with children with either generalized anxiety, separation anxiety, or social anxiety disorder (Birmaher et al. 2003; Research Unit on Pediatric Psychopharmacology [RUPP] Anxiety Study Group 2001); one with children with GAD (Rynn et al. 2001); and two with children with social anxiety disorder (Beidel 2007; Wagner et al. 2004). Thus, none informs on the psychopharmacology of SAD specifically; however, in the Research Unit on Pediatric Psychopharmacology's large 8-week study, fluvoxamine efficacy was not restricted or specific to any single disorder (RUPP Anxiety Study Group 2001). Of clinical relevance is that patient improvement on the SSRI, relative to placebo, was detectable after 3 weeks of treatment.

Because efficacy and side-effect differences across the SSRIs are not likely, the clinician must rely on other considerations when making a choice of medication. If cost is a major consideration, the generic form of fluoxetine might be considered as a first choice. Fluoxetine is relatively long-acting. Although this characteristic is advantageous when adherence to daily medication is unlikely, it may present disadvantages if side effects emerge, because these are more likely to linger after medication cessation than with short-acting preparations.

Behavioral disinhibition, which can be severe (outbursts, nastiness, rages, impulsive behavior), is not rare in children treated with SSRIs. Therefore, initiating treatment with a short-acting SSRI is sensible. If the family is unreliable in giving the medication to the child, and the child has no significant side effects when taking the short-acting compound, a switch to a long-acting SSRI is reasonable. Dosage varies across children, however, and there is no standard to guide maximum doses. Some children respond to minimal doses; consequently, the initial dose should be very low (e.g., daily doses of 2 mg of fluoxetine or 6.25 mg of sertraline). Other children require relatively high doses. Gradual increments offer the opportunity to establish the lowest dose at which side effects emerge. Some benefit is typically apparent within 3–4 weeks, with further benefit with continued treatment.

Determining how long the child should continue taking medication is difficult. Because Susan has been plagued by anxiety for a long time, a treatment goal would be to have her experience an extended symptom-free period. If treatment with an SSRI is helpful, treatment for at least 6 months seems indicated. Discontinuation of medication should preferably occur during a nonstressful period, such as during the summer when there is no school. Medication reduction should be gradual, to allow for observation of symptom recurrence and reinstitution if needed of the full effective dose prior to clinical relapse. After total discontinuation, the child should be followed, because a lag of several weeks or a few months between drug cessation and relapse is not unusual.

Some clinicians wonder whether a SSRI should be recommended for a child, in view of reports that SSRIs are associated with a twofold increase in risk for suicidal ideation compared to placebo (approximately 4% vs. 2%). Importantly, however, no suicide occurred in the very large population treated. The continuing controversy over interpretation of these observations (Klein 2006; Vasa et al. 2006) has led to a black box warning. The message is that clinicians need to be aware of the potential for suicidal thoughts occurring in an occasional child and to monitor the child accordingly, but the findings should not preclude treatment when it is indicated.

Clinical care of any one patient does not rely exclusively on published studies but is also determined by clinical experience. The children in studies of SSRIs did not receive other interventions, except in one study with socially anxious children (Beidel et al. 2007), and in only one study was there a few weeks' delay to ensure the stability of the anxiety diagnosis before treatment implementation (RUPP Anxiety Study Group 2001). However, my recommendation is to attempt behavioral treatment before initiating medication for treating SAD. Even a child with severe separation anxiety symptoms, such as Susan, might experience great improvement from systematic behavioral treatment that emphasizes exposure and focuses on both the parents and the child.

Furthermore, psychosocial treatment with the family usually optimizes the benefits of medication in children with SAD. Details of such efforts are not offered because this discussion is about psychopharmacology. My recommendation to use behavioral treatment prior to medication does not reflect a bias against medication for children with psychiatric disorders. This recommendation is specific to children with separation anxiety. For example, in the case of attention-deficit/hyperactivity disorder, I do not hold this view at all.

Integrative Perspective

Andrea M. Victor, Ph.D.
Gail A. Bernstein, M.D.

DIAGNOSTIC FORMULATION

Susan meets DSM-IV-TR criteria for separation anxiety disorder because of her excessive distress regarding separating from parents, excessive worry that an untoward event will lead to separation (e.g., fear that her mother will forget her at school or be in an accident), refusal to go to school, fear of sleeping alone, complaints of physical symptoms, and onset before age 18 years. A precipitant for her anxiety symptoms may be her mother's recent return to work. Susan is exhibiting excessive anxiety during times of separation from her parents, as well as in anticipation of separation. The focus of Susan's worries revolves around the fear of something bad happening to her (i.e., she will fall asleep and never wake up) or her parents (i.e., they will be swept up in a tornado) that would prevent her from seeing them again. These worries are interfering with Susan's ability to attend school. Approximately 75% of children with SAD exhibit school refusal (Masi et al. 2001). Currently, Susan does not meet criteria for a comorbid diagnosis. She is endorsing other worries (i.e., not being smart enough, peer relationship issues, family finances), but they are not impairing enough to meet criteria for GAD. These additional anxiety symptoms should be closely monitored.

The clinician needs to differentiate SAD from other anxiety disorders, which requires understanding what a child fears will occur when he or she is separated from parents. Children with SAD specifically fear that something bad will happen to them or their parents and will result in permanent separation. Children with other anxiety disorders may also fear being away from their parents but for different reasons. For example, children with social phobia may fear being away from their parents due to the difficulties the children have in social situations. Children with GAD often worry about their own safety and the safety of their family members, but this typically does not interfere with separation from family. The Anxiety Disorders Interview Schedule for DSM-IV, Child Version (Silverman and Albano 1996), is a semistructured interview that can be administered to the parent and/or child to aid in diagnostic clarification among anxiety disorders.

Verduin and Kendall (2003) found that children (ages 8–13 years) with SAD had a greater mean number of comorbid diagnoses than did children with GAD and/or social phobia. The most common comorbid diagnoses in children with SAD were GAD in 74%, specific phobia in 58%, attention-deficit/hyperactivity disorder in 22%, social phobia in 20%, and oppositional defiant disorder in 12%. A comorbid mood disorder was significantly less likely in children with SAD (2%) than in children with a primary diagnosis of GAD (17%) or social phobia (15%).

DSM-IV-TR DIAGNOSIS

Axis I   309.21 Separation anxiety disorder

Axis II   No diagnosis

Axis III   No medical difficulties

Axis IV   Moderate psychosocial stressors: mother's recent return to work; school refusal

Axis V   Global Assessment of Functioning=49 (current)

TREATMENT RECOMMENDATIONS

Effective treatment of children with SAD often requires a multimodal approach that may include psychoeducation, school consultation, CBT, and pharmacotherapy (Connolly et al. 2007). Susan will likely require all components listed above because of the severity of her symptoms and the impact of her anxiety on her daily functioning at home and school. The initial treatment plan suggests that Susan would benefit from a trial of CBT. If Susan shows minimal progress after several weeks of CBT alone, then pharmacotherapy could be considered to decrease anxiety and thus facilitate the CBT process. Progress during CBT is based on the child's level of success in participating in the planned exposure hierarchy.

CBT has been demonstrated to be efficacious for treating children with SAD (Eisen and Schaefer 2005; Masi et al. 2001). CBT is typically time limited, with a focus on present symptoms and psychoeducation. Parents need assistance in understanding the nature of their child's anxiety, and they benefit when their concerns are validated and self-blame is minimized. During the initial sessions of CBT, time is spent educating the parent and child about the behaviors that maintain SAD over time (e.g., avoidance of anxiety-provoking situations) and the treatment approaches (e.g., thought identification, cognitive modification, behavioral exposures) that are effective in alleviating anxiety.

Children with SAD often report fearful thoughts related to anxiety-provoking situations (e.g., attending school, being away from parents, going to sleep). Commonly expressed anxious thoughts include "Mom will forget me at school," "Mom will get in a car accident and I will never see her again," and "I will get kidnapped and never see my parents again." These anxious thoughts cause children to demonstrate behaviors (e.g., school refusal) in attempts to prevent separation from their parents. Children with SAD believe that these negative outcomes have a high likelihood of occurring; therefore, treatment involves challenging these thoughts through behavioral exposure exercises.

During CBT, the therapist works with the child and parents to develop plans for the child to confront the feared situations through exposures. The treatment team needs to develop a hierarchy of exposures that is tailored to the needs of an individual child. The hierarchy consists of a detailed list of feared situations ordered from least anxiety provoking (e.g., being in a different room than the mother) to most anxiety provoking (e.g., attending a full day of school). The child then practices each exposure, beginning with the least anxiety-provoking situation. The goal of exposures is to decrease the child's anxiety by challenging the child's current beliefs and helping the child develop new, more accurate beliefs about the feared situations. The child's anxious responses gradually dissipate as the feared situation is endured for longer periods of time and the feared outcome does not occur. Praise and rewards are used to help motivate the child to engage in exposures.

Pharmacotherapy is considered if the child shows minimal improvement in symptoms with CBT alone. Pharmacotherapy and CBT may be implemented together when the child's symptoms are significantly interfering with his or her daily functioning and result in a crisis at home or school (e.g., child refuses to attend school). SSRIs are the first choice of psychotropic medications to treat children with SAD (AACAP Work Group on Quality Issues 2007). Two randomized, controlled clinical trials have demonstrated that SSRIs are efficacious and safe in treating children and adolescents with anxiety disorders, including SAD (Birmaher et al. 2003; RUPP Anxiety Study Group 2001). Other possible medications to treat children with SAD are tricyclic antidepressants and benzodiazepines. Tricyclic antidepressants are generally not tolerated as well as SSRIs in children; the former may result in cardiovascular effects and are dangerous in overdose. Benzodiazepines are recommended only for short-term use due to the possibility of tolerance and dependence. Benzodiazepines can be used in combination with an SSRI or tricyclic antidepressant until the effects of the antidepressant are apparent.

REFERENCES

Beidel DC, Turner SM, Sallee FR, et al: SET-C versus fluoxetine in the treatment of childhood social phobia. J Am Acad Child Adolesc Psychiatry 46:1622–1632, 2007

Birmaher B, Axelson DA, Monk K, et al: Fluoxetine for the treatment of childhood anxiety disorders. J Am Acad Child Adolesc Psychiatry 42:415–423, 2003

Choate ML, Pincus DB, Eyberg SM, et al: Parent-Child Interaction Therapy for Treatment of Separation Anxiety Disorder in Young Children: a pilot study. Cognitive and Behavioral Practice 12:126–135, 2005

Connolly SD, Bernstein GA, Work Group on Quality Issues: Practice parameter for the assessment and treatment of children and adolescents with anxiety disorders. J Am Acad Child Adolesc Psychiatry 46:267–283, 2007

Eisen AR, Schaefer CE: Separation Anxiety in Children and Adolescents: An Individualized Approach to Assessment and Treatment. New York, Guilford, 2005

Furr JM, Tiwari S, Suveg C, et al: Anxiety disorders in children and adolescents, in Handbook of Anxiety and Anxiety Disorders. Edited by Antony M, Stein M. New York, Oxford University Press, 2008, pp 636–656

Kendall PC: Treating anxiety disorders in youth: results of a randomized clinical trial. J Consult Clin Psychol 62:100–110, 1994

Kendall PC, Hedtke K: Cognitive-Behavioral Therapy for Anxious Children: Therapist Manual, 3rd Edition. Ardmore, PA, Workbook Publishing, 2006a

Kendall PC, Hedtke K: Coping Cat Workbook, 2nd Edition. Ardmore, PA, Workbook Publishing, 2006b

Kendall PC, Southam-Gerow MA: Long-term follow-up of a cognitive-behavioral therapy for anxiety-disordered youth. J Consult Clin Psychol 64:724–730, 1996

Kendall PC, Flannery-Schroeder E, Panichelli-Mindel S, et al: Therapy for youths with anxiety disorders: a second randomized clinical trial. J Consult Clin Psychol 65:366–380, 1997

Kendall PC, Safford S, Flannery-Schroeder E, et al: Child anxiety treatment: outcomes in adolescence and impact on substance use and depression at 7.4-year follow-up. J Consult Clin Psychol 72:276–287, 2004

Kendall PC, Robin J, Hedtke K, et al: Considering CBT with anxious youth? Think exposures. Cogn Behav Pract 12:136–150, 2005

Klein DF: The flawed basis for FDA post-marketing safety decisions: the example of anti-depressants and children. Neuropsychopharmacology 31:689–699, 2006

Masi G, Mucci M, Millepiedi S: Separation anxiety disorder in children and adolescents: epidemiology, diagnosis, and management. CNS Drugs 15:93–104, 2001

Pine DS, Klein RG: Anxiety disorder, in Rutter's Child and Adolescent Psychiatry, 5th Edition. Edited by Rutter M, Bishop D, Pine D, et al. London, Blackwell Science, 2008, pp 628–647

Pine DS, Klein RG, Roberson-Nay R, et al: Response to 5% carbon dioxide in children and adolescents: relationship to panic disorder in parents and anxiety disorders in subjects. Arch Gen Psychiatry 62:73–80, 2005

Research Unit on Pediatric Psychopharmacology Anxiety Study Group: Fluvoxamine for the treatment of anxiety disorders in children and adolescents. N Engl J Med 344:1279–1285, 2001

Rynn MA, Siqueland L, Rickels K, et al: Placebo-controlled trial of sertraline in the treatment of children with generalized anxiety disorder. Am J Psychiatry 158:2008–2014, 2001

Silverman WK, Albano AM: Anxiety Disorders Interview Schedule for DSM-IV, Child Version, Child and Parent Interview Schedules. San Antonio, TX, Psychological Corporation, 1996

Vasa RA, Carlino AR, Pine DS, et al: Pharmacotherapy of depressed children and adolescents: current issues and potential directions. Biol Psychiatry 59:1021–1028, 2006

Verduin TL, Kendall PC: Differential occurrence of comorbidity within childhood anxiety disorders. J Clin Child Adolesc Psychol 32:290–295, 2003

Wagner KD, Berard R, Stein MB, et al: A multicenter, randomized, double-blind, placebo-controlled trial of paroxetine in children and adolescents with social anxiety disorder. Arch Gen Psychiatry 61:1153–1162, 2004

■ CHAPTER 4 ■

Chatterbox at Home

Selective Mutism

Bruce Black, M.D.

CASE PRESENTATION

IDENTIFYING INFORMATION

Emily, age 5 years 2 months, lives with her parents, her 7-year-old sister, and 2-year-old brother.

CHIEF COMPLAINT

Emily was brought in by her parents, who reported that "Emily does not speak in most social situations outside our home or with strangers in our home."

HISTORY OF PRESENT ILLNESS

Emily's parents report that Emily "has always been this way." They became increasingly concerned when she started her third year of preschool and still had never spoken in school. She started preschool at age 3 years 2 months and did not speak at school for the entire year. She was described as generally withdrawn, isolated, and reluctant to participate in most activities. The following year, she attended a different preschool and was placed in a prekindergarten class. Initially, she was withdrawn and isolative, but after several months, she

Bruce Black, M.D., is Founder and Director of Comprehensive Psychiatric Associates in Wellesley, Massachusetts, and Assistant Professor of Psychiatry at the Tufts University School of Medicine in Boston, Massachusetts (for complete biographical information, see "About the Contributors," p. 613).

gradually began to join in play and participate in group activities, still not speaking. She had one-on-one playdates at her house and spoke freely to her classmates while at home, but continued not to speak to them in school. At birthday parties, including her own, she did not speak to anyone. Several times in the late fall, she whispered to two classmates and a young teaching assistant on the playground. However, after returning from Christmas vacation, she did not speak to anyone at school for the remainder of the year.

During the summer after that second year of preschool, in response to her parents' frequent pleas, Emily promised them that she would speak in preschool in the fall. Although she returned to the same prekindergarten with the same teachers, most of her classmates had entered kindergarten in other schools. After 1 month, she still had not spoken to anyone. Her parents and teachers felt that she was becoming progressively more inhibited and withdrawn. The lead teacher in the classroom reportedly "nagged" Emily to speak to her, asking her direct questions and then saying, "I know you can tell me." Her parents also frequently encouraged her to speak. Both teachers and parents offered her rewards if she would speak in school, but with no impact.

Emily has never spoken to unfamiliar adults; is markedly reluctant to speak to extended family members, even at home; and does not speak to her parents in public places "if she [thinks] someone might hear her." She is very reluctant to participate in any activities in which she might draw attention to herself. For example, she asked to join a friend's T-ball team. As a parent reports, "Emily did fine in the practice and warm-ups, where everyone was doing the same thing and no one was paying attention to her, but at game time she refused to go up to bat and did not respond in the outfield even when the ball hit her."

Emily has seen three different child psychotherapists, without apparent benefit. Her parents report that the psychotherapists "played with Emily and tried to get her to speak to them" but did not offer the parents any advice on what they could do to help Emily speak. One of the psychotherapists reportedly told the parents that selective mutism is caused by trauma and that Emily must have been traumatized, despite their lack of awareness of any traumatic events, or, if not, that she could not be suffering from "true selective mutism."

A speech therapist attempted to work with Emily in school, but Emily would not speak to her. (She did speak to the speech therapist freely after the therapist spent several hours playing with her in her home. The therapist characterized her speech and language functioning in that setting as developmentally appropriate and unremarkable.)

Emily has mild phobias (dogs, water) that do not meet the criteria for simple phobia because of a lack of impairment. Her history does not suggest depression, elimination disorders, or any other psychiatric or developmental difficulties.

Past Psychiatric History

As described above.

Medical History

Her medical history is unremarkable.

Developmental History

Emily's developmental history is otherwise unremarkable.

Social History

Emily is the middle of three children in an intact family. Both parents work as professionals. Emily has no known history of traumatic events.

Family History

Emily's mother described herself as "very shy" as a child but said she "outgrew" her shyness by adolescence. She was not mute. Emily's maternal aunt was also very shy as a child. Emily's maternal grandfather was overanxious and alcoholic, as were several maternal cousins. The family's psychiatric history is otherwise unremarkable.

Mental Status Examination

Emily was unobtrusively observed talking and playing with her mother and 7-year-old sister in the clinic waiting room. Her speech and language functioning appeared to be grossly normal. Her affect and the form and content of her speech and play were unremarkable. Her parents were then instructed to take her into my office while I was out of the room and to sit on a couch and look through *I SPY*, a children's hidden-picture book. After they had been in my office for 5–10 minutes, I entered the room but pretended to take no notice of them and avoided looking at them. Emily continued to talk freely with her family and was quite animated in her enjoyment of finding hidden pictures in the book. I then began to gradually increase my attention toward her, first glancing occasionally toward her, then moving my chair gradually in her direction, then making comments on her activity ("Wow, Emily's good at 'I Spy'") without looking toward her, then making momentary eye contact, then making comments directly to her ("You sure are good at that") and asking simple questions ("I love *I SPY* books, don't you?"). As my attention and attempts to interact with Emily gradually increased, she appeared increasingly tense and apprehensive, avoided my gaze, looked frequently to her mother, and stopped speaking. She made no verbal reply to my comments or questions.

In addition to performing the clinical interview and examination, I obtained further details of Emily's clinical history through the use of standardized parent and teacher questionnaires and symptom rating scales, supplemented with specific selective mutism questionnaires (Black 2001a, 2001b).

COMMENTARIES

Psychotherapeutic Perspective

Anne Marie Albano, Ph.D., A.B.P.P.

DIAGNOSTIC FORMULATION

Emily's case description is not atypical for young children with selective mutism. As is evident in the case report, Emily's development appears normal in all respects except for her voluntary production of speech in situations involving unfamiliar adults and children. No significant medical or learning issues have been reported, and the parents deny any history of trauma. Indeed, early speculations on the etiology of "elective mutism," the DSM precursor to selective mutism, suggested that a history of trauma may precede the diagnosis. However, research on selective mutism does not support this theory. More likely, Emily is experiencing an early and extreme form of social anxiety disorder (Albano et al. 2003). Older children and adolescents who have social anxiety disorder tend to actively avoid social situations in which they may be the focus of attention and potential negative evaluation. Parents often encourage their children or teenagers with social anxiety disorder to engage in social situations, including attending school and social events, but older youths struggle against these activities and may engage in active avoidance, arguments, and fleeing (escape) from situations that they are forced to attend. For Emily, at her tender age, the only recourse against being in a situation where she feels excessive anxiety and the discomfort of being the focus of attention is to stay mute. This behavior is akin to the "freeze" response in the "fight, flight, or freeze"

Anne Marie Albano, Ph.D, A.B.P.P., is Associate Professor of Clinical Psychology in the Division of Child and Adolescent Psychiatry, and Director of Columbia University Clinic for Anxiety and Related Disorders at Columbia University in New York, New York (for complete biographical information, see "About the Contributors," p. 613).

mechanisms that developed throughout evolution and are deeply rooted in neurobiological mechanisms of survival. Hence, the assessment of selective mutism warrants a thorough evaluation of anxiety and the child's ability to manage challenging situations.

A thorough assessment of a child with selective mutism involves a careful review of the child's developmental history, a clinical evaluation, and possibly a speech and language evaluation (Albano and Hayward 2004). In Emily's case, the speech therapist reported developmentally appropriate and unremarkable speech. Additionally, intelligence testing may be indicated, typically in the form of a nonverbal evaluation (e.g., Peabody Picture Vocabulary Test—Third Edition; Dunn and Dunn 1997), along with tests examining graphomotor abilities, receptive language, and audition. These evaluative strategies are recommended to screen for any potential speech, hearing, or learning issue that may have an impact on the child's speech production.

Many parents of children with selective mutism can provide a videotape or audiotape of the child's speech in the home setting so the therapist can see and hear the child interacting with others. In lieu of a tape sample, observation of the child in multiple settings and with familiar and unfamiliar people will likewise provide good information about the child's response to others and the process of shutting down and becoming mute. Suggested settings for observation include the classroom or a school setting, the therapist's waiting room, and a play situation. Much like what was reported in the case description, the clinician will observe Emily's speech and interaction habits when Emily is comfortable with her family, and then the pattern of shutting down when unfamiliar people are introduced into the environment and eventually approach her to speak. Also of importance is observation of the parental reactions to the introduction of other people into the room, to see how they interact with Emily in these situations.

Because Emily is too young for a child-focused diagnostic evaluation, in our clinic we would administer a semistructured interview to her parents to evaluate the full range of Emily's anxiety and related disorders of childhood. The Anxiety Disorders Interview Schedule for DSM-IV, Parent Version (Silverman and Albano 1996), could be administered to the parents and supplemented with a behavioral observation as described above. In addition, the parent versions of the Fear Survey Schedule for Children—Revised (Shore and Rapport 1998), the Multidimensional Anxiety Scale for Children (March et al. 1997), and a rating scale such as the Child Behavior Checklist (including the Teacher Report Form; Achenbach 1991) would allow the clinician a comprehensive view of the child's functioning.

Diagnostic Impression

Emily presents with a family history of shyness and anxiety in her mother and mother's relatives. In addition, Emily evidences mild fears of dogs and water, and demonstrates an inhibited temperament in her preschool settings. Inhibited temperament, such as that evidenced by Emily, has been identified as a risk factor for anxiety disorders (Hayward et al. 1998; Rosenbaum et al. 1991). As noted in the case summary, Emily does speak to peers during playdates at her house, and she did converse with her speech therapist during a home visit. Hence, she presents with a vulnerability to anxiety, as indicated by family history and description of her temperament, and she evidences anxiety and avoidance of performing (speaking) in settings outside of her home.

DSM-IV-TR DIAGNOSIS

Axis I   313.23 Selective mutism
            300.23 Social phobia
Axis II   None
Axis III   None apparent
            Screen for verbal intelligence and evaluate for the presence of any learning issue
Axis IV   Repeating preschool and not being promoted to kindergarten with same-age peers due to failure to speak in school
Axis V   Global Assessment of Functioning=55
            Currently experiencing moderate impairment at school and with peers

TREATMENT RECOMMENDATIONS

One can only guess that Emily's parents are somewhat skeptical about psychotherapy, because their three prior attempts in treatment for Emily were unsuccessful. When children are very young, as in Emily's case, the treatment plan must involve a predominantly parent- or family-focused intervention. At present, evidence-based psychosocial treatments for young children with selective mutism or anxiety are still in development. However, given the large and consistent evidence base for the treatment of anxiety disorders in school-age children and adolescents (see Silverman et al. 2008) and the impressive research support for parent-focused treatments for young children with disruptive behavior disorders, Emily's best chances for success lie within a parent-focused, operant-based approach to working with her anxiety and resistance to speaking outside of her home.

    One of the first steps in treatment is to conduct a functional analysis of when and where Emily's speaking occurs or desists. This analysis must also involve a careful assessment of what the people around Emily do in response to her speaking or not speaking. As noted in the case description, her parents and teachers have cajoled, bribed, and pleaded with Emily. Children with social anxiety fear any attention, so the amount of attention given to begging and trying to bribe Emily into speaking may overwhelm her. Furthermore, her interactions with peers, especially how other children react to her in various situations, should be examined. Treatment then should begin with psychoeducation for the parents and instruction in the application of reinforcement principles, specifically in how to shape Emily's speech production. When working with young children, I often use the principles and procedures found in *Parent-Child Interaction Therapy* (Hembree-Kigin and McNeil 1995) and *Parenting the Strong-Willed Child* (Forehand and Long 2002). These parent-focused programs provide straightforward, practical information and practice in shaping desirable behavior and extinguishing undesirable behavior. Also, rather than using rewards or bribes with children, parents can be taught the proper use of naturally occurring reinforcers that already exist in the child's world. For example, a 4-year-old child with selective mutism was shaped to speak in external situations using his favorite cereal. Each morning, this child ate a certain cereal product in a special favorite cup. One day, the cereal and cup were gone, and only plain cereal was available at home. However, when he came to the clinic, both the cup and cereal were in the therapist's office. Throughout the sessions, when he spoke, he was given pieces of the cereal dropped into his cup, and over time, the cereal also became available in his classroom and other social settings. The judicious use of this reinforcer worked very well to shape his speaking behavior.

It is recommended that in addition to working with the parents in shaping the child's behavior and using reinforcement in an appropriate and powerful manner, the clinician provide psychoeducation for the teacher and school personnel. The clinician may design the least burdensome and unobtrusive method for the teacher to use in the classroom. When a child who has been mute speaks in class, the immediate impulse is to give lots of praise to the child in an attempt at reinforcement. However, the child typically experiences this type of attention as overwhelming, so the focus with school personnel is to teach them to be warm and subtle in their reinforcement, and to gradually shape the child's speaking behavior over time. The teacher can create a "speaking card," an index card that the teacher tapes on the young child's desk and marks with a check or smiley face whenever the child makes an utterance. After receiving a certain number of checks, the child earns a reinforcer in the classroom that day (e.g., gets to feed the class fish; is at the head of the line for recess), and at the end of the day, the card goes home with the child for continuity and communication to the parents.

If shaping and other operant procedures are not met with success within a reasonable time period (4–5 weeks for speaking to be occurring on a regular basis), I recommend a careful examination to determine what factors are impeding the therapy process. Family factors must also be considered in treatment-refractory cases, to find out whether the parents are unable for some reason to follow through with the behavioral approach. More intensive family approaches with a focus on the parents' issues and resistances should be explored. Some parents report that they cannot "deprive" the child of desired reinforcers or otherwise cannot work through the initial phase of treatment when the child is becoming familiar with the behavioral methods and may be upset with the parents for sticking to the program ("If you ask the waiter for the ice cream, then you can have it; if not, we can try again another time").

A referral to a child psychiatrist for a medication evaluation should be considered in refractory cases. Evidence supports the use of medications in children with selective mutism and related anxiety disorders (Black and Uhde 1994). The combination of operant procedures and medication is indicated for children who are resistant to psychosocial treatment for various reasons, such as comorbidity, severity of the mutism, length of time that the child has not spoken, and severity of the child's anxiety.

Parents may also benefit from patient and family advocacy agencies that focus specifically on selective mutism and anxiety disorders in youth. Often, parents who have struggled with and helped their children to overcome this problem can offer their support and guidance. Three national organizations, listed below, can often link families with family support services and treatment providers in their local areas.

> The Selective Mutism Group (http://www.selectivemutism.org), part of the Childhood Anxiety Network, is a nonprofit organization dedicated to providing information, resources, and support to those impacted by a child with the anxiety disorder known as selective mutism.

> The mission of the Selective Mutism Foundation (http://www.selective mutismfoundation.org) is to promote further research, advocacy, social acceptance, and the understanding of selective mutism as a debilitating disorder.

> The Anxiety Disorders Association of America (http://www.adaa.org/ GettingHelp/FocusOn/children&Adolescents/SM.asp) is "a national nonprofit organization dedicated to the prevention, treatment, and cure of anxiety disorders and to improving the lives of all people who suffer from them."

Psychopharmacologic Perspective

Courtney Pierce Keeton, Ph.D.
John T. Walkup, M.D.

DIAGNOSTIC FORMULATION

Emily demonstrates the hallmark symptom of selective mutism: a persistent failure to speak in new and public settings such as school and the playground despite speaking normally in familiar settings such as her home. Emily's mutism in multiple settings reflects an overwhelming anxious response elicited by unfamiliar social situations. That she has "always been this way" suggests an early onset consistent with an inhibited temperament, which is a risk factor for anxiety. The family history of shyness points to both a genetic vulnerability and an environment that supports an anxious response to social stimuli that may include parental support for social inhibition or modeling of inhibited behavior.

DSM-IV-TR DIAGNOSIS

Axis I   313.23 Selective mutism
            Rule out social phobia
Axis II   No diagnosis
Axis III   None
Axis IV   Educational problems
            Social problems
Axis V   Global Assessment of Functioning=51

Rationale for Diagnosis

Emily meets criteria for selective mutism and possibly social phobia. Additional questioning will determine the extent to which Emily is more globally socially avoidant in social situations because of fear of embarrassment.

Courtney Pierce Keeton, Ph.D., is Instructor of Psychiatry and Behavioral Sciences in the Division of Child and Adolescent Psychiatry at Johns Hopkins Medical Institutions in Baltimore, Maryland.

John T. Walkup, M.D., is Associate Professor of Psychiatry and Behavioral Sciences and Deputy Director of the Division of Child and Adolescent Psychiatry at Johns Hopkins Medical Institutions, Baltimore, Maryland; and Medical Director of the Research Unit of Pediatric Psychopharmacology.

For complete biographical information, see "About the Contributors," p. 613.

Lack of speaking in social situations can sometimes be attributed to a pervasive developmental disorder or a communication disorder. Pervasive developmental disorder is unlikely in Emily's case due to observations of normal social interactions with parents, appropriate reciprocal interactions with siblings and peers at home, and the absence of stereotyped interests and behavior. Similarly, a communication disorder, such as a receptive or expressive language deficit, is ruled out based on her normal communication in the home. The lack of a history of trauma excludes the possibility that her mutism is a symptom of posttraumatic stress disorder.

EPIDEMIOLOGY

Selective mutism affects less than 1% of school-age children (Bergman et al. 2002). The majority of children with selective mutism also meet criteria for social phobia. The clinical picture may be further complicated by the presence of simple phobias, separation anxiety disorder, oppositional defiant disorder, or speech and language problems (Sharp et al. 2007). Up to 70% of children with selective mutism have an immediate family member with a history of social phobia (Black and Uhde 1995). No evidence is available to suggest that selective mutism is caused by traumatic events.

COMORBIDITY

Like the majority of children with selective mutism, Emily exhibits symptoms of social phobia. Social phobia is characterized by fear and avoidance associated with social and performance situations in which embarrassment may occur (e.g., playing in a T-ball game). Other conditions may also co-occur.

SCREENING/DIAGNOSTIC TOOLS

The diagnosis of selective mutism requires a review of medical and psychiatric symptoms, as well as cognitive, audiological, and speech and language function (Dow et al. 1995). Rating scales support diagnostic impressions and monitor symptom change over time. Additionally, parents and teachers are encouraged to record a child's behavioral changes, such as increasing nonverbal behaviors (e.g., eye contact) and speech in all contexts.

TREATMENT RECOMMENDATIONS

Psychoeducation is recommended to teach Emily's family about potential genetic, biological, and psychosocial contributors to symptom severity; available treatment options; and appropriate expectancies for improvement. Behavioral therapy involving Emily, her parents, and schoolteachers should include a functional analysis of behavior, gradual reinforcement of verbal and appropriate social interaction, and ignoring avoidance behavior including mutism.

Pharmacotherapy with a selective serotonin reuptake inhibitor (SSRI) is also suggested for Emily.

RATIONALE FOR TREATMENT CHOICES

Before treatment is initiated, Emily's family would benefit from education about selective mutism and explanation about why previous assessments and treatments failed. A behavioral or cognitive-behavioral intervention with a knowledgeable and experienced clinician is recommended because these treatments are useful for children with selective mutism and are considered the first-line treatment (Cohen et al. 2006). Medication typically is not the first-choice intervention for young children with selective mutism but is commonly used when psychosocial interventions prove inadequate or ineffective. Medication may be a first-line treatment in early-onset and severe selective mutism to facilitate engagement in psychosocial interventions.

Large-scale treatment studies of children with selective mutism have not been conducted. Information regarding pharmacologic treatment comes from a small double-blind placebo-controlled trial (Black and Uhde 1994) and from case studies or case series (see Kumpulainen 2002). The rationale for SSRI treatment is based on the efficacy of these agents for childhood anxiety disorders, including selective mutism (Reinblatt and Riddle 2007; Seidel and Walkup 2006); the failure of nonmedication interventions to consistently demonstrate significant benefits; and the fact that social and academic impairments are associated with chronic mutism. Several case studies demonstrate clinical benefits and minimal risks for patients taking SSRIs. Interestingly, some studies have noted that early-onset selective mutism is more treatment responsive than late-onset selective mutism (e.g., Dummit et al. 1996).

PSYCHOPHARMACOLOGIC TREATMENT

For children as young as Emily, few data are available to guide medication choice or a titration schedule for SSRIs. In general, the child should receive a low dose of SSRI, often as low as 25%–50% of adult starting doses for anxiety or depression. The dose of medication can be increased every 5–7 days over the first month of treatment to maximize treatment response while minimizing side effects. Although some children respond well to low doses, other children will require higher doses. For example, in the absence of side effects and continued symptoms, upward adjustment after the first month of treatment to fluoxetine 20–30 mg/day, fluvoxamine 100–150 mg/day, sertraline 100–150 mg/day, or citalopram 30–40 mg/day is warranted to achieve a high-quality response. Further upward adjustment is possible for those children who remain symptomatic but have demonstrated improvement with previous doses and minimal side effects. Close monitoring for both benefit and side effects is required in this age group. Common side effects include behavioral activation, gastrointestinal problems, and headaches.

PLAN IF MEDICATION TREATMENT FAILS

If children do not respond as expected to medication and psychosocial treatment, a review of the evaluation or a consultation may be useful. For children whose diagnosis of selective mutism is confirmed after reevaluation, more aggressive pharmacologic treatment may be indicated. A child who is unresponsive or only partially responsive to low or medium adult doses of an SSRI may be given higher doses if he or she has few or no side effects. If dose increases are not possible because of side effects and treatment response is minimal, switching to another SSRI is a possible next step. Given the absence of a clear evidence base, pharmacologic algorithms for refractory or partially responsive depression or anxiety may serve as a guide to the treatment of youth with selective mutism.

Integrative Perspective

Bruce Black, M.D.

DIAGNOSTIC FORMULATION

Emily's history is quite typical of children with the diagnosis of selective mutism (Black and Uhde 1992, 1995). Selective mutism generally has an early onset, either coincidental with or preceded by other signs of heightened anxiety and behavioral inhibition in social settings (Black 1996; Black et al. 1997). Parents often report that their child "has always been this way," and onset is nearly always apparent by kindergarten. Concurrent symptoms of social anxiety and limitations in social interactions are usually present, and virtually all children with selective mutism also meet diagnostic criteria for social anxiety disorder. Approximately 30% of children with selective mutism will meet diagnostic criteria for another DSM-IV-TR anxiety disorder (other than social anxiety disorder), although this was not true in Emily's case. Elimination disorders, particularly associated with marked anxiety about toileting, are not uncommon.

DSM-IV-TR DIAGNOSIS

Axis I   313.23 Selective mutism
            300.23 Social phobia

Axis II   No diagnosis

Axis III   None

Axis IV   None

Axis V   Global Assessment of Functioning=55 (on admission)
          Global Assessment of Functioning=95 (at discharge)

TREATMENT RECOMMENDATIONS

Parent behavioral counseling and treatment with fluoxetine were recommended. Fluoxetine was started at a dosage of 2 mg/day (0.5 mL fluoxetine oral solution). Within 10 days, the parents reported that Emily seemed "a little happier about school, more positive in general." After 4 weeks, her teacher reported that she was participating more in school and had spoken to two peers. Although Emily's parents reported that she seemed somewhat more restless and "hyper" since starting medication, they did not feel this was a problem, and Emily was otherwise tolerating the medication well, without apparent adverse effects. The dosage of fluoxetine was increased to 4 mg/day. Emily's nonverbal participation in school continued to progress steadily, and her parents noted that she was markedly less inhibited and speaking to them more freely and more loudly in public places.

Behavioral counseling focused on systematic desensitization through graduated exposure, beginning with situations in which Emily was already able to speak or seemed likely to be able to speak, and then very gradually introducing stimuli to provoke anxiety (and mutism). Simultaneously, her teachers and parents were instructed to stop asking, begging, or pressuring Emily to speak and, in fact, to avoid discussing her lack of speech with her completely. At about the same time the medication was started, Emily's mother began going into the preschool classroom with Emily after school was out, when no one else in the classroom, and spending time playing with her and covertly encouraging verbal interaction. The quantity and volume of Emily's speech with her mother in the classroom was initially very limited but began to increase steadily after about 4 weeks.

After 6 weeks, the dosage of Emily's fluoxetine was increased to 6 mg/day. The restlessness that had been noted soon after Emily started the medication was reported to increase noticeably after each increase in dosage, particularly with the increase to 6 mg/day, but her parents continued to feel that this was not a problem and was of minimal concern relative to what they perceived to be very significant therapeutic benefits. After 8 weeks, Emily was observed talking to two classmates on the preschool playground. A young teaching assistant from Emily's classroom, with whom Emily had never spoken at school, visited her at home, and Emily "talked her ear off." Her preschool teacher began to walk in and out of the classroom while Emily was playing and talking with her mother in their after-school sessions. The teacher was instructed to avoid interacting or even looking toward Emily during these incursions. Emily initially appeared apprehensive and stopped speaking to her mother while the teacher was in the room; however, this reaction seemed to pass within a few days, and Emily resumed speaking to her mother freely. The teacher gradually began to increase her attention toward Emily during these sessions.

After 10 weeks of taking medication, Emily was talking to everyone at school and had spoken in a loud voice in front of a group at circle time. Four weeks later, she was described as "a little chatterbox" at school. Because of concerns regarding her persistent restlessness and somewhat increased oppositional behaviors, the fluoxetine dose was decreased to 4 mg. She continued to do well, and the restlessness and increased oppositional behaviors improved. She was described as increasingly comfortable interacting with and speaking with unfamiliar adults at home and in public places. Her fears of dogs and water resolved. After about 11 months of taking medication, Emily began full-day kindergarten without any difficulty. The summer after kindergarten, she attended two different day camp programs and had no difficulty speaking freely and interacting with peers and adults. She began first grade without difficulty. After 2 months in first grade, the fluoxetine dose was decreased to 2 mg for 2 months, then to 1 mg for 2 months, and then discontinued. Her parents noted mild increases in "moodiness" after each dose decrease and after discontinuation, but these changes resolved within 1–2 weeks. At follow-up 3 months into second grade, Emily continued to do well and was described as happy, sociable, and not noticeably more shy or inhibited than her peers.

DISCUSSION

Fluoxetine has been shown to be effective in the treatment of selective mutism in one small double-blind, placebo-controlled treatment study (Black and Uhde 1994). In clinical practice, about one-third of children seem to show marked improvement, about one-third show clear benefit but with continued significant impairment and only slow improvement in inhibition and mutism, and about one-third show little apparent benefit. Younger children may respond better to medication than older children. Even in those children with a marked decrease in inhibition, progression to full speech may not occur for 3–5 months after starting medication. Behavioral "activation," restlessness, and increased oppositional behavior are common side effects of medication, occurring in about 50%–70% of children taking fluoxetine. Usually, these changes are not of significant concern. They may be more pronounced in children with coexisting attention-deficit/hyperactivity disorder (ADHD), although determining if such symptoms are medication effects or symptoms of comorbid ADHD may sometimes be difficult. Occasionally, grossly excessive disinhibition (engaging in socially inappropriate behaviors, such as a kindergarten girl "mooning" her class) or excessive risk-taking behaviors in previously overly cautious children may occur. For children advanced enough in school that sustained attention and focus may sometimes be expected (usually not before second or third grade), treatment-related distractibility and difficulty focusing on academic tasks may be severe enough to impact academic progress. All of these side effects are generally dose related and very infrequently lead to medication discontinuation. When distractibility or difficulty focusing is of significant concern, yet continued antianxiety treatment seems necessary, switching to clomipramine may be helpful.

An optimal therapeutic dose and length of treatment have not been established for fluoxetine. A low starting dosage (2–4 mg/day) is recommended, with gradual dose increases as tolerated. Many young children respond well at dosages in the range of 4–6 mg/day, whereas older children may benefit from increases in dosage up to 10 mg/day. Longer periods of treatment (1–2 years following symptom remission) and very gradual dose tapering (over 4–6 months) may be associated with a better prognosis after medication discontinuation. Nevertheless, many children who have responded well to medication do relapse after the medication is reduced or eliminated, demonstrating increased inhibition and decreased speech (although rarely does a child return to complete mutism after speaking while taking medication), and often negative mood changes such as irritability or dysphoria. Children with a more robust treatment response seem to have a better course of tapering and discontinuing medication than do children who have benefited from medication but remain significantly inhibited.

Although behavioral treatment approaches for selective mutism have not been well studied, they generally seem to be helpful, and the combination of behavioral treatment and medication may be more effective than either treatment alone. For milder cases of selective mutism or for children who may be showing signs of progress without treatment, behavioral treatment alone should be tried before instituting medication. Both systematic desensitization and behavioral modification with defined goals and reinforcements may be useful. Systematic desensitization with graduated exposure, as used with Emily, was described earlier in this commentary. This approach generally does not require the provision of extraneous rewards, because the increased social interaction, particularly social speech, is intrinsically quite rewarding. The graduated exposure may often call for considerable creativity and perseverance on the part of the clinician and parents in determining how to keep moving forward. Although a more direct behavioral modification approach with specific goals (e.g., talk to Mom in the classroom when no one else is present, or whisper "good morning" to the teacher) and rewards may be helpful for some children with selective mutism, for many children, any discussion of their mutism or of taking steps to decrease it is so anxiety provoking that it may be aversive and produce increased anxiety and inhibition or a marked oppositional response or both. Whatever approach is taken by the adults, "nagging" or pressuring a child to speak generally increases inhibition, is counterproductive, and should absolutely be avoided. Avoiding this behavior may be difficult for many parents and teachers and may need to be strongly and frequently encouraged by the clinician. Nonbehavioral treatment approaches such as play therapy or non-goal-oriented parent or family counseling do not appear to be of any benefit in reducing symptoms of selective mutism.

REFERENCES

Achenbach TM: Manual for the Child Behavior Checklist/4–18 and 1991 Profile. Burlington, VT, University of Vermont Department of Psychiatry, 1991

Albano AM, Hayward C: The developmental psychopathology approach to understanding and treating social anxiety disorder, in Phobic and Anxiety Disorders: A Clinician's Guide to Effective Psychosocial and Pharmacological Interventions. Edited by Ollendick TH, March JS. New York, Oxford University Press, 2004, pp 198–235

Albano AM, Chorpita BF, Barlow DH: Anxiety disorders, in Child Psychopathology, 2nd Edition. Edited by Mash EJ, Barkley RA. New York, Guilford, 2003, pp 279–329

Bergman L, Piacentini J, McCracken J: Prevalence and description of selective mutism in a school-based sample. J Am Acad Child Adolesc Psychiatry 41:938–946, 2002

Black B: Social anxiety and selective mutism, in American Psychiatric Press Review of Psychiatry, Vol 15. Edited by Dickstein LJ, Oldham JM, Riba MB. Washington, DC, American Psychiatric Press, 1996, pp 469–496

Black B: Questionnaire for parents (SM supplement). 2001a. Available at: http://wellpsych.com/SM_parent_qstnr.pdf. Accessed July 2, 2008.

Black B: School questionnaire (SM supplement). 2001b. Available at: http://www.wellpsych.com/SM_school_qstnr.pdf. Accessed July 2, 2008.

Black B, Uhde TW: Elective mutism as a variant of social phobia. J Am Acad Child Adolesc Psychiatry 31:1090–1094, 1992

Black B, Uhde TW: Treatment of elective mutism with fluoxetine: a double-blind, placebo-controlled study. J Am Acad Child Adolesc Psychiatry 33:1000–1006, 1994

Black B, Uhde TW: Psychiatric characteristics of children with selective mutism: a pilot study. J Am Acad Child Adolesc Psychiatry 34:847–856, 1995

Black B, Leonard HL, Rapoport JL: Specific phobia, panic disorders, social phobia, and selective mutism, in Textbook of Child and Adolescent Psychiatry, 2nd Edition. Edited by Wiener JM. Washington, DC, American Psychiatric Press, 1997, pp 491–506

Cohen SL, Chavira DA, Stein MB: Practitioner review: psychosocial interventions for children with selective mutism: a critical evaluation of the literature from 1990–2005. J Child Psychol Psychiatry 47:1085–1097, 2006

Dow SP, Sonies BC, Scheib D, et al: Practical guidelines for the assessment and treatment of selective mutism. J Am Acad Child Adolesc Psychiatry 34:836–846, 1995

Dummit ES, Klein RG, Tancer NK, et al: Fluoxetine treatment of children with selective mutism: an open trial. J Am Acad Child Adolesc Psychiatry 35:615–621, 1996

Dunn LM, Dunn LM: Peabody Picture Vocabulary Test, 3rd Edition. Circle Pines, MN, American Guidance Service, 1997

Forehand R, Long NJ: Parenting the Strong-Willed Child. Lincolnwood, IL, NTC Publishing Group, 2002

Hayward C, Killen J, Kraemer H, et al: Linking self-reported childhood behavioral inhibition to adolescent social phobia. J Am Acad Child Adolesc Psychiatry 37:1308–1316, 1998

Hembree-Kigin T, McNeil CB: Parent-Child Interaction Therapy. New York, Plenum, 1995

Kumpulainen K: Phenomenology and treatment of selective mutism. CNS Drugs 16:175–180, 2002

March JS, Parker JD, Sullivan K, et al: The Multidimensional Anxiety Scale for Children (MASC): factor structure, reliability and validity. J Am Acad Child Adolesc Psychiatry 36:554–565, 1997

Reinblatt S, Riddle M: The pharmacological management of childhood anxiety disorders: a review. Psychopharmacology (Berl) 191:67–86, 2007

Rosenbaum JF, Biederman J, Hirshfeld DR, et al: Behavioral inhibition in children: a possible precursor to panic disorder or social phobia. J Clin Psychiatry 52:5–9, 1991

Seidel L, Walkup JT: Selective serotonin reuptake inhibitor use in the treatment of the pediatric non-obsessive-compulsive disorder anxiety disorders. J Child Adolesc Psychopharmacol 16:171–179, 2006

Sharp WG, Sherman C, Gross AM: Selective mutism and anxiety: a review of the current conceptualization of the disorder. J Anxiety Disord 21:568–579, 2007

Shore GN, Rapport MD: The Fear Survey Schedule for Children—Revised (FSSC-HI): ethnocultural variations in children's fearfulness. J Anxiety Disord 12:437–461, 1998

Silverman WK, Albano AM: The Anxiety Disorders Interview Schedule for DSM-IV, Child and Parent Versions. New York, Oxford University Press, 1996

Silverman WK, Pina AA, Viswesvaran C: Evidence-based psychosocial treatments for phobic and anxiety disorders in children and adolescents. J Clin Child Adolesc Psychol 37:105–130, 2008

■ CHAPTER 5 ■

Everything Bothers Her

Major Depressive Disorder

John S. March, M.D., M.P.H.

CASE PRESENTATION

IDENTIFYING INFORMATION

Sally is a 13-year-old eighth grader referred for a psychiatric evaluation by her pediatrician. She lives with her parents and her brother.

CHIEF COMPLAINT

Sally reports that she is "feeling really low due to trouble with my friends."

HISTORY OF PRESENT ILLNESS

Sally reports that she has been feeling down since seventh grade, claiming, "It all started when I had a big fight with my best friend, Karen. After that, all my friends turned against me." Eventually, she and Karen reconciled, but by that time Sally felt much more insecure in her friendships. In spite of these problems, she finished the year with a B+ average. Over the summer, she spent most of her time at home "just watching TV." Her parents were concerned and encouraged her to get in touch with friends, but she said, "They're probably all away," and did not contact them.

When school started this year, Sally was hopeful that things would be better. She spent time with her friends but often worried whether they liked her.

John S. March, M.D., M.P.H., is Professor of Psychiatry and Chief of Child and Adolescent Psychiatry at Duke University Medical Center in Durham, North Carolina (for complete biographical information, see "About the Contributors," p. 613).

Her mother noticed a cycle in which Sally worried about whether her friends still liked her and "pestered them," and this behavior led to her friends backing off a bit. Sally also began to struggle in school during the semester. She complained of "spacing out" while in class or doing homework. Although she maintained her grades, she required significantly more time and effort than previously. Sally also began to have difficulty falling asleep at night. Before falling asleep, she worried about her friends and how she was falling behind in school. She had difficulty getting out of bed in the morning because she was so tired, had stomachaches, and was worried about whom she would talk to at school. During this same time, she had a bigger appetite and often craved sweets or junk food.

In the late fall, because of their concern about Sally's increased isolation, sleep schedule, and falling grades, Sally's parents took her to her primary care doctor. After asking Sally several questions, the doctor explained that she had depression and recommended that she start medication. He prescribed fluoxetine. By the time she was taking 20 mg/day, her mood had brightened and her worries had been decreasing. Her symptoms did not alleviate completely, however, and she continued to have trouble with her attention, so her primary care doctor gradually increased the doseage to 50 mg/day. At this dosage, her anxiety and depression improved a great deal, but Sally experienced minimal benefits for her social problems, self-esteem, and attention. She had also gained 12 lbs. Her primary care doctor recommended paroxetine and referred her to a local therapist. Because Sally's symptoms had not resolved after 3 months of treatment with paroxetine and weekly supportive psychotherapy, her primary care doctor referred her for this evaluation.

Past Psychiatric History

In kindergarten and first grade, Sally had a tough time starting school. She worried about her parents getting hurt or forgetting to pick her up; she had anticipatory distress, reluctance to go to school, and reluctance to be alone at home; and she had associated physical symptoms, especially fear of vomiting. These symptoms resolved midway through first grade and did not return. She has always been a bit shy with peers and adults but always socially appropriate.

Sally occasionally had difficulty with attention in school. Her mother explained that past report cards often had comments calling her "dreamy," but because she had always received very good grades, her parents had not been particularly concerned. She had never been overactive, impulsive, or disobedient. When Sally was asked about her attention, she laughed and said, "I always zone out! My friends have been calling me 'space cadet' since we knew what it meant." She and her mother also have noticed that occasionally she gets lost in conversations. She does not have a history of any other affective or anxiety disorders or further eating or sleep difficulties. Additionally, she and her mother deny disruptive behavior or learning difficulties; elimination problems; psychiatric, personality, or substance abuse disorders; tics; or obsessive-compulsive spectrum disorders.

MEDICAL HISTORY

Sally has no contributory medical problems. She is not sexually active and has a good understanding of the risk of sexually transmitted disease.

DEVELOPMENTAL HISTORY

Sally was delivered at 38 weeks by cesarean section, due to her mother's pre-eclampsia and fetal distress. Otherwise, her development was unremarkable.

SOCIAL HISTORY

The family has moved several times because of her father's job. After the most recent move 4 years ago, the family enrolled Sally at a small private school that would be more "nurturing and provide Sally with individual attention." The family's functioning is remarkable for mild family conflict over how best to handle Sally's social difficulties and her normative to elevated sibling conflict with her younger brother, Adam.

FAMILY HISTORY

A brief, two-generational family history of psychiatric illness reveals major depressive disorder (MDD) in Sally's father, mother, mother's sibling, and maternal grandmother, and obsessive-compulsive disorder in Sally's maternal grandfather.

MENTAL STATUS EXAMINATION

Sally presented as a casually dressed, mildly overweight youngster who was cooperative with the interview. Her speech was normal in rate, tone, and volume. Her psychomotor status was marked by considerable fidgeting. Sally described her mood as "good." Sally's affect was euthymic. Her thoughts were logical and goal directed. There was no evidence of thought blocking, insertion, or deletion, or ideas of reference. Sally's thought content was remarkable for themes noted above. No perceptual abnormalities were noted. Her sensorium was clear, cognitive functions were grossly intact, and insight was preserved. Sally denied current suicidality or homicidality.

SCREENING QUESTIONNAIRES

Sally and her parents filled out a set of rating scales in advance of their visit. On the Children's Depression Inventory (CDI; Kovacs 1985), Sally endorsed items indicating negative self-esteem and interpersonal conflicts; her total CDI score of 30 indicates moderate to severe depression. On the Multidimensional Anxiety Scale for Children (MASC; March et al. 1997b), Sally endorsed items indicating elevated social anxiety, again scoring in the moderate to severe range. On the Conners' Teacher Rating Scale—Revised (Conners et al. 1998b), Sally's teacher endorsed items indicating attention-deficit/hyperactivity disorder (ADHD). On the Conners' Parent Rating Scale—Revised (Conners et al. 1998a), Sally's parents endorsed items indicating social problems, psychosomatic concerns, and ADHD. Sally did not endorse any items suggesting psychopathology on the Child and Adolescent Trauma Survey (March et al. 1997a, 1998) or the MASC Children Obsessive-Compulsive Screen (March 1997). On a family measure administered to both Sally and her mother, the family scored high in family affiliation, medium in family control and parent-child conflict, and low in family conflict. The Stages of Change Index (McConnaughy et al. 1983) indicated that Sally had some motivation to change but reluctance as well.

COMMENTARIES

Psychotherapeutic Perspective

Greg Clarke, Ph.D.

DIAGNOSTIC FORMULATION

Diagnoses to rule out for Sally are major depression or dysthymia, social anxiety and/or generalized anxiety, and ADHD. The case presentation suggests the following for the period before Sally started pharmacotherapy and psychotherapy:

- *Fairly clear symptoms of major depression*—predominant depressive mood, feeling down since seventh grade (despite euthymic affect at current assessment); anhedonia; social withdrawal over the summer; a considerable increase in appetite, particularly for sweets; difficulty falling asleep, particularly initial insomnia; and diminished ability to think and concentrate (she

---

Greg Clarke, Ph.D., is with Kaiser Permanente Center for Health Research in Portland, Oregon (for complete biographical information, see "About the Contributors," p. 613).

had this difficulty prior to the episode but it appears to have worsened, as reflected by the comment that more effort was needed to complete homework)

- *Unclear or partial major depression symptoms*—feelings of fatigue or diminished energy (this is mentioned only in context of an insomnia consequence); thoughts of worthlessness as reflected in her social anxieties about peer acceptance; and considerable fidgeting during the interview, which might be evidence of psychomotor agitation (note: might also be ADHD symptom)
- *Fully absent symptoms of major depression*—no mention of thoughts of death or suicide

ASSESSMENT

Self-report depression scales, such as the Center for Epidemiologic Studies Depression Scale (Radloff 1991), the Beck Depression Inventory (Beck et al. 1986), or the administered CDI, are useful for screening and for gauging therapy progress, but have limited usefulness as diagnostic tools. Adult respondent instruments, such as the Child Behavior Checklist (Achenbach and Edelbrock 1983) or Conners' Teacher/Parent Rating Scales (Conners et al. 1998a, 1998b), have similar advantages and drawbacks. I would administer these scales for confirmation and/or to illuminate other areas for review, as well as to set a baseline for evaluating treatment progress, but I would not rely on them for an initial diagnosis. My primary diagnostic information would come from a clinical interview to gauge the presence, severity, and duration of the symptoms of the provisional diagnoses listed above. I would model my interview on one of the semistructured psychiatric interviews, such as the Children's Schedule for Affective Disorders and Schizophrenia—Present and Lifetime Version (K-SADS-PL; Kaufman et al. 1996), although I would not feel as compelled to adhere to the administration as rigidly as required in clinical trials.

The limited information provided in this case presentation does not permit a clear differential diagnosis. More in-depth interviewing would be necessary to disentangle candidate diagnoses, clarify how persistent and impairing the symptoms are, and so forth. However, my provisional diagnoses follow.

DSM-IV-TR DIAGNOSIS

Axis I   296.35 Major depressive disorder, in partial remission (Strong family loading makes this diagnosis the most likely.)

300.02 Generalized anxiety disorder (GAD), current (GAD cannot be diagnosed if present wholly within the context of a major depression episode, so the temporal and clinical overlap between GAD and major depression must be clarified.)

314.01 or 314.00 ADHD (It is unclear whether this is the combined or inattentive type, current.)

309.21 Separation anxiety, past history

Axis II   No evident personality disorders

Axis III   No evident medical disorders

Axis IV   Family is intact and fairly well functioning.
Peer relations are more troublesome. Her social skills are immature and inadequate to initiate and maintain appropriate levels of peer relations.

Axis V   Global Assessment of Functioning (or in this case, Children's Global Assessment Scale score)= 55–60

TREATMENT RECOMMENDATIONS

Sally has received an initial course of antidepressant medication at a therapeutic dose, with a subsequent dose increase and the addition of nonspecific supportive psychotherapy in response to residual symptoms and a failure to return to premorbid functioning. This is a reasonable progression of stepped therapy akin to that being tested in the Texas Children's Medication Algorithm Project (Hughes et al. 1999). The most important goal is to assist Sally to recover as completely as possible, because quick recovery appears to provide the greatest protection against future recurrences of depression (Pintor et al. 2003), which will be a significant concern for Sally, given her first major depression onset in adolescence, her significant psychiatric comorbidity, and her strong family history for mood disorder. The recent switch to another antidepressant may have been an attempt to achieve more complete remission and/or to reduce pharmacotherapy-induced weight gain. This medication switch should be monitored carefully for evidence of major depression relapse.

One possible strategy for improving Sally's major depression treatment regimen would be the addition of an evidence-based psychotherapy, such as cognitive-behavioral therapy (CBT; Brent et al. 1997) or interpersonal therapy for adolescents (IPT-A; Mufson et al. 2004). The results of the Treatment for Adolescents with Depression Study (March et al. 2004) suggest that CBT added to pharmacotherapy yields significant additional improvement. Adding IPT-A in particular might assist with psychosocial recovery.

Sally has an anxiety disorder in addition to depression. Fortunately, both selective serotonin reuptake inhibitors (SSRIs) and CBT have a track record with anxiety disorder as well as depression (Seidel and Walkup 2006). However, Sally might benefit from additional anxiety-focused CBT components, such as exposure/response prevention, relaxation training, and systematic desensitization (Cartwright-Hatton et al. 2004).

Stimulant pharmacotherapy for ADHD also seems indicated. However, as a nonprescribing psychologist specializing in mood disorders, I would seek the input of a child psychiatrist specializing in this treatment modality. Particular concerns would include the advisability of polypharmacy (stimulants and SSRIs) and the possibility that adding ADHD-specific behavioral therapy would be overwhelming at this time.

Psychopharmacologic Perspective

Graham J. Emslie, M.D.

DIAGNOSTIC FORMULATION

From a psychopharmacologic perspective, the case described raises many important issues, including both diagnostic and treatment challenges. The patient is a 13-year-old female living with her parents and younger brother. She has a prior history of anxiety (primarily separation and social anxiety) and attention problems. Beginning in seventh grade, she had what appears to have been a minor depression with partial remission. Clearly, this adolescent has multiple characteristics that make her at risk for depression: family history of depression (two first-degree and two second-degree relatives) and comorbid conditions (anxiety and attention problems, as well as a minor depression) during seventh grade. During eighth grade, she had a major depressive episode, which was treated with two SSRIs (both of adequate duration and dosage) and supportive therapy, which resulted in partial remission of her depression. Probable sequelae from the depression include increased social difficulties, increased school problems, decreased self-esteem, and sleep difficulties. At the time of the referral she had moderate depression, increased social anxiety, and attention difficulties.

This case illustrates the importance of accurate diagnosis, consideration of interactions of comorbid conditions, causes and consequences of illness, and the need for a rational, evidence-based approach to treatment.

Graham J. Emslie, M.D., is Professor and Charles E. and Sarah M. Seay Chair in Child Psychiatry, and Chief of the Child and Adolescent Psychiatry Division at University of Texas Southwestern Medical Center at Dallas and Children's Medical Center of Dallas in Dallas, Texas (for complete biographical information, see "About the Contributors," p. 613).

DIAGNOSIS

Sally's case is described beautifully, includes all the elements of a complete evaluation (e.g., present and past history of symptoms, developmental history, social history, family psychiatric history, and mental status examination), and utilizes well-validated scales. However, an exact diagnosis cannot be made from the information provided. That said, the information provided is probably more than is usually obtained, and I suspect that the inferred diagnosis is probably correct.

DSM-IV-TR provides specific diagnostic criteria for separation anxiety disorder, ADHD, and major depressive disorder. For example, on the basis of the information presented, I presume the patient does not meet criteria for ADHD, combined type, although it is possible. According to DSM-IV-TR, to be diagnosed with ADHD, inattentive type, Sally must have six to nine of the criterion symptoms, with onset prior to age 7. To be diagnosed with MDD, she must have at least five of the nine symptoms. If she does not meet these criteria, does it matter if she is one symptom away from meeting full criteria for these disorders? I think not, although no controlled treatment trials have been recommended for subsyndromal disorders, so discussion of treatment options would have to take this factor into account. The scales mentioned in Sally's case are screening measures, not diagnostic measures. I recommend the following two clinician-administered scales to determine the presence of current ADHD and MDD criterion symptoms: the ADHD Rating Scale (Zhang et al. 2005) and the Quick Inventory of Depressive Symptomatology (Rush et al. 2003), both of which include all criterion symptoms. Further assessment would be needed to determine if Sally's level of impairment meets criteria.

The presence of comorbid conditions raises several important concerns requiring consideration in pharmacologic management. In clinical samples, 70%–80% of adolescents with MDD have at least one comorbid psychiatric disorder, so this is a frequent clinical issue that has to be addressed. Failure to identify comorbid conditions is a frequent cause of treatment failure. Identifying comorbid conditions in acute situations may be difficult due to the acuity of the primary disorder; therefore, comorbid conditions need to be continually assessed as treatment progresses. The question is whether the two disorders are separate (e.g., whether ADHD onset occurred 6–7 years prior to MDD). Even if the disorders are separate, one needs to consider how they influence each other (e.g., ADHD leading to discouragement in school and subsequent depression, or MDD preceding substance use disorder). In some situations, the issue is whether the patient has two disorders or simply overlapping symptoms (e.g., severe ADHD and conduct disorder vs. bipolar disorder). At times, prolonged mood or thought disorders will result in neurocognitive deficits that can be indistinguishable from ADHD. In these cases, however, the onset of the

ADHD symptoms would follow the onset of the primary disorder (in this case, MDD). The associations between anxiety and depression are even more complex, because they appear to have a developmental progression, with anxiety disorder occurring earlier and depression later in some individuals.

Finally, in the assessment prior to treatment, the clinician needs to consider both precipitants and consequences of the disorder. Sally had some social difficulties prior to the onset of depression, yet the depression worsened the problem with social withdrawal. Even if her depression is treated, it is unreasonable to assume that social relatedness would automatically return to premorbid baseline. The same is true for the patient's difficulties with self-esteem, attention, and sleep.

DSM-IV-TR DIAGNOSIS

Axis I   296.22 Major depressive disorder
            314.00 ADHD, predominantly inattentive type
Axis II   Deferred
Axis III   None
Axis IV   Education problems
            Social problems
Axis V   Global Assessment of Functioning=58

TREATMENT RECOMMENDATIONS

PRIMARY DISORDER (DEPRESSION)

Treatment recommendations for Sally are relatively straightforward if the assessment provided above is accurate. Treatment guidelines and algorithms for treatment of depression, ADHD, and anxiety are available (Birmaher et al. 2007; Cheung et al. 2007; Connolly et al. 2007; Hughes et al. 2007; Pliszka and AACAP Work Group on Quality Issues 2007). Generally, the guidelines synthesize the increasing evidence base, both what is known empirically and what is lacking in adequate data, to allow clinicians choices.

The focus of this commentary is on psychopharmacologic management, which is only one component of an intervention and is unlikely to be effective without a well-established physician-patient-family relationship. Although the therapeutic alliance is a well-known contributor to positive outcome, it is frequently neglected.

Psychopharmacologic treatment focuses on strategic management of the primary disorder, including assessment of side effects, management of comorbid conditions, and management of associated symptoms. Typically, precipitants and consequences of the disorders do not require psychopharmacologic management, although there may be some exceptions. In addition, rational medication management generally involves one intervention at a time (with exceptions), with a preference for monotherapy. Finally, increasing evidence indicates that measured care (i.e., care in which the clinician systematically measures symptoms being treated, functioning, and adverse effects across time) improves outcome (Trivedi et al. 2007).

If it is assumed that Sally has MDD (first episode) and has had two adequate trials of an SSRI, and this current trial has not resulted in remission, then the choices are to switch or to augment. A recent National Institute of Mental Health–funded large adult treatment trial exemplifies this approach (Rush et al. 2006; Trivedi et al. 2006) (for further discussion, see Hughes et al. 2007). For adolescents, current recommendations are to switch to a non-SSRI or to augment with lithium or bupropion. Other options would rely entirely on adult data. Generally, switching is for minimal responders or nonresponders or for patients experiencing side effects, and augmentation is for patients who feel they have some response they wish to maintain but not quite full response or remission. One caveat is that distinguishing side effects from continued or worsening depression can be difficult. For example, antidepressants may cause apathy, sleep disturbance, or appetite changes, but these symptoms are also present in depression, making the distinction between ongoing or worsening symptoms (due to insufficient treatment) versus side effects of medication difficult.

Comorbid Condition (ADHD)

In Sally's case, the clinician would consider treatment of possible comorbid ADHD, using the treatment guidelines for ADHD, with the most effective treatment being a stimulant. If one initiates only one intervention at a time, as recommended above, the initial question, then, would be which intervention to initiate first: treating the comorbid ADHD or changing the depression treatment.

Associated Symptoms

Occasionally, pharmacologic management is used to treat associated symptoms that may require treatment until the primary disorder is treated. Often, such symptoms are not direct criterion symptoms of the primary disorder (e.g., aggression in a patient with MDD), but even criterion symptoms sometimes require additional treatment (e.g., severe sleep disturbance, severe irritability). The general rule is to stop these treatments once the underlying disorder improves. Thus, the first treatment is to treat the underlying disorder, but this treatment may be insufficient, so another medication may be added for the specific concern. Some data from studies of adults with depression and insomnia suggest that treatment with a hypnotic and an antidepressant is superior to an antidepressant alone in reducing symptoms (Fava et al. 2006).

CONTINUATION TREATMENT

Continuation treatment for 6–9 months following response is recommended for treatment of depression. In addition, during continuation therapy, aggressive treatment of residual symptoms is recommended because of an increased chance of relapse. Treatment of residual symptoms can be with pharmacology and/or with specific psychotherapies (e.g., CBT, IPT-A).

In summary, accurate diagnosis and assessment are essential; treatment should be rational, systematic, and sequential; and different modalities of treatment should be integrated as needed to achieve an optimal outcome.

Integrative Perspective

John S. March, M.D., M.P.H.

DIAGNOSTIC FORMULATION

Above, I presented Sally's case in a traditional narrative format, beginning with the history of her present illness that follows the chief complaint. The following medical approach to psychodiagnosis is another way to present her history, however, and demonstrates how I actually work.

A MEDICAL APPROACH TO PSYCHODIAGNOSIS

Careful, symptom-focused interviewing about Sally's current difficulties reveals that Sally meets DSM-IV-TR diagnostic criteria for major depression, which has been present for approximately 6 months, as her primary diagnosis. Prominent mood symptoms include depressed mood most of the day, as well as irritable mood when stressed or provoked. Prominent neurovegetative symptoms include weight gain (excess eating as a coping behavior), insomnia, diminished ability to think or concentrate, and fatigue. Like most young persons with moderate to severe MDD, Sally experiences these symptoms at home, with peers, and at school. Although she has had normative transient suicideal ideation, Sally has not been overtly suicidal or homicidal.

The diagnostic interview also establishes that Sally meets DSM-IV-TR diagnostic criteria for anxiety disorder not otherwise specified (NOS), with broadly based anxiety symptoms involving physical symptoms, social anxiety, and reliance on anxiety-driven approach/avoidance coping strategies that nevertheless do not meet full diagnostic criteria for one of the more discrete anxiety syndromes. Sally shows considerable discomfort in social situations, particularly with peers, that is difficult to disentangle from MDD.

Depression and anxiety clearly interact, and this interaction needs to be addressed in treatment. It appears that Sally is intolerant of being alone and that when she feels anxious (or bored), her preferred activity (not unusual in girls her age, but nonetheless clearly excessive in her case) to relieve emotional distress is interacting socially with her friends. When pursuing social contact, she often drives others away by "harassing" them, thereby increasing social anxiety, which in turn prompts anxiety-driven seeking of reassurance about "whether they like me" from parents, teachers, and friends. Thus, Sally's proximity seeking drives social rejection, which in turn drives isolation, more desperate social behaviors, and further alienation of friends, parents, and teachers, keeping the overall process going around and around.

Lastly, Sally meets DSM-IV-TR diagnostic criteria for a previously undiagnosed ADHD, inattentive type, as manifested by a context-dependent mix of poor attention and concentration. Sally's ADHD symptoms, which preceded her depression, are present primarily when she is bored and are exacerbated when she is socially anxious. Importantly, Sally's ADHD symptoms cause problems with peers and in school. Problematic attention and concentration symptoms include easy distractibility to auditory or visual cues; poor problem-solving skills, especially in social situations; and difficulties with sustained attention, especially under low–stimulus salience conditions.

This alternative, medical symptom–focused evaluation more closely resembles the history and physical (H and P) format that I have used as a family physician and pediatric psychiatrist. It is intended to illustrate a particular way of using the medical model to drive clinical interviewing and decision making in the practice of pediatric psychiatry (March and Ollendick 2004). My standard medical model interview draws on two well-established approaches—evidence-based medicine (March et al. 2005) and functional analysis of behavior as the platform for implementing cognitive-behavioral psychotherapy (Silverman and Kurtines 1996)—and places a third—the narrative approach to psychiatric illness—in the context of the illnesses that are driving the patient's story.

Medical interviewing begins with a few identifying demographic characteristics and a presenting complaint that lead to a heightened prior probability of a particular primary diagnosis. For example, a 58-year-old man who presents in the emergency room with acute-onset crushing chest pain would likely receive a tentative diagnosis of unstable angina or acute myocardial infarction. The goal of a medical interview would be to review the signs and symptoms associated with occlusive coronary artery disease and look for common comorbidities that would complicate the primary diagnosis. For example, the interviewer would ask about known risk factors or features suggesting atherosclerotic vascular disease, hypertension, congestive heart failure, or an arrhythmia.

In Sally's case, her age, gender, and presenting complaint are consistent with a probable diagnosis of depression complicated by anxiety and disruptive behavior. Drawing upon rating scale data completed prior to the visit, I confirm my initial impressions and refine the diagnostic evaluation with presumptive diagnoses of MDD, social anxiety disorder, and possibly ADHD and oppositional defiant disorder. From the medical interview, it is clear that Sally meets DSM-IV-TR criteria for MDD (these are listed up front) and also for anxiety disorder NOS (a mix of generalized and social anxiety disorder symptoms). From the perspective of functional analysis of behavior (Silverman and Kurtines 1996), the interaction between negative affectivity (depression and anxiety) and problematic peer and family relationships is clearly specified as a target for intervention.

Once it has been established that Sally meets the diagnostic criteria for inattentive-subtype ADHD, the rest of the differential diagnosis (analogous to panic disorder, chest wall pain, or gallbladder disease, among others, in our gentleman with chest pain) is dispensed with by exception.

Unlike the narrative approach, which puts relationship disturbances and other risk factors up front, the medical approach assumes that the illness drives the patient's story, and that risk and protective factors make it more or less likely that the patient will improve with the appropriate interventions (Hamilton 2004, 2005).

DSM-IV-TR DIAGNOSIS

Axis I   296.22 Major depressive disorder, single episode, moderate

          300.00 Anxiety disorder not otherwise specified

          314.00 ADHD, predominantly inattentive type

Axis II   No diagnosis

Axis III None

Axis IV   Mild stressors

Axis V   Global Assessment of Functioning=60 (current month)

          Global Assessment of Functioning=50 (this year)

TREATMENT RECOMMENDATIONS

Treatment recommendations are built around the need for additional assessments, recommendations for psychosocial interventions, medication management, and both pedagogic and behavioral interventions in school. Importantly, the interventions of choice are explicitly evidence based (Kratochvil et al. 2002, 2006; Ollendick and March 2004; Weersing and Brent 2006) and can easily be integrated (March and Wells 2003).

Psychotherapy

The empirical literature strongly suggests that Sally will do best if her symptom picture is skillfully addressed using proven psychosocial interventions that are tightly linked to their target symptoms (Hibbs and Jensen 2005). To a large extent, the therapist in this model functions as a coach or mentor to implement a treatment that operates both at the psychological level (learning new skills) and on the somatic substrate of the disorder. In this sense, the recommended interventions are usefully seen as analogous to diet and exercise in diabetes. In this context, I would recommend CBT for depression and anxiety management training. A number of books and treatment manuals are helpful references for clinicians using CBT treatments (e.g., Curry et al. 2005; Kendall 2000) or for patients themselves (Brantley 2005; Burns 1980, 1999; McQuaid and Carmona 2004).

The therapist using CBT will need to incorporate several themes emerging from the literature on depression (behavioral activation, cognitive restructuring, conflict reduction), anxiety (exposure, cognitive restructuring, positive self-reinforcement), and parent training for ADHD (management of oppositional behavior) in a fashion that is developmentally sensitive and appropriate to the targets identified in the functional behavioral analysis. In this context, CBT is something like physical therapy in that it uses overlearning strategies that are tightly coupled to their targets to address the psychosocial and somatic targets of interest and, in so doing, integrates easily with pharmacologic management.

Sally should be encouraged to participate in social activities away from school, such as a drama club or sport, to help broaden her friendship networks. Irrespective of setting, the spiral of using friends to dampen negative affectivity, which in turn drives social isolation and more negative affectivity, needs to be an early target of treatment.

As outlined particularly well by Rapee et al. (2000a, 2000b), elements of parent management training will be useful to modify the negative reinforcement cycles that perpetuate the oppositional behaviors that are a manifestation of both ADHD and maladaptive coping with anxiety and depression. Additionally, a book by Chansky (2004) can be very helpful for parents.

Diet and exercise consultation might help Sally shed excess weight. Exercise may also benefit Sally by helping to reduce depression and maintain treatment gains.

Medications

Even with skillful CBT, Sally is unlikely to make significant progress without pharmacotherapy, at least for the time being. When conducting medication trials, the therapy team needs to pay careful attention to the dose-response and time-response characteristics of whatever compound is being tried across all important domains of outcome. In this context, I recommend the following, in the stated order: Sally should discontinue paroxetine, which has clearly been associated with excessive weight gain and inadequate response. She should then be given a trial of atomoxetine for ADHD (Biederman et al. 2002; Kratochvil et al. 2005), inattentive type, with comorbid anxiety and depressive symptoms. With withdrawal from paroxetine and initiation of atomoxetine, Sally needs to be carefully monitored for increased suicidal ideation/behaviors and other adverse events, including cardiovascular reactions.

Medication management covers both anxiety and depression and may facilitate the implementation of CBT, as well as add to its effectiveness. In turn, CBT may protect against relapse when medications are withdrawn. Of particular importance, medications alone may increase the suicidal event rate (Hammad et al. 2006; Kratochvil et al. 2006), and receiving concomitant CBT may reduce if not eliminate this risk while improving overall outcome (March et al. 2006). When CBT is combined with medications for treatment, close monitoring by a multidisciplinary team easily satisfies the monitoring requirements of good clinical practice. In Sally's case, working with parents and coordination with the school are important aspects of implementing the outlined treatment strategy, which can be conducted entirely on an outpatient basis.

ACADEMIC PERFORMANCE

Sally is doing well in school, but work has been more challenging because of her poor attention. With the permission of her family, her therapist should update the school about Sally's treatment so that teachers will be aware and so they might help with the cognitive-behavioral interventions.

CODA

Sally's case closely matches the most common presentation of chronic mixed anxiety and depressive illness in youth, namely the chronic waxing and waning symptoms with both homotypic and heterotypic continuity (Costello et al. 2004). By following the evaluation format and treatment approaches outlined in this report, in our hands, Sally would have a 50% probability of remission within 4 months of starting treatment and a 90% chance of making substantial improvement.

REFERENCES

Achenbach TM, Edelbrock CS: Manual for the Child Behavior Checklist. Burlington, University of Vermont, Department of Psychology, 1983

Beck AT, Steer RA, Brown GK: Beck Depression Inventory, 2nd Edition. San Antonio, TX, Psychological Corporation, 1986

Biederman J, Heiligenstein JH, Faries DE, et al: Efficacy of atomoxetine versus placebo in school-age girls with attention-deficit/hyperactivity disorder. Pediatrics 110:e75, 2002

Birmaher B, Brent D, AACAP Work Group on Quality Issues, et al: Practice parameter for the assessment and treatment of children and adolescents with depressive disorders. J Am Acad Child Adolesc Psychiatry 46:1503–1526, 2007

Brantley J: Calming Your Anxious Mind: How Mindfulness and Compassion Can Free You From Anxiety, Fear, and Panic. Oakland, CA, New Harbinger, 2005

Brent DA, Holder D, Kolko D, et al: A clinical psychotherapy trial for adolescent depression comparing cognitive, family, and supportive therapy. Arch Gen Psychiatry 54:877–885, 1997

Burns D: Feeling Good: The New Mood Therapy. New York, Penguin, 1980

Burns D: The Feeling Good Handbook. New York, Penguin, 1999

Cartwright-Hatton S, Roberts C, Chitsabesan P, et al: Systematic review of the efficacy of cognitive behaviour therapies for childhood and adolescent anxiety disorders. Br J Clin Psychol 43:421–436, 2004

Chansky TE: Freeing Your Child From Anxiety: Powerful, Practical Strategies to Overcome Your Child's Fears, Phobias and Worries. New York, Crown, 2004

Cheung AH, Zuckerbrot RA, Jensen PS, et al; GLAD-PC Steering Group: Guidelines for Adolescent Depression in Primary Care (GLAD-PC), II: treatment and ongoing management. Pediatrics 120:e1313–e1326, 2007

Conners CK, Sitarenios G, Parker JD, et al: The revised Conners' Parent Rating Scale (CPRS-R): factor structure, reliability, and criterion validity. J Abnorm Child Psychol 26:257–268, 1998a

Conners CK, Sitarenios G, Parker JD, et al: Revision and restandardization of the Conners' Teacher Rating Scale (CTRS-R): factor structure, reliability, and criterion validity. J Abnorm Child Psychol 26:279–291, 1998b

Connolly SD, Bernstein GA; Work Group on Quality Issues: Practice parameter for the assessment and treatment of children and adolescents with anxiety disorders. J Am Acad Child Adolesc Psychiatry 46:267–283, 2007

Costello EJ, Egger HL, Angold A: The developmental epidemiology of anxiety disorders, in Phobic and Anxiety Disorders in Children and Adolescents: A Clinician's Guide to Effective Psychosocial and Pharmacological Interventions. Edited by Ollendick TH, March JS. New York, Oxford University Press, 2004, pp 61–91

Curry JF, Wells KC, Brent DA, et al: Treatment for Adolescents with Depression Study (TADS). Cognitive Behavior Therapy Manual. Introduction, Rationale, and Adolescent Sessions. Durham, NC, Duke University Medical Center, 2005

Fava M, McCall WV, Krystal A, et al: Eszopiclone coadministered with fluoxetine in patients with insomnia coexisting with major depressive disorder. Biol Psychiatry 59:1052–1060, 2006

Hamilton JD: Evidence-based thinking and the alliance with parents. J Am Acad Child Adolesc Psychiatry 43:105–108, 2004

Hamilton J: Clinicians' guide to evidence-based practice. J Am Acad Child Adolesc Psychiatry 44:494–498, 2005

Hammad TA, Laughren T, Racoosin J: Suicidality in pediatric patients treated with antidepressant drugs. Arch Gen Psychiatry 63:332–339, 2006

Hibbs E, Jensen P: Psychosocial Treatments for Child and Adolescent Disorders, 2nd Edition. Washington, DC, American Psychological Association, 2005

Hughes CW, Emslie GJ, Crismon ML, et al: The Texas Children's Medication Algorithm Project: report of the Texas Consensus Conference Panel on Medication treatment of Childhood Major Depressive Disorder. J Am Acad Child Adolesc Psychiatry 38:1442–1454, 1999

Hughes CW, Emslie GJ, Crismon ML, et al; Texas Consensus Conference Panel on Medication Treatment of Childhood Major Depressive Disorder: Texas Children's Medication Algorithm Project: update from Texas Consensus Conference Panel on Medication Treatment of Childhood Major Depressive Disorder. J Am Acad Child Adolesc Psychiatry 46:667–686, 2007

Kaufman J, Birmaher B, Brent DA, et al: Schedule for Affective Disorders and Schizophrenia for School-Age Children—Present and Lifetime Version (K-SADS-PL): initial reliability and validity data. J Am Acad Child Adolesc Psychiatry 36:980–988, 1997

Kendall PC: Child and Adolescent Therapy: Cognitive-Behavioral Procedures, 3rd Edition. New York, Guilford, 2005

Kovacs M: The Children's Depression Inventory (CDI). Psychopharmacol Bull 21:995–998, 1985

Kratochvil CJ, Harrington MJ, Burke WJ, et al: Pharmacotherapy of childhood anxiety disorders. Curr Psychiatry Rep 4:264–269, 2002

Kratochvil CJ, Newcorn JH, Arnold LE, et al: Atomoxetine alone or combined with fluoxetine for treating ADHD with comorbid depressive or anxiety symptoms. J Am Acad Child Adolesc Psychiatry 44:915–924, 2005

Kratochvil CJ, Vitiello B, Walkup J, et al: Selective serotonin reuptake inhibitors in pediatric depression: is the balance between benefits and risks favorable? J Child Adolesc Psychopharmacol 16:11–24, 2006

March JS: Manual for the Multidimensional Anxiety Scale for Children (MASC). North Tonawanda, NY, Multi-Health Systems, 1997

March JS, Ollendick TH: Integrated psychosocial and pharmacological treatment, in Phobic and Anxiety Disorders in Children and Adolescents: A Clinician's Guide to Effective Psychosocial and Pharmacological Interventions. Edited by Ollendick TH, March JS. New York, Oxford University Press, 2004, pp 141–172

March J, Wells K: Combining medication and psychotherapy, in Pediatric Psychopharmacology: Principles and Practice. Edited by Martin A, Scahill L, Charney DS, et al. London, Oxford University Press, 2003, pp 326–346

March J, Amaya-Jackson L, Terry R, et al: Post-traumatic stress in children and adolescents after an industrial fire. J Am Acad Child Adolesc Psychiatry 36:1080–1088, 1997a

March JS, Parker JD, Sullivan K, et al: The Multidimensional Anxiety Scale for Children (MASC): factor structure, reliability, and validity. J Am Acad Child Adolesc Psychiatry 36:554–565, 1997b

March JS, Amaya-Jackson L, Murray MC, et al: Cognitive-behavioral psychotherapy for children and adolescents with posttraumatic stress disorder after a single-incident stressor. J Am Acad Child Adolesc Psychiatry 37:585–593, 1998

March J, Silva S, Petrycki S, et al: Fluoxetine, cognitive-behavioral therapy, and their combination for adolescents with depression: Treatment for Adolescents with Depression Study (TADS) randomized controlled trial. JAMA 292:807–820, 2004

March JS, Chrisman A, Breland-Noble A, et al: Using and teaching evidence-based medicine: the Duke University child and adolescent psychiatry model. Child Adolesc Psychiatr Clin N Am 14:273–296, 2005

March J, Silva S, Vitiello B: The Treatment for Adolescents with Depression Study (TADS): methods and message at 12 weeks. J Am Acad Child Adolesc Psychiatry 45:1393–1403, 2006

McConnaughy EA, Prochaska JO, Velicer WF: Stages of change in psychotherapy measurement and sample profiles. Psychotherapy: Theory, Research, and Practice 20:368–375, 1983

McQuaid J, Carmona P: Peaceful Mind: Using Mindfulness and Cognitive Behavioral Psychology to Overcome Depression. Oakland, CA, New Harbinger, 2004

Mufson L, Dorta KP, Wickramaratne P, et al: A randomized effectiveness trial of interpersonal psychotherapy for depressed adolescents. Arch Gen Psychiatry 61:577–584, 2004

Ollendick TH, March JS: Phobic and Anxiety Disorders: A Clinician's Guide to Effective Psychosocial and Pharmacological Interventions. New York, Oxford University Press, 2004

Pintor L, Gasto C, Navarro V, et al: Relapse of major depression after complete and partial remission during a 2-year follow-up. J Affect Disord 73:237–244, 2003

Pliszka S; AACAP Work Group on Quality Issues: Practice parameter for the assessment and treatment of children and adolescents with attention-deficit/hyperactivity disorder. J Am Acad Child Adolesc Psychiatry 46:894–921, 2007

Radloff LS: The use of the Center for Epidemiologic Studies Depression Scale in adolescents and young adults. J Youth Adolesc 20:149–166, 1991

Rapee R, Spense S, Cobham V, et al: Helping Your Anxious Child: A Step-by-Step Guide for Parents. Oakland, CA, New Harbinger, 2000a

Rapee R, Wignal A, Hudson J, et al: Treating Anxious Children and Adolescents: An Evidence Based Approach. Oakland, CA, New Harbinger, 2000b

Rush AJ, Trivedi MH, Ibrahim HM, et al: The 16-item Quick Inventory of Depressive Symptomatology (QIDS), clinician rating (QIDS-C), and self-report (QIDS-SR): a psychometric evaluation in patients with chronic major depression. Biol Psychiatry 54:573–583, 2003

Rush AJ, Trivedi MH, Wisniewski SR, et al: Bupropion-SR, sertraline, or venlafaxine-XR after failure of SSRIs for depression. N Engl J Med 354:1231–1242, 2006

Seidel L, Walkup JT: Selective serotonin reuptake inhibitor use in the treatment of the pediatric non-obsessive-compulsive disorder anxiety disorders. J Child Adolesc Psychopharmacol 16:171–179, 2006

Silverman W, Kurtines W: Anxiety and Phobic Disorders: A Pragmatic Approach. New York, Plenum, 1996

Trivedi MH, Fava M, Wisniewski SR, et al; Star*D Study Team: Medication augmentation after the failure of SSRIs for depression. N Engl J Med 354:1243–1252, 2006

Trivedi MH, Rush AJ, Gaynes BN, et al: Maximizing the adequacy of medication treatment in controlled trials and clinical practice: STAR*D measurement-based care. Neuropsychopharmacology 32:2479–2489, 2007

Weersing VR, Brent DA: Cognitive behavioral therapy for depression in youth. Child Adolesc Psychiatr Clin N Am 15:939–957, 2006

Zhang S, Faries DE, Vowles M, et al: ADHD Rating Scale IV: psychometric properties from a multinational study as a clinician-administered instrument. Int J Methods Psychiatr Res 14:186–201, 2005

■ CHAPTER 6 ■

Excessively Silly

Bipolar Disorder

Mary Kay Gill, R.N., M.S.N., J.D.
Boris Birmaher, M.D.

CASE PRESENTATION

IDENTIFYING INFORMATION

Heather is a 9-year-old girl who lives with her biological mother, 11-year-old sister, and 81-year-old maternal grandfather in a suburban area. Her parents are divorced, and Heather sees her biological father infrequently. She is enrolled in the third grade at a local private school.

CHIEF COMPLAINT

According to Heather's mother, over the past few months, Heather has been very irritable and nervous, she has not been sleeping well, and teachers have been complaining about Heather's excessive silliness at school.

HISTORY OF PRESENT ILLNESS

Heather's mother described Heather as a generally happy child, who gets along well with her sister, grandfather, and mother. She is well liked at school and

Mary Kay Gill, R.N., M.S.N., J.D., is Program Coordinator of Course and Outcome for Bipolar Youth and Longitudinal Assessment of Manic Symptoms at Western Psychiatric Institute and Clinic at the University of Pittsburgh Medical Center in Pittsburgh, Pennsylvania.

Boris Birmaher, M.D., is Endowed Chair in Early-Onset Bipolar Disease and Professor of Psychiatry at the University of Pittsburgh School of Medicine in Pittsburgh, Pennsylvania.

For complete biographical information, see "About the Contributors," p. 613.

has several friends in the neighborhood. However, for the past 3–4 months, according to the mother, Heather's mood has been mostly "up." Heather frequently laughs and giggles for no apparent reason. At school, she giggles so much that she is unable to recite the morning prayer and Pledge of Allegiance. Heather's mother said that teachers have complained about Heather's excessive silliness and describe times when she talks so fast that she is difficult to understand. Her mother reported that Heather has so much energy that she sometimes takes 2–3 hours to fall asleep, and when she awakens at 6 A.M., she is energetic and does not appear to be tired despite sleeping 2–3 hours less than usual. Her mother also reported that at times Heather talks so fast and jumps from one subject to another so quickly that it is hard to follow what Heather is saying. Heather tells her mother that her "thoughts are going around and around in her head." She has been learning Bible verses at school and sometimes walks around the house chanting Bible verses and is unable to stop. Heather is focused on becoming a singer, actress, or model and keeps asking her mother to find out how she can get on the television program *Star Search*. Her mother described Heather as being quite insistent about appearing on television and said that Heather really believes she will be a "star." She is slightly hypersexual and crawls onto adults' laps in a flirtatious manner and has begun kissing her mother on the mouth, which is very unusual for Heather. Heather has been more irritable over the past few months with a low frustration tolerance, at times "exploding" when she cannot have what she wants. She has been more argumentative and at times aggressive with her older sister. Heather and her mother denied that Heather has suicidal and homicidal ideations. Her mother reported that the above-noted symptoms last from 3 to 7 days a week, with minimal euthymic periods. Heather's mother is unaware of any event that may have precipitated this change in Heather's mood and behavior.

Both Heather and her mother denied current depressive symptoms. However, Heather has experienced two episodes of major depression in the past (see "Past Psychiatric History," below).

In addition to the previously mentioned manic symptoms, Heather also has anxiety symptoms. Over the past 7–8 months, Heather has experienced 10 panic attacks. She endorsed all associated symptoms, including shortness of breath, palpitations, sweating, shaking, choking, chest pain, nausea, dizziness, derealization/depersonalization, fear of losing control, fear of dying, numbness/tingling, and chills and hot flushes. She stated that each attack lasts for about 20 minutes. Some of the panic attacks have been unexpected. Both Heather and her mother denied that these symptoms are impairing or that Heather has changed her behavior in response to the attacks.

Heather and her mother endorsed current symptoms of separation anxiety disorder (SAD). Heather stated that "ever since I can remember," she has not liked to be separated from her mother. Heather stated that when her mother is away from home, Heather often worries that her mother will "have an accident, not come back, or run away." Heather also stated that she worries every day that she herself will be killed or kidnapped. She stated that she does not have a tantrum or cry when her mother leaves the house but that she always begs her mother to stay home. She admitted that during the last school year, she pretended to be sick on several occasions to stay home with her mom. Heather often follows her mother from room to room when they are at home together. On most nights, Heather cannot sleep alone and sleeps with her mother. Heather also reported having nightmares, almost every night, involving a separation theme.

Heather reported having had symptoms of generalized anxiety disorder (GAD) for the past 4 years. Her mother indicated that Heather worries more than other children her age and that Heather has multiple worries about things happening at home and school most days of the week. The worries are about future and past events. Heather stated that she cannot control her worries, and her mother reported that Heather experiences many physical symptoms of GAD on most days. Her mother stated that Heather is very self-conscious, worries a lot about competence, and needs much reassurance. Heather has recently been especially worried about her school performance and has been extremely anxious when taking tests, saying that her mind "goes blank" during the test.

Both mother and daughter denied symptoms of other psychiatric disorders, including psychotic disorders, disruptive behavior disorders, obsessive-compulsive disorder, posttraumatic stress disorder, and substance abuse. Heather has no history of physical or sexual abuse.

Past Psychiatric History

Heather has had two past episodes of depression. One episode occurred when she was age 5 and lasted for 8 months; the second and more serious occurred when she was age 8 and lasted for 7 months. Both episodes met diagnostic criteria for major depressive episode. During the second episode, Heather told her mother that she felt "like she wanted to cut herself." She had taken the scissors and thought about cutting her throat. In addition to suicidal ideation, Heather endorsed feeling sad most of the day, every day; not being interested in her usual activities; having difficulty falling asleep and feeling tired during the day; loss of appetite; inability to concentrate; and decreased self-esteem. Heather denied ever having attempted suicide. The first episode of depression subsided without treatment. For the second episode, Heather was treated with cognitive-behavioral therapy (CBT) for 7–8 months. Heather was also treated with paroxetine 10 mg/day for 4–6 weeks, but her mother discontinued this medication, stating that it made Heather "worse." While taking paroxetine, Heather began to experience panic attacks, which persisted after the medication was discontinued.

Heather's mother also reported that prior to the onset of depressive symptoms, Heather exhibited symptoms of attention-deficit/hyperactivity disorder (ADHD), inattentive type. These symptoms included having difficulty paying attention to tasks, being easily distracted, being forgetful, frequently losing her belongings, having difficulty following through with instructions, and fidgeting. Her mother reported that these symptoms are persistent but become much worse when Heather's mood becomes silly or "up."

SUBSTANCE ABUSE HISTORY

Heather has no history of substance abuse.

MEDICAL HISTORY

Heather has no significant medical problems.

DEVELOPMENTAL HISTORY

Heather's mother reported that she used no medication, alcohol, cigarettes, or illicit drugs during her pregnancy. She reported that the pregnancy, labor and delivery, and postnatal period were within normal limits. She also stated that Heather's developmental milestones were reached early.

SOCIAL HISTORY

Heather lives with her biological mother, 11-year-old sister, and 81-year-old grandfather. Her biological mother has full custody, and her biological father has limited involvement with Heather. He has weekly supervised visits with Heather, although recently Heather has not wished to see her father. Her mother described Heather's father as alcoholic and added that he has been verbally abusive to Heather in the past.

Heather is enrolled in the third grade at a local private school. Her mother reported that Heather is a good student, although recently her grades have been affected by her manic symptoms. According to her mother, although Heather is usually "popular" with peers and has no problems with making friends, she started a new school this year and has not yet established any close friendships.

FAMILY HISTORY

Heather's mother has been diagnosed with bipolar I disorder, social phobia, posttraumatic stress disorder, panic disorder, and alcohol dependence. She was treated for postpartum depression after Heather's birth and has had multiple psychiatric hospitalizations.

Heather's father has a history of major depressive disorder (MDD), as well as alcohol and cocaine dependence.

Heather's 11-year-old sister has been diagnosed with bipolar I disorder and anxiety disorder not otherwise specified.

MENTAL STATUS EXAMINATION

Heather is a 9-year-old girl who appeared her stated age. She was dressed provocatively, wearing a sheer animal print blouse, which exposed part of her midriff, and a bright scarf.

Heather was friendly, outgoing, and cooperative with the interview. She was distractible but seemed to make an effort to pay attention to questions. She was very talkative and at times drifted to an unrelated topic, but she responded well to redirection. Heather was restless and fidgeted in her seat and had more difficulty staying in her seat as the interview progressed. She described her mood as "good" and "happy," and her affect was congruent. Her speech was rapid at times but not pressured. Heather denied auditory or visual hallucinations. She denied current suicidal or homicidal ideation. Heather was aware that she has been getting into trouble at school because she is "too silly" and has "too much energy inside" but stated that she cannot control this behavior.

COMMENTARIES

Psychotherapeutic Perspective

Mary A. Fristad, Ph.D., A.B.P.P.

DIAGNOSTIC FORMULATION

The assessment of bipolar disorder should include a detailed, longitudinal summation of the onset, offset, and duration of manic and depressive symptoms in relation to stressful life events, a medical history (including psychotropic and other medication utilization), a developmental history, assessment of school ad-

Mary A. Fristad, Ph.D., A.B.P.P., is Professor of Psychiatry and Psychology and Director of Research and Psychological Services in the Division of Child and Adolescent Psychiatry at The Ohio State University in Columbus, Ohio (for complete biographical information, see "About the Contributors," p. 613).

justment, and a three-generational family history; information regarding symptoms should be elicited from both the child and the parent (Danner et al. 2009; Kowatch et al. 2005a; Quinn and Fristad 2004). Heather's case meets these criteria. Self-report inventories, such as the Child Mania Rating Scale (Pavuluri et al. 2006) and the General Behavior Inventory (Depue et al. 1989; Youngstrom et al. 2001), are effective screening devices, and rating scales are useful to document symptom severity, but neither can be used to make a diagnosis of bipolar disorder (Danner et al. 2009). However, mood rating scales and self-report inventories—clinician-rated forms completed during office visits and mood charts that Heather and/or her mother complete at home—are useful to monitor treatment response and to track changes in diagnosis.

Heather's presentation illustrates several features common to childhood-onset bipolar spectrum disorders (bipolar I, bipolar II; cyclothymia, bipolar disorder not otherwise specified). First, she has multiple symptoms of anxiety, including panic, SAD, and GAD. Second, her symptoms manifested at an early age, with her first depressive episode notable by age 5. Third, when treated with a selective serotonin reuptake inhibitor (SSRI) for a depressive episode, Heather deteriorated. Fourth, Heather appears to have preexisting ADHD, inattentive type, the symptoms of which appear worse when Heather is manic. Clear exacerbation of the "overlap" symptoms of distractibility and increased goal-directed activity is needed to count these as symptoms of both ADHD and bipolar disorder. Fifth, Heather has a significant family history. Her father has a history of MDD, and her mother and sister have been diagnosed with bipolar I disorder.

Heather has had two past episodes of depression. Currently, she is exhibiting manic symptoms, including both euphoric and irritable mood, grandiosity, decreased need for sleep, increased talkativeness, flight of ideas, distractibility, psychomotor agitation, and hypersexuality.

DSM-IV-TR DIAGNOSIS

Axis I   296.42 Bipolar I disorder, most recent episode manic, moderate

             314.00 ADHD, predominantly inattentive type

             309.21 Separation anxiety disorder

             300.02 Generalized anxiety disorder

Axis II   None

Axis III   None

Axis IV   Poor relationship with father, who has been verbally abusive in the past and is diagnosed with alcohol and cocaine dependence

             Mother has had multiple psychiatric hospitalizations and is diagnosed with alcohol dependence (although there is no indication of current problems)

Axis V   Global Assessment of Functioning=55
Currently experiencing moderate impairment at school and home, questionable with peers

TREATMENT RECOMMENDATIONS

First, Heather should receive a medication evaluation (as discussed by Kowatch, in his commentary later in this chapter). Second, Heather and her family should begin psychoeducational psychotherapy. Three formats have been tested for children her age: individual family psychoeducation (Fristad 2006), multifamily psychoeducation groups (Fristad et al. 2003), and the RAINBOW program (Pavuluri et al. 2004). These three programs have common elements: 1) education about mood disorders and their management and 2) skill building in emotion regulation, communication, and problem solving (Lofthouse and Fristad 2004). Heather and her mother might first participate in a multi-family group and then follow up in individual family therapy, or they might begin immediately with the latter, depending on what services are available in their community. Group and individual family interventions have different pragmatic and clinical advantages and disadvantages (Fristad 2006). Heather and her family should work with a therapist familiar with childhood-onset bipolar disorder to avoid the many misattributions about symptoms that can occur when a therapist does not have such knowledge (Mackinaw-Koons and Fristad 2004). Heather has had suicidal ideation previously; this should be carefully monitored throughout treatment.

The stability of Heather's mother and sister needs to be considered. Because multiple family members with bipolar disorder can all be stressors for one another (family mood charting can illustrate this), all family members in the home should receive comprehensive care. Family sessions can address how members can cope best with their own symptoms and the stressors inherent in the home. As a part of this approach, Heather and her family should be assisted in establishing family routines around meals and sleep.

Heather is currently estranged from her father, who may not be stable currently. Inviting him to a family therapy session might provide an opportunity to assist him in resuming active treatment for his substance abuse and depression.

Heather's psychotherapy should also address her anxiety symptoms. Comorbid anxiety disorders are a negative predictor of outcome (DelBello et al. 2007), so minimizing their impact will be critical to her overall success. CBT is recommended to treat both SAD and GAD. If CBT successfully reduces Heather's anxiety, medications (SSRIs) to target anxiety can be avoided, which is desirable because SSRIs can trigger manic symptoms. Also, her ADHD, inattentive type, should be targeted. Medication management of her inattentive symptoms may be required after her mood is stabilized. Heather and her family will also need to understand how these symptoms typically manifest and how they can be managed at home.

As part of Heather's psychosocial intervention, school-based functioning should be monitored. Heather historically has been a good student and has done well with academics, behavior, and social interactions. However, these areas of functioning have been affected by her current illness. Additionally, her ADHD, inattentive type, quite likely impacts her school performance negatively. Thus, communication between the mental health team, family, and school professionals may be helpful to generate an intervention strategy for Heather at school. In particular, I recommend providing school staff with educational material (see http://www.bpkids.org for sample handouts) and deciding on a prearranged "cool-off" setting, the use of which either Heather's teacher or Heather can initiate.

Finally, Heather's mother may benefit from joining an online support group (see http://www.bpkids.org). Heather, her sister, and her mother may all benefit from learning more about their disorders (a book list is provided in "Resources" in Fristad and Goldberg Arnold 2004).

If these interventions are not successful in ameliorating Heather's symptoms, medication readjustment should be considered. Additionally, Heather and her mother should work with their therapist to update treatment goals (Fristad and Goldberg Arnold 2004, pp. 153–155) and continue to implement and test the efficacy of interventions they devise collaboratively in therapy.

Psychopharmacologic Perspective

Robert A. Kowatch, M.D., Ph.D.

DIAGNOSTIC FORMULATION

What is most interesting about Heather is that if she were age 19 rather than age 9, no one would question the diagnosis of bipolar disorder. She presents with 3- to 7-day periods of elevated/euphoric moods, pressured speech, increased energy, decreased need for sleep, racing thoughts, grandiosity,

---

Robert A. Kowatch, M.D., Ph.D., is Professor of Psychiatry and Pediatrics and Director of Psychiatry Research at Cincinnati Children's Hospital Medical Center in Cincinnati, Ohio (for complete biographical information, see "About the Contributors," p. 613).

increased goal-directed behavior, and hypersexuality. This patient meets DSM-IV-TR criteria for a current manic episode, with six out of seven symptoms for mania. These symptoms last 3–7 days a week and have caused significant impairment; the patient's teachers have complained about the patient's excessive silliness in class. Heather meets DSM-IV-TR criteria for bipolar I disorder, nonpsychotic, current episode manic. Her presentation is characteristic of what Geller et al. (2000) described as prepubertal and early-onset bipolar disorder. A meta-analysis of the phenomenology and clinical characteristics of mania in children found that the majority of children and adolescents with bipolar disorder present with periods of increased energy (mania or hypomania), accompanied by irritability, distractibility, pressured speech, grandiosity, racing thoughts, decreased need for sleep, and euphoria/elation (Kowatch et al. 2005b). Heather clearly fits this pattern.

Heather also meets DSM-IV-TR criteria for panic disorder, SAD, GAD, and ADHD. Anxiety disorders and ADHD are frequently comorbid with bipolar disorders in children and adolescents (Axelson et al. 2006; Geller et al. 2004; Wozniak et al. 1995). Comorbid panic disorder in bipolar children and adolescents has been found to increase the odds of making a serious suicide attempt by a factor of 4 (Goldstein et al. 2005). Before Heather had a manic episode, she had two separate episodes of major depression, one at age 5 years and another at age 7. Episodes of major depression at a young age are also characteristic of early-onset bipolar disorder (Geller et al. 1994). The family history is significant for a first-degree relative (biological mother) with bipolar I disorder, which increases the likelihood that the patient will have a bipolar disorder by a factor of 5 (Youngstrom and Duax 2005). The patient's mother also has three comorbid anxiety disorders, which are also common in adults with bipolar disorder (Freeman et al. 2002).

DSM-IV-TR DIAGNOSIS

Axis I   296.43 Bipolar I disorder, severe without psychotic features, most recent episode manic

314.00 ADHD, predominantly inattentive type

300.01 Panic disorder without agoraphobia

309.21 Separation anxiety disorder

300.02 Generalized anxiety disorder

Axis II   None

Axis III   None

Axis IV   Mild—problems with primary support group (divorced parents)

Axis V   Global Assessment of Functioning=50

Serious symptoms

TREATMENT RECOMMENDATIONS

The first goal of treating any patient with mania is to stabilize the person's mood with either a traditional mood stabilizer, such as lithium or valproate, or an atypical antipsychotic (McClellan et al. 2007). No strong data are available to recommend a traditional mood stabilizer over an atypical antipsychotic in children and adolescents. Clinically, the atypical antipsychotics work more quickly and have a larger therapeutic effect than do traditional mood stabilizers. However, many safety issues remain unresolved about the long-term use of atypical antipsychotics in children and adolescents (Correll and Carlson 2006).

The majority of children and adolescents with bipolar disorder require combination pharmacotherapy for mood stabilization, but the data on combination treatment are limited (Findling et al. 2003; Kowatch et al. 2003). In the only double-blind, placebo-controlled study of an atypical antipsychotic for the treatment of adolescents with bipolar disorder, quetiapine in combination with divalproex resulted in a greater reduction of manic symptoms than did divalproex monotherapy, suggesting that the combination of a mood stabilizer and an atypical antipsychotic is more effective than a mood stabilizer alone for the treatment of adolescent mania. In this study, the dosage of quetiapine was titrated to 450 mg/day in 7 days and was well tolerated (DelBello et al. 2002).

Two other pharmacologic treatment issues with Heather are her comorbid ADHD and anxiety disorders. Treatment of children with bipolar disorder and co-occurring ADHD requires mood stabilization with a traditional mood stabilizer or an atypical antipsychotic prior to initiating stimulant medications (Biederman et al. 1999). A randomized controlled trial of 40 children and adolescents with bipolar disorder and ADHD demonstrated that low-dose mixed-salts amphetamine can be safely and effectively used for treatment of comorbid ADHD symptoms following mood stabilization with divalproex (Scheffer et al. 2005). Sustained-release psychostimulants may be more effective at reducing rebound symptoms in children and adolescents with bipolar disorder. A typical dosage of such stimulants for a child with bipolar disorder and ADHD would be 36–54 mg/day of methylphenidate (Concerta) or 10–20 mg/day of amphetamine (Adderall XR).

Comorbid anxiety disorders can be treated using psychotherapy, medications, or both. Among the psychosocial treatments, CBT has been found efficacious for the treatment of social phobia, SAD, and GAD, and for obsessive-compulsive and posttraumatic stress disorders (March 1995; March et al. 1998). The SSRIs have also been found to be efficacious for the treatment of anxiety disorders (Birmaher et al. 2003), but caution should be used because these agents may trigger manic, mixed, or rapid cycling episodes in patients with bipolar disorder. Therefore, in most cases, particularly in patients with bipolar I disorder, before attempting to use SSRIs to alleviate the anxiety disorder, the clinician should first stabilize the bipolar disorder with a traditional mood stabilizer or atypical antipsychotic.

Most traditional psychotherapeutic interventions have not been systematically studied in children and adolescents with bipolar disorder, but patient and family education and therapy are frequently very effective. It is very helpful to educate children and adolescents and their families and teachers about bipolar illness, the importance of medication compliance, and the need for regular monitoring of mood stabilizer serum levels and other laboratory measures. Instructing patients and/or their parents to keep a daily record of the level of depressive and manic symptoms (mood charting) is a tool that may help monitor symptom presence and recurrence. Several groups have demonstrated the efficacy of family therapy for the treatment of bipolar children and adolescents and their families (Fristad 2006; Miklowitz et al. 2004). Other psychosocial tactics that are useful with these patients include 1) minimizing periods of overstimulation, 2) maintaining good sleep hygiene, 3) addressing issues of medication nonadherence immediately, 4) discussing the risk of substance abuse with the patient and family, and 5) encouraging mood charting by the patient and parent. The following are useful print resources for parents:

- *New Hope for Children and Teens With Bipolar Disorder: Your Friendly, Authoritative Guide to the Latest in Traditional and Complementary Solutions* (Birmaher 2004)
- *Raising a Moody Child: How to Cope With Depression and Bipolar Disorder* (Fristad and Goldberg Arnold 2004)

Bipolar disorder in children and adolescents is increasingly recognized as a serious and prevalent mood disorder that requires early recognition and intervention. Like diabetes, bipolar disorder tends to be a chronic disorder in children and adolescents and is best managed with supportive and educational therapies that involve the patient and family. Increased recognition, diagnosis, and treatment of children and adolescents with bipolar disorder will improve the outcome for these patients and their families.

Integrative Perspective

Mary Kay Gill, R.N., M.S.N., J.D.
Boris Birmaher, M.D.

DIAGNOSTIC FORMULATION

BIPOLAR I DISORDER, CURRENT EPISODE MANIC

Heather initially presented with recurrent MDD with melancholic symptom-atology. These symptoms and her family history of bipolar disorder increased her risk to develop bipolar disorder (Strober and Carlson 1982). In fact, a few years after she experienced depression, she developed symptoms of mania that included lack of need for sleep, increased energy, pressured speech, and hy-persexuality, as well as extreme silliness and excessive fantasies that are beyond what is expected for her developmental age. Heather's symptoms of bipolar dis-order have been fluctuating rapidly, making her diagnosis and treatment diffi-cult. In addition, as is common in children with bipolar disorder (Axelson et al. 2006; Birmaher et al. 2006; Pavuluri et al. 2005), Heather has had increased ir-ritability, aggression, and oppositional behaviors, which may have been easily misdiagnosed as oppositional defiant disorder. However, these symptoms mainly appear (or worsen) in the context of her mood symptomatology. Be-cause no other psychiatric or medical illnesses can account for Heather's mood fluctuation and lability, the clinician made a diagnosis of bipolar I disorder, current episode manic. However, for other patients, a clinician should con-sider additional factors, such as substance or steroid use or ongoing physical or sexual abuse, because these factors may confound the clinical picture.

ATTENTION-DEFICIT/HYPERACTIVITY DISORDER, INATTENTIVE TYPE

Because Heather has a history of chronic inattention, which predated the onset of her mood symptoms, the physician diagnosed ADHD, inattentive type. These symptoms worsened during the periods of depression and mania, but they con-tinued during her euthymic periods. Comorbid ADHD is frequently diagnosed in youth with bipolar disorder (Axelson et al. 2006; Kowatch et al. 2005a; Pavu-luri et al. 2006). This diagnosis poses a challenge for the diagnosis of bipolar dis-order, however, because many ADHD symptoms overlap with the symptoms of mania and hypomania. Clinicians should be alert for the following, which may suggest the presence of bipolar disorder: the symptoms of ADHD fluctuate over time, the ADHD symptoms worsen or do not respond to treatment with stimu-lants, the child has a significantly decreased need for sleep (not only sleep problems encountered at the beginning of the night, as is typical in children with ADHD), and the patient displays hypersexuality that is not attributable to exposure to sexual abuse or sexual situations. Although a patient's attentional problems may be the prodromal symptoms of bipolar disorder and not necessarily the symptoms of another diagnosis, further research in this area is warranted.

ANXIETY DISORDERS

Because Heather's panic attacks were not impairing her functioning, only a rule-out diagnosis of panic disorder without agoraphobia was given. Anxiety disorders are common in youth and adults with bipolar disorder (Axelson et al. 2006; Kowatch et al. 2005a, 2005b; Pavuluri et al. 2005). In fact, some anxiety disorders, particularly panic disorder and bipolar disorder, appear to have a specific association (Birmaher et al. 2002). This is important, because currently the best available pharmacologic treatment for anxiety in children is an SSRI (Birmaher et al. 1994), which may destabilize the mood of a patient with bipolar disorder. Of course, patients with anxiety may be offered treatment with psychotherapies, which have been found efficacious for the management of anxiety disorders in children and adolescents (Connolly et al. 2007).

DSM-IV-TR DIAGNOSIS

Axis I   296.40 Bipolar I disorder, most recent episode manic

           314.00 ADHD, predominantly inattentive type

           309.21 Separation anxiety disorder

           300.02 Generalized anxiety disorder

Axis II   None

Axis III   None

Axis IV   Problems with primary support group: minimal contact with father

Axis V   Global Assessment of Functioning (in this case, Children's Global Assessment Scale)=55

TREATMENT RECOMMENDATIONS

The treatment of bipolar disorder is divided into acute and maintenance (to prevent recurrences). The treatment varies depending on the severity of the symptoms and whether the patient has depression, mania, hypomania, mixed or rapid cycling episodes, and/or psychotic features (Birmaher et al. 2006; Kowatch et al. 2005a; Pavuluri et al. 2005). Also, the clinician together with the patient and parents should decide if the symptoms are amenable to treatment in an outpatient clinic or if inpatient or partial hospitalization is necessary.

In addition to pharmacotherapy for patients, all patients and their families require education and psychotherapy to help them to understand and cope with their acute and chronic symptoms, the fact that the illness is chronic and quite possibly lifelong, and the "side effects" of the illness, such as conflicts, poor academic performance, behavior problems, and problems with the law. Moreover, bipolar disorder runs in families, and family members may also have other psychiatric disorders (e.g., substance abuse). Therefore, the treatment of children with bipolar disorder should include their families, and, if warranted, other family members should be referred for appropriate treatment (Birmaher et al. 2006; Pavuluri et al. 2005).

Additionally, the patient's comorbid disorders, ongoing problems at school, and interpersonal problems should be addressed. However, as discussed below, the comorbid disorders usually should be addressed after the mood disorder has been stabilized.

The treatment of choice for a child with acute mania involves the use of mood stabilizers, including an atypical antipsychotic (Kowatch et al. 2005a; Pavuluri et al. 2005). Because a considerable amount of time is often needed for the beneficial effects of lithium or valproate to become apparent, use of an atypical antipsychotic agent is preferable in patients with acute symptoms that are affecting their psychosocial functioning and especially in those patients with agitation, psychosis, or behaviors that may harm others or themselves. These medications work quickly, and some of their side effects, such as sedation, may be advantageous to control a patient's behaviors.

As noted in the case presentation, Heather was not severely manic or agitated. After appropriate laboratory tests (e.g., creatinine, blood urea nitrogen, electrolytes, thyroid function tests, urinalyses) were conducted, the clinician decided to start treatment with a slow-release lithium formulation (Eskalith CR). The dosage of lithium was gradually increased to 225 mg in the morning and 450 mg at bedtime, and her lithium blood levels were 0.76 mEq/L. Heather's symptoms improved over the following 1–2 months, but as commonly seen in children with bipolar disorder (Birmaher et al. 2006), she developed depression and auditory hallucinations. She heard voices threatening to kill her or her family. After appropriate blood work (fasting glucose and lipid profile, liver function tests, complete blood count with differential) was done and Heather's body mass index and waist circumference were measured, the clinician added quetiapine 150 mg/day at bedtime. However, 2 weeks later, Heather's psychosis worsened and she began to experience suicidal ideation with a plan. At this time, Heather was hospitalized. During the inpatient hospitalization, the dosage of quetiapine was increased to 500 mg/day and the lithium levels were optimized to 1.0 mEq/L. After 2 weeks, Heather's symptoms improved and she was discharged from the hospital.

During her follow-up, Heather's anxiety symptoms were successfully managed through CBT. However, because ADHD, inattentive type, continued to affect her school performance and self-esteem and induced significant conflicts at home, a long-acting stimulant was added. As others have demonstrated, stimulant treatment of ADHD is necessary for some youths with bipolar disorder to improve their comorbid ADHD symptoms (Scheffer et al. 2005). In general, after the mood symptoms have been under control, children and adolescents tolerate well the addition of stimulants to their mood stabilizers.

While being treating with quetiapine for several months, Heather gained a considerable amount of weight that was not controlled by her dieting efforts. In light of this bothersome side effect and the fact that Heather's mood had been stable for several months, the quetiapine was slowly tapered and discontinued. Subsequently, Heather again developed a moderate depression. Although no randomized controlled trials have been done with lamotrigine in youth, anecdotal evidence indicates that lamotrigine is effective for the treatment of depressive or anxiety symptoms (Kowatch et al. 2005a; Pavuluri et al. 2005). Thus, lamotrigine (100 mg twice a day) was added to Heather's lithium. She has tolerated the lamotrigine well, and for the last year her symptoms have been under good control.

Although evidence indicates that family-focused therapy (FFT) is an effective treatment for adolescents and adults with bipolar disorder (Miklowitz et al. 2004; Pavuluri et al. 2005), studies of FFT in children have not been reported. This type of psychotherapy appears to increase the patient's adherence to treatment (a problem frequently encountered in patients with bipolar disorder), decrease family conflict, increase the patient's and family's coping skills, and reduce the risk for further depression and hospitalizations. In light of this, Heather and her family were treated with 15 sessions of FFT, with good results.

REFERENCES

Axelson D, Birmaher B, Strober M, et al: Phenomenology of children and adolescents with bipolar spectrum disorders. Arch Gen Psychiatry 63:1139–1148, 2006

Biederman J, Mick E, Prince J, et al: Systematic chart review of the pharmacologic treatment of comorbid attention deficit hyperactivity disorder in youth with bipolar disorder. J Child Adolesc Psychopharmacol 9:247–256, 1999

Birmaher B: New Hope for Children and Teens With Bipolar Disorder: Your Friendly, Authoritative Guide to the Latest in Traditional and Complementary Solutions. New York, Three Rivers Press, 2004

Birmaher B, Waterman GS, Ryan ND, et al: Fluoxetine for childhood anxiety disorder. J Am Acad Child Adolesc Psychiatry 33:993–999, 1994

Birmaher B, Kennah A, Brent D, et al: Is bipolar disorder specifically associated with panic disorder in youths? J Clin Psychiatry 63:414–419, 2002

Birmaher B, Axelson DA, Monk K, et al: Fluoxetine for the treatment of childhood anxiety disorders. J Am Acad Child Adolesc Psychiatry 42:415–423, 2003

Birmaher B, Axelson D, Strober M, et al: Clinical course of children and adolescents with bipolar spectrum disorders. Arch Gen Psychiatry 63:175–183, 2006

Connolly SD, Bernstein GA, Work Group on Quality Issues: Practice parameter for the assessment and treatment of children and adolescents with anxiety disorders. J Am Acad Child Adolesc Psychiatry 46:267–283, 2007

Correll CU, Carlson HE: Endocrine and metabolic adverse effects of psychotropic medications in children and adolescents. J Am Acad Child Adolesc Psychiatry 45:771–791, 2006

Danner S, Young ME, Fristad MA: Assessment of bipolar disorder in children, in Assessing Childhood Psychopathology and Developmental Disabilities. Edited by Matson J, Andrasik F, Matson ML. New York, Springer, 2009, pp 273–308

DelBello M, Schwiers M, Rosenberg HL, et al: Quetiapine as adjunctive treatment for adolescent mania associated with bipolar disorder. J Am Acad Child Adolesc Psychiatry 41:1216–1223, 2002

DelBello MP, Hanseman D, Adler CM, et al: Twelve-month outcome of adolescents with bipolar disorder following first hospitalization for a manic or mixed episode. Am J Psychiatry 164:582–590, 2007

Depue RA, Krauss S, Spoont MR, et al: General Behavior Inventory identification of unipolar and bipolar affective conditions in a nonclinical university population. J Abnorm Psychol 98:117–126, 1989

Findling RL, McNamara NK, Gracious BL, et al: Combination lithium and divalproex sodium in pediatric bipolarity. J Am Acad Child Adolesc Psychiatry 42:895–901, 2003

Freeman MP, Freeman SA, McElroy SL: The comorbidity of bipolar and anxiety disorders: prevalence, psychobiology, and treatment issues. J Affect Disord 68:1–23, 2002

Fristad MA: Psychoeducational treatment for school-aged children with bipolar disorder. Dev Psychopathol 18:1289–1306, 2006

Fristad MA, Goldberg Arnold JS: Raising a Moody Child: How to Cope With Depression and Bipolar Disorder. New York, Guilford, 2004

Fristad MA, Gavazzi SM, Mackinaw-Koons B: Family psychoeducation: an adjunctive intervention for children with bipolar disorder. Biol Psychiatry 53:1000–1008, 2003

Geller B, Fox LW, Clark KA: Rate and predictors of prepubertal bipolarity during follow-up of 6- to 12-year-old depressed children. J Am Acad Child Adolesc Psychiatry 33:461–468, 1994

Geller B, Zimerman B, Williams M, et al: Diagnostic characteristics of 93 cases of a prepubertal and early adolescent bipolar disorder phenotype by gender, puberty and comorbid attention deficit hyperactivity disorder. J Child Adolesc Psychopharmacol 10:157–164, 2000

Geller B, Tillman R, Craney JL, et al: Four-year prospective outcome and natural history of mania in children with a prepubertal and early adolescent bipolar disorder phenotype. Arch Gen Psychiatry 61:459–467, 2004

Goldstein TR, Birmaher B, Axelson D, et al: History of suicide attempts in pediatric bipolar disorder: factors associated with increased risk. Bipolar Disord 7:525–535, 2005

Kowatch RA, Sethuraman G, Hume JH, et al: Combination pharmacotherapy in children and adolescents with bipolar disorder. Biol Psychiatry 53:978–984, 2003

Kowatch RA, Fristad M, Birmaher B, et al; Child Psychiatric Workgroup on Bipolar Disorder: Treatment guidelines for children and adolescents with bipolar disorder. J Am Acad Child Adolesc Psychiatry 44:213–235, 2005a

Kowatch RA, Youngstrom EA, Danielyan A, et al: Review and meta-analysis of the phenomenology and clinical characteristics of mania in children and adolescents. Bipolar Disord 7:483–496, 2005b

Lofthouse N, Fristad MA: Psychosocial interventions for children with bipolar disorder. Clin Child Fam Psychol Rev 7:71–88, 2004

Mackinaw-Koons B, Fristad MA: Children with bipolar disorder: how to break down barriers and work effectively together. Prof Psychol Res Pr 35:481–484, 2004

March JS: Cognitive-behavioral psychotherapy for children and adolescents with OCD: a review and recommendations for treatment. J Am Acad Child Adolesc Psychiatry 34:7–18, 1995

March JS, Amaya-Jackson L, Murray MC, et al: Cognitive-behavioral psychotherapy for children and adolescents with posttraumatic stress disorder after a single-incident stressor. J Am Acad Child Adolesc Psychiatry 37:585–593, 1998

McClellan J, Kowatch R, Findling RL; Work Group on Quality Issues: Practice parameter for the assessment and treatment of children and adolescents with bipolar disorder. J Am Acad Child Adolesc Psychiatry 46:107–125, 2007

Miklowitz D, George E, Axelson DA, et al: Family focused treatment for adolescents with bipolar disorder. J Affect Disord 82 (suppl 1):S113–S128, 2004

Pavuluri MN, Graczyk PA, Henry DB, et al: Child- and family-focused cognitive behavioral therapy for pediatric bipolar disorder: development and preliminary results. J Am Acad Child Adolesc Psychiatry 43:528–537, 2004

Pavuluri MN, Birmaher B, Naylor MW: Pediatric bipolar disorder: a review of the past 10 years. J Am Acad Child Adolesc Psychiatry 44:846–871, 2005

Pavuluri MN, Henry DB, Devineni B, et al: Child Mania Rating Scale: development, reliability, and validity. J Am Acad Child Adolesc Psychiatry 45:550–560, 2006

Quinn C, Fristad MA: Defining and identifying early-onset bipolar spectrum disorder. Curr Psychiatry Rep 6:101–107, 2004

Scheffer RE, Kowatch RA, Carmody T, et al: Randomized placebo-controlled trial of mixed amphetamine salts for symptoms of comorbid ADHD in pediatric bipolar disorder following mood stabilization with divalproex sodium. Am J Psychiatry 162:58–64, 2005

Strober M, Carlson G: Bipolar illness in adolescents with major depression. Arch Gen Psychiatry 39:549–555, 1982

Wozniak J, Biederman J, Kiely K, et al: Mania-like symptoms suggestive of childhood-onset bipolar disorder in clinically referred children. J Am Acad Child Adolesc Psychiatry 34:867–876, 1995

Youngstrom EA, Duax J: Evidence-based assessment of pediatric bipolar disorder, part I: base rate and family history. J Am Acad Child Adolesc Psychiatry 44:712–717, 2005

Youngstrom EA, Findling RL, Danielson CK, et al: Discriminative validity of parent report of hypomanic and depressive symptoms on the General Behavior Inventory. Psychol Assess 13:267–276, 2001

■ CHAPTER 7 ■

Life of the Party

Chronic Marijuana Use

Paula Riggs, M.D.

CASE PRESENTATION

IDENTIFYING INFORMATION

Brad is a 17-year-old seeking outpatient treatment for his marijuana abuse.

CHIEF COMPLAINT

Brad reported, "I hit my girlfriend when I was high. She was pressuring me to get a job, but I said that I couldn't because I'm a 'pothead.' I never thought of my marijuana use as a problem, but it scared me when I hit her."

HISTORY OF PRESENT ILLNESS

Brad arrived at a scheduled clinic intake appointment on time; he was dressed in jeans, a white T-shirt, and high-top basketball shoes. He says that he began experimenting with marijuana at age 14 and has been smoking daily for the past year, escalating to multiple times daily after his mom "kicked him out of the house" about 8 months ago and he started living with three male room-mates.

Brad says that he never considered his drug use a problem because the only thing he uses is marijuana and he is "not that into other drugs or alcohol." He

Paula Riggs, M.D., is Associate Professor of Psychiatry at the University of Colorado School of Medicine in Denver, Colorado (for complete biographical information, see "About the Contributors," p. 613).

does think that he is "addicted" to marijuana and is not sure that he could quit even if he wanted to. He adds that "smoking weed is the way I cope with everything; I don't feel normal if I'm not high." He also acknowledges a growing number of problems in his life related to his escalating use in the past year, including relationship problems with his mother and girlfriend, problems with school, and job loss. He also reports that marijuana makes him "lazy" and unmotivated. The immediate precipitant for seeking treatment is the loss of control over his aggression (hitting his girlfriend) last week, coupled with fears that his girlfriend will break up with him if he does not get treatment now.

Brad endorsed initial insomnia, which has been a chronic problem as far back as he can remember, and states that he has a normal appetite.

PAST PSYCHIATRIC HISTORY

Brad denies undergoing mental health or substance abuse treatment previously. He says he was diagnosed with attention-deficit/hyperactivity disorder (ADHD) in second grade by his pediatrician (teacher referral), who recommended medication. However, because his mother "didn't believe in drugging kids," he never started on medication. His mother has always described him as extremely "hyper," even as a baby, much more so than his brother.

As far back as Brad can remember, he has always gotten into trouble for talking and disrupting class activities. He recalls having been very fidgety as early as first and second grade, being poorly organized and distractible, and having difficulty concentrating and staying focused. He adds that he has always been a "major procrastinator"; has trouble "finishing" things; and is "very, very impatient" and easily frustrated. He denies current or past depression, anxiety disorder, and psychosis. He says that his appetite is normal. Although he reports always having had trouble "winding down" to go to sleep, he denies periods of requiring significantly less sleep than usual or other symptoms of mania. He usually smokes marijuana at bedtime to help him go to sleep.

SUBSTANCE USE HISTORY

Brad began smoking cigarettes at age 11 and currently smokes three-fourths of a pack per day. He began smoking marijuana with his older brother (1½ years older) when he was 14 and progressed to daily smoking by age 15. He escalated to multiple-times-daily use about 8 months ago after his mother "kicked him out" of the house because she continued to find drug paraphernalia and bags of marijuana in his room after he lied about "quitting." He began living with three male roommates, all of whom smoke and "deal" marijuana. He began drinking alcohol at "parties" at age 15. He says that his normal pattern of drinking is to get drunk with his friends or roommates on Friday and Saturday nights (drinking seven to eight beers over the course of an evening). He has never been a daily drinker and denies ever experiencing withdrawal symptoms. He has driven a car while intoxicated on alcohol and marijuana on several occasions but has not been stopped for driving while impaired or driving under the influence. He denies the use of any other drugs more than five times in his lifetime. He has tried Ecstasy twice and cocaine (intranasally) three times in the past year.

MEDICAL HISTORY

Brad denies significant medical illness. He has a history of environmental and seasonal allergies. He has had no surgeries. He has a small 1-cm well-healed scar lateral to his right eyebrow—the result of his having fallen off his bicycle at age 10. He reports no loss of consciousness in that fall and denies other head injuries or seizures.

DEVELOPMENTAL HISTORY

To Brad's knowledge, he is the product of a normal pregnancy and delivery and he had no delays in developmental milestones. His mother smoked cigarettes during the pregnancy but did not drink alcohol or use other drugs to his knowledge. He was a B/C student in elementary school, with worsening grades in middle school. Chronic truancy, failing grades, and drug use at school led to his transfer to an alternative high school in ninth grade. He dropped out of high school when he turned 17, but he plans to get his GED so he can get into culinary school next fall.

SOCIAL HISTORY

Brad says that his father was always "very strict" and verbally abusive to Brad, his brother, and his mother. He would "get mad over nothing, especially if he was drunk." His parents separated about 4 months ago and are going through a divorce. Brad has spoken with his father once on the phone since his father moved out. He says he has never been close to his father. He has always been closer to his mother, but increasing conflicts related to his drug use have seriously strained his relationship with his mother in the past year.

FAMILY HISTORY

Brad's father had alcohol dependence and is in recovery. He has been abstinent for the past year. His mother was dependent on nicotine and quit smoking a year ago when his father stopped drinking. His older brother, age 19, is currently in jail for possessing and selling methamphetamine; he also has alcohol abuse and cannabis dependence.

MENTAL STATUS EXAMINATION

Brad was alert and oriented to person, place, and time. He is tall, with a lean athletic build. He absentmindedly drummed his pencil on the table intermittently throughout the interview. He was somewhat distractible during the interview but engaged with good eye contact.

Affect

Brad's affect was appropriate, with a normal range, and he appeared euthymic.

Mood

Brad denied depression and he rated his mood as 2 when asked to rate his mood on a 1–10 scale, given the anchor points 1 = *no depression* and 10 = *suicidal, hopeless.*

Memory and Attention

Brad had some difficulty with short-term working memory on the digit span task but was able to complete the task accurately with slight prompting on the second attempt.

Thought Content/Amount

Brad denied any psychotic symptoms and appeared not to have racing thoughts or a thought disorder.

COMMENTARIES

Psychotherapeutic Perspective

Yifrah Kaminer, M.D., M.B.A.

DIAGNOSTIC FORMULATION

Brad meets criteria for marijuana dependence with physiological dependence, as evidenced by increased tolerance during a 12-month period. Important activities are impaired by Brad's continued use, and he has continued use despite

Yifrah Kaminer, M.D., M.B.A., is Professor of Psychiatry in the Department of Psychiatry and Alcohol Research Center, and Codirector of Research in the Division of Child and Adolescent Psychiatry at the University of Connecticut Health Center in Farmington, Connecticut (for complete biographical information, see "About the Contributors," p. 613).

Preparation of this commentary was supported by National Institute on Alcohol Abuse and Alcoholism grant K24 AA013442-02 (Dr. Yifrah Kaminer).

knowledge of associated problems. He has alcohol abuse problems, as evidenced by driving under the influence several times. ADHD needs to be ruled out. The information about Brad's ADHD is based on past history and confirms a lifetime diagnosis. However, to confirm a present ADHD diagnosis, the clinician needs to repeat the assessment of comorbid psychiatric disorders after a drug-free period of at least 2 weeks. The rationale is to prevent confusion with masked symptomatology attributed to drug use or potential withdrawal symptoms from marijuana (see "Treatment Recommendations" below).

DSM-IV-TR DIAGNOSIS

Axis I   304.30 Cannabis dependence with physiological dependence

305.00 Alcohol abuse

Rule out ADHD

Rule out intermittent explosive disorder

Rule out oppositional defiant disorder

Axis II   None

Axis III   None

Axis IV   Problems with primary support group (i.e., family, friends)

Educational problems (i.e., school dropout)

Occupational problems (i.e., unemployed)

Housing problem (i.e., out of family home, resides with drug dealers, unknown ability to financially sustain self but most probably unable to unless involved in drug dealing)

Axis V   Global Assessment of Functioning=45 (serious impairment in all parameters indicated on Axis IV)

TREATMENT RECOMMENDATIONS

Adolescents with substance use disorders (SUDs) constitute a heterogeneous population characterized by differences in the type/combination of substance(s) used, severity of use, consequences, and presence of comorbid psychiatric disorders. Marijuana is the most common illicit substance used by adolescents diagnosed with SUD in the United States. The majority of adolescents with cannabis use disorders are diagnosed with one or more comorbid psychiatric disorders (Dennis et al. 2004). Clinical consensus suggests that comorbid disorders in youth should be treated simultaneously (Kaminer and Bukstein 2008). However, although this approach is clinically sensible and has been examined in adults, it has not yet been empirically tested in adolescents.

DSM-based diagnostic formulation is not sufficient to determine a patient's severity of use. The clinician needs to complete a more comprehensive assessment of the severity of the adolescent's substance abuse and other domains before making decisions regarding the following: 1) placement in an appropriate treatment setting as delineated by the American Society of Addiction Medicine's *ASAM Patient Placement Criteria for the Treatment of Substance-Related Disorders*, 2nd Edition, Revised (ASAM PPC-2R; Mee-Lee et al. 2001) and 2) an optimal treatment plan, which may include a singular treatment modality or integrated treatment modalities (Bukstein et al. 2005).

Necessary information is missing from Brad's case presentation. Additional questions include but are not limited to the following: When was the last time Brad used drugs or alcohol? How much (i.e., quantity) does he use? How does he pay for rent and for his marijuana? Has he been involved in illegal activity to generate income? Was the physical abuse of his girlfriend a single episode, or is there a pattern of physical abuse? Does Brad have friends who do not use drugs? Several instruments, such as the Teen Addiction Severity Index (Kaminer et al. 1991), a commonly used multidimensional (i.e., alcohol, other substances, school, employment, family, peer social, legal, and psychiatric) semistructured interview, can be used to gather comprehensive information and assess a patient's severity of dysfunction in these domains.

Several interesting facts are included in Brad's case description. First, because it is highly unusual for an adolescent to seek treatment when there is no legal contingency attached, Brad's seeking help indicates motivation for treatment. However, this will be his first episode of treatment after 2 years of daily intensive drug use. Adolescents often are not ready to engage in treatment and change drug use during a first attempt to recover. The Problem Recognition Questionnaire (Cady et al. 1996) can be used to measure pretreatment readiness to change marijuana use.

Second, the lack of a diagnosis of marijuana withdrawal in DSM-IV (and DSM-IV-TR) is problematic given the accumulating evidence that individuals experience withdrawal symptoms. If Brad does respond to treatment and stop his heavy marijuana use, he will likely manifest withdrawal symptoms. Withdrawal syndrome is indicated by a cluster of 6 or more out of 22 symptoms from the Marijuana Withdrawal Symptom Checklist, such as irritability, craving, mental cloudiness, decreased appetite, weight loss, and insomnia and marijuana dreams (Budney et al. 1999). A decision regarding placement in a treatment setting needs to take the patient's motivation and a potential withdrawal syndrome into consideration (Mee-Lee et al. 2001).

Third, presently Brad lacks a support system because his family forced him out of his home. Therefore, the clinician needs to determine whether Brad has any non-drug-using friends or other family members who could provide him with basic needs (i.e., shelter, food), at least during the treatment and continued care phase.

ASAM PPC-2R provides a "crosswalk" of levels of care and dimensions that is used to determine an appropriate setting for a patient based on the individual's placement on the dimensions. The following levels of care are available for adolescents: early intervention; outpatient treatment; intensive outpatient treatment/partial hospitalization; residential/intensive inpatient treatment (clinically managed low-intensity residential; medium-intensity residential; high-intensity residential/inpatient treatment); and medically managed intensive inpatient treatment.

Intensive outpatient treatment may be appropriate for Brad, according to his placement on dimension 1, acute intoxication and/or withdrawal potential; dimension 3, emotional, behavioral, or cognitive conditions and complications—as evidenced by Brad's mild to moderate impairment in social functioning, ability to self-care, and course of illness predictive of frequent monitoring or interventions (e.g., including drug urinalysis and psychotherapy); dimension 5, relapse, continued use, or continued problem potential—as evidenced by Brad's significant risk of continued use or relapse; and dimension 6, recovery environment—as evidenced by Brad's environment that is impeding recovery. A major concern is Brad's need to change living arrangements to stay away from apartment mates who use and deal drugs. He can either return home, which needs to be negotiated with his parents; find a home with a nonuser; or as a last resort move to a higher level of care, which in his case would be clinically managed low-intensity residential treatment.

As noted in ASAM PPC-2R, an indicated level of care may not exist or be accessible in a patient's community. Also, there are treatment menu variations in programs within the same level. The treatment-pivotal components that are recommended for Brad include integration of personal and family or community reinforcement interventions complemented by periodic drug urinalysis (Liddle and Rowe 2006). For example, on the personal level, the recommended intervention includes cognitive-behavioral therapy (CBT) for handling high-risk situations for drug use and for providing skills to enhance anger management, as well as motivational interviewing to improve engagement. All interventions may rely on the treatment manuals developed for the Cannabis Youth Treatment study (Dennis et al. 2004), which can be downloaded free of charge from http://www.kap.samhsa.gov/products/manuals/cyt. Finally, the clinician needs to evaluate the necessity of and resources available for consulting Brad on school, employment, peer relationship, anger management, and potential legal issues.

Treatment of Brad's psychiatric comorbidity should be provided regardless of the level of care. Nevertheless, the clinician needs to determine whether such treatment is available in the assigned level of care or program given feasibility of resources. Alternatives need to be addressed if psychopharmacologic treatment for ADHD is necessary.

Psychopharmacologic Perspective

Oscar G. Bukstein, M.D., M.P.H.

DIAGNOSTIC FORMULATION

Brad's marijuana use is clearly the focus of his presentation. His self-referred status is the exception to the rule, because most youth are taken for evaluation and treatment of substance use problems by their parents or other authority figures. Similarly, Brad acknowledges problems with his marijuana use and displays some motivation and reported desire for treatment, which are not typical of most adolescents with similar problems.

Despite Brad's experimentation with Ecstasy, cocaine, and perhaps other drugs, only tobacco, marijuana, and alcohol have sufficient use histories that constitute maladaptive patterns of use leading to clinically significant impairment or distress and that meet other DSM-IV-TR criteria for a SUD. Distinguishing between diagnoses of abuse and dependence is important because a diagnosis of dependence predicts a prognosis with a more chronic course: *abuse* connotes use of the specific substance plus consequences, whereas *dependence* refers to significant physical adaptation of the user to the substance in the form of physiological symptoms such as tolerance and withdrawal and/ or compulsive use behaviors. If criteria for both are met, the individual is given a dependence diagnosis.

TOBACCO

Brad reports an early onset of tobacco (cigarette) use, currently at three-fourths of a pack per day. At this level of daily use, Brad would likely manifest some withdrawal symptoms after cessation of cigarette use. Largely because tobacco becomes a legal substance for individuals at age 18 and because of the relatively short duration of use, adolescents rarely suffer from consequences of use or endorse other dependence symptoms except occasional attempts to quit. Brad is likely not to be motivated to quit.

Oscar G. Bukstein, M.D., M.P.H., is Associate Professor of Psychiatry at the University of Pittsburgh School of Medicine in Pittsburgh, Pennsylvania (for complete biographical information, see "About the Contributors," p. 613).

ALCOHOL

Brad endorses a relatively common adolescent pattern of binge drinking two times a week. His endorsement of driving while intoxicated fulfills DSM-IV-TR criterion 2 of alcohol abuse ("recurrent substance use in situations in which it is physically hazardous"). He reports no other consequences or symptoms of alcohol dependence.

MARIJUANA

Brad's endorsement of problems in his life related to escalating marijuana use in the past year includes relationship problems with his mother and girlfriend, aggression (in effect, DSM-IV-TR substance abuse criterion 4: "continued substance use despite having persistent or recurrent social or interpersonal problems caused or exacerbated by the effects of the substance"), and problems with school and job loss (i.e., DSM-IV-TR substance abuse criterion 1: "failure to fulfill major role obligations at work, school, or home"). These consequences of use support a marijuana *abuse* diagnosis.

However, a dependence diagnosis is supported by Brad's reported inability to quit (i.e., DSM-IV-TR substance dependence criterion 4: "a persistent desire or unsuccessful efforts to cut down or control substance use") and his belief that marijuana use makes him unmotivated and "lazy," and possibly aggressive (i.e., DSM-IV-TR substance dependence criterion 7: "continued despite knowledge of having a persistent...physical or psychological problem that is likely to have been caused or exacerbated by the substance"). According to available information, therefore, Brad meets only two out of the needed three criteria for dependence.

Although Brad meets criteria for cannabis abuse, many adolescents are "diagnostic orphans" in that they meet one or two dependence criteria while meeting no abuse criteria. Studies of adolescents with alcohol use disorders indicate that these adolescents appear to be more similar to those youth with full dependence criteria in terms of course.

Given Brad's claims about being "addicted" or lacking control of use, he may or may not meet the following DSM-IV-TR dependence criteria: criterion 3, "the substance is often taken in larger amounts or over a longer period than was intended"; criterion 5, "a great deal of time is spent in activities necessary to obtain the substance..., use the substance..., or recover from its effects"; and criterion 6, "important social, occupational, or recreational activities are given up or reduced because of substance use."

For all youth reporting substance use or suspected of substance use, inquiry into each of the SUD criteria for both abuse and dependence is essential for making the correct diagnosis. Although not part of diagnosis, ascertainment of quantity and frequency of use is also important. With tobacco and alcohol, this is relatively straightforward. However, determination of quantity of use is often difficulty with cannabis because the drug is often shared, the potency of the drug varies, and the drug is used on multiple occasions through the day.

OTHER COMORBID PSYCHIATRIC DISORDERS

Brad's report of a history of ADHD and some current symptoms (a "major procrastinator"; has trouble "finishing" things; impatience; observed distractibility and difficulty with short-term memory during the interview) suggest a probable current diagnosis of ADHD, which is not surprising given the frequent comorbidity of ADHD in adolescents being treated for SUDs. ADHD is commonly associated with conduct disorder and/or oppositional defiant disorder, but the case presentation does not give information about the presence or absence of symptoms or behaviors meeting these disruptive behavior disorder criteria.

Although Brad denies other common psychiatric comorbidities with SUD, such as depression, bipolar disorder, and anxiety disorder(s), screening for these disorders is essential to any comprehensive diagnostic evaluation.

DSM-IV-TR DIAGNOSIS

Axis I   305.20 Cannabis abuse; rule out dependence
           305.00 Alcohol abuse
           Rule out ADHD
Axis II   No diagnosis
Axis III   Cigarette smoking
Axis IV   Problems with primary support group: conflict with mother
           Problems related to social environment: conflict with girlfriend
           Educational problems: dropped out of school
           Vocational problems: job loss
Axis V   Global Assessment of Functioning=55 (current)

Prior to or concurrent with the development of a treatment plan, the clinician should further clarify Brad's diagnoses by 1) asking additional questions about cannabis dependence criteria; 2) using ADHD rating scales for self and other informant (parent, teacher); and 3) screening for or surveying for other deviant behaviors, such as antisocial behaviors, sexual history, and other risk-taking behaviors.

TREATMENT RECOMMENDATIONS

Brad's motivation, insight, and absence of previous treatment for SUDs suggest that a lower level of care, such as outpatient or intensive outpatient treatment, might be sufficient. Drug and alcohol treatment professionals often use specific adolescent criteria developed by the ASAM (Mee-Lee et al. 2001) to assist in determining level of care. The "Practice Parameter for the Assessment and Treatment of Children and Adolescents With Substance Use Disorders," developed by the American Academy of Child and Adolescent Psychiatry, offers a guide to basic principles of treatment (Bukstein et al. 2005). Pertaining to assessment, the use of toxicologic methods (e.g., urine drug screens) both at baseline assessment and ongoing during treatment is an important element, designed to provide an objective check on adolescent self-report. Despite the presence of comorbid disorders, adolescents with SUDs should receive specific treatment for their substance use. Adolescent treatment results in decreased heavy drinking, marijuana and other illicit drug use, and criminal involvement, as well as improved psychological adjustment and school performance (Hser et al. 2001). Because longer duration of treatment is associated with several favorable outcomes, maintaining adolescents in some form of treatment for 90 days or more appears optimal. In terms of empirical support for specific treatment modalities, family therapy and CBT, both alone and with motivational enhancement, have been shown to be efficacious (Bukstein et al. 2005; Liddle and Rowe 2006; Monti et al. 2001). Community reinforcement approaches utilizing contingency contracting and vouchers also appear to be promising (Henggeler et al. 2007).

In treating an adolescent with SUD(s), the clinician should develop a treatment plan that utilizes modalities that target 1) motivation and engagement; 2) family involvement to improve supervision, monitoring, and communication between parents and adolescent; 3) problem-solving skills and social skills, as well as relapse prevention; 4) comorbid psychiatric disorders through psychosocial and/or medication treatments; 5) social ecology in terms of increasing prosocial behaviors, peer relationships, and academic functioning; and 6) adequate duration of treatment and follow-up care (Bukstein et al. 2005). Self-support groups such as Alcoholics Anonymous and Narcotics Anonymous can be encouraged as adjuncts to the modalities above.

Although no specific pharmacotherapies have been developed to target marijuana use disorders, clinicians should always consider appropriate pharmacologic treatment of comorbid psychiatric disorders. The potential diagnosis of ADHD in Brad's case should prompt consideration of medication management (Waxmonsky and Wilens 2005). In adolescents with ADHD and active SUD symptoms and behaviors, nonstimulant agents (atomoxetine or bupropion) are preferable to stimulants, given the absence of more substantial evidence of stimulant efficacy in this population. For patients with poor response to nonstimulant agents, stable treatment, and/or merely a history of SUD or recreational/experimental substance use (assuming nonamphetamine SUD), the use of extended-release or longer-acting stimulants with lower abuse liability and diversion potential is recommended.

Integrative Perspective

Paula Riggs, M.D.

DIAGNOSTIC FORMULATION

Brad, age 17, meets DSM-IV-TR diagnostic criteria for cannabis dependence, nicotine dependence, alcohol abuse, and ADHD, combined type. Although he knew he was "addicted" to marijuana, he did not think of his marijuana use as a problem (precontemplation) until he hit his girlfriend while high during an argument last week. In retrospect, he has been able to achieve some additional insight about the relationship of his escalating marijuana use in the past year and worsening motivation, inability to follow through on obligations, and increasing academic and psychosocial/relationship problems (contemplation), which precipitated seeking treatment at this time (action).

A number of therapeutic modalities—behavioral, family based, and cognitive behavioral—have been shown to have efficacy for treating adolescent SUDs (Whitmore and Riggs 2006). Brad's older age, level of cognitive ability, insight, and treatment seeking, as well as limited current family involvement, indicate that he would likely do well with individual CBT, with its empathic, motivational enhancement approach (Riggs et al. 2007).

Brad is unlikely to benefit optimally from substance abuse treatment unless his ADHD symptoms (e.g., frustration intolerance, impulsivity, poor attention and concentration) are treated concurrently. Because he has no prior history of treatment for ADHD, including no history of psychostimulant abuse or diversion, a long-acting psychostimulant such as osmotic-release methylphenidate (OROS-MPH) should be considered as first-line treatment. Longer-acting psychostimulants (especially those developed to decrease likelihood of diversion) have similar efficacy but lower abuse liability than do shorter-acting psychostimulant formulations. Moreover, a once-daily dosing regimen will enhance medication compliance. Patient education, close monitoring of adverse side effects and target symptom response, and compliance with substance abuse treatment are important given the limitations of current research on the safety and efficacy of psychostimulants for ADHD in nonabstinent adolescents.

DSM-IV-TR DIAGNOSIS

Axis I   304.30 Cannabis dependence

           305.00 Alcohol abuse

           305.1 Nicotine dependence

           314.01 ADHD, combined type

Axis II   Deferred

Axis III   Environmental allergies (mild, seasonal)

Axis IV   Unemployment; primary relationship problem

Axis V   Global Assessment of Functioning=52 (current)

TREATMENT RECOMMENDATIONS

SUBSTANCE USE DISORDERS

Brad should begin a 16-week course of individual, manual-standardized CBT (for substance abuse), which may include up to three or more sessions with his family or girlfriend if clinically indicated. Brad's self-reported drug use should be evaluated on a weekly basis and documented by timeline follow-back procedures. Self-reported drug use has been shown to be a valid measure in adolescents when confidentiality is assured. However, urine samples for drug screening should also be obtained weekly as a biological measure to validate self-reported use and as a clinical outcome measure.

ATTENTION-DEFICIT/HYPERACTIVITY DISORDER

Although abstinence from substance use is ideal before initiation of pharmacotherapy for ADHD, it is often not a realistic goal. Achieving success in drug treatment is difficult under any circumstance but much less likely if one has an untreated Axis I mental disorder such as ADHD (present in 30%–50% of substance-abusing adolescents) with symptoms that include impulsivity, poor concentration, distractibility, and frustration intolerance. Treatment recommendations for Brad include titrating the dosage of OROS-MPH to 72 mg/day over a 2-week period, concurrent with starting CBT for the SUD. A baseline and weekly DSM-IV-TR ADHD symptom checklist should be administered to evaluate and document target symptom response to medication and to facilitate optimal dosage titration. Weekly assessment of both drug use and adverse side effects will help determine potential adverse interactions between medication and drug use in a patient who has not yet achieved abstinence.

REFERENCES

Budney AJ, Novy PL, Hughes JR: Marijuana withdrawal among adults seeking treatment for marijuana dependence. Addiction 94:1311–1322, 1999

Bukstein OG, Bernet W, Arnold V, et al; Work Group on Quality Issues: Practice parameter for the assessment and treatment of children and adolescents with substance use disorders. J Am Acad Child Adolesc Psychiatry 44:609–621, 2005

Cady M, Winters KC, Jordan DA, et al: Measuring treatment readiness for adolescent drug abusers. J Child Adolesc Subst Abuse 5:73–91, 1996

Dennis ML, Godley SH, Diamond G, et al: The Cannabis Youth Treatment (CYT) Study: main findings from two randomized trials. J Subst Abuse Treat 27:197–213, 2004

Henggeler SW, Chapman JE, Rowland MD, et al: If you build it, they will come: statewide practitioner interest in contingency management for youths. J Subst Abuse Treat 32:121–131, 2007

Hser YI, Grella CE, Hubbard RL, et al: An evaluation of drug treatments for adolescents in four U.S. cities. Arch Gen Psychiatry 58:689–695, 2001

Kaminer Y, Bukstein OG: Adolescent Substance Abuse: Psychiatric Comorbidity and High-Risk Behavior. New York, Routledge/Francis & Taylor, 2008

Kaminer Y, Bukstein O, Tarter RE: The Teen Addiction Severity Index (T-ASI): rationale and reliability. Int J Addict 26:219–226, 1991

Liddle HA, Rowe CL: Adolescent Substance Abuse: Research and Clinical Advances. Cambridge, UK, Cambridge University Press, 2006

Mee-Lee D, Shulman GD, Fishman M, et al: American Society of Addiction Medicine Patient Placement Criteria for the Treatment of Substance-Related Disorders, 2nd Edition, Revised. Chevy Chase, MD, American Society of Addiction Medicine, 2001

Monti PM, Colby SM, O'Leary TA: Adolescents, Alcohol, and Substance Abuse: Reaching Teens Through Brief Interventions. New York, Guilford, 2001

Riggs PD, Mikulich-Gilbertson SK, Lohman ML, et al: A randomized controlled trial of fluoxetine and CBT in adolescents with major depression, behavior problems and substance use disorders. Arch Pediatr Adolesc Med 161:1026–1034, 2007

Waxmonsky JG, Wilens TE: Pharmacotherapy of adolescent substance use disorders: a review of the literature. J Child Adolesc Psychopharmacol 15:810–825, 2005

Whitmore EA, Riggs PD: Developmentally informed diagnostic and treatment considerations in comorbid conditions, in Adolescent Substance Abuse: Research and Clinical Advances. Edited by Liddle HA, Rowe CL. Cambridge, UK, Cambridge University Press, 2006, pp 264–283

■ CHAPTER 8 ■

My Mind Is Breaking

Psychosis

Julia W. Tossell, M.D.
Judith L. Rapoport, M.D.

CASE PRESENTATION

IDENTIFYING INFORMATION

Ashley is a 12-year-old girl who lives with her parents and two siblings.

CHIEF COMPLAINT

The parents report, "Our daughter is very confused and thinks everyone is going to die."

HISTORY OF PRESENT ILLNESS

Over the last several months, Ashley has been having periods of weeping in her room, and often has trouble falling asleep at bedtime. Her parents began to receive calls from her teachers, reporting that Ashley was turning in her assignments late or not at all, and that she seemed both sad and absentminded in

Julia W. Tossell, M.D., is Staff Clinician in the Child Psychiatry Branch at the National Institute of Mental Health in Bethesda, Maryland.

Judith L. Rapoport, M.D., is Chief of the Child Psychiatry Branch at the National Institute of Mental Health in Bethesda, Maryland.

For complete biographical information, see "About the Contributors," p. 613.

The patient described in this chapter is not based on any individual, but rather reflects the breadth of clinical experience obtained during research into childhood-onset schizophrenia at the National Institute of Mental Health since the early 1990s.

school. Her older brother told their parents that he had walked past Ashley's room and seen her apparently talking to someone he could not see and laughing aloud for no reason. When he went in to talk to her, she told him, "I think my mind is breaking," and then ordered him out of her room. A few days later, Ashley's mother got an urgent call at work from the guidance counselor at the school. Ashley had asked permission to go to the bathroom but had not returned to her classroom. She had been found standing in the hallway outside her classroom, mute, but with a terrified expression on her face. When questioned, she had muttered, "Where am I?…I can't do what 'they' tell me to do…Everyone is going to die…"

The next day, Ashley was seen by her pediatrician, who noted that Ashley took a long time to answer his questions, responded with monosyllabic answers, spent a lot of time looking around the room with a frightened expression, and burst into laughter for no apparent reason. A comprehensive physical evaluation by her pediatrician and then by a child neurologist, including brain magnetic resonance imaging and electroencephalography, showed no abnormalities. Ashley was given a referral to a child and adolescent psychiatrist, who scheduled an appointment for 2 weeks later.

In the interim, Ashley stopped attending school and spent most of her days in her bedroom, where she alternated between sleeping and lying inert on her bed. She refused most of her meals and lost 10 lbs. She occasionally accepted a drink or a small snack if it was given to her in a package that she could open by herself. Most nights she was awake, alternating between laughing aloud and repeating apparently random phrases with intervals of wordless weeping.

Past Psychiatric History

Ashley had been diagnosed with attention-deficit/hyperactivity disorder (ADHD), inattentive type, at age 5½ years, when she entered kindergarten. She was treated with several stimulants without significant benefit.

When Ashley was age 11, her family noted a change in her usual demeanor. She had always been a quiet and reserved child, preferring to spend her free time with her two close girlfriends, but she began to spend less time with them and more time alone in her room. She was less interested in playing with her 8-year-old sister, with whom she had been particularly close. These changes, while notable, were not alarming to her parents. They attributed the changes to her entry into adolescence and recalled that her well-adjusted 15-year-old brother had also become quieter as he approached adolescence.

Substance Abuse History

Ashley has no history of substance abuse.

MEDICAL HISTORY

Ashley was the product of a normal spontaneous vaginal delivery at term. She had no chronic illnesses and no history of hospitalizations or head trauma with loss of consciousness.

DEVELOPMENTAL HISTORY

All of Ashley's milestones were at the later end of the normal range. She had speech therapy in first through third grades for a mild expressive language disorder. Her elementary school's consulting psychologist considered that Ashley might have pervasive developmental disorder not otherwise specified, in view of her language delay and her social reticence around peers, but did not make the diagnosis because Ashley did very well in one-on-one situations with children her age and had two close girlfriends.

SOCIAL HISTORY

Ashley lives with both parents, her older brother, and her younger sister. Her father is a college graduate with a master's degree in software engineering. Her mother has an associate's degree and works as an office manager for a medical practice.

Ashley had attended her local elementary and middle schools, participating in weekly group speech and language therapy. She had enjoyed riding her bike but avoided team sports because her physical clumsiness got in the way of her performance. She had been involved in Girl Scouts and Sunday school, both of which she enjoyed, and where she had been well accepted by the other children despite her quietness.

When Ashley stopped attending school, her mother took a leave of absence from work to care for her, but the loss of income was beginning to cause tension between Ashley's parents.

FAMILY HISTORY

Ashley's father was successfully treated for unipolar depression as a young adult. One grandfather was described as "probably an alcoholic," and several elderly relatives were described as "strange…loners."

MENTAL STATUS EXAMINATION

At her first meeting with the child and adolescent psychiatrist, Ashley answered some questions "yes" or "no," but she ignored others completely. She sat rigid in her chair, with few body movements or gestures, and rarely looked at the doctor. At times, she gazed at the ceiling but would not describe what she was looking at. She nodded "yes" when asked whether she was hearing voices, whether they talked to each other about her, and whether they gave her commands. When asked if she could do things other kids could not do, she briefly smiled and nodded but refused to give further details. She acknowledged feeling sad most of the time, uninterested in her usual activities, and being awake much of the night listening to the voices, which she heard both inside her head and with her ears. She had some thoughts that she would be better off if she were dead but denied any specific plans to hurt herself or other people. She denied racing thoughts or feelings of elation and reported feeling very tired as a consequence of her limited sleep duration. Her speech was never pressured, her activity level was never elevated, and her usual modest demeanor never changed.

INITIAL TREATMENT WITH THE PSYCHIATRIST

The child and adolescent psychiatrist diagnosed Ashley as having a depression with psychotic features; ADHD, inattentive type; and expressive language disorder. She prescribed sertraline at an initial dosage of 25 mg/day. After taking sertraline 50 mg/day for 1 week, Ashley found that her sleep improved in duration, but otherwise there were no significant changes as the clinician increased the dosage to 150 mg/day. At that point, the doctor decided to add an antipsychotic medication, choosing aripiprazole because of its benign side-effect profile. Ashley continued taking a regimen of sertraline 150 mg/day and aripiprazole 20 mg/day for 2 months, with no significant improvement. The psychiatrist revised the diagnosis.

COMMENTARIES

Psychopharmacologic Perspective

Sanjiv Kumra, M.D., M.S.
Kathryn R. Cullen, M.D.

DIAGNOSTIC FORMULATION

This vignette describes Ashley, age 12, a girl with a history of premorbid dysfunction who gradually develops a constellation of cognitive and emotional deficits affecting hedonic capacity, volition and drive, affect, productivity of thought and speech, behavioral monitoring, and perception. These symptoms are associated with impaired function with family, peers, school, and self-care. Although the differential diagnosis of psychotic symptoms in youth includes major depressive disorder, several aspects of the case presentation suggest that this formulation may not entirely capture the complexity of Ashley's difficulties. Although childhood-onset schizophrenia is rare (Beitchman 1985) and potentially a more severe variant of the adult-onset disorder (Frazier et al. 2007), several reasons suggest that this diagnosis should be considered for Ashley.

Careful clinical assessment is pivotal in establishing an accurate diagnosis in youths with psychosis. To date, phenomenological studies suggest that the clinical presentation of schizophrenia in children and adolescents is on a continuum with adult-onset schizophrenia (McKenna et al. 1994).

Negative symptoms frequently appear during the prodromal phase of schizophrenia, are associated with cognitive impairments, and account for a substantial degree of the psychosocial disability in youth with the disorder (Lencz et al. 2004). Three negative symptoms—affective flattening, alogia, and avolition—are often difficult to recognize and to evaluate in children and adolescents be-

Sanjiv Kumra, M.D., M.S., is Associate Professor of Psychiatry and Chief of the Division of Child Psychiatry in the Department of Psychiatry at the University of Minnesota in Minneapolis, Minnesota.

Kathryn R. Cullen, M.D., is Assistant Professor in the Child Psychiatry Division in the Department of Psychiatry at the University of Minnesota Medical School in Minneapolis, Minnesota.

For complete biographical information, see "About the Contributors," p. 613.

cause they occur on a continuum with normality, are relatively nonspecific, and may be due to other factors (including positive symptoms of schizophrenia and depression). Ashley is described by her parents as having several negative symptoms, including anhedonia, which are manifested by "spending less time with her friends and more time alone in her room," long periods of "sleeping and lying inert on her bed," "refusing meals," and replying in a "monosyllabic" fashion to questions. The changes in Ashley's behavior do not appear to reflect chronic environmental understimulation, demoralization, or medication effects. In contrast to Ashley, most teenagers with depression typically present with intense painful affect and irritability. Ashley's lack of other affective symptoms (e.g., racing thoughts, feelings of elation, pressured speech, elevated activity level, change in demeanor) does not support a diagnosis of bipolar disorder.

Several other features of Ashley's presentation are alarming and suggest a re-evaluation of her referral diagnosis. Disorganized thinking, or formal thought disorder, is an important feature of schizophrenia in youth (Caplan et al. 2000). Thought disorder is frequently manifested, as in this case vignette, by tangentiality and derailment of thought processes. These problems in thought processes are frequently associated with grossly disorganized behaviors; Ashley was observed to "laugh aloud for no reason" and "stand in the hallway, mute, with a terrified expression on her face," which suggests inappropriate affect. Inappropriate affect is one of the defining features of the disorganized type of schizophrenia and one of the most difficult treatment targets for therapy. The disorganization in Ashley's thought processes may account for why she is noted to have difficulties in performing activities of daily living, such as going to the bathroom, and why she eventually stopped attending school. Ashley's difficulties in school may also reflect cognitive deficits in attention, memory, and executive processes that are frequently evident in children and adolescents with schizophrenia.

In youth with schizophrenia, hallucinations may occur in any sensory modality, but auditory hallucinations are by far the most common (Russell 1994). In the case of Ashley, initial evidence that she is responding to auditory hallucinations is noted by her brother, who observed that she was "apparently talking to someone I could not see, and laughing aloud for no reason." Later, when questioned by a psychiatrist, Ashley admitted to hearing voices that "talk to each other about me and give commands." Parents of children with schizophrenia may have difficulty precisely defining the onset of psychotic symptoms, because many children recognize that their psychotic symptoms are unusual and may be reluctant to share these experiences with others. Also, a majority of youth with schizophrenia have poor insight regarding the presence of their psychotic illness.

Key diagnoses to consider in the differential diagnosis of psychotic symptoms in a child or adolescent include mood disorders (bipolar disorder, depression), anxiety disorders (obsessive-compulsive disorder, posttraumatic stress disorder, generalized anxiety disorder), pervasive developmental disorders, drug abuse disorders, and general medical conditions (McKenna et al. 1994). In Ashley's case, signs of an emotional disturbance have been present for a continuous period of at least 6 months, and during that time period she has had greater than 1 month of active phase symptoms: negative symptoms (social withdrawal, apathy, self-neglect), disorganization (thinking and behaviors), and distortion of reality (e.g., hallucinations). Ashley's developmental history reveals a number of prepsychotic abnormalities in terms of speech deficits and delays, motor clumsiness, and transient features of pervasive developmental disorder (e.g., social anxiety). Several clinical studies have confirmed these premorbid deficits are more exaggerated in patients with childhood-onset schizophrenia (Hollis 2003). Also, the majority of children with schizophrenia have a history of ADHD during the premorbid phase of the disorder (Hollis 2003). A prodromal phase of schizophrenia, characterized by social withdrawal, disorganized behavior, affective symptoms, deterioration in self-care, worsening school performance, and idiosyncratic behavior associated with a decline in baseline functioning (Lencz et al. 2004), is also apparent from Ashley's history. Recognition of childhood-onset schizophrenia remains problematic; children and adolescents may receive many other diagnoses before a diagnosis of schizophrenia is given, and a mean of 2.0 years passes between onset of psychotic symptoms and diagnosis (Frazier et al. 2007).

Although the precipitants for Ashley's psychotic episode remain unclear from the case description, an increased risk of schizophrenia has been found in association with substance misuse, in particular with amphetamine and marijuana usage (Kumra 2007). However, epidemiological data suggest that a sharp rise in the incidence of schizophrenia coincides with the onset of pubertal changes; therefore, brain maturational changes may somehow "trigger" the onset of the disorder (Pantelis et al. 2007). The fact that several of Ashley's elderly relatives were described as "strange...loners" is interesting. Schizophrenia is a highly heritable condition, and relatives of patients with childhood-onset schizophrenia frequently have been reported to have a higher risk for schizophrenia spectrum disorders and avoidant personality disorder (Asarnow et al. 2001).

DSM-IV-TR DIAGNOSIS

Axis I   295.10 Schizophrenia, disorganized type
Axis II   No diagnosis
Axis III   None
Axis IV   Educational problems
Axis V   Global Assessment of Functioning=25 (current)

TREATMENT RECOMMENDATIONS

Increasing evidence indicates that compared with later-onset schizophrenia, childhood-onset schizophrenia is associated with worse outcomes, possibly reflecting the negative impact of the illness during a critical period of brain development. Ashley's initial treatment plan should focus on acute symptom amelioration and improvement in functional achievement in terms of academics and social skills (Kumra et al. 2008). The majority of youth with childhood-onset schizophrenia benefit from multiple treatment strategies to address symptomatology, comorbid conditions, and other psychosocial and developmental issues. Although pharmacotherapy remains the cornerstone of treatment, psychosocial treatments (e.g., family interventions, social skills training) and special education placement should also be considered for Ashley. However, empirical data supporting the use of nonpharmacologic treatments in this population are limited.

Some data suggest that youth with schizophrenia may be less treatment responsive than adults with typical-onset schizophrenia and have a greater incidence of adverse effects when exposed to antipsychotic medications. Given that Ashley has experienced minimal improvement on a combination of sertraline and aripiprazole, the clinician might consider discontinuing the sertraline and pushing the dosage of aripiprazole to 30 mg/day, if permissible. If Ashley experiences no significant improvement in positive symptoms, consideration should be given to switching to a different antipsychotic, such as risperidone or quetiapine. Because these medications are likely to be associated with some degree of appetite stimulation and weight gain, the parents should be given some type of healthy lifestyle teaching to limit these potential problems in Ashley. After at least two trials of standard, first-line antipsychotic medication, the clinician should consider prescribing medications such as olanzapine or clozapine, which have a higher risk of side effects. Clozapine is the only antipsychotic consistently shown to be effective for treatment-resistant cases (Findling et al. 2007).

Integrative Perspective

Julia W. Tossell, M.D.
Judith L. Rapoport, M.D.

DIAGNOSTIC FORMULATION

Ashley became ill at a time of both biological (early puberty) and social (transition from elementary to middle school) stress. The presence of some "strange" relatives in the family suggests the possibility of genetic loading for psychotic spectrum disorders. Finally, her parents' response to Ashley's illness was colored by their feelings about her father's experience with a mental illness.

Before making the diagnosis of depression with psychotic features, Ashley's psychiatrist also considered bipolar disorder, schizophrenia, and schizoaffective disorder. However, Ashley showed no symptoms of mania other than a possible grandiose delusional system, and thus a diagnosis of bipolar disorder was ruled out. Her negative symptoms could equally represent depression or the flatness and apathy of schizophrenia. However, very early-onset schizophrenia is extremely rare, and pediatric mood disorders are less rare (Calderoni et al. 2001; McKenna et al. 1994; Murray et al. 2004). The clinician's decision to start with a working diagnosis of psychotic depression was a good place to begin.

After further evaluation of Ashley's clinical presentation, course, family history, and lack of response to treatment, the psychiatrist revised the diagnosis to schizophrenia. Children with very early-onset schizophrenia have a high rate of comorbid psychiatric conditions: language delay, ADHD, and social anxiety are common, and pervasive developmental disorders are not unusual (Nicolson et al. 2000; Rapoport et al. 2005; Schaeffer and Ross 2002; Sporn et al. 2004).

Helpful rating instruments, for purposes of both diagnostic clarification and monitoring of treatment response, include the Schedule for Affective Disorders and Schizophrenia for School-Age Children—Present and Lifetime Version (Kaufman et al. 1997), Children's Global Assessment Scale (Shaffer et al. 1983), Brief Psychiatric Rating Scale for Children (Overall and Pfefferbaum 1982), Bunney-Hamburg Psychosis Rating Scale (Bunney and Hamburg 1963), Scale for the Assessment of Positive Symptoms (Andreasen 1984), and Scale for the Assessment of Negative Symptoms (Andreasen 1983). The Autism Screening Questionnaire (Berument et al. 1999) is helpful in assessing for comorbid pervasive developmental disorders.

DSM-IV-TR DIAGNOSIS

Axis I   295.10 Schizophrenia, disorganized type

Axis II   None

Axis III   None

Axis IV   Educational problems

Axis V   Global Assessment of Functioning=30 (current)

TREATMENT RECOMMENDATIONS

After Ashley did not respond to her regimen of sertraline and aripiprazole, the psychiatrist cross-tapered to quetiapine. Ashley took quetiapine 300 mg twice a day for 8 weeks. Although she no longer insisted that her food be presented to her in an intact package and regained approximately 5 lbs, Ashley was otherwise unchanged. After consulting with colleagues, the psychiatrist began the process of discontinuing the quetiapine and starting Ashley on clozapine.

Clozapine is not used as a first-line antipsychotic in many countries, because of its many potential serious side effects (including neutropenia, elevated glucose, obesity, metabolic syndrome, seizures, and myocarditis) (C. M. Young and Findling 2004; C. R. Young et al. 1998). The monitoring system required for safe administration of clozapine poses its own burden on the child and the family (Novartis 2005). However, clozapine may be uniquely efficacious for otherwise treatment-resistant schizophrenia in both children and adults and has an important role in their treating (Kranzler et al. 2005, 2006; Lewis et al. 2006; Shaw et al. 2006).

While Ashley was taking 150 mg/day of clozapine, her family noted a subtle but definite improvement in Ashley, who seemed to be less involved in responding to her unusual internal stimuli. By week 6, Ashley was taking 300 mg/day of clozapine. She was speaking in brief sentences, sometimes initiating conversations with the family, sleeping well at night, and staying awake during the daytime. She commented spontaneously that "this medicine helps me feel better." At this point, the local public school convened an individualized education program meeting to begin the process of identifying an appropriate school placement for Ashley.

Ashley's parents began to explore services offered by their state and county, and were greatly relieved to accept the help of a part-time home health aide provided by the county. They looked into Social Security Disability Insurance benefits but found that even with the mother not working, the family's income was too high to qualify. With the support of the psychiatrist, who helped them sort through their concerns about possibly stigmatizing Ashley, the parents decided to disclose Ashley's diagnosis to their extended family and their church community. Both family and church members reacted with expressions of support and offers to help with child care for Ashley and her younger sister. The guidance counselor at the younger sister's school gave Ashley's parents a referral to an after-school support group for healthy siblings of ill children, and Ashley's mother provided the needed transportation so that the child could participate.

A sleep-deprived electroencephalogram at week 6 of clozapine treatment showed that Ashley had occasional epileptiform discharges, which the neurologist felt did not require treatment (Haring et al. 1994). The electrocardiogram at week 6 showed borderline QTc elevation. Ashley was seen by a pediatric cardiologist, and an echocardiogram was obtained. The results were normal. The cardiologist recommended that any future clozapine dosage increases be done in tandem with frequent electrocardiograms.

Ashley's mother usually took Ashley for her weekly complete blood count with differential in the morning, because that time of day fit best into her mother's schedule. At week 9, Ashley's absolute neutrophil count had fallen from its usual value (ranging between 2.2 and 3.4) to 1.7, below the acceptable level for continued clozapine treatment. Clozapine was held, and another complete blood count was drawn the next day, but in the afternoon. This absolute neutrophil count was 2.6, and clozapine treatment was continued. However, because of the low value, Ashley would require weekly blood count monitoring for the first 12 months of clozapine treatment, instead of moving to alternate-week monitoring after the first 6 months of treatment. The psychiatrist explained to Ashley's parents that diurnal variation in blood counts is normal (Esposito et al. 2006) and advised that all future blood draws be done in the afternoon. She also mentioned that raising the white blood and absolute neutrophil counts with lithium was a possibility for the future, should the afternoon absolute neutrophil count hover at the lower end of the acceptable range, but that she hoped to avoid this option because of the many serious side effects of lithium (Newcomer 2006).

By the sixth month of clozapine treatment, Ashley had gained 40 lbs. The psychiatrist discussed with Ashley's parents the many risks associated with this weight gain. The parents contacted the nutritionist in their pediatrician's practice, who helped them with menu planning for Ashley. The family also began to take regular evening walks to help Ashley improve her fitness level and burn more calories. The psychiatrist decided to wait and see if this new regimen helped Ashley return to a healthier weight before prescribing an off-label medication that might help her lose weight (Morrison et al. 2002; Nickel et al. 2005).

After 12 months of taking clozapine 300 mg/day, Ashley was seeing the psychiatrist for monthly "medication management" visits. She was enrolled in a self-enclosed special education classroom at a public school several miles from her home, joining the mainstream children for physical education and lunch. Her one-on-one aide assisted both with her academics and in negotiating the complexities of the cafeteria, the gym, and the bus. Although Ashley still hallucinated, she was usually able to ignore the hallucinations during school and while around other people. Propranolol 20 mg three times a day relieved her moderate akathisia.

In addition to the visits with Ashley's psychiatrist, the whole family met twice a month with a family therapist, who helped them confront the practical implications and the psychological stresses posed by Ashley's serious chronic illness.

REFERENCES

Andreasen NC: The Scale for the Assessment of Negative Symptoms. Iowa City, University of Iowa Press, 1983

Andreasen NC: The Scale for the Assessment of Positive Symptoms. Iowa City, University of Iowa Press, 1984

Asarnow RF, Nuechterlein KH, Fogelson D, et al: Schizophrenia and schizophrenia-spectrum personality disorders in the first-degree relatives of children with schizophrenia: the UCLA Family Study. Arch Gen Psychiatry 58:581–588, 2001

Beitchman JH: Childhood schizophrenia. A review and comparison with adult-onset schizophrenia. Psychiatr Clin North Am 8:793–814, 1985

Berument SK, Rutter M, Lord C, et al: Autism Screening Questionnaire: diagnostic validity. Br J Psychiatry 175:444–451, 1999

Bunney WE Jr, Hamburg DA: Methods for reliable longitudinal observation of behavior. Arch Gen Psychiatry 9:280–294, 1963

Calderoni D, Wudarsky M, Bhangoo R, et al: Differentiating childhood-onset schizophrenia from psychotic mood disorders. J Am Acad Child Adolesc Psychiatry 40:1190–1196, 2001

Caplan R, Guthrie D, Tang B, et al: Thought disorder in childhood schizophrenia: replication and update of concept. J Am Acad Child Adolesc Psychiatry 39:771–778, 2000

Esposito D, Chouinard G, Hardy P, et al: Successful initiation of clozapine treatment despite morning pseudoneutropenia. Int J Neuropsychopharmacol 9:489–491, 2006

Findling RL, Frazier JA, Gerbino-Rosen G, et al: Is there a role for clozapine in the treatment of children and adolescents? J Am Acad Child Adolesc Psychiatry 46:423–428, 2007

Frazier JA, McClellan J, Findling RL, et al: Treatment of early onset schizophrenia spectrum disorders (TEOSS): demographic and clinical characteristics. J Am Acad Child Adolesc Psychiatry 46:979–988, 2007

Haring C, Neudorfer C, Schwitzer J, et al: EEG alterations in patients treated with clozapine in relation to plasma levels. Psychopharmacology (Berl) 114:97–100, 1994

Hollis C: Developmental precursors of child- and adolescent-onset schizophrenia and affective psychoses: diagnostic specificity and continuity with symptom dimensions. Br J Psychiatry 182:37–44, 2003

Kaufman J, Birmaher B, Brent D, et al: Schedule for Affective Disorders and Schizophrenia for School-Age Children—Present and Lifetime Version (K-SADS-PL): initial reliability and validity data. J Am Acad Child Adolesc Psychiatry 36:980–988, 1997

Kranzler H, Roofeh D, Gerbino-Rosen G, et al: Clozapine: its impact on aggressive behavior among children and adolescents with schizophrenia. J Am Acad Child Adolesc Psychiatry 44:55–63, 2005

Kranzler HN, Kester HM, Gerbino-Rosen G, et al: Treatment-refractory schizophrenia in children and adolescents: an update on clozapine and other pharmacologic interventions. Child Adolesc Psychiatr Clin N Am 15:135–159, 2006

Kumra S: Schizophrenia and cannabis use. Minn Med 90:36–38, 2007

Kumra S, Oberstar JV, Sikich L, et al: Efficacy and tolerability of second-generation antipsychotics in children and adolescents with schizophrenia. Schizophr Bull 34:60–71, 2008

Lencz T, Smith CW, Auther A, et al: Nonspecific and attenuated negative symptoms in patients at clinical high-risk for schizophrenia. Schizophr Res 68:37–48, 2004

Lewis SW, Barnes TR, Davies L, et al: Randomized controlled trial of effect of prescription of clozapine versus other second-generation antipsychotic drugs in resistant schizophrenia. Schizophr Bull 32:715–723, 2006

McKenna K, Gordon CT, Lenane M, et al: Looking for childhood-onset schizophrenia: the first 71 cases screened. J Am Acad Child Adolesc Psychiatry 33:636–644, 1994

Morrison JA, Cottingham EM, Barton BA: Metformin for weight loss in pediatric patients taking psychotropic drugs. Am J Psychiatry 159:655–657, 2002

Murray RM, Sham P, Van Os J, et al: A developmental model for similarities and dissimilarities between schizophrenia and bipolar disorder. Schizophr Res 71:405–416, 2004

Newcomer JW: Medical risk in patients with bipolar disorder and schizophrenia. J Clin Psychiatry 67 (suppl 9):25–30; discussion 36–42, 2006

Nickel MK, Nickel C, Muehlbacher M, et al: Influence of topiramate on olanzapine-related adiposity in women: a random, double-blind, placebo-controlled study. J Clin Psychopharmacol 25:211–217, 2005

Nicolson R, Lenane M, Singaracharlu S, et al: Premorbid speech and language impairments in childhood-onset schizophrenia: association with risk factors. Am J Psychiatry 157:794–800, 2000

Novartis [changes to the prescribing information for Clozaril (clozapine) tablets]. East Hanover, NJ, Novartis, 2005

Overall JE, Pfefferbaum B: The Brief Psychiatric Rating Scale for Children. Psychopharmacol Bull 18:10–16, 1982

Pantelis C, Velakoulis D, Wood SJ, et al: Neuroimaging and emerging psychotic disorders: the Melbourne ultra-high risk studies. Int Rev Psychiatry 19:371–381, 2007

Rapoport JL, Addington AM, Frangou S: The neurodevelopmental model of schizophrenia: update 2005. Mol Psychiatry 10:434–449, 2005

Russell AT: The clinical presentation of childhood-onset schizophrenia. Schizophr Bull 20:631–646, 1994

Schaeffer JL, Ross RG: Childhood-onset schizophrenia: premorbid and prodromal diagnostic and treatment histories. J Am Acad Child Adolesc Psychiatry 41:538–545, 2002

Shaffer D, Gould MS, Brasic J, et al: A children's global assessment scale (CGAS). Arch Gen Psychiatry 40:1228–1231, 1983

Shaw P, Sporn A, Gogtay N, et al: Childhood-onset schizophrenia: a double-blind, randomized clozapine-olanzapine comparison. Arch Gen Psychiatry 63:721–730, 2006

Sporn AL, Addington AM, Gogtay N, et al: Pervasive developmental disorder and childhood-onset schizophrenia: comorbid disorder or a phenotypic variant of a very early onset illness? Biol Psychiatry 55:989–994, 2004

Young CM, Findling RL: Pharmacologic treatment of adolescent and child schizophrenia. Expert Rev Neurother 4:53–60, 2004

Young CR, Bowers MB Jr, Mazure CM: Management of the adverse effects of clozapine. Schizophr Bull 24:381–390, 1998

■ CHAPTER 9 ■

She Just Won't Eat a Thing

Anorexia Nervosa

E. Blake Finkelson, B.A.
B. Timothy Walsh, M.D.

CASE PRESENTATION

IDENTIFYING INFORMATION

Caroline is a 16-year-old high school junior who lives with her mother.

CHIEF COMPLAINT

Caroline presented for outpatient treatment after an admission to a specialized eating disorders inpatient program. She had been brought to the unit because, according to her mother, "It has gone too far; she just won't eat a thing."

HISTORY OF PRESENT ILLNESS

Although Caroline has a history of dieting and exercising excessively since she was 13 years old, she maintained a stable but low weight with the help of a nu-

E. Blake Finkelson, B.A., is a doctoral student in clinical psychology and a graduate research assistant in the Children, Families and Cultures (CFC) Laboratory at the Catholic University of America, Washington, D.C.

B. Timothy Walsh, M.D., is Ruane Professor of Pediatric Psychopharmacology in the Department of Psychiatry in the College of Physicians and Surgeons at Columbia University, and Director of the Division of Clinical Therapeutics at New York State Psychiatric Institute in New York, New York.

For complete biographical information, see "About the Contributors," p. 613.

tritionist until this past winter, when she entered a national karate tournament. Before the competition was to start, her teacher encouraged her to intensify her workouts to make a lower weight class. Caroline decided to resume "respectable workouts," including hundreds of push-ups and hours of aerobic exercises, and started watching what she ate "to be a better competitor and to feel better about myself." She thought her weight loss "didn't show" because of water retention, and she restricted food intake even further, at times eating only lettuce during the day. She lied to her mother and nutritionist about what she was eating and falsified her food diary.

In the 4 months prior to her admission to the hospital, she became even more rigid about her food intake, eating no more than 600 kcal/day. She would not let anyone else prepare her food, yet she enjoyed cooking for others and collecting recipes. Her eating habits had become ritualized; she cut her food into very small pieces, moved them around on her plate, and chewed each bite 20 times before swallowing. She exercised secretly and felt self-conscious leaving the house on days when she had not done her quota of crunches.

Over the past 6 months, Caroline had intermittent low-mood states, reporting that "some days I feel numb." Other symptoms included fatigue, occasional dizziness on standing, trouble concentrating in class, decreased interest in activities, a tendency to isolate from others, disrupted sleep (awakening three or four times per night), anxiety, and feelings of guilt ("whenever I eat"). For 2 months, she "just [didn't] want to wake up in the morning," but she denied ever planning to hurt herself. She said she did not want to die but just wanted some end to her current situation. She also endorsed recent onset of symptoms such as the need to wash her hands for a full 10 minutes after eating and the need to re–color coordinate her closet a couple times a week.

HOSPITAL COURSE

Because of her low weight, medical complications, and rapid worsening of symptoms, Caroline was admitted to the adolescent medicine service of her local general hospital. Fortunately, this unit had substantial experience in the care of adolescents with eating disorders.

An initial medical evaluation revealed that Caroline had significant orthostatic hypotension and low serum levels of potassium and sodium. No other medical complications of anorexia nervosa were detected, and there was no indication of other significant medical illnesses that might be contributing to her weight loss (Walsh 2005). Caroline was given intravenous fluids for 24 hours to assist rehydration and to correct the electrolyte disturbances. She was given a standard hospital diet containing 1,800 kcal, to which she objected strenuously, feeling that any more than 1,000 kcal/day would be far too much. The medical and nursing staff assured Caroline that this diet was absolutely required to assure her physical stability, and made it clear that she would not be able to leave the hospital until she was able to consume the prescribed diet.

Caroline and her parents met with a child and adolescent psychiatrist with expertise in eating disorders who would treat her after discharge. Accompanied by the attending adolescent medicine physician, the psychiatrist emphasized to Caroline and her family that Caroline had a very serious disorder that sometimes results in death (Sullivan 1995) and that should be treated aggressively. The physicians and family reviewed a range of options for treatment after discharge. Caroline remained in the hospital for 1 week and was given a diet of 1,800 kcal/day. Her electrolytes normalized, and her symptoms of orthostatic hypotension abated. After a week in the hospital, she had gained 4 lbs and was discharged at 90 lbs.

Past Psychiatric History

Caroline reported that her struggle with food, body image, and weight began around age 12, during the decline of her parents' marriage, a time of much "yelling and silence, but not much in between." Her father was always angry, and her mother was often sad. The patient noticed a decline in her mother's appetite, especially during family dinners, and "in support" of her mother, Caroline also began eating less during meals. However, when she was alone, she turned to food as "a comfort thing," sneaking junk food into her room late at night. She gained about 12 lbs that year and reached her adult height, 5 ft 4 in, and highest lifetime weight, 136 lbs.

The summer after her thirteenth birthday, Caroline's parents divorced and she was "forced" to move to another town with her mother. Upon starting her new school, Caroline felt pressure to make new friends and maintain her status as an athlete. She decided to take control of her eating and to "shape up." She set a goal of eliminating "all body fat via exercising and cutting out nonessential food groups." Four months into the new school year, Caroline had become the only eighth grader to make varsity soccer, was training for her black belt in karate, was maintaining straight A's, and had dropped from 134 lbs to 120 lbs. She was proud of losing "what my mom called 'my baby-fat'" and enjoyed the positive attention she received from peers. Caroline continued to eat "healthy" and to "push myself to the limit" in sports. By the end of the school year, she had achieved her goal weight of 115 lbs but felt that she could stand to lose just a little more. She set out to see "how little I really needed to eat." A typical day would include three fruits, 4 oz of juice, ½ cup of cereal with skim milk, a plate of lettuce, and "maybe" one slice of bread. Whenever she felt that she had eaten too much, she made herself vomit. She recalls feeling guilty and ashamed after purging but less so than after digesting a full meal.

Around this time, friends begin to express concern, but Caroline believed they were jealous. At 102 lbs, Caroline was certain she did not have a problem.

She stopped menstruating but rationalized, "This happens to many athletes." She noticed she was having more thoughts about food; her mother became concerned and threatened to send Caroline "to a shrink." Caroline increased her food intake slightly, and her weight rose to 105 lbs. On her pediatrician's recommendation, she started to see a nutritionist, who helped her maintain this weight until the middle of the school year.

RELEVANT MEDICAL HISTORY

Menarche occurred at age 12. The patient was amenorrheic for 5 months at age 14 and has not menstruated in the past 6 months. At a recent emergency room visit, she had a low pulse (30–40 beats/minute) and was told that her electrolytes were abnormal. The patient has also noted that her hair has begun falling out.

DEVELOPMENTAL HISTORY

Caroline was on target for meeting developmental milestones.

SOCIAL HISTORY

Caroline is an only child whose parents divorced when Caroline was age 13. She lives with her mother, an attorney, and only sees her father, a stockbroker, once a month. Her father remarried last year, around the time of her relapse. He is now an avid marathon runner.

Caroline is a junior in high school and an A student in honors classes. She is a star athlete (currently suspended from participation) at school, has a black belt in karate, speaks fluent Spanish and French, and is teaching herself Norwegian. She is well regarded by her peers but feels that she has not developed a true close circle of friends since changing schools at age 13.

FAMILY HISTORY

Caroline's mother believes that she was depressed when living with her ex-husband but was never treated. She contends that she has never been critical of her daughter's figure but is intensely critical of her own and obsessed with maintaining a size zero. She reports, "I am a vegetarian and don't eat large quantities of food." Caroline's father is recovering from alcoholism and has been sober for 3 years.

MENTAL STATUS EXAMINATION

At 5 ft 4 in and 90 lbs, the patient is a markedly thin young woman despite wearing numerous layers of sweaters. Initially, the patient reported no distress about her current weight and agreed to hospitalization only to appease her mother. She explained that everyone is overreacting and pinched the skin on her stomach in an attempt to validate this point. The patient defended her status, saying that she has "not made myself sick" in over 2 years and described her current eating and exercise regimen as "healthy."

Initially, she denied anxiety and depression, but she stated that she is troubled by her current appearance and behavior and is terrified of recovery. She reported that she is constantly distracted and exhausted from food-focused thoughts and frightened "that this might kill me." She reported an intense "fear of all foods" and of reaching "triple digits," and she expressed that she is certain that she gains weight more rapidly than other people do. The patient believes she can best recover at her own pace and feels that 99 lbs is a good goal weight. There was no evidence of thought disorder, and apart from distortions in her body image and attitudes about eating, health, and weight, her overall judgment and insight appeared intact.

COMMENTARIES

Psychotherapeutic Perspective

Daniel le Grange, Ph.D.

DIAGNOSTIC FORMULATION

Caroline is a 16-year-old high school junior, a straight-A student, presenting with a 4-year history of food, body image, and weight concerns. Menarche occurred at age 12, when Caroline weighed 136 lbs and had reached her adult height of 5 ft 4 in (body mass index [BMI]=23.3, <90th percentile for age and sex). At presentation, she weighed 90 lbs (BMI=15.4, <5th percentile for age and sex) and had secondary amenorrhea (6 months in duration). Caroline has a history of exercising excessively, and although she is a good athlete at school, she also engages in episodes of intense workouts at home (e.g., hundreds of push-ups and hours of aerobic exercises in one time period). She has a history of at least one recent visit to an emergency room, where she presented with a low pulse (30–40 beats/minute) and abnormal electrolytes, and in the past month, she was admitted for

Daniel le Grange, Ph.D., is Associate Professor of Psychiatry in the Department of Psychiatry, Section for Child and Adolescent Psychiatry, and Director of the Eating Disorders Program at The University of Chicago in Chicago, Illinois (for complete biographical information, see "About the Contributors," p. 613).

1 week to a specialized inpatient eating disorders unit after eating <600 kcal/day and weighing 86 lbs. At this admission, Caroline presented with significant orthostatic hypotension and low serum levels of potassium and sodium, but no indication of any other significant medical illness. She was discharged after medical stabilization and having gained 4 lbs on a daily intake of 1,800 kcal.

Caroline denied purging in the past 2 years, although she endorsed past subjective binge eating episodes followed by self-induced vomiting. The frequency of these episodes could not be established. At present, she demonstrated marked fear of certain foods and weight gain. She also reported eating rituals, such as cutting her food into small pieces and having to chew each bite 20 times before swallowing. No other symptoms of ritualistic behaviors were endorsed. Caroline showed little appreciation of the severity of her medical status. However, she acknowledged that constant food-focused thoughts are distracting. She stated that her ideal weight is 99 lbs. Caroline endorsed intermittent low-mood states over the past 6 months, complaining of feeling fatigued, poor concentration in class, decreased interest in activities, social isolation, and disrupted sleep (frequent awakening after falling asleep). In addition, she reported not wanting to wake up in the morning but did not endorse any suicidal ideation.

Caroline is an only child of two professional parents. Her mother endorsed some eating disorder symptoms, and her dad is recovering from alcoholism. Caroline described her parents as having had marital difficulties around the time that her eating difficulties began. Her parents divorced soon after Caroline turned age 13, at which time she and her mother moved to another town. Caroline has not been successful at making friends in her new school, even though this move was more than 3 years ago. Her latest relapse in eating disorder symptoms coincided with her father's remarrying. Caroline visits with her father once per month, but the degree to which he is involved in her current treatment, which includes an outpatient clinician and a nutritionist, is not known. The case presentation does not report whether Caroline is taking any psychotropic medicines at this time.

RATIONALE FOR DIAGNOSIS

Caroline meets all four DSM-IV-TR criteria for a diagnosis of anorexia nervosa: not maintaining weight at or above a minimally normal weight for age and gender, fear of gaining weight, denial of the seriousness of current low body weight, and amenorrhea for at least three consecutive menstrual cycles. She meets the criterion for the restricting type of anorexia nervosa, as opposed to the binge-eating/purging type, because during the current episode, there is no evidence of regular objective binge eating episodes or purging behavior. However, both abnormal electrolytes on examination and a history of excessive exercise should allow the clinician to revise the current subtyping, if deemed appropriate. A majority of patients with anorexia nervosa also present with some anxiety and/or mood disturbances, which are usually side effects of severe starvation. Caroline endorses several symptoms in keeping with a diagnosis of a mood disorder, as well as some significant obsessive-compulsive behaviors. Both mood disorder and obsessive-compulsive disorder frequently co-occur with anorexia nervosa. Further inquiry should allow the clinician to establish whether either of these disorders is a primary diagnosis.

In addition to conducting a clinical interview, the clinician should administer the Eating Disorder Examination (Fairburn and Cooper 1993), the "gold standard" assessment tool to confirm an eating disorder diagnosis. This instrument is a structured interview that takes a trained interviewer about 1 hour to administer.

DSM-IV-TR DIAGNOSIS

Axis I   307.1 Anorexia nervosa, restricting type
          Rule out mood disorder
          Rule out obsessive-compulsive disorder
Axis II   None
Axis III Amenorrhea
Axis IV   Parents' divorce, father's remarriage
Axis V   Global Assessment of Functioning=61–70

TREATMENT RECOMMENDATIONS

The ideal treatment team for anorexia nervosa would comprise the following: a therapist (psychologist, child and adolescent psychiatrist, or other mental health professional) to conduct family-based treatment (FBT), a child and adolescent psychiatrist to rule out mood disorder or obsessive-compulsive disorder and manage any comorbid disorder, and a pediatrician to monitor Caroline's medical status for outpatient treatment. Such a team is most effective if all members are part of a dedicated eating disorders service and participate in weekly case reviews. The therapist will record the patient's weight at the outset of each meeting, with the outcome setting the tone for each session, whereas the pediatrician will monitor a gown weight at each visit.

FBT should be adjusted to accommodate the fact that Caroline 1) is an only child and 2) lives essentially in a single-parent family. Nevertheless, the therapist should consider whether and how the father and his spouse might be involved in treatment. This involvement will depend on 1) the amicability of the parents' divorce, 2) the nature of Caroline's relationship with her father and his spouse, and 3) the distance involved (unable to establish from case description). The therapist's initial recommendations are for parental supervision of all meals and for the patient to remain home for about 2 weeks. Involving the mother's parents in these tasks, if possible, should be considered. Given indications of the mother's concerns with her own weight, the therapist should assess the extent to which this is an issue and address it from the outset.

FBT has been shown to be the most promising therapy for adolescents with anorexia nervosa. Several randomized controlled trials have demonstrated that parents are a resource in restoring their adolescent's weight and helping to put the adolescent back on track with development (Eisler et al. 1997, 2000, 2007; le Grange et al. 1992; Lock et al. 2005, 2006; Robin et al. 1994, 1999; Russell et al. 1987). FBT is conducted in an outpatient setting, is theoretically agnostic, and makes no assumptions about the etiology of the eating disorder. Instead, it attempts to capitalize on the strengths that parents bring to the recovery of their offspring. Interventions focus initially on weight restoration before turning to psychosocial or developmental concerns. FBT has been manualized and consists of three clearly demarcated phases (Le Grange 1999; Lock et al. 2001).

PHASE 1: PARENTAL CONTROL OF WEIGHT RESTORATION

During phase 1 (sessions 1–10), the therapist focuses on the dangers of severe malnutrition associated with anorexia nervosa and emphasizes the need for parents to take immediate action to reverse this process. The therapist carefully reviews the development of the eating disorder, while highlighting the devastating effects that anorexia nervosa has had on the patient's medical and psychological well-being. The therapist stresses these concerns to support the development of a parental alliance around the goal of weight restoration. To avoid counterproductive adolescent-parent power struggles over eating, the parent is advised to refrain from engaging in *any* discussions about eating, while showing sympathy for the adolescent's struggle.

During this phase, a family meal is typically conducted at the second treatment session. This session allows the therapist to observe the interaction patterns around eating and help parents find ways to succeed in having the patient eat more than she intended. It also allows the therapist to convey support to the patient, given the difficulty of eating. Throughout this phase, the therapist continues to carefully review with the parents the weekly efforts around helping their daughter gain weight, while showing the patient support and understanding for her struggle around this issue.

PHASE 2: RETURNING CONTROL OVER EATING
BACK TO THE ADOLESCENT

The therapist transitions to phase 2 (sessions 11–16) after 1) the patient clearly accepts her parents' expectations for adequate food intake and 2) steady weight gain is evident. The parents are encouraged to help their child take more control over her own eating once the patient and the parents demonstrate less anxiety around mealtimes and regarding the goal of weight gain. Also during this stage of treatment, the parents are asked to begin to encourage their daughter to engage in other adolescent activities, such as socializing with friends. Before the patient participates in other activities, the parents must feel reassured that these would not provide opportunities for exercising or skipping a meal.

PHASE 3: ADOLESCENT DEVELOPMENT AND TREATMENT TERMINATION

When the patient is maintaining a healthy weight on her own, the treatment focus shifts away from the eating disorder. During phase 3 (sessions 17–20), the therapist examines the impact that anorexia nervosa has had on establishing a healthy adolescent identity, considering that the patient's development might have been severely interrupted by the eating disorder. The therapist reviews the stages of adolescent development: concerns associated with puberty, worries about peer relationships, and struggles regarding independence from the family and establishing significant relationships outside the family.

Involving divorced parents or assisting single parents in FBT is outlined in detail in the treatment manual (Lock et al. 2001). Should FBT not be effective with a specific family, the only other psychotherapy option that is supported by some research evidence is ego-oriented individual therapy (Robin et al. 1994, 1999).

Psychopharmacologic Perspective

Angela S. Guarda, M.D.

DIAGNOSTIC FORMULATION

Caroline is a 16-year-old girl who presents with a BMI of 15.4 and classic anorexia nervosa of the binge-purge type of less than 3 years' duration. Her eating disorder behaviors include restricting her food intake, exercising excessively, and self-induced vomiting. She also meets criteria for a depressive episode and has had a recent increase in both depressive and obsessional symptomatology in the setting of increased weight loss. Caroline's premorbid history is significant for perfectionism and high academic achievement. Her family history is

Angela S. Guarda, M.D., is Associate Professor of Psychiatry and Behavioral Sciences at the Johns Hopkins School of Medicine in Baltimore, Maryland (for complete biographical information, see "About the Contributors," p. 613).

notable for a possible episode of depression, her mother's restrained eating and weight concern, and her father's driven exercise behavior. Life stressors include parental divorce around the age at onset of the eating disorder, a recent move, adjustment to a new school, and her father's remarriage.

Anorexia nervosa is a driven behavioral syndrome characterized by dieting to the point of starvation in the context of an increasingly overvalued fear of fatness. As the disorder progresses, preoccupation with food and weight escalates into a consuming passion, accompanied by a narrowing and stereotyping of the behavioral repertoire. Excessive time is spent engaging in ritualized eating and exercise behaviors, and social isolation and avoidance of social eating settings increase. Poor insight, rationalization, and lying to disguise anorectic behaviors are typical. Patients are ambivalent about recovery and repeatedly subvert attempts by others to encourage them to gain weight. All of these characteristics are evident in Caroline's case.

Predisposing risk factors for anorexia nervosa include both genetic vulnerability and environmental factors. Perfectionistic and obsessional traits are overrepresented in at-risk families, and young girls who develop anorexia nervosa are often academic and athletic overachievers whose parents are accomplished professionals. Onset is usually in adolescence, and the disorder exhibits a markedly female predominance that is possibly related to pubertal hormonal changes and increases in body fat distribution in young girls. Caroline's initial weight loss was socially reinforced by her peers. This positive feedback coupled with the life stressors mentioned above and involvement in competitive sports (varsity soccer and karate) may have escalated her food restriction and exercise. As weight loss progresses, physiological and psychological complications of starvation, including delayed gastric transit times, early satiety, and increased depressive and obsessional symptomatology, are believed to contribute to sustaining disordered behavior and cognitions. Episodic binge eating can emerge as a consequence of the prolonged starved state, and purging behaviors, such as self-induced vomiting in Caroline's case, can result in potentially life-threatening electrolyte imbalances. Although Caroline denies recent vomiting, her hypokalemia suggests that she is still engaging in this behavior.

Frequent comorbid psychiatric conditions include depression and anxiety disorders. Starvation can cause a syndrome identical to major depression, making it difficult to determine if the depression is primary and truly comorbid or is secondary to Caroline's starved state. Because her depression worsened in the 6 months prior to hospitalization, while her weight was at its lowest, the depression may be a consequence of her starved state. If so, her mood is expected to normalize with refeeding and weight gain, which would support an initial diagnosis of depression not otherwise specified rather than major depression. Nevertheless, the family history of possible depression in her mother raises the possibility that Caroline may benefit from treatment with an antidepressant, especially if her mood remains low once her nutritional status is corrected.

DSM–IV–TR DIAGNOSIS

Axis I   307.1 Anorexia nervosa, binge-eating/purging type

311 Depressive disorder, not otherwise specified (likely secondary to starvation)

Axis II   No diagnosis (perfectionistic and obsessional personality traits)

Axis III Malnutrition

Secondary amenorrhea

Orthostatic hypotension

Dehydration

Hypokalemia and hyponatremia

Axis IV   Parental divorce, remarriage of parent, move, new school

Axis V   Global Asssessment of Functioning=40 (current) (Past year=60)

The diagnosis of anorexia nervosa is made on clinical grounds. Exhaustive medical workups to rule out other etiologies of weight loss are not indicated when criteria are met, unless other characteristics raise suspicion for a medical differential diagnosis. Amenorrhea, although still included as a diagnostic criterion in DSM-IV-TR, does not apply in premenarchal girls and is a consequence of starvation. Amenorrhea is increasingly believed to be a poor diagnostic differentiator or indicator of case severity.

Because denial of illness and minimization of symptoms is typical of patients with anorexia nervosa, collateral information from family members regarding the patient's eating and exercise behavior as well as preoccupation with weight and shape is helpful in distinguishing this disorder from other psychiatric conditions that may result in weight loss (e.g., anorexia of depression, anxiety disorders that affect feeding). Most patients with anorexia nervosa endorse a desired weight or maximum tolerable weight in the anorectic range (BMI<18). The most commonly used self-report screening tool for anorexia nervosa is the Eating Attitudes Test (Garner et al. 1982), which has acceptable reliability and validity but can yield false positives. A simpler five-question screening tool is the SCOFF (Morgan et al. 1999), which is similar to the CAGE questionnaire (Ewing 1984), used for alcohol abuse.

TREATMENT RECOMMENDATIONS

The treatment of adolescent anorexia nervosa is primarily behavioral rather than pharmacologic and has two phases: weight restoration and relapse pre-

vention. The initial focus is on helping patients block eating disordered behaviors, normalizing food intake, and restoring weight. Following weight
restoration, interventions should target relapse prevention. As in other behavioral conditions (e.g., substance abuse), relapse is the norm rather than the exception, but the long-term prognosis for the majority of adolescent cases with
less than a 3-year history is good with specialty treatment.

Some empirical evidence suggests that family therapy is superior to individual therapy in treating adolescents with anorexia nervosa. Family therapy
focuses on assisting parents to feed their child by appropriately enforcing consequences and rewards based on the child's eating and exercise behavior,
rather than focusing on understanding or interpreting the behavior, or searching for "root causes." Separated family therapy (parent training), in which the
therapist meets with the parents separately from the patient, is as effective as
conjoint family therapy, in which parents and patient are treated together as a
unit, and may be advisable in Caroline's case given the recent parental divorce.
When parents' behavior unwittingly reinforces a patient's anorectic beliefs, as
in Caroline's mother's vegetarianism and "fat talk" as well as Caroline's father's
running behavior, it is helpful to encourage parents to curtail these behaviors
and to model balanced eating and exercise. Sessions occur weekly. Parents are
instructed to avoid openly disagreeing about treatment-related issues in front of
the patient and to support the treatment team by presenting a united front
against the disorder. Clear expectations for progress are stipulated (e.g., ½- to 1-
lb weight gain per week until weight is restored), and the patient is weighed
routinely at each session. Failure to progress or medical instability (e.g., serious
or repeated electrolyte imbalances, syncope, seizures, severe bradycardia, prolonged electrocardiographic QT interval, continued weight loss) is reason for
inpatient hospitalization, preferably in a behavioral specialty program for the
treatment of eating disorders. Such programs are able to weight restore the majority of patients with anorexia nervosa, using behavioral and group therapy approaches.

Pharmacologic treatment for anorexia nervosa has proven to be a challenge, with no consistent empirical evidence supporting efficacy in promoting
weight gain, targeting eating disordered cognitions, or improving depressive or
obsessional symptoms. Few randomized controlled trials of medication interventions have been performed, and none of these were completed specifically
in children. Although some adult trials have included adolescents, published
data have not analyzed adolescent outcomes separately.

Controlled studies in adults have more commonly addressed the effect of
medication on weight restoration than on the relapse prevention phase of treatment. These studies have encountered methodological challenges specific to
this disorder. As a result of the high lethality of anorexia nervosa, ethical issues

surround use of a placebo control arm, so most pharmacologic studies have used medication as an adjunct to behavioral interventions, making it more difficult to detect a treatment effect. Because the disorder is relatively uncommon, sample sizes have tended to be small and studies underpowered. Furthermore, the ego-syntonic nature of the disorder presents significant obstacles to subject recruitment, randomization, and adherence. Patients commonly avoid treatment, refuse randomization to whichever treatment arm they perceive as more intensive, or drop out early.

Agents studied have included drugs used to treat comorbid anxiety or depression, drugs known to address rigid or idiosyncratic thought content in other disorders, and drugs known to affect weight or appetite. Early studies of antidepressants focused on tricyclics; however, these agents have rarely been used since the advent of selective serotonin reuptake inhibitors (SSRIs) because of the tricyclics' associated cardiac risks, as well as other less serious but bothersome side effects. The most extensively studied SSRI in anorexia nervosa is fluoxetine; however, overall results have been disappointing. Both a case-control longitudinal study of 33 patients (Strober et al. 1997) and a double-blind, randomized controlled study of 31 subjects found that adjunctive fluoxetine in underweight hospitalized inpatients treated in a behavioral program did not improve outcome or weight gain (Attia et al. 1998). A recent larger study of fluoxetine for relapse prevention in weight-restored patients also revealed no superiority for drug versus placebo (Walsh et al. 2006), despite an earlier study suggesting efficacy (Kaye et al. 2001). Although Caroline presents with depressive symptomatology and her mother has a history of a possible untreated depression, little empirical evidence is available to suggest that treatment with an antidepressant while Caroline is still underweight will improve her prognosis. If her mood remains low with weight restoration, a trial of an antidepressant may be warranted.

Studies of other pharmacologic agents, including cyproheptadine, zinc, lithium, tetrahydrocannabinol, naltrexone, cisapride, and recombinant growth hormone, have shown no effect or only marginal effects over placebo. Furthermore, some of these drugs are associated with serious side effects (e.g., arrhythmia, transaminitis) that negate potential usefulness. Recently, there has been growing interest in the atypical neuroleptics both to augment weight gain and to decrease eating disordered preoccupations because overvalued fear of fatness can reach near-delusional proportions in patients with anorexia nervosa. Several case reports indicate favorable responses to these agents, especially to olanzapine (see Steffen et al. 2006 for a review). At least two randomized, double-blind, controlled trials are currently in progress but have encountered difficulty in terms of patient recruitment and adherence for some of the reasons outlined above. Therefore, neuroleptics cannot be recommended at this time for the treatment of anorexia nervosa given their side-effect profile, especially in the adolescent population.

In summary, little evidence is available to guide pharmacologic interventions for anorexia nervosa. This is a behavioral condition for which behavioral treatments, especially family-based interventions, are the most effective treatment available for younger patients. Parent training is often effective in patients who are restoring weight. When weight restoration fails or when the patient is medically unstable, admission to a behavioral specialty program is the preferred course of action. The use of medication for relapse prevention remains largely uncharted and should be the focus of future randomized controlled studies. Judicious use of SSRIs may be indicated in weight-restored patients who continue to exhibit significant mood and anxiety symptoms or in patients with a strong family history of these conditions. The potential role of atypical neuroleptics in promoting weight gain or treating the cognitive disturbances that characterize the condition remains to be clarified.

Integrative Perspective

B. Timothy Walsh, M.D.
E. Blake Finkelson, B.A.

DIAGNOSTIC FORMULATION

Caroline presents with characteristic features of anorexia nervosa, including a refusal to maintain her body weight at a minimally normal weight and an intense fear of gaining weight. She exhibits a serious distortion in her view of her body, believing that weighing 99 lbs would be fine, and she has developed amenorrhea since the beginning of her illness.

Caroline exhibits a number of problems that, although not required for the diagnosis of anorexia nervosa, are commonly present in those with this eating disorder. Her multiple layers of clothing indicate significant cold intolerance, and it is likely that her body temperature is below normal. She reports hair loss and electrolyte disturbances. Her pulse and blood pressure were unusually low at an emergency room visit, and she has experienced dizziness upon standing, likely due to orthostatic hypotension.

Her history suggests that Caroline currently has the restricting type of anorexia nervosa, because she reports that she severely restricts her caloric intake but does not regularly engage in either binge eating or any form of purging behavior, such as self-induced vomiting or the misuse of laxatives or diuretics. However,

Caroline also describes recent electrolyte disturbances, which occur more commonly among those who engage in these behaviors, and she admits that she "made herself sick" for over 2 years. Therefore, the clinician should consider that Caroline may actually have the binge-eating/purging type of anorexia nervosa but that she is reluctant to admit the purging behavior (Walsh and Satir 2005).

Although numerous theories have been advanced, ranging from the psychoanalytic through the biological, the fundamental cause of anorexia nervosa remains unknown (Walsh 2003). Caroline exhibits a number of premorbid characteristics, such as competitive athleticism and perfectionism, which are likely associated with an increased risk of developing the disorder. Also, some currently unidentified genetic influences — possibly including traits such as perfectionism — likely impact an individual's risk of developing the disorder. Indeed, Caroline's history indicates that her mother struggled with her own disordered eating attitudes and behaviors and Caroline's father, a recovering alcoholic, now engages in intensive exercise. Cultural, developmental, and environmental factors presumably interact to trigger the onset of anorexia nervosa among vulnerable individuals.

The occurrence of comorbid disorders is common in anorexia nervosa. High levels of anxiety and depression are often present and are sometimes sufficiently severe to fulfill diagnostic criteria for a specific syndrome (Halmi et al. 1991). Although Caroline appears to meet criteria for major depressive disorder, her depressive symptoms did not become manifest until after the onset of her eating disorder and have always remitted at normal weight, suggesting that her mood disorder may be weight related. Caroline's ritualistic behavior with regard to food is commonly associated with anorexia nervosa but has been well described in accounts of human starvation resulting from war or privation. Although some of her compulsive behavior patterns, such as rearranging her closet, do not seem food related and may suggest a possible diagnosis of obsessive-compulsive disorder, they do not interfere with her functioning or cause distress. Therefore, the clinician may decide to assign only the diagnosis of anorexia nervosa and reserve judgment about the presence of major depressive disorder or obsessive-compulsive disorder until Caroline's nutritional status has been addressed.

DSM-IV-TR DIAGNOSIS

Axis I   307.1 Anorexia nervosa, restrictive subtype
          Rule out major depressive disorder
Axis II   Deferred
Axis III Malnutrition, amenorrhea
Axis IV   Family conflict
Axis V   Global Assessment of Functioning=50

TREATMENT RECOMMENDATIONS

INITIAL OUTPATIENT TREATMENT

During the discussion with the child and adolescent psychiatrist, Caroline's mother decided to request a 2-week emergency family medical leave from her job so she could be home full-time with Caroline, and Caroline's father agreed to spend Monday, Wednesday, and Friday evenings with Caroline. The next day, Caroline's mother made a breakfast for herself and Caroline, including cereal with whole milk and a bagel with cream cheese, and insisted that Caroline remain in the kitchen until the meal was completed. Despite Caroline's tears and anger, her mother remained firm, and after an hour Caroline finished her breakfast. This became the pattern over the next week: Caroline resisted mightily, but under her mother's consistent approach, the intensity of her protests began to wane and her weight increased 2 lbs. Caroline's father joined them for evening meals and was wholeheartedly supportive of the mother's plans. Together, they met weekly with the psychiatrist, who helped them work through problems, assured Caroline that her parents' intensive involvement was only a temporary stage of treatment, and encouraged them to continue their good work together.

After 10 days, Caroline had gained 5 lbs, and the child and adolescent psychiatrist and Caroline's pediatrician agreed that she could return to school. Her mother returned to work but continued to have breakfast and dinner with Caroline, spelled by her father several times per week, and arranged for the school nurse to have lunch with Caroline.

Although Caroline's weight continued to rise slowly, the return to school was not without problems. Caroline's teachers found her to be moody, and Caroline had trouble explaining her problem to her classmates. At the weekly meeting with the psychiatrist, Caroline's mother asked whether medication might be of use for these symptoms. The psychiatrist indicated that she was reluctant to prescribe medication at this point and explained to Caroline's parents that the available evidence suggests that antidepressant medication is not of substantial benefit for patients with anorexia nervosa, either when patients are underweight or when the drugs are used to prevent relapse (Attia et al. 1998; Walsh et al. 2006). Despite her occasional moodiness, Caroline's affect and her interaction with her parents were, on the whole, improving, as typically occurs with weight normalization (Meehan et al. 2006). The psychiatrist mentioned that there were some recent hints that atypical antipsychotic medication might assist some patients to gain weight, but definitive studies had not been reported, and, in any case, Caroline was gaining weight at a satisfactory pace (Bissada et al. 2008).

Moving Ahead

Over the next 3 months, Caroline's weight continued to rise, eventually reaching 115 lbs, and Caroline was given increasing freedom to choose her own meals. With a hint of relief, Caroline reported to her mother that she had gotten her period for the first time in months. Caroline's pediatrician and psychiatrist agreed that the intense efforts to gain weight could be relaxed. Caroline was allowed to rejoin the soccer team but with the clear understanding that any weight loss would be promptly followed by a return of the restrictions on her eating and participation in sports.

As Caroline's recovery continued, the psychiatrist began to discuss other issues with her and her parents, such as Caroline's discomfort with her father's new family and her anxieties about dating. Caroline also acknowledged that on a few occasions, she had overeaten and induced vomiting. The doctor praised Caroline's willingness to discuss these problems openly, and suggested that together they monitor these issues and attempt to address them in their regular visits. The doctor mentioned that in the event that the binge eating and vomiting became more frequent, they should discuss additional treatment interventions, such as individual cognitive-behavioral therapy (CBT) and the use of antidepressant medication. The development of full-blown bulimia nervosa sometimes occurs after individuals have recovered from anorexia nervosa, and extensive work with young adults has found that both CBT and antidepressant medication, specifically fluoxetine at 60 mg/day, can be effective (Walsh 2003).

Follow-Up

Two years after her hospital admission, Caroline had maintained her weight at about 118 lbs and was menstruating regularly. Her academic performance was solid, though not exceptional, and she was a standout on the varsity soccer team. She continued to have thoughts that she was too fat and avoided desserts, but she was able to resist the impulse to diet. She continues to see the psychiatrist every few months to review these symptoms and to discuss her plans to apply to college.

REFERENCES

Attia E, Haiman C, Walsh BT, et al: Does fluoxetine augment the inpatient treatment of anorexia nervosa? Am J Psychiatry 155:548–551, 1998

Bissada H, Tasca GA, Barber AM, et al: Olanzapine in the treatment of low body weight and obsessive thinking in women with anorexia nervosa: a randomized, double-blind, placebo-controlled trial. Am J Psychiatry 165:1281–1288, 2008

Eisler I, Dare C, Russell GFM, et al: Family and individual therapy in anorexia nervosa: a 5-year follow-up. Arch Gen Psychiatry 54:1025–1030, 1997

Eisler I, Dare C, Hodes M, et al: Family therapy for adolescent anorexia nervosa: the results of a controlled comparison of two family interventions. J Child Psychol Psychiatry 41:727–736, 2000

Eisler I, Simic M, Russell GFM, et al: A randomized controlled treatment trial of two forms of family therapy in adolescent anorexia nervosa: a five-year follow-up. J Child Psychol Psychiatry 48:552–560, 2007

Ewing JA: Detecting alcoholism: the CAGE questionnaire. JAMA 252:1905–1907, 1984

Fairburn CG, Cooper Z: The Eating Disorder Examination, 12th Edition, in Binge Eating: Nature, Assessment and Treatment. Edited by Fairburn CG, Wilson GT. New York, Guilford, 1993, pp 317–355

Garner DM, Olmsted MP, Bohr Y, et al: The Eating Attitudes Test: psychometric features and clinical correlates. Psychol Med 12:871–878, 1982

Halmi KA, Eckert E, Marchi P, et al: Comorbidity of psychiatric diagnoses in anorexia nervosa. Arch Gen Psychiatry 48:712–718, 1991

Kaye WH, Nagata T, Weltzin TE, et al: Double-blind placebo-controlled administration of fluoxetine in restricting- and restricting-purging-type anorexia nervosa. Biol Psychiatry 49:644–652, 2001

Le Grange D: Family therapy for adolescent anorexia nervosa. J Clin Psychol 5:727–740, 1999

Le Grange D, Eisler I, Dare C, et al: Evaluation of family therapy in anorexia nervosa: a pilot study. Int J Eat Disord 12:347–357, 1992

Lock J, le Grange D, Agras WS, et al: Treatment Manual for Anorexia Nervosa: A Family Based Approach. New York, Guilford, 2001

Lock J, Agras WS, Bryson S, et al: A comparison of short- and long-term family therapy for adolescent anorexia nervosa. J Am Acad Child Adolesc Psychiatry 44:632–639, 2005

Lock J, Couturier J, Agras WS: Comparison of long-term outcomes in adolescents with anorexia nervosa treated with family therapy. J Am Acad Child Adolesc Psychiatry 45:666–672, 2006

Meehan KG, Loeb KL, Roberto CA, et al: Mood change during weight restoration in anorexia nervosa. Int J Eat Disord 39:587–589, 2006

Morgan JF, Reid F, Lacey JH: The SCOFF questionnaire: assessment of a new screening tool for eating disorders. BMJ 319:1467–1468, 1999

Robin AL, Siegel PT, Koepke T, et al: Family therapy versus individual therapy for adolescent females with anorexia nervosa. J Dev Behav Pediatr 15:111–116, 1994

Robin AL, Siegel PT, Moye AW, et al: A controlled comparison of family versus individual therapy for adolescents with anorexia nervosa. J Am Acad Child Adolesc Psychiatry 38:1482–1489, 1999

Russell GFM, Szmukler GI, Dare C, et al: An evaluation of family therapy in anorexia nervosa and bulimia nervosa. Arch Gen Psychiatry 44:1047–1056, 1987

Steffen KJ, Roerig JL, Mitchell JE, et al: Emerging drugs for eating disorder treatment. Expert Opin Emerg Drugs 11:315–336, 2006

Strober M, Freeman R, DeAntonio M, et al: Does adjunctive fluoxetine influence the post-hospital course of restrictor-type anorexia nervosa? A 24-month prospective, longitudinal followup and comparison with historical controls. Psychopharmacol Bull 33:425–431, 1997

Sullivan PF: Mortality in anorexia nervosa. Am J Psychiatry 152:1073–1074, 1995

Walsh BT: Eating disorders, in Psychiatry, 2nd Edition. Edited by Tasman A, Kay J, Lieberman JA. London, Wiley, 2003, pp 1501–1518

Walsh BT: Eating disorders, in Harrison's Principles of Internal Medicine, 16th Edition. Edited by Kasper DL, Braunwald E, Fauci AS, et al. New York, McGraw-Hill, 2005, pp 430–433

Walsh BT, Satir DA: Diagnostic issues in the assessment of patients with eating disorders, in Assessment of Eating Disorders. Edited by Mitchell J, Peterson C. New York, Guilford, 2005, pp 1–16

Walsh BT, Kaplan AS, Attia E, et al: Fluoxetine after weight restoration in anorexia nervosa: a randomized controlled trial. JAMA 295:2605–2612, 2006

■ CHAPTER 10 ■

The Blinker

Tourette's Disorder

Daniel A. Gorman, M.D., F.R.C.P.C.
Bradley S. Peterson, M.D.

CASE PRESENTATION

IDENTIFYING INFORMATION

Justin is an 11-year-old who lives with his parents and his 13-year-old sister. He is in a regular sixth-grade class at the local public school.

CHIEF COMPLAINT

Justin was referred by his pediatrician for a psychiatric consultation because of repetitive behaviors and emotional distress. At the first consultation session, only Justin's parents met with the psychiatrist, and the parents sat far apart on the couch. The tension between them was immediately evident, and their manner of interacting was a forced cordiality. They described their concerns, with Justin's mother doing most of the talking.

Daniel A. Gorman, M.D., F.R.C.P.C., is Staff Psychiatrist in the Neuropsychiatry Program at The Hospital for Sick Children, and Assistant Professor in the Department of Psychiatry at the University of Toronto in Toronto, Ontario, Canada.

Bradley S. Peterson, M.D., is Suzanne Crosby Murphy Professor in Pediatric Neuropsychiatry and Director of Magnetic Resonance Imaging Research in the Department of Psychiatry at Columbia University/New York State Psychiatric Institute in New York, New York.

For complete biographical information, see "About the Contributors," p. 613.

HISTORY OF PRESENT ILLNESS

Justin's mother explained that when Justin was 6 years old, he started blinking more forcefully and frequently than usual. It was spring, and his parents thought he was having seasonal allergies. They treated him with a nonprescription allergy medication, and the exaggerated blinking improved over the next several weeks. When it returned a few months later, however, they took him to see his pediatrician, who referred him to an ophthalmologist. Although the ophthalmologist thought Justin might have a mild blepharitis, she actually saw little clinical evidence of this. Nonetheless, she treated him with a lubricant and an antibiotic cream, and the blinking improved for a couple of months before worsening again. Several months later, Justin also started sniffing frequently, which was followed by increased nose wrinkling, mouth stretching, and throat clearing. His parents took him back to his pediatrician, who performed a complete physical examination, including a detailed neurological examination. The results were normal, other than the repetitive behaviors themselves, and the pediatrician reassured the family that Justin just had some "nervous twitches" and would grow out of them.

Over the past 5 years, however, Justin's repetitive behaviors have become more numerous, frequent, and forceful. Additional behaviors have included snorting, head shaking, shoulder shrugging, and finger snapping. These behaviors usually do not interfere directly with his activities, except they slow him down when he is doing schoolwork. For example, when he reads he may lose his place because of his head shaking, and his writing is interrupted by the urge to put down his pencil and snap his fingers. Justin is often unaware that he is making the movements or noises, but sometimes he feels them coming on and can suppress them temporarily. He has also become increasingly self-conscious about them, and although he has many friends at school, a couple of boys have started to make fun of him. They imitate his blinking and call him "bobblehead" and "Miss Piggy" in reference to his head shaking and snorting, respectively.

Recently, Justin came home from school in tears. His movements and noises had been worsening over the past few months, and they had been particularly severe that day. When his mother asked him what was wrong, he shouted, "I can't live with this! I wish I was never born!" The next morning his mother called the pediatrician, who saw him later that week. The repetitive behaviors did not seem much worse to the pediatrician than at Justin's last appointment 6 months before, and again the neurological examination was otherwise normal. Because Justin seemed so distressed, however, the pediatrician referred him to a child psychiatrist.

The psychiatrist asked Justin's parents if anything else might be upsetting Justin. A long pause ensued before Justin's father finally said, "Things haven't been so good between my wife and me lately." Several months earlier, Justin's mother had learned that her husband was having an affair with a colleague at work. They have tried not to argue in front of their children, but they know the children sense that something is wrong.

When asked about his schoolwork, Justin's parents said that he has been struggling. In the past he was generally a B student, but this year he has been getting more C's and some D's. His teacher has commented that Justin often does not listen in class, and his parents find that he needs close supervision to complete his homework. He does not have trouble staying seated in a restaurant or movie theater, but he frequently gets up from doing homework to go to the bathroom or get a snack. He fidgets sometimes but is not particularly squirmy or overactive. Reading is especially challenging for him, and he often has to reread a sentence a few times to make sure he understands it.

Justin's parents did not think he had any obsessive-compulsive symptoms, but when Justin himself was interviewed in the second consultation session, he revealed that he has several. For example, when he is walking and turns one way, he feels the need to turn the opposite way "to make it even." He often re-ties his shoelaces several times so that the level of tightness is the same for both feet, and he adjusts his socks repeatedly so that they come up to the same level on his calf. He also has an intrusive thought that his parents will be killed in a car accident.

Neither Justin nor his parents expressed any other major concerns. His parents have found him to be somewhat more withdrawn over the past few months, but his eating and sleeping habits are good, and he still enjoys a variety of activities, including ice hockey, karate, watching TV, and playing video games. Other than that day when he came home from school in tears, he has not voiced thoughts of not wanting to live. He can be a bit of a worrier and needs more preparation than his sister to manage transitions, but he responds well to reassurance. He does not tend to be oppositional or defiant and has no history of aggression or conduct problems. He has not been exposed to alcohol or drugs and has no history of trauma. He has no history of psychotic symptoms.

MEDICAL HISTORY

Justin's physical health has generally been good. His parents report that between the ages of 7 and 10, he had a few episodes of strep throat, confirmed by culture, and was treated each time with antibiotics. They do not think his repetitive behaviors were particularly worse around the time of those episodes. He has asthma, for which he occasionally uses an inhaler. Otherwise, he takes no medications. His hearing and vision were both tested recently and found to be normal.

DEVELOPMENTAL HISTORY

The pregnancy with Justin was uncomplicated, but the labor was prolonged, and forceps were required. Upon delivery, Justin had some difficulty breathing and was monitored in the neonatal nursery for a couple of days before being discharged home with his parents. Justin's mother describes him as an "awesome" baby who was interactive and fed and slept well. His language and gross motor development have been normal, but his fine motor skills are weaker than his sister's, and his parents describe his handwriting as "atrocious."

SOCIAL HISTORY

Justin's parents have been married for almost 16 years. His father works for an insurance company, and his mother is a teacher. They were "college sweethearts" and married shortly after graduation, but over the years they have drifted apart emotionally, and since Justin's mother discovered the affair, they have been discussing separation. Justin's sister is described as an "overachiever" and a "hard act to follow" for Justin; she is a straight-A student, excels at sports, and is popular with her classmates. Justin is described as "less intense" than his sister and "a little sensitive," but until his tics became much worse a few months ago, he was doing reasonably well socially and academically. He makes friends easily, and his friends' parents have often commented on how polite and well behaved he is when he visits. Although his parents wish he would push himself more academically, he has always been happy to earn B's. The recent slip in his grades has discouraged him, however, and his attitude about school has deteriorated.

FAMILY HISTORY

Justin's parents initially denied any family history of psychiatric illness. On further inquiry, however, Justin's father reported that he has had a long-standing facial twitch that used to be more severe, as well as several "habits" such as blowing on his fingers, biting his lips, and cracking his knuckles. In addition, Justin's mother describes herself as an "anxious person" and a "perfectionist," and she has a number of counting rituals and checking behaviors.

MENTAL STATUS EXAMINATION

On mental status examination, Justin was shy but cooperative. Although he exhibited frequent blinking and head shaking, as well as occasional throat clearing and snorting, he was not generally restless or fidgety. His affect was initially anxious and constricted, but he became more relaxed and expressive as the interview progressed, smiling and laughing at appropriate moments. He described his mood as usually "normal," except he feels "sad" when classmates tease him. Sometimes his repetitive behaviors bother him so much that he wishes he were dead, but he has never thought seriously about killing himself. His thought content was notable for themes of low self-esteem; he feels that he is "weird" and "bad at school." He also endorsed some obsessive-compulsive symptoms, as described previously.

COMMENTARIES

Psychotherapeutic Perspective

Douglas W. Woods, Ph.D.
Christine A. Conelea, M.S.

DIAGNOSTIC FORMULATION

Justin's symptom presentation is consistent with an Axis I diagnosis of Tourette's disorder, which is characterized by the presence of multiple motor and one or more vocal tics for at least 1 year. Because of the elevated comorbidity rates found in those with Tourette's disorder, additional diagnostic work should be done to assess and differentially diagnose attention-deficit/hyperactivity disorder (ADHD), obsessive-compulsive disorder (OCD), and major depression.

Justin meets DSM-IV-TR criteria for Tourette's disorder given his multiple motor tics (i.e., blinking, mouth stretching, head shaking, shoulder shrugging, and finger snapping) and vocal tics (i.e., sniffing, throat clearing, and snorting), at least some of which have been present for more than 12 months. Justin's presentation is characteristic of Tourette's disorder, with an onset between ages 4 and 6, a changing tic repertoire, and symptom worsening through pre- to mid-adolescence (Leckman et al. 1999). Justin also describes a premonitory urge, which is an unpleasant feeling or sensation preceding a tic that frequently occurs in those with Tourette's disorder. The Yale Global Tic Severity Scale (Leckman et al. 1989) and the Premonitory Urge for Tics Scale (Woods et al. 2005) would be useful to assess the severity of Justin's Tourette's disorder and premonitory urge, respectively.

Various factors may have contributed to the onset or maintenance of Justin's Tourette's disorder. Suggestive of a strong genetic component, Justin's father appears to have an undiagnosed tic disorder, and his mother may have OCD (see Pauls 2003 for a review). Given the lack of documented temporal correspondence between the repeated strep infections and tic onset/exacerba-

---

Douglas W. Woods, Ph.D., is Associate Professor and Director of Clinical Training at the University of Wisconsin–Milwaukee in Milwaukee, Wisconsin.

Christine A. Conelea, M.S., is a graduate student in the the Clinical Psychology Doctoral Program at University of Wisconsin–Milwaukee in Milwaukee, Wisconsin.

For complete biographical information, see "About the Contributors," p. 613.

tion, a diagnosis of pediatric autoimmune neuropsychiatric disorder associated with streptococcal infection (PANDAS) is unlikely (Church et al. 2003).

In addition to the potential etiological factors, a number of variables may be responsible for Justin's current symptom exacerbation. First, given that stress often makes tics worse (Bornstein et al. 1990), the relational difficulties between Justin and his parents, the marital stress between Justin's parents, and the negative school environment stemming from peer teasing and declining school performance may contribute to tic exacerbation. Second, it is possible that the tics themselves are being strengthened by the reduction of the aversive premonitory urge following tic occurrences. This negative reinforcement hypothesis is believed to maintain, in part, some tics (Himle et al. 2006).

Efforts should also be made to clarify possible comorbid diagnoses. Justin reported a number of repetitive behaviors (e.g., evening up, adjusting socks, retying shoelaces) that could be classified as either complex tics related to Tourette's disorder or compulsions related to OCD. The distinction between the two is not always clear, but generally, repetitive behaviors preceded by either physiological signs of anxiety or specific aversive cognitions (e.g., "something bad will happen to me") are more consistent with an OCD diagnosis, whereas repetitive behaviors preceded by a vague tension or somatic sensation are more consistent with a Tourette's disorder diagnosis (Miguel et al. 1997). For example, if Justin's repetitive behaviors are preceded by the intrusive thoughts of harm coming to his parents, the symptoms may be consistent with an OCD diagnosis.

Justin appeared to be exhibiting dysphoric mood, although it did not appear to have risen to the level of a major depression diagnosis. Given the temporal relationships, a variety of psychosocial factors likely contribute to the negative mood, including parental marital problems, falling grades, teasing because of tics, frustration with the uncontrollability of the tics, and possible problems with OCD.

Symptoms of ADHD were suggested, but the clinician should consider how the tics, possible OCD symptoms, and potential mood concerns may be contributing to Justin's difficulties in sustaining attention while listening in class, reading, and doing homework. The clinician also should assess for a potential undiagnosed learning disability, which often co-occurs in individuals with Tourette's disorder.

DSM-IV-TR DIAGNOSIS

Axis I   307.23 Tourette's disorder
          Rule out ADHD
          Rule out obsessive-compulsive disorder
          Rule out major depressive disorder

Axis II   None
Axis III   None
Axis IV   Discord with parents
           Parental marital problems
           Academic problems
           Discord with classmates
Axis V   Global Assessment of Functioning=61 (current)

TREATMENT RECOMMENDATIONS

Assuming that Justin has only a Tourette's disorder diagnosis, treatment would follow a three-pronged approach: psychoeducation about Tourette's disorder, implementation of strategies to reduce tic-exacerbating events in Justin's environment, and incorporation of specific methods to successfully manage tics. Psychoeducation about the phenomenology, etiology, onset, course, and comorbid conditions associated with Tourette's disorder would be provided to Justin and his parents. Such education may be useful in decreasing family stress about the nature of the disorder, normalizing Justin's experiences to some extent, and providing hope for successful management.

Following a comprehensive behavioral assessment of how various environmental factors impact Justin's tic expression, efforts to reduce the impact of tic-exacerbating events in Justin's environment would be implemented. Based on the case description, interventions would include family therapy to overcome communication difficulties between Justin and his parents, marital therapy to decrease the stress-inducing marital conflicts, teacher and peer education about Tourette's disorder to decrease negative perceptions and improve social functioning (Woods et al. 2003), stress management training to help Justin cope with stress-inducing situations, and elimination of any potentially rewarding social consequences Justin gets as a result of tics (e.g., removal from teasing peers or of a difficult homework assignment, statements of concern following a particularly noticeable tic).

The final element of treatment would involve specific tic management procedures. Given the mild to moderate nature of Justin's tics, we would begin with a course of habit reversal training. Habit reversal training is a type of behavioral therapy that has been shown to be effective for reducing tics in several small randomized controlled trials (see Himle et al. 2006 for a review) and has been manualized (Woods 2001). Habit reversal training involves awareness training, competing response training, and social support training. Awareness training consists of describing the tic and early warning signs of tic occurrence (e.g., sensations or behaviors preceding a tic), detecting tic occurrences, and identifying high-risk tic situations (Woods 2001). Competing response training consists of teaching the child to engage in another behavior for a period of time (i.e., 1 minute) contingent on tic occurrence or associated early warning signs. Social support training involves teaching a significant other in the patient's life (usually a parent in the case of a child) to praise the successful use of competing response exercises and to prompt the child to use a competing response when such a response is not implemented upon a tic occurrence.

Should behavioral therapy be ineffective or only partially effective at reducing tic occurrences, we would refer the patient for a medication evaluation. Likewise, if Justin's tics were substantially more severe, such that he was at risk of injuring himself or others, or if he were avoiding social situations due to the tics, a medication referral would be recommended prior to behavior therapy.

Psychopharmacologic Perspective

Barbara J. Coffey, M.D., M.S.

DIAGNOSTIC FORMULATION

In summary, Justin is an 11-year-old boy with a 5-year history of multiple motor and vocal tics, consistent with a diagnosis of Tourette's disorder. In addition, he has a history of inattention in school, fidgetiness, restlessness, and difficulty completing homework assignments, which is suggestive of ADHD. He has repetitive behaviors, such as redoing, intrusive thoughts, and a need for symmetry/evening up, which are suggestive of OCD; because time spent on and/or level of distress about these behaviors is not specified in the history, it is not clear whether Justin would meet criteria for the full disorder or a subthreshold condition, either of which is common in clinically referred youth with Tourette's disorder (Coffey et al. 2000b). Other symptoms of concern include difficulty with reading, weak fine motor skills, and poor handwriting, which raise the possibility of a reading disorder and/or developmental coordination disorder. Justin's tendency to worry suggests the possibility of a generalized anxiety disorder. Finally, Justin is described as somewhat withdrawn in the past few

Barbara J. Coffey, M.D., M.S., is Director of the Institute for Tourette and Tic Disorders at the New York University Child Study Center, and Associate Professor in the Department of Child and Adolescent Psychiatry at the New York University School of Medicine in New York, New York (for complete biographical information, see "About the Contributors," p. 613).

months, with evidence of significant distress and sadness about the social impact of his tics, and perhaps about the conflict and distance between his parents, as evidenced by his statement that he wishes he were dead. Thus, an adjustment disorder with depressed mood or mixed anxiety and depressed mood should also be considered in the differential diagnosis.

From a biopsychosocial perspective, Justin's present illness may have several biological contributors. Given the protracted labor, forceps delivery, and early respiratory distress, Justin's early neurological development could have been rendered vulnerable, contributing to the development of Tourette's disorder; evidence suggests that prenatal and perinatal factors such as birth trauma can influence the onset and severity of tics (Leckman et al. 1990). The family history of probable Tourette's disorder in the father, and an anxiety disorder, possibly OCD, in the mother suggests a genetic diathesis for the development of a tic disorder or Tourette's disorder in Justin (Pauls 2003). From an epidemiological perspective, as reported in several studies, Justin is presenting at a time in life when Tourette's disorder severity is at its peak: around age 10–11 years (Leckman et al. 1998). From a general medical perspective, Justin's history of asthma and possible seasonal allergy could manifest in signs of throat clearing, sniffing, and coughing, which could also contribute to the tic symptoms. Finally, given no reported increase in repetitive behaviors with laboratory-documented streptococcal infection, a diagnosis of PANDAS is unlikely.

Several important psychosocial factors contribute to the formulation. From the psychological perspective, history indicates that Justin is a typically developing 11-year-old, with many friendships, age-appropriate interests, solid intelligence, and good academic performance in the past. However, despite his strengths and apparent coping abilities to date, Justin is now showing emotional distress and loss of self-esteem as a result of problems in three areas: social (e.g., being teased by peers), academic (e.g., difficulty completing schoolwork), and emotional (e.g., parents' marital problems).

DSM-IV-TR DIAGNOSIS

Axis I   307.23 Tourette's disorder

300.3 Obsessive-compulsive disorder, full versus subthreshold

314.00 ADHD, predominantly inattentive type

315.4 Developmental coordination disorder

Rule out generalized anxiety disorder

Rule out adjustment disorder with depressed mood or mixed anxiety and depressed mood

Rule out reading disorder

Axis II   None present

Axis III   Streptococcal pharyngitis, past, in remission
           Asthma
           Rule out seasonal/environmental allergies
Axis IV   Level of psychosocial stressors is moderate to high: social issues (i.e.,
           teasing by peers); decline in academic performance; parental con-
           flict, including extramarital affair
Axis V   Global Assessment of Functioning=55 (current)

SUGGESTED DIAGNOSTIC ASSESSMENT TOOLS

Instruments that can facilitate assessment of level of severity of Justin's primary
symptoms:

1. *Tics:* The Yale Global Tic Severity Scale (Leckman et al. 1989) is a clinician-administered continuous scale that includes measures of domains of
   tic number, frequency, intensity, complexity, and interference, as well as a
   tic-related impairment scale.
2. *OCD symptoms:* The Children's Yale-Brown Obsessive Compulsive Scale
   (Scahill et al. 1997) is a clinician-rated measure of obsessive-compulsive
   symptoms.
3. *ADHD:* The Swanson, Nolan, and Pelham Rating Scale, 4th Edition
   (SNAP-IV; Swanson 1992), is a rating scale for ADHD based on DSM-IV
   symptoms, as rated by parent or teacher.
4. *Anxiety:* The Multidimensional Anxiety Scale for Children (March et al.
   1997) is a validated, multidimensional self-report of anxiety symptoms.
5. *Depressed mood:* The Children's Depression Rating Scale—Revised
   (Poznanski et al. 1985) is a clinician-rated scale used as a screening and
   diagnostic tool and a measure of severity of depression in children.

TREATMENT RECOMMENDATIONS

Tourette's disorder and associated comorbid disorders are optimally treated
with a multimodal treatment approach, using a combination of psychoeducation, parent guidance and support, consultation to the teacher(s), and pharmacologic and psychotherapeutic interventions (Jankovic 2001).

Justin and his parents need to be educated regarding the nature, phenomenology, comorbidity (particularly with OCD and ADHD), and expected
course and outcome of Tourette's disorder. Family referral to the Tourette Syndrome Association, a nationally based advocacy, research, and support group,
is indicated, as it is for all newly diagnosed children and families.

An additional evaluation that might help to clarify the differential diagnosis
would be a neuropsychological screen to rule out a reading disorder or other

processing disorder, given Justin's difficulty with reading and his recent academic decline. Neuropsychological testing could also provide information on whether Justin might have evidence of impairment in executive functioning, given his difficulty completing homework assignments and his distractibility.

From the pharmacologic perspective, the only medications labeled with an indication for Tourette's disorder are haloperidol and pimozide. However, given their relative risk, particularly in long-term treatment, for significant adverse effects such as tardive dyskinesia, cognitive blunting, and weight gain, they are usually not recommended for first-line use in patients with mild to moderate tic symptoms. Instead, first-line treatment of mild to moderate Tourette's disorder is usually with an α-adrenergic agonist, such as clonidine or guanfacine. Substantial evidence supports their efficacy in the treatment of Tourette's and chronic tic disorders, despite the fact they are prescribed off-label (Scahill et al. 2006). Clonidine or guanfacine would have the additional benefit of reducing Justin's restlessness and fidgetiness. The primary adverse effect is sedation, which can be mitigated by initiating treatment with low doses and slow titration.

Other pharmacologic options to consider, assuming that the diagnosis of inattentive-type ADHD is confirmed, include the addition of a stimulant to the α-adrenergic agonist to address the selective vigilance component, because the α-adrenergic agents do not target this symptom. One study demonstrated that a combination of methylphenidate and clonidine was beneficial in reducing both ADHD symptoms and tics in children ages 7–14 with ADHD and chronic tic disorders (Tourette's Syndrome Study Group 2002). If this strategy is not effective, consideration of a switch to atomoxetine should be given, because evidence indicates that this selective norepinephrine reuptake inhibitor is also efficacious in reducing both ADHD and tics in youth with ADHD and chronic tics (Allen et al. 2005).

Psychotherapeutic interventions to be considered include behavioral intervention therapy for tics (also known as habit reversal therapy), which is supported by a growing evidence base as having efficacy in treatment of tic disorders (Wilhelm et al. 2003). Justin's parents should also be offered a couples evaluation and potential therapy to address their marital conflicts, which are undoubtedly having an impact on Justin.

Finally, consultation with Justin's teacher is indicated, so as to develop and implement an individualized education program tailored to Justin's specific needs upon completion of the neuropsychological testing. At the very least, Justin needs extended time on homework and classroom assignments to address his repeating behaviors.

Integrative Perspective

Daniel A. Gorman, M.D., F.R.C.P.C.
Bradley S. Peterson, M.D.

DIAGNOSTIC FORMULATION

Justin's repetitive behaviors have a number of features that are characteristic of tics and distinguish them from other types of abnormal movements. Tics are sudden, rapid, recurrent, nonrhythmic, stereotyped movements or vocalizations that appear purposeless. In contrast with tremor, choreoathetosis, ballismus, and myoclonus, tics may be voluntarily suppressed for brief periods. Like many older children and adults who have tic disorders, Justin sometimes experiences a premonitory urge—that is, a feeling of tension or discomfort that precedes the tic and is located in the body part where the tic occurs. He can resist this urge temporarily, but eventually he must give in to it by performing the tic. Other abnormal movements that can be voluntarily suppressed for brief periods include akathisia, stereotypies, and compulsions, but Justin's history does not suggest any of these conditions. Akathisia is a feeling of motor restlessness that is usually located in the lower extremities and often leads to frequent pacing, whereas tics generally first appear in the face, head, and shoulders before sometimes progressing in a rostral-caudal pattern. Stereotypies tend to be more rhythmic than tics and are typically both self-stimulating and anxiety reducing. Compulsions are of much longer duration than tics, appear more purposeful and goal directed, and are often performed in response to an obsessive thought. The diagnosis of a tic disorder is further supported by Justin's neurological examination, which is normal except for the repetitive behaviors themselves.

Once the repetitive behaviors are identified as tics, the next step in diagnosis is to determine the type of tic disorder. Justin has a history of multiple motor tics (blinking, nose wrinkling, mouth stretching, head shaking, shoulder shrugging, finger snapping) and vocal tics (sniffing, throat clearing, snorting), with onset before age 18 years. Because his tics occur many times per day and have persisted for more than 1 year without a tic-free period of more than 3 consecutive months, they are considered chronic. A history of chronic motor *or* vocal tics, *but not both*, suggests a diagnosis of chronic motor or vocal tic disorder, whereas a history of chronic motor *and* vocal tics, as in Justin's case, suggests a diagnosis of Tourette's disorder. Finally, medical evaluation by Justin's pediatrician revealed no evidence of a general medical condition that might be responsible for his tics, and Justin has not been taking any medications or using other substances that could be causing them. Thus, Justin meets full DSM-IV-TR criteria for Tourette's disorder.

In contrast with DSM-IV criteria, DSM-IV-TR criteria for Tourette's disorder no longer require that the disturbance cause marked distress or significant impairment in functioning. Indeed, many individuals who have Tourette's disorder are not bothered by the tics themselves, although comorbid conditions may cause them more problems. Justin's tics, however, have been distressing and impairing. They have interfered with his ability to complete schoolwork and contributed to social difficulties, such as being teased by peers. His self-esteem has suffered, and he has even had passive suicidal thoughts.

Family and twin studies indicate that Tourette's disorder has a strong genetic basis and is related to chronic motor or vocal tic disorder and OCD. It is not surprising, therefore, that Justin's father has a history of a chronic facial tic as well as some tic-related habits, and that Justin's mother has a number of obsessive-compulsive and other anxiety symptoms. In addition to Justin's genetic vulnerability, however, epigenetic and environmental factors contributed to the phenotypic expression of his tics (Spessot and Peterson 2006). Tourette's disorder is up to nine times more common in males than in females, likely because of neuroendocrine factors. In addition, Justin has a history of perinatal complications and multiple group A β-hemolytic streptococcal infections, both of which have been associated with Tourette's disorder. Psychosocial stressors also appear to affect tic severity, at least in the short term, and the recent worsening of Justin's tics may be related to the tension in his parents' marriage.

A majority of individuals who present clinically with Tourette's disorder have one or more comorbid conditions, particularly ADHD, OCD, and learning disorders. Justin's parents and teacher are concerned about Justin's difficulty paying attention, but this problem could have several possible sources, and further assessment is required to narrow the differential diagnosis. One possibility is that Justin is distracted by his tics or by his efforts to suppress them. Second, Justin may have primary attentional difficulties consistent with ADHD, predominantly inattentive type, and this can be evaluated further with standardized instruments such as the SNAP-IV completed by his parents and teacher (Swanson 1992). Third, Justin's obsessive-compulsive symptoms may be interfering with task completion; for example, his tendency to reread sentences several times may in fact represent a compulsion. Finally, Justin's inattention may be related to a specific learning disorder, which can be determined only by conducting a detailed psychoeducational assessment; this would include at least cognitive testing with the Wechsler Intelligence Scale for Children, 4th Edition (Wechsler 2003), as well as academic testing in reading, spelling, written expression, and mathematics.

DSM-IV-TR DIAGNOSIS

Axis I   307.23 Tourette's disorder
              Rule out ADHD, predominantly inattentive type
              Rule out obsessive-compulsive disorder
              Rule out learning disorder
Axis II   No diagnosis
Axis III   Asthma
Axis IV   Parents' marital problems
              Academic problems
              Teasing by classmates
Axis V   Global Assessment of Functioning=60 (current)

TREATMENT RECOMMENDATIONS

Justin and his parents should be educated about Tourette's disorder, with particular emphasis on the involuntary nature of tics, the natural course of the disorder (Coffey et al. 2000a), and the common comorbidities (Gaze et al. 2006). Because tics are involuntary and can be suppressed only temporarily, Justin's parents and other caregivers should avoid telling him to stop his tics. Rather, the tics should be viewed as a form of individual variation and generally ignored. The natural course of Tourette's disorder, as well as chronic motor or vocal tic disorder, is that the tics typically have their onset around age 5–6 years and gradually worsen during middle childhood, reaching peak severity at age 10–11 years on average. During adolescence, however, most individuals with a chronic tic disorder experience a substantial improvement in their tics, such that by early adulthood, the tics are mild or have disappeared altogether. Only a minority of patients continue to experience moderate or severe tics into adulthood. Superimposed on this long-term course is a waxing and waning of tics over time scales ranging from minutes to months.

Treating tics with medication is indicated when the tics themselves are causing significant distress or impairment in academic, social, or vocational functioning. Justin is at the age when tics are typically at their worst, and knowing that they are likely to improve on their own over the next decade may influence the clinician and family to hold off on using medication to suppress them. Moreover, providing information about Tourette's disorder and implementing psychosocial interventions to support Justin's self-esteem may relieve his distress associated with the tics and obviate the need for medication. If these measures are insufficient, however, then treatment with an α-adrenergic agonist (clonidine or guanfacine) could be considered. Atypical and typical neuroleptics are likely to bring about greater improvement in tics, but because of their more serious adverse effects, they are reserved for individuals whose tics are markedly distressing or impairing or have not improved sufficiently with an α-adrenergic agonist (Scahill et al. 2006).

Comorbid conditions often cause more distress and impairment than the tics themselves and should be addressed accordingly. Furthermore, although tics are likely to subside during adolescence, ADHD and especially OCD symptoms may become even more impairing over time. Long-term monitoring is therefore essential, even when the tics improve. If further evaluation of Justin supports a diagnosis of ADHD, predominantly inattentive type, then treating him with a stimulant should be considered. Because of their efficacy and safety profiles, stimulants are considered the first-line medication treatment for ADHD in individuals with or without tics (Pliszka et al. 2006). Although stimulants may exacerbate tics in certain individuals with ADHD and a tic disorder, several studies have found no group differences in tic exacerbation between patients treated with stimulants and those who received placebo (Scahill et al. 2006). If Justin's tics do worsen with stimulants, however, appropriate alternatives include α-adrenergic agonists, atomoxetine, bupropion, and tricyclic antidepressants. The α-adrenergic agonists generally do not improve inattentive symptoms, but they are helpful for hyperactive-impulsive symptoms as well as tics. In addition, the combination of an α-adrenergic agonist and a stimulant was found to be more effective for ADHD symptoms than either medication alone in children with both ADHD and tics (Tourette's Syndrome Study Group 2002).

To address Justin's obsessive-compulsive symptoms, the clinician could consider cognitive-behavioral therapy or treatment with a selective serotonin reuptake inhibitor (SSRI). Both treatments, particularly when used together, have been shown to be effective in children with OCD (Pediatric OCD Treatment Study Team 2004), although an SSRI used alone may be less effective for pediatric OCD in the presence of a comorbid tic disorder (March et al. 2007). Any learning difficulties that Justin is found to have should be addressed with appropriate educational interventions at school, often formalized in an individualized education program. Finally, because tension between Justin's parents is having a negative influence on family functioning, as well as on Justin's emotional well-being and possibly his tics, marital or family therapy should be recommended.

REFERENCES

Allen AJ, Kurlan RM, Gilbert DL, et al: Atomoxetine treatment in children and adolescents with ADHD and comorbid tic disorders. Neurology 65:1941–1949, 2005

Bornstein RA, Stefl ME, Hammond L: A survey of Tourette syndrome patients and their families: the 1987 Ohio Tourette Survey. J Neuropsychiatry Clin Neurosci 2:275–281, 1990

Church AJ, Dale RC, Lees AJ, et al: Tourette's syndrome: a cross sectional study to examine the PANDAS hypothesis. J Neurol Neurosurg Psychiatry 74:601–607, 2003

Coffey BJ, Biederman J, Geller DA, et al: The course of Tourette's disorder: a literature review. Harv Rev Psychiatry 8:192–198, 2000a

Coffey BJ, Biederman J, Spencer T, et al: Informativeness of structured diagnostic interviews in the identification of Tourette's disorder in referred youth. J Nerv Ment Dis 188:583–588, 2000b

Gaze C, Kepley HO, Walkup JT: Co-occurring psychiatric disorder in children and adolescents with Tourette syndrome. J Child Neurol 21:657–664, 2006

Himle MB, Woods DW, Piacentini JC, et al: Brief review of habit reversal training for Tourette syndrome. J Child Neurol 21:719–725, 2006

Jankovic J: Tourette's syndrome. N Engl J Med 345:1184–1192, 2001

Leckman JF, Riddle MA, Hardin MT, et al: The Yale Global Tic Severity Scale: initial testing of a clinician-rated scale of tic severity. J Am Acad Child Adolesc Psychiatry 28:566–573, 1989

Leckman JF, Dolnansky ES, Hardin MT, et al: Perinatal factors in the expression of Tourette's syndrome: an exploratory study. J Am Acad Child Adolesc Psychiatry 29:220–226, 1990

Leckman JF, Zhang H, Vitale A, et al: Course of tic severity in Tourette syndrome: the first two decades. Pediatrics 102:14–19, 1998

Leckman JF, King RA, Cohen DJ: Tics and tic disorders, in Tourette's Syndrome—Tics, Obsessions, Compulsions: Developmental Psychopathology and Clinical Care. Edited by Leckman JF, Cohen DJ. Hoboken, NJ, Wiley, 1999, pp 23–42

March JS, Parker JD, Sullivan K, et al: The Multidimensional Anxiety Scale for Children (MASC): factor structure, reliability, and validity. J Am Acad Child Adolesc Psychiatry 36:554–565, 1997

March JS, Franklin ME, Leonard H, et al: Tics moderate treatment outcome with sertraline but not cognitive-behavior therapy in pediatric obsessive-compulsive disorder. Biol Psychiatry 61:344–347, 2007

Miguel EC, Baer L, Coffey BJ, et al: Phenomenological differences appearing with repetitive behaviors in obsessive-compulsive disorder and Gilles de la Tourette's syndrome. Br J Psychiatry 170:140–145, 1997

Pauls DL: An update on the genetics of Gilles de la Tourette syndrome. J Psychosom Res 55:7–12, 2003

Pediatric OCD Treatment Study Team: Cognitive-behavior therapy, sertraline, and their combination for children and adolescents with obsessive-compulsive disorder: the Pediatric OCD Treatment Study (POTS) randomized controlled trial. JAMA 292:1969–1976, 2004

Pliszka SR, Crismon ML, Hughes CW, et al; Texas Consensus Conference Panel on Pharmacotherapy of Childhood Attention Deficit Hyperactivity Disorder: The Texas Children's Medication Algorithm Project: revision of the algorithm for pharmacotherapy of attention-deficit/hyperactivity disorder. J Am Acad Child Adolesc Psychiatry 45:642–657, 2006

Poznanski EO, Freeman LN, Mokros H: Children's Depression Rating Scale—Revised. Psychopharmacol Bull 21:979–989, 1985

Scahill L, Riddle MA, McSwiggin-Hardin M, et al: Children's Yale-Brown Obsessive Compulsive Scale: reliability and validity. J Am Acad Child Adolesc Psychiatry 36:844–852, 1997

Scahill L, Erenberg G, Berlin CM Jr, et al: Contemporary assessment and pharmacotherapy of Tourette syndrome. NeuroRx 3:192–206, 2006

Spessot AL, Peterson BS: Tourette syndrome: a multifactorial, developmental psychopathology, in Manual of Developmental Psychopathology, 2nd Edition, Vol 3. Edited by Cicchetti D, Cohen DJ. New York, Wiley, 2006, pp 436–469

Swanson JM: School-Based Assessments and Interventions for ADD Students. Irvine, CA, KC Publications, 1992

Tourette's Syndrome Study Group: Treatment of ADHD in children with tics: a randomized controlled trial. Neurology 58:527–536, 2002

Wechsler D: The Wechsler Intelligence Scale for Children, 4th Edition. San Antonio, TX, Psychological Corporation, 2003

Wilhelm S, Deckersbach T, Coffey BJ, et al: Habit reversal versus supportive therapy for Tourette's disorder: a randomized controlled trial. Am J Psychiatry 160:1175–1177, 2003

Woods DW: Habit reversal treatment manual for tic disorders, in Tic Disorders, Trichotillomania and Other Repetitive Disorders: Behavioral Approaches to Analysis and Treatment. Edited by Woods DW, Miltenberger RG. Boston, MA, Kluwer Academic, 2001, pp 97–132

Woods DW, Koch M, Miltenberger RG: The impact of tic severity on the effects of peer education about Tourette's syndrome. J Dev Phys Disabil 15:67–78, 2003

Woods DW, Piacentini J, Himle MB, et al: Premonitory Urge for Tics Scale (PUTS): initial psychometric results and examination of the premonitory urge phenomenon in youths with tic disorders. J Dev Behav Pediatr 26:397–403, 2005

■ CHAPTER 11 ■

She Never Falls Asleep

Disordered Sleep in an Adolescent

Ronald E. Dahl, M.D.
Allison G. Harvey, Ph.D.

CASE PRESENTATION

IDENTIFYING INFORMATION

Kim is a 15-year-old female currently in tenth grade attending a large public high school. She is the oldest of three siblings and lives with both parents and her younger siblings in a city apartment.

CHIEF COMPLAINT

Kim complains of an inability to sleep.

HISTORY OF PRESENT ILLNESS

Since childhood, Kim has been anxious and "prone to worry." The presenting complaint is a multiple-year history of difficulty falling asleep. The sleep problem has become significantly worse over the past 2 years, beginning in the fall of her freshman year. Over the past few months, the problem has intensified still further, and over the past 2 weeks, she has missed multiple days of school

Ronald E. Dahl, M.D., is Staunton Professor of Psychiatry and Pediatrics and Professor of Psychology at the University of Pittsburgh in Pittsburgh, Pennsylvania.

Allison G. Harvey, Ph.D., is Associate Professor of Clinical Psychology and Director of the Sleep and Psychological Disorders Laboratory at the University of California, Berkeley.

For complete biographical information, see "About the Contributors," p. 613.

and experienced increasingly negative affect (especially feelings of frustration and hopelessness about the sleep problems).

Kim's sleep problem started after a summer holiday in which Kim adopted a schedule of going to bed at 2:00 A.M. and waking at noon or 1:00 P.M. On returning to school in the fall, she tried to revert to a 10:00 P.M. bedtime but found that she would lie awake for 3–4 hours, finally falling asleep at 1:00–1:30 A.M. While trying to get to sleep, Kim experienced considerable anxiety, distress, and worry. Her worries included concerns that insufficient sleep would make it difficult to concentrate at school the next day and would have a negative effect on her appearance (looking tired); she also worried about which of her friends really liked her and whether the boy she secretly liked thought badly about her and would never ask her out. During her ninth-grade academic year, Kim never really managed to establish a regular sleep-wake schedule.

The following summer, Kim reverted back to the 2:00 A.M. to noon sleep-wake schedule and was much happier and also noticed she was a bit less worried. However, 1 week before the new school year commenced, the problems recurred and seemed, if anything, of greater intensity than the previous year. She was increasingly worried about the consequences of not being able to sleep (e.g., that she would not be able to concentrate at school and that she would look tired and unattractive). In addition, she worried that the academic demands of the next grade would be more difficult and that her high school grades would not allow her to get into college. She was often unable to get to sleep until 3:00 A.M. Once asleep, however, she slept deeply.

Kim presented for treatment 4 weeks into the new school year. Daily sleep diaries kept for 14 days indicated a difference between her weekday and weekend sleep-wake patterns. Although she reported that she aims to get into bed at 9:30 P.M. on school nights, she often does not get into bed until 11:30 P.M. Kim reported that she hates lying in bed awake because of the associated anxiety and worry, so she avoids bedtime by chatting to her friends over the Internet or via her cell phone and text messages. She eventually falls asleep between midnight and 2:00 A.M. To catch the school bus at 6:45 A.M., she needs to wake at 6:00 A.M. She has considerable difficulty getting up at this time and reported falling asleep in classes and having difficulty concentrating at school. On several occasions, she has missed school because of difficulty getting up.

Kim and her parents have seen multiple doctors and specialists and tried a wide range of remedies, including melatonin, relaxation exercises, and an herbal remedy. At one point, the pediatrician tried a prescription for clonidine to be given at bedtime. Except for transient periods of improvement, none of the treatment approaches have made a significant impact on the problem.

To cope with her daytime tiredness, Kim started to drink coffee last year when she arrived home from school so she could complete her homework.

Past Psychiatric History

Kim has a history consistent with generalized anxiety disorder but has not been diagnosed previously.

Substance Abuse History

Kim has no substance abuse history.

Medical History

Kim has a history of medically unexplained bouts of abdominal pain.

Developmental History

Kim was a shy and anxious child. She has a history of separation anxiety when starting school and difficulty making friends in some new social situations.

Social History

Kim has missed several days of school and been tardy multiple times from oversleeping in the morning. Her parents both left school at age 16, so they place a strong emphasis on academic achievement. They have always stressed the importance of their children doing well in school and hold clear expectations regarding college and beyond.

Family History

Kim's father and maternal grandmother have had depression, and her mother has been treated for panic disorder.

Mental Status Examination

Kim is poised and bright but is noticeably anxious and tired.

COMMENTARIES

Psychotherapeutic Perspective

Jodi A. Mindell, Ph.D., C.B.S.M.

DIAGNOSTIC FORMULATION

Insomnia is relatively common in adolescents. Prevalence rates for insomnia in adolescents range from 6% to 39%. In a study of adolescents in the United Kingdom, France, Germany, and Spain, Ohayon et al. (2000) found that 4% had met DSM-IV criteria for insomnia in the past 30 days. Of these adolescents, approximately half were designated as having primary insomnia, 27% had insomnia related to a psychiatric condition, 12% had insomnia associated with substance use, and 7% had insomnia related to a medical condition. In a more recent study of over 1,000 adolescents (ages 13–16 years) in the United States, utilizing DSM-IV-TR criteria, Johnson et al. (2006) found a lifetime prevalence of primary insomnia of 10.7%, with a median age at onset of 11 years. In addition, 52.8% reported having a comorbid psychiatric condition.

Difficulty initiating or maintaining sleep is the hallmark feature of insomnia. Kim appears to meet the DSM-IV-TR diagnostic criteria for primary insomnia, because 1) she has a predominant complaint of difficulty initiating or maintaining sleep for at least 1 month; 2) the sleep disturbance and associated daytime fatigue are causing her clinically significant distress and school impairment; 3) although she is anxious, the sleep disturbance does not appear to be occurring exclusively during the course of another mental disorder, in this case generalized anxiety disorder; and 4) the sleep disturbance is not due to the direct physiological effects of a substance (although drug testing may be appropriate as a rule-out for an adolescent patient) or a general medical condition.

The one diagnostic criterion that Kim may not meet is that the sleep disturbance must *not* occur exclusively during the course of a circadian rhythm sleep disorder. Kim very likely has a circadian rhythm sleep disorder, namely delayed sleep phase type. The DSM-IV-TR criteria for a circadian rhythm

Jodi A. Mindell, Ph.D., C.B.S.M., is Professor of Psychology at Saint Joseph's University, Professor of Pediatrics at the University of Pennsylvania School of Medicine, and Associate Director of the Sleep Center at The Children's Hospital of Philadelphia in Philadelphia, Pennsylvania (for complete biographical information, see "About the Contributors," p. 613).

sleep disorder include "a persistent or recurrent pattern of sleep disruption leading to excessive sleepiness or insomnia that is due to a mismatch between the sleep-wake schedule required by a person's environment and his or her circadian sleep-wake pattern," as well as criteria 2 and 4 listed above. In addition, delayed sleep phase type requires "a persistent pattern of late sleep onset and late awakening time, with an inability to fall asleep and awaken at a desired earlier time." This sleep disturbance is quite common in adolescents, affecting approximately 7% of teenagers, given the commonly experienced phase delay that occurs postpuberty (American Academy of Sleep Medicine 2005).

Clinically, an easy way to differentiate whether an individual has primary insomnia or circadian rhythm sleep disorder, delayed sleep phase type, is to determine whether the person has difficulties falling asleep no matter what time he or she goes to bed (insomnia) or whether the individual has little difficulty falling asleep if bedtime is set to the natural fall-asleep time (delayed sleep phase syndrome). Kim appears to meet the criteria established above for circadian rhythm sleep disorder. Furthermore, the lack of difficulties once she falls asleep also supports delayed sleep phase type rather than insomnia. Further evaluation of this differential diagnosis is necessary. Another sleep disorder that is in the differential diagnosis is restless legs syndrome, but that appears less likely given the information provided about Kim.

Furthermore, Kim has been having increased difficulties in the past 2 years. This increase in symptoms likely coincides with changes in her pubertal status. Research indicates a delaying of the circadian clock by approximately 2 hours following puberty (Mindell and Owens 2003). Kim's natural tendency to have a delayed internal clock is demonstrated by her summer sleep schedule (sleeping from 2:00 A.M. to noon). This shift in her internal clock is also likely exacerbated by her tendency to worry and be anxious, making it even more difficult for her to fall asleep at bedtime.

DSM-IV-TR DIAGNOSIS

Axis I   307.42 Primary insomnia (pending further evaluation)

   327.31 Circadian rhythm sleep disorder, delayed sleep phase type (pending further evaluation)

   300.02 Generalized anxiety disorder (pending further evaluation)

Axis II   No diagnosis

Axis III None

Axis IV   None

Axis V   Global Assessment of Functioning=70

TREATMENT RECOMMENDATIONS

As described below, a number of treatment recommendations can be made in the case of Kim to treat both the primary insomnia and the likely concomitant circadian rhythm sleep disorder, delayed sleep phase type. For a more thorough coverage of treatment of insomnia and circadian rhythm sleep disorder, see Mindell and Owens (2003).

SLEEP SCHEDULE

Kim should establish a more consistent sleep schedule that is similar on both weekdays and weekends. This sleep schedule should maximize her sleep and not allow her to shift her circadian clock on weekends. For example, an appropriate recommendation would be for Kim to maintain a weekday sleep schedule of midnight to 6:00 A.M. and a weekend schedule of midnight to 9:00 A.M. If her bedtime during the week is moved to her more natural fall-asleep time, sleep pressure will increase, resulting in her falling asleep faster and decreasing the association of "tossing and turning" with lying in bed. At first, she will likely be sleepy in the morning on school days, given only 6 hours in bed; however, once she is falling asleep more quickly, her bedtime can be gradually moved earlier in 15-minute increments. Allowing a 9:00 A.M. wake time on weekends will enable Kim to get 9 hours of sleep on weekends, without letting her internal clock shift too much.

INSTITUTING BEDTIME ROUTINE AND LIMITING ELECTRONICS IN BEDROOM

A common sleep hygiene recommendation is to establish a relaxing bedtime routine. Such a routine signals the body that it is time to transition to sleep. Bedtime routines should not include electronics, such as television viewing, talking on the phone, or instant messaging. Currently, Kim is in the habit of chatting to her friends via the Internet, on the phone, and by instant messaging. Such behaviors are highly engaging and stimulating, thus interfering with the ability to fall asleep.

CUTTING CAFFEINE

Research has clearly indicated that late-day caffeine intake can interfere with falling asleep and staying asleep. Kim's late-day caffeine intake is likely contributing to her difficulties sleeping.

MORNING BRIGHT LIGHT EXPOSURE

To entrain the internal clock to an earlier time, exposure to morning bright light can be beneficial. Bright light exposure can be achieved through the use of a light box. This treatment would entail 20–30 minutes of exposure to high lux light in the early morning.

MANAGING ANXIETY

A referral for psychotherapy for anxiety is appropriate in the case of Kim. A bi-directional relationship exists between sleep disturbances and anxiety. For example, sleep disturbances are a diagnostic criterion for anxiety and can perpetuate anxious behaviors (Mindell 2003). Similarly, anxiety can contribute to difficulties falling asleep and staying asleep. In a study by Iwawaki and Sarmany-Schuller (2001), a negative relationship was found between anxiety level and sleep duration for adolescents (12–16 years), with a later bedtime and shorter sleep duration related to higher levels of anxiety.

CONCLUSIONS

Kim is a 15-year-old youth with a several-year history of difficulty falling asleep at bedtime and anxiety. A circadian rhythm sleep disorder, delayed sleep phase type, is likely contributing to her sleep difficulties. A comprehensive treatment plan that targets her negative sleep habits, shifted internal clock, and anxious thoughts will likely lead to significant improvements in her sleep.

Psychopharmacologic Perspective

Judith A. Owens, M.D., M.P.H., D'A.B.S.M.

DIAGNOSTIC FORMULATION

Kim presents with a constellation of symptoms consistent with a primary diagnosis of circadian rhythm sleep disorder, delayed sleep phase type, compounded by primary insomnia. The delayed sleep phase type of circadian rhythm sleep disorder is characterized by an intractable and persistent delay in both sleep onset and morning wake times of several hours, relative to the desired and/or accept-

Judith A. Owens, M.D., M.P.H., D'A.B.S.M., is Associate Professor of Pediatrics at Brown Medical School, and Director of the Pediatric Sleep Disorders Clinic at Hasbro Children's Hospital and of the Learning, Attention, and Behavior Program at Rhode Island Hospital in Providence, Rhode Island (for complete biographical information, see "About the Contributors," p. 613).

able sleep period. This often results in symptoms of secondary sleep-onset insomnia (i.e., the individual develops conditioned anxiety around difficulty falling or staying asleep, which leads to heightened physiological and emotional arousal and further compromises the ability to sleep) and extreme difficulty waking at the desired time. However, the patient typically has little or no sleep-onset delay when following his or her preferred sleep schedule. Circadian rhythm sleep disorder, delayed sleep phase type, frequently causes significant functional impairment and social distress, as well as depression, and often leads to academic problems related to tardiness and absenteeism. Secondary dependence on alertness-enhancing substances (e.g., caffeine, stimulants) may develop. Although genetic and physiological factors clearly have a role, many of these patients also have comorbid psychiatric conditions (anxiety, school avoidance), which further compound the issue and compromise adherence to treatment.

The diagnosis of circadian rhythm sleep disorder, delayed sleep phase type, is based on a patient's clinical history, including a detailed sleep history of preferred fall-asleep and wake times, and predictable periods of relative sleepiness and alertness throughout the day. Other possible causes of delayed sleep onset—restless legs syndrome, excessive caffeine use, poor sleep hygiene, voluntary sleep curtailment, and substance abuse—should be excluded. A 7- to 14-day sleep diary is often helpful in identifying sleep patterns over time; actigraphy (in which a small computerized device is attached to the wrist to measure body movements over time, to differentiate between sleep and wake times, and to provide estimations of sleep onset latency and total sleep duration) can also be useful in delineating sleep patterns. Physiological measures (salivary melatonin levels, nadir core body temperature) are currently not typically used clinically, and polysomnography is not routinely indicated.

DSM-IV-TR DIAGNOSIS

Axis I   327.31 Circadian rhythm sleep disorder, delayed sleep phase type
            307.42 Primary insomnia
Axis II   None
Axis III   None
Axis IV   None
Axis V   Global Assessment of Functioning=70

TREATMENT RECOMMENDATIONS

The treatment of circadian rhythm sleep disorder, delayed sleep phase type, typically involves one or more of the following interventions: resetting the circadian clock by manipulating sleep-wake schedules, having phototherapy in the morning, and taking an oral melatonin supplement in the evening. For patients with less than a 4-hour delay (the difference between desired and actual sleep onset times), a "phase advance" is usually recommended, in which a designated wake time is set (i.e., 7:00 A.M.) with no provision for sleeping later on weekends or taking naps, and then bedtime is progressively advanced from the current sleep onset time in 20-minute increments every few days until the desired bedtime is reached. Chronotherapy is generally reserved for patients with more severe delays (greater than 4–6 hours); this intervention involves delaying bedtime and wake time by 2 hours each day (or 3 hours every 2 days), depending on a preset "window" for sleeping (i.e., 8 hours), and moving "forward" around the clock until the desired bedtime is reached.

Phototherapy involves timed morning light exposure, which is intended to decrease melatonin levels and enhance alertness, as well as avoidance of bright light in the evening. Early morning light exposure of 2,000–10,000 lux, usually in the form of a light box, for 1–3 hours is the ideal recommendation, although shorter intervals may also be used for practical purposes. Broad-spectrum light is generally recommended, although some evidence indicates that blue-green light may have optimal phase-advancing effects. Patients should avoid gazing directly into the light and exercise caution regarding comcomitant use of photosensitizing medications.

Melatonin, a hormone secreted by the pineal gland in response to darkness, is one of the most powerful biological sleep signals. The mechanism of action of commercially available melatonin is to augment the secretion of endogenous pineal hormone; the plasma levels of exogenous melatonin peak within 1 hour of administration. Melatonin has both chronobiotic (circadian phase–shifting) and mild hypnotic (sleep-inducing) effects; the sedating effects tend to be optimal when endogenous melatonin levels are low. Because of the mild sedation associated with melatonin, it is often used clinically at bedtime in doses of 2.5–3 mg in older children and 5–6 mg in adolescents to reduce sleep onset latency; however, studies in adults suggest that the optimal phase-shifting effect may be produced by small amounts of melatonin (0.3–0.5 mg) 5–7 hours before sleep onset. Although melatonin is generally considered to be safe, potential side effects include increased blood pressure, headache, dizziness, nausea, lowering of seizure threshold, and potential suppression of the hypothalamic-gonadal axis such that precocious puberty can occur if melatonin is abruptly withdrawn in a prepubertal child. Because melatonin is not regulated by the U.S. Food and Drug Administration, the commercially available formulations tend to vary in strength and purity.

Finally, treatment of circadian rhythm sleep disorder, delayed sleep phase type, requires education of both the patient and caregivers regarding sleep physiology and the rationale behind the treatment strategies. Good sleep hygiene (i.e., avoidance of naps and caffeine) and a regular sleep-wake schedule on weekdays and weekends are key; secondary conditioned insomnia is most appropriately managed with behavioral interventions targeted toward reversing the association between bed and wakefulness with such techniques as using the bed for sleep only and getting out of bed if unable to fall asleep (stimulus control), restricting time in bed to the actual time asleep (sleep restriction), and relaxation techniques to reduce anxiety. Issues potentially confounding treatment compliance, such as comorbid psychopathology, school avoidance, and secondary gain, should be explored and addressed. Given that many patients with this disorder have an inherent tendency toward a delayed sleep phase and often readily "drift" to later bedtimes and wake times, the clinician also needs to discuss relapse management.

Integrative Perspective

Ronald E. Dahl, M.D.
Allison G. Harvey, Ph.D.

DIAGNOSTIC FORMULATION

Kim's case highlights a not unusual overlap of possible diagnoses that include insomnia; circadian rhythm sleep disorder, delayed sleep phase type; and sleep problems secondary to anxiety or depression. From both diagnostic and etiological perspectives, disentangling these domains in adolescents can be extremely difficult, for several reasons:

- Difficulty falling asleep is an extremely common component of both depression and anxiety disorders in youth.
- Bedtime worries and ruminations (and erratic sleep-wake schedules) are also common features of affective disorders in adolescents and are also major underpinnings to the development of insomnia.
- Late bedtimes on school nights (and even later sleep schedules on weekends and holidays, with catch-up sleep obtained by sleeping in extremely late) can lead to a delayed sleep phase type of circadian rhythm sleep disorder in many adolescents, and this pattern is often exacerbated by sleep onset difficulties.
- Many of the so-called coping behaviors individuals use to deal with this pattern of problems are distraction strategies (to avoid lying in bed worrying and ruminating about stressful thoughts and images), such as late-night use of the Internet, media, and so forth, which can further delay habitual bed-

time. Then, coffee and other stimulants are often used to deal with daytime fatigue and tiredness, but these can fuel a vicious cycle in which the person has trouble going to sleep at bedtime.

- Among anxious and worried youth, overconcern about getting enough sleep can fuel greater performance anxiety at bedtime, in a classic model of developing chronic insomnia.
- More generally, sleep and vigilance represent opponent processes. Because sleep is in essence a turning off of awareness and responsiveness to the external environment, states of vigilance and anxiety are antithetical to going to sleep.

Kim meets criteria for generalized anxiety disorder and primary insomnia, and probably meets criteria for circadian rhythm sleep disorder, delayed sleep phase type. Given the epidemiological and clinical data—approximately 75% of youth with anxiety or depression will give a history of significant difficulties falling asleep (Ryan et al. 1987)—it should not be surprising to find that Kim's history indicates that she has had symptoms of both disorders.

Given the overlapping diagnoses (and the bidirectional effects of sleep and mood), a strong case can be made to initiate treatment targeting both the sleep and sleep-wake schedule difficulties. The initial goal is to improve sleep, using a behavioral intervention, and see how much positive impact the improvement in sleep can have on Kim's affect and motivation.

DSM-IV-TR DIAGNOSIS

Axis I   307.42 Primary insomnia

327.31 Circadian rhythm sleep disorder, delayed sleep phase type

300.02 Generalized anxiety disorder

Axis II   None

Axis III   None

Axis IV   None

Axis V   Global Assessment of Functioning=62 (current)

TREATMENT RECOMMENDATIONS

The treatment of choice for Kim's case is a multiple-component psychological intervention that aims to 1) assist Kim in finding her own motivation for making changes to improve her sleep, 2) provide education about sleep, 3) regularize the sleep-wake schedule with stimulus control, 4) address Kim's worry, and 5) work toward a presleep routine that does not include media use and socializing with friends.

Before describing each of the components, we emphasize the importance of a thorough assessment. The initial assessment of a patient suffering from insomnia should start with a thorough clinical interview with the patient and his or her family members to obtain information about the duration, frequency, and severity of nighttime sleep disturbance, including estimates of the key sleep parameters: sleep onset latency, number of awakenings after sleep onset, total amount of time awake after sleep onset, total sleep time, and an estimate of sleep quality. This information should encompass weekday and weekend schedules; the regularity of the schedule; the average schedule; the onset and duration of the insomnia and the type of symptoms (i.e., sleep onset, sleep maintenance, early morning or late morning awaking problem, or any combination of these); the daytime correlates and consequences of insomnia; and the parental responses to the insomnia. In addition, the clinician needs to obtain information about prescription and over-the-counter medications and conduct a screen for the presence of psychiatric disorders and medical problems (including other sleep disorders). The patient should be asked to complete a sleep diary each morning, as soon as possible after waking, for 1–2 weeks; this diary provides a wealth of information, including an insight into the night-to-night variability in sleeping difficulty and sleep-wake patterns and the presence of circadian rhythm disorders, such as the delayed sleep phase type. An assessment should also include an exploration of the patient's fears, because fear, distress, or any cognitive or emotional cue that prevents an overall sense of safety is likely to be antithetical to sleep (because sleep onset requires turning off awareness, responsiveness, and vigilance). Adolescents can get into the habit of mentally reviewing or replaying worrisome thoughts about or memories of stressful events. Some youth with stressful memories or specific fears manage to avoid these thoughts during the day through distracting activities, but at night—especially when the youth is trying to fall asleep—the lack of distractors can result in rumination on these thoughts.

This treatment is typically delivered in six weekly 50-minute sessions. Between sessions, home projects aim to ensure generalizability of session content to the patient's life. Progress is monitored with daily sleep diaries.

PROVIDING THE MOTIVATION

Many sleep-incompatible or sleep-interfering behaviors used by Kim are rewarding (e.g., text messaging with friends into the night and freely surfing the Internet after parents have gone to bed). Moreover, as children move into adolescence, parental influence over bedtime and bedroom activities wanes. Hence, we begin treatment with a motivational component designed to assist Kim to find her internal motivation for enhancing her sleep. This component involves exploring the pros and cons of change, supporting Kim's self-efficacy, eliciting "self-motivational statements," generating solutions to potential barriers to change, and identifying social supports for change.

SLEEP AND CIRCADIAN EDUCATION

By increasing knowledge, the educational component helps target specific factors and behaviors that interfere with good sleep. This is particularly important as children move into adolescence, a period in which multiple sleep-interfering factors converge, causing a tendency to shift toward later bedtimes and increased autonomy to decide on bedtimes. Education about the circadian rhythm is critical on the basis of evidence that adolescence is characterized by a biological change toward a delayed sleep phase, a key feature of Kim's sleep-wake cycle. This intervention component has two aims: to correct unhelpful sleep habits while developing new healthy sleep habits and to maintain these new healthier habits. Thus, we addressed the following in treating Kim: 1) the use of electronic devices in the bedroom during the presleep period, 2) the vastly different sleep-wake schedules that Kim adopts on weekdays relative to weekends and holidays, 3) daytime naps and caffeine use, and 4) the need for exposure to bright light in the morning (i.e., outdoor sunshine or bright artificial light) to counter phase delay in circadian rhythm. After the initial session, the following steps were used to correct Kim's habits: behavioral contracts and monitoring healthy sleep behaviors and sleep-unfriendly behaviors on a daily basis. The maintenance of healthy habits was achieved by regular check-ins on progress throughout the remaining sessions and by including targets of change from this component in the later relapse prevention component.

STIMULUS CONTROL

Stimulus control aims to regularize the sleep-wake cycle and reverse maladaptive conditioning regarding the bed and not sleeping by limiting sleep-incompatible behaviors within the bedroom environment, while increasing cues for sleep-compatible behaviors. The stimulus control component involves providing a detailed rationale for and assisting the patient to 1) use the bed and bedroom only for sleep (and not for TV watching or text messaging); 2) get out of bed and go to another room when unable to fall asleep or to return to sleep within approximately 15–20 minutes, and return to bed only when sleepy again; and 3) arise in the morning at the same time (no later than +2 hours on weekends), and gradually move toward a regular schedule 7 days a week (Bootzin and Stevens 2005). We encourage anxious youth, when they are out of bed because they are unable to fall asleep, to engage in a diary writing task. The goal of this activity is to reduce the attraction of sleep-interfering activities, such as the Internet and television.

BEDTIME WORRY, RUMINATION, AND VIGILANCE

Kim's bedtime worry, rumination, and vigilance need to be addressed. Vigilance and worry interfere with sleep because they activate distress and physiological arousal (Espie 2002; Harvey 2002). This treatment component includes 1) diary writing or scheduling a "worry period" to encourage the processing of worries several hours prior to bedtime; 2) creating a "to do" list prior to getting into bed to reduce worrying about future plans or events; 3) training to disengage from presleep worry and redirect attention to pleasant (distracting) imagery; 4) demonstrating the adverse consequences of thought suppression while in bed; and 5) scheduling a presleep wind-down period prior to bedtime. Our approach to reducing vigilance with Kim was two-pronged: 1) to provide education and increased awareness of vigilance and 2) to provide training on actively directing attention to deactivating stimuli in the bedroom environment.

TARGETING MEDIA USE AND SOCIAL ACTIVITIES

A central issue influencing bedtime for Kim has been the use of electronic media (e.g., Internet, cell phone) for entertainment and social interaction at night. To achieve earlier sleep onset, we created a behavioral contract in which Kim voluntarily *chose* a time for turning off all access to these devices.

RELAPSE PREVENTION

The goal of relapse prevention is to consolidate and maximize maintenance of gains and to set the child and parent on a trajectory for continued improvement. This goal is guided by an individualized summary of learning and achievements. Areas needing further intervention are addressed by setting specific goals and creating a specific plan for achieving each goal (see Dahl 1996; Dahl and Lewin 2002).

ALTERNATIVE TREATMENTS

If initial treatments do not work, there are four considerations for a next-step approach:

1. If the adolescent is on a very late schedule and unable to gradually move sleep onset to an earlier time, the clinician can suggest a chronotherapy intervention of delaying sleep onset by 3 hours a night, gradually going around the clock until sleep lines up at 10 P.M. Although this intervention sounds cumbersome and a bit radical, it can work extremely well because while staying up on a series of 27-hour days, the patient is able to go to sleep more quickly and can reorganize all of the sleep habits and associations during the intervention (for a more detailed description, see Dahl 1998).
2. The clinician can administer a focused intervention for the anxiety (and/or depression).
3. Because anxiety, depression, and insomnia are likely to be mutually maintaining, the clinician can attempt administering the sleep-focused and anxiety-focused interventions concurrently.

4. The clinician can prescribe medications for the patient's insomnia, anxiety, or depression.

REFERENCES

American Academy of Sleep Medicine: International Classification of Sleep Disorders, 2nd Edition. Westchester, IL, American Academy of Sleep Medicine, 2005

Bootzin RR, Stevens SJ: Adolescents, substance abuse, and the treatment of insomnia and daytime sleepiness. Clin Psychol Rev 25:629–644, 2005

Dahl RE: The regulation of sleep and arousal: development and psychopathology. Dev Psychopathol 8:3–27, 1996

Dahl RE: Common sleep problems in children, in Sleep Disorders. Edited by Poceta JS, Mitler MM. Totowa, NJ, Humana Press, 1998, pp 161–186

Dahl RE, Lewin DS: Pathways to adolescent health sleep regulation and behavior. J Adolesc Health 31:175–184, 2002

Espie CA: Insomnia: conceptual issues in the development, persistence, and treatment of sleep disorder in adults. Annu Rev Psychol 53:215–243, 2002

Harvey AG: A cognitive model of insomnia. Behav Res Ther 40:869–894, 2002

Iwawaki S, Sarmany-Schuller I: Cross-cultural (Japan-Slovakia) comparison of some aspects of sleeping patterns and anxiety. Stud Psychol (Bratisl) 43:215–224, 2001

Johnson EO, Roth T, Schultz L, et al: Epidemiology of DSM-IV insomnia in adolescence: lifetime prevalence, chronicity, and an emergent gender difference. Pediatrics 117:e247–e256, 2006

Mindell JA: Insomnia in children and adolescents, in Insomnia: Principles and Management. Edited by Szuba MP, Kloss JD, Dinges D. Cambridge, UK, Cambridge University Press, 2003, pp 125–135

Mindell JA, Owens J: A Clinical Guide to Pediatric Sleep: Diagnosis and Management of Sleep Problems. Philadelphia, PA, Lippincott Williams & Wilkins, 2003

Ohayon MM, Roberts RE, Zulley J, et al: Prevalence and patterns of problematic sleep among older adolescents. J Am Acad Child Adolesc Psychiatry 39:1549–1556, 2000

Ryan ND, Puig-Antich J, Ambrosini P, et al: The clinical picture of major depression in children and adolescents. Arch Gen Psychiatry 44:854–861, 1987

■ CHAPTER 12 ■

The World Is a Very Dirty Place

Obsessive-Compulsive Disorder

Susan E. Swedo, M.D.

CASE PRESENTATION

IDENTIFYING INFORMATION

Andy is an athletic 8-year-old who was thriving in second grade before he began having complaints of "not being able to stay clean."

CHIEF COMPLAINT

Andy's parents brought Andy to the clinic to discuss his recent behavior changes.

HISTORY OF PRESENT ILLNESS

Andy's mother and father accompanied him to the appointment and reported that Andy's symptoms began 1 week earlier, on a Saturday morning, when he refused to get dressed because he had "nothing clean" to wear. His mother had just finished doing Andy's laundry, so she went to get the basket of freshly washed clothes. When she entered Andy's bedroom, his mother was shocked to see that he had strewn clothes all over the floor of the room, and was even more surprised when he explained, "They're all dirty. I can't wear them!" His mother knew that the clothes could not be dirty because she had taken away all of Andy's soiled clothes the previous evening; however, since he was so clearly upset by the situ-

Susan E. Swedo, M.D., is Tenured Investigator in the National Institute of Mental Health Intramural Research Program, and Chief of the Pediatrics and Developmental Neuropsychiatry Branch at the National Institute of Mental Health in Bethesda, Maryland (for complete biographical information, see "About the Contributors," p. 613).

ation, his mother decided not to confront the irrational behavior, and she simply told Andy to choose a clean outfit from the laundry basket. Andy pulled the sleeves of his pajamas down over his hands and proceeded to pick through the basket, discarding one garment after another because of "dirt" or "a stain." In exasperation, his mother finally chose an outfit for him and ordered him to put it on "right this minute" and go downstairs to breakfast. Andy began to cry (not typical for him at all) but agreed to get dressed. He appeared for breakfast 25 minutes later, wearing one of his older brother's shirts over his pajamas. He explained that he had tried to put on the outfit his mother had chosen but had dropped it on the floor and it had become "too dirty" to wear. Andy's younger sister broke into laughter at this explanation, which provoked further tears from Andy. His mother finally convinced him to sit down at the breakfast table and eat. She noticed that Andy pulled his pajama sleeves down over his hands before picking up his cereal spoon and then ate only one bite of cereal and another of toast before declaring that he "wasn't really that hungry" and asked to be excused from the table. Andy remained in his room for the rest of the day, refusing lunch because "I'm just not hungry" but joining the family at dinner for only a few minutes before asking to be excused "to watch the TV show you promised I could see tonight."

Andy's parents were not overly concerned by his behavior on Saturday, because he often spent hours in his room, playing video games and watching TV. However, on Sunday morning, after another battle over "dirty" and "clean" clothes and his refusal to eat brunch because "I'm still not hungry," Andy's parents became concerned that something was wrong. Their concerns mounted further when Andy refused his best friend's invitation to play at the park because "The park is filthy! I'll never be able to get clean if I go there." His parents felt that something was definitely wrong.

Andy's parents scheduled an appointment with his pediatrician on Monday morning. The physician took a careful history, which revealed that Andy was not only concerned about wanting to stay clean but also fearful that his food was contaminated ("Dirt could have fallen onto my plate"), which was why he had refused to eat any meals over the weekend. Andy also complained of feeling ill: "My head hurts this morning and my stomach hurt all weekend." The pediatrician's diagnosis was obsessive-compulsive disorder (OCD), manifested as contamination fears and avoidance rituals. He told Andy that he must start eating and drinking again, and suggested that Andy try bottled water and Ensure or another canned meal replacement because "they're manufactured under sterile conditions" and would be safe from contamination. He also recommended that Andy start treatment immediately with a selective serotonin reuptake inhibitor (SSRI), but after hearing of the potential risks of therapy, Andy's parents opted to hold off on treatment until they could obtain a second opinion. Fortunately, Andy's physician was able to secure an appointment for later that week with an experienced child psychiatrist.

Andy entered the psychiatrist's office reluctantly and pretended not to see the doctor's outstretched hand. He perched on the edge of the chair, fidgeting constantly and glancing anxiously about the room. After a few moments, he got up and went to stand by the window, staring glumly outside. Andy's parents reported that his symptoms had worsened over the course of the week, with the contamination fears generalizing to the point that the whole house had become "dirty." Andy's brother and sister seemed to have become a source of contamination, and Andy refused to leave his bedroom unless they were away at school. Even then, Andy would venture no further than the hallway bathroom, where he spent 30–45 minutes at a time washing his hands to rid them of imagined contaminants. His food contamination fears had worsened to the point that his mother had to wash the bottles and cans in front of him and then hand them to Andy using a "Cleanest" (Kleenex) tissue. Andy used a series of tissues to wipe down each bottle or can before opening it, and then took only a few swallows before worrying that a speck of dirt could have fallen into the drink and made it "dirty." His mother felt that he was getting sufficient fluids and calories, however, because she offered the drinks and supplements frequently.

PAST PSYCHIATRIC HISTORY

The psychiatrist takes a complete psychiatric history from Andy's parents. The history reveals only that Andy has been quite happy throughout his young life.

SUBSTANCE ABUSE HISTORY

Andy has no history of substance abuse.

MEDICAL HISTORY

The complete medical history reveals that Andy has always been quite healthy. The only abnormality noted on physical examination was slight left-sided cervical lymphadenopathy and mild erythema of the oropharynx, prompting Andy's physician to obtain a rapid strep test, which was negative.

DEVELOPMENTAL HISTORY

Andy is on target for meeting developmental milestones.

SOCIAL HISTORY

Andy lives with his parents, brother, and sister.

FAMILY HISTORY

His family medical history was positive for depression in his mother's sisters and maternal grandmother, and a paternal uncle was reported to have Tourette's disorder. Andy's older brother had seen a physician for an eyeblink tic when he was 7 years old, but it had resolved spontaneously after a few months and he now had no symptoms. The family had no history of OCD, although the father recalled a brief period of excessive worries (a need for symmetry and concerns about harm coming to his parents) when he was "just about Andy's age."

MENTAL STATUS EXAMINATION

Andy is a pleasant, cooperative boy who appeared his stated age and developmental stage. During the examination, he appeared somewhat sad and anxious, but he answered questions willingly, with normal rate and volume of speech. He denied any perceptual abnormalities. His intelligence seemed to be average to above average. His insight was good, and his judgment was without obvious impairments.

COMMENTARIES

Psychotherapeutic Perspective

John Piacentini, Ph.D., A.B.P.P.

DIAGNOSTIC FORMULATION

Andy's presenting complaints of germ and dirt fears are consistent with a diagnosis of OCD. In fact, contamination-related obsessions and compulsions are among the most common symptoms of OCD in childhood. Andy's fear of contamination is not limited to one specific setting or item but has generalized from clothing and food to the whole house, including other family members, and beyond (e.g., the park). Such generalization is also common, and Andy's case demonstrates that the illness may progress from subclinical to near incapacitation in relatively rapid fashion.

DSM-IV-TR requires that for a diagnosis of OCD, a person's symptoms must be time-consuming (1 hour or more per day) or cause marked distress or

John Piacentini, Ph.D., A.B.P.P., is Professor of Psychiatry and Biobehavioral Sciences at the David Geffen School of Medicine, and Director of the Child OCD, Anxiety, and Tic Disorders Program at the Semel Institute for Neuroscience and Human Behavior at the University of California, Los Angeles (for complete biographical information, see "About the Contributors," p. 613).

significant functional interference. Although the total time taken by Andy's symptoms is not specified, both distress (crying, physical complaints) and interference (refusing playdates, staying in his room, not eating) are apparent. Andy's limited insight into his symptoms is not atypical; DSM-IV-TR does not require that children recognize their symptoms as excessive or unreasonable.

In addition, the medical history and examination did not identify any medical explanations for Andy's symptoms. Andy's sudden onset in conjunction with evidence of a recent sore throat suggests that his symptoms may have been triggered by an autoimmune reaction to a streptococcal infection (pediatric autoimmune neuropsychiatric disorders associated with streptococcus, or PANDAS) (Murphy et al. 2004). However, the negative strep test did not support this hypothesis. Andy's symptoms also do not appear better accounted for by another psychiatric disorder. Among the most common differential diagnoses for OCD in children and adolescents are generalized anxiety disorder, tic disorders, and pervasive developmental disorder. In contrast to patients with OCD, patients with generalized anxiety disorder tend to have worries that are more related to real-life concerns and, with the possible exception of excessive reassurance seeking, are not accompanied by ritualistic behaviors. Distinguishing complex motor tics from OCD-related compulsions (e.g., tapping, counting, arranging) can be difficult, especially given the common co-occurrence of the two disorders. Tics are often expressed in response to premonitory sensory urges and can be distinguished from the obsessions underlying ritualizing. In contrast to the ego-dystonic nature of obsessions, the perseverative thoughts and behaviors associated with pervasive developmental disorder have a more syntonic and functional nature. Pervasive developmental disorder is also characterized by social functioning deficits not found in OCD.

OCD is reasonably common in childhood, with a lifetime prevalence of 1.0%–2.5% and a mean onset age of about 8–11 years (Rapoport et al. 2000). Although comorbidity is common, Andy's presentation does not suggest the presence of any concurrent psychiatric problems. However, this may be a function of his young age, and Andy remains at increased risk for the development of additional disorders (most likely another anxiety disorder, depressive disorder, or tic disorder) over time. Family history of subclinical OCD in the father and tic disorders in other family members provides additional confidence in Andy's diagnosis, given the family genetics of these disorders.

Accurate evaluation of OCD requires a careful developmental and illness history. Although Andy's parents first noted his OCD symptoms a week before his evaluation, these, or similar, symptoms likely were present at a subclinical level for a longer period of time. The Children's Yale-Brown Obsessive Compulsive Scale (CY-BOCS; Scahill et al. 1997) is a semistructured clinician-rated instrument used to establish OCD severity and provide a comprehensive list of current and past symptoms. The CY-BOCS takes 30–45 minutes to administer and provides a psychometrically sound method for assessing symptom improvement over the course of treatment. As seen in Andy's case, OCD often negatively impacts psychosocial functioning. Similar to the CY-BOCS, the Child Obsessive-Compulsive Impact Scales—Revised (Piacentini et al. 2007b) are brief parallel parent- and child-report rating scales that can be used to document baseline OCD-related impairment and improvement over time. Documentation of past or current psychiatric comorbidity, using a clinical interview, such as the Anxiety Disorders Interview Schedule for DSM-IV, Parent Version (Silverman and Albano 1996), or a parent-report measure, such as the Child Behavior Checklist (Achenbach 1991), is also important, given the extent to which these other symptoms might impact OCD treatment or require their own intervention.

DSM–IV-TR DIAGNOSIS

Axis I   300.3 Obsessive-compulsive disorder
Axis II   No diagnosis
Axis III No diagnosis
Axis IV   None
Axis V   Global Assessment of Functioning=53 (current)

TREATMENT RECOMMENDATIONS

At present, exposure-based cognitive-behavioral therapy (CBT) and pharmacologic intervention with serotonin reuptake inhibitors are the only empirically supported treatments for OCD in children and adolescents (Barrett et al. 2008; Pediatric OCD Treatment Study Team 2004). Expert consensus recommends exposure-based CBT as the first-line treatment of choice for young children with OCD (March et al. 1997). Given Andy's young age, recent onset, and lack of comorbid disturbance or developmental issues, the likelihood of a positive response to this treatment approach is very good. However, should CBT provide insufficient benefit, then medication should be considered as an adjunctive intervention. Consensus also suggests that treatment should involve Andy's parents and perhaps other family members as well.

Based on Andy's healthy premorbid functioning, psychological or neurological testing or other forms of adjunctive psychotherapy are not presently indicated. School intervention, typically based on the extent to which symptoms interfere with academic or social functioning in this setting, does not appear warranted in Andy's case, although this could change.

CBT for OCD is based on the observation that ritualistic behaviors, including avoidance, are negatively reinforced by their ability to reduce obsession-triggered distress (Foa and Kozac 1986). For example, the more effective compulsive hand washing is at reducing contamination fears, the more likely the child will engage in this behavior over time. In addition, engaging in the compulsion does not provide the child with an opportunity to challenge or disprove the obsession (e.g., "these germs won't really hurt me"), thereby further strengthening the connection between obsession and compulsion (the so-called obsessive-compulsive cycle). Exposure-based CBT seeks to break this cycle by encouraging children to resist the urge to ritualize (response prevention) in the face of obsession-triggered distress (Piacentini and Langley 2004).

The most effective CBT interventions for childhood OCD are multicomponent and supplement exposure plus response prevention with psychoeducation about the disorder, a behavioral reward system to enhance treatment compliance, and, for an older child or adolescent, cognitive restructuring aimed at teaching the individual to more critically challenge his or her obsessive thoughts (Piacentini et al. 2007a). Treatment progresses in a gradual fashion, according to a symptom hierarchy, with milder symptoms exposed initially, followed by more difficult exposures as treatment progresses. For example, Andy's therapist might initially ask him to briefly touch his fingertip to a "contaminated" T-shirt. Although Andy might have difficulty resisting washing at first, this distress typically diminishes relatively quickly via autonomic habituation. Through repeated exposures, Andy will learn that nothing bad happens if he does not wash (i.e., the feared consequences of not washing are not going to occur). Although exposures are typically developed and initially practiced during therapeutic sessions, most treatment gains accrue from repeated practice in the natural environment. Parental involvement in treatment focuses on eliminating family accommodation of symptoms (e.g., participating in the child's rituals or fostering avoidance of feared situations or objects) because this accommodation runs directly counter to the goals of exposure plus response prevention. For children who are about age 9 or younger or who have cognitive impairment, treatment may be more effective when presented in a play format. Younger children also commonly require greater parental involvement in therapy, which involves training the parent to serve as an adjunct therapist in the home setting.

Psychopharmacologic Perspective

Mark A. Riddle, M.D.

DIAGNOSTIC FORMULATION

As the second-opinion consultant to both Andy's parents and the pediatrician, the psychiatrist needs first to establish a diagnosis and formulation before proceeding to treatment. The information provided about this 8-year-old boy suggests a diagnosis of OCD. Andy presents with rather severe obsessions (thoughts about dirt and filth) and compulsions (refusal to wear clean clothes because "they are dirty," refusal to play in the park because it "is filthy," and refusal to eat because "dirt could have fallen onto my plate"), all of which focus on contamination. These symptoms are distressing and impairing and have already required parental accommodation. Prior to the onset of his OCD symptoms, Andy was described as quite healthy and happy. Although DSM-IV-TR does not provide a duration criterion for OCD, the very recent onset—just 1 week ago—is noteworthy. Nothing in the case presentation suggests the diagnosis of any other psychiatric disorder or medical condition, other than perhaps a sore throat with a negative strep test.

No confirmatory tests are available for OCD. Symptoms of OCD commonly wax and wane in severity; rating scales can be useful for following the severity of symptoms over time. The most commonly used rating scales are the child-completed Leyton Obsessional Inventory—Child Version (Berg et al. 1986) and the clinician-completed CY-BOCS (Scahill et al. 1997).

Andy appears to be a high-functioning boy from a high-functioning family. The parents' response to the rapid onset of rather severe OCD symptoms appears to be thoughtful and helpful. In terms of possible genetic vulnerabilities, the younger brother has a history of a transient eyeblink tic, and the father had a brief period as a boy of excessive worries that included "a need for symmetry," which could be considered an obsessive-compulsive symptom. The extended maternal family has a history of depression, and the paternal family has a his-

---

Mark A. Riddle, M.D., is Professor of Psychiatry and Pediatrics and Director of the Division of Child and Adolescent Psychiatry at the Johns Hopkins University School of Medicine; and Vice President for Psychiatric Sciences at the Kennedy Krieger Institute in Baltimore, Maryland (for complete biographical information, see "About the Contributors," p. 613).

tory of Tourette's disorder. Given that early-onset OCD (before age 18) runs in families (Nestadt et al. 2000) and is associated with tic (Grados et al. 2001) and anxiety disorders (Nestadt et al. 2001), the formulation in this case would favor age-appropriate expression of a genetic vulnerability. Also, given the transient nature of the father's and brother's symptoms, combined with Andy's quite recent symptom onset, caution is indicated regarding prediction of course and prognosis.

DSM-IV-TR DIAGNOSIS

Axis I   300.3 Obsessive-compulsive disorder

Axis II   None

Axis III   Sore throat

Axis IV   No psychosocial or environmental problems

Axis V   Global Assessment of Functioning=60 (current) (past year=90)

TREATMENT RECOMMENDATIONS

The first step in treatment is illness education. OCD is a relatively common disorder, with a lifetime prevalence of 0.5%–2.0% (Towbin and Riddle 2007). When young children receive an OCD diagnosis, parents are usually quite concerned about etiology, confirmatory tests, course of illness, and prognosis. Reassurance that the child or parent did not do something to cause the OCD is obviously important. If the formulation includes genetic vulnerability, concerns about future generations are obvious. Prognosis is difficult to address when the symptoms have been present for only 1 week. However, the prognosis for OCD is quite favorable—many children have a complete remission, and severity is likely to wane even if symptoms continue. Finally, genetic vulnerability is probably complex and should not affect decisions about having additional children.

The next step in treatment is acute stabilization and crisis management, if necessary. The biggest concern with Andy was his refusal to eat for several days because of contamination concerns. Fortunately, he was responsive to the pediatrician's simple and skillful intervention.

The next step is to decide whether further treatment is needed. Some clinicians might recommend a "watchful waiting" approach, given that the symptoms have been present for only about a week and might be transient (i.e., self-limited). Although situations occur in which watchful waiting is appropriate, the severity of Andy's symptoms warrants a more assertive treatment plan.

Two evidence-based, short-term treatments can be used for OCD: CBT and medication, specifically SSRIs. Both are moderately effective in relieving the symptoms of OCD. In a recent meta-analysis of six placebo-controlled studies of SSRIs for OCD involving more than 700 participants, the rate of response was 52% in the SSRI-treated group and 32% in the placebo group (Bridge et al. 2007).

In addition to the two evidence-based treatments, CBT and SSRIs, another important component of treatment is parent counseling regarding optimal approaches to managing a child's OCD symptoms. Helping parents find a comfortable and effective balance between accommodating to their child's symptoms and setting firm limits on impairing symptoms can be a daunting clinical challenge. Even the best of parents who have a child with impairing OCD find it difficult to manage their child's behaviors without expert support and advice.

No treatment is effective unless the child and parents accept the treatment. Even medication, which is a passive treatment, can be undermined by lack of compliance. Thus, for Andy, given his parents' stated concerns about the potential risks of medication, CBT might be the most effective first-line treatment. Most CBT therapists accept patients as young as 7 or 8 years old. Careful therapist selection, based on the therapist's experience and skills, is very important. In the best study to date of CBT for OCD in children (Pediatric OCD Treatment Study Team 2004), the CBT therapists at one site had a treatment effect that was more than three times greater than the effect at the other site.

If high-quality CBT is not available or has been tried and found ineffective, treatment with an SSRI is indicated. Six SSRIs are available in the United States: citalopram, escitalopram, fluoxetine, fluvoxamine, paroxetine, and sertraline. No evidence supports any differences among them in terms of efficacy; however, various characteristics of these medications may influence choice. Three SSRIs—fluvoxamine, fluoxetine, and sertraline—are approved by the U.S. Food and Drug Administration for OCD in children. All but citalopram and escitalopram have generic forms available and are less expensive. Fluoxetine has a very long half-life, which is an advantage when a dose is missed but a disadvantage when changing medicines. Paroxetine has nonlinear kinetics, which makes for nonlinear relationships between dose and blood levels (Findling et al. 1999).

For maximizing potential therapeutic benefits, several general principles regarding use of SSRIs in children are noteworthy. Children and families can be assured that side effects, when present, are generally mild. Rare potential major side effects—suicidal ideation or attempts, onset of mania in vulnerable children, and impairing sexual dysfunction—need to be described during the consent process. Standard practice includes low initial dosing followed by gradual increases in the context of regular monitoring of therapeutic response and side effects. Treatment at the highest tolerated dosage for 6–8 weeks is needed before declaring a medication ineffective (Towbin and

Riddle 2007). Although some early data suggested that higher doses of SSRIs were needed to successfully treat adults with OCD, placebo-controlled studies of SSRIs for OCD in children and adolescents have not indicated that higher doses are needed for youth. Doses needed to treat OCD, depression, and various anxiety disorders are generally the same.

Limited research data are available to guide medication treatment for children with OCD if the initial SSRI is not effective. The two most commonly used strategies are to switch to another SSRI or to augment with another medication. The most common augmenter, especially for children who have tics and/or a family history of tics, is a low-dose neuroleptic (McDougle et al. 2000).

Integrative Perspective

Susan E. Swedo, M.D.

DIAGNOSTIC FORMULATION

The pediatrician was right about the diagnosis—Andy has OCD. Although Andy's parents have provided a comprehensive history of the preceding week, they might not be aware of the full extent of Andy's symptoms, particularly his obsessional thoughts, and Andy needs to be engaged in the diagnostic assessment. The CY-BOCS (Scahill 1997) is a useful tool in this regard. Often, children are too embarrassed by the "silly" or "crazy" content of their obsessional thoughts to share them with their parents, and the CY-BOCS provides a matter-of-fact means for children to reveal their hidden thoughts and worries. Children are often reassured by the checklist, saying, "If my symptom is on your checklist, it must not be too weird." The Multidimensional Anxiety Scale for Children (March et al. 1997) is another useful tool in the diagnostic workup of children with OCD, because it can reveal the presence of another anxiety disorder that might have been obscured by the OCD. All children with OCD should be evaluated for depression, which can occur either as a result of demoralization from the unrelenting obsessive-compulsive symptoms or as a comorbid condition (up to 60% of childhood cases) (Leonard et al. 2005). Andy's psychiatrist ascertained that he did not have depressive symptoms at the time of the initial evaluation.

Often, as in Andy's case, the past history becomes crucial in determining the most appropriate course of treatment for children with OCD. Andy's symptoms of the past week were an escalation of long-standing obsessive-compulsive symptoms and anxieties. A supportive interview revealed that Andy has actually been having symptoms since the beginning of the school year. Initially, the only source of contamination was a boy who had bullied Andy in his class-room. Andy devised an extensive avoidance scheme that he was able to insti-tute without anyone becoming aware of the reasons behind his behaviors. For example, he asked to be seated at the front of the classroom so he could "see the board better," but he really just wanted to sit as far away from the bully as pos-sible. At lunchtime and during recess, Andy would hide in the bathroom until the bully had left the lunchroom or playground, and then Andy would return to the classroom by a circuitous route, avoiding any places that the bully might have stepped. The past history revealed that the food contamination also had started several weeks earlier, as a generalization of the contamination of the school lunchroom. In retrospect, Andy's mother realized that Andy had ini-tially been eating a huge snack as soon as he got home from school (because he had not been able to eat at school), but about 6–8 weeks ago, he started going straight to the bathroom when he got home and then heading into his bed-room to change his clothes. Andy confessed that he was doing these rituals to "get the dirt off" before eating a snack or the evening meal.

Despite careful probing, the psychiatrist could not determine what had caused the symptoms to escalate so abruptly over the weekend. The symptoms might have been triggered by another bout of teasing that Andy suffered at school on Friday, or they might have worsened because Andy was feeling phys-ically ill. Andy blamed the escalation of his food contamination fears on the pe-diatrician's attempts to reassure him: "If the doctor thinks that I need to have special, 'sterile' food, I figured that meant the regular food really was dirty." This phenomenon is common in OCD. Parents and clinicians are trying to make things better for the affected child but inadvertently reinforce the obses-sional fear.

DSM-IV-TR DIAGNOSIS

Axis I   300.3 Obsessive-compulsive disorder
Axis II   None
Axis III   Recovering from recent episode of pharyngitis
Axis IV   No problems of the social environment, education system, or primary
           support group
Axis V   Global Assessment of Functioning=58 (current)

TREATMENT RECOMMENDATIONS

The ideal treatment for Andy's symptoms would be a combination of medica-tion and CBT, specifically use of an SSRI and exposure with response prevention therapy (Pediatric OCD Treatment Study Team 2004). The combination is very effective, particularly with contamination fears and washing-cleaning rituals, and should provide Andy with significant relief. Many parents, like Andy's, are concerned about using SSRIs in children because of the black box warning about suicidal behaviors. However, among children with anxiety disorders, the risk/benefit ratio clearly favors use of SSRIs, because the children with beneficial effects far outnumber those with adverse side effects (and suicidality does not appear to be increased among children receiving SSRIs for anxiety disorders) (March et al. 2006). Many children balk at participating in behavior therapy; they are concerned that the treatment will be too difficult or will not help their symptoms. Allowing the children to take control of their therapy, such as encouraging them to be "detectives" in ferreting out hidden obsessional concerns or having them determine which symptoms should be targeted first, will increase the chances that they will participate willingly and improve the chances that the behavioral therapy will succeed.

If Andy's symptoms really did begin acutely, the psychiatrist would need to determine whether Andy meets criteria for the PANDAS subgroup (Swedo et al. 1998). In that case, the previous medical history would be negative or perhaps reveal a short-lived subclinical episode in the past. If Andy's symptoms were triggered by a streptococcal infection, the review of symptoms might reveal enuresis, increased daytime urinary frequency, or the recent onset of nightmares and other sleep disturbances. The psychiatric history would often be positive for irritability and personality changes; recent-onset separation anxiety disorder; hyperactivity, impulsivity, and attentional difficulties; and/or depressive symptoms (Swedo et al. 1998, 2004). If a constellation of such symptoms was present, PANDAS might be a consideration. However, the subgroup is defined by a longitudinal association between streptococcal infections and neuropsychiatric symptom exacerbations, so the "diagnosis" could not be definitive at this time. The psychiatrist should examine Andy to determine whether or not he has choreiform movements, which are present in more than 90% of acutely ill children in the PANDAS subgroup (Swedo et al. 2004). The psychiatrist should obtain another throat culture, because rapid strep tests are not 100% accurate, and an untreated strep infection not only complicates the neuropsychiatric symptoms, but also puts the child at risk for rheumatic fever and other post-streptococcal sequelae.

Treatment of a positive throat culture would be warranted, but otherwise, management of obsessive-compulsive symptoms in the PANDAS subgroup is the same as for other cases of OCD—a combination of SSRI medication and CBT. Given that Andy's contamination fears are preventing him from eating, a course of immunomodulatory therapy might be considered, even during this first episode, if the symptom profile was completely consistent with the

PANDAS criteria (Perlmutter et al. 1999). However, such treatments typically should be reserved for severely ill children and are not yet considered to be first-line therapy even for that group.

In summary, the clinical history is of paramount importance in the diagnosis of OCD in children and adolescents. The acuity of symptom onset, course of disease progression, and presence of comorbid signs and symptoms all aid the clinician in determining whether the child has OCD, and if so, which subtype is most likely.

REFERENCES

Achenbach TM: Manual for the Child Behavior Checklist/4–18 and 1991 Profile. Burlington, VT, University of Vermont Department of Psychiatry, 1991

Barrett P, Farrell L, Pina A, et al: Evidence-based psychosocial treatments for child and adolescent OCD. J Clin Child Adolesc Psychol 37:131–155, 2008

Berg CJ, Rapoport JL, Flament M: The Leyton Obsessional Inventory—Child Version. J Am Acad Child Psychiatry 25:84–91, 1986

Bridge JA, Iyengar S, Salary CB, et al: Clinical response and risk for reported suicidal ideation and suicide attempts in pediatric antidepressant treatment: a meta-analysis of randomized controlled trials. JAMA 297:1683–1696, 2007

Findling RL, Reed MD, Myers C, et al: Paroxetine pharmacokinetics in depressed children and adolescents. J Am Acad Child Adolesc Psychiatry 38:952–959, 1999

Foa EB, Kozak MJ: Emotional processing of fear: exposure to correct information. Psychol Bull 99:20–35, 1986

Grados MA, Riddle MA, Samuels JF, et al: The familial phenotype of obsessive-compulsive disorder in relation to tic disorders: the Hopkins OCD family study. Biol Psychiatry 50:559–565, 2001

Leonard HL, Ale CM, Freeman JB, et al: Obsessive-compulsive disorder. Child Adolesc Psychiatr Clin N Am 14:727–744, 2005

March JS, Parker JD, Sullivan K, et al: The Multidimensional Anxiety Scale for Children (MASC): factor structure, reliability and validity. J Am Acad Child Adolesc Psychiatry 36:554–565, 1997

March JS, Klee BJ, Kremer CM: Treatment benefit and risk of suicidality in multicenter, randomized, controlled trials of sertraline in children and adolescents. J Child Adolesc Psychopharmacol 16:91–102, 2006

McDougle CJ, Epperson CN, Pelton GH, et al: A double-blind, placebo-controlled study of risperidone addition in serotonin reuptake inhibitor–refractory obsessive-compulsive disorder. Arch Gen Psychiatry 57:794–801, 2000

Murphy TK, Sajid M, Soto O, et al: Detecting pediatric autoimmune neuropsychiatric disorders associated with streptococcus in children with obsessive-compulsive disorder and tics. Biol Psychiatry 55:61–68, 2004

Nestadt G, Lan T, Samuels J, et al: Complex segregation analysis provides compelling evidence for a major gene underlying obsessive-compulsive disorder and for heterogeneity by sex. Am J Hum Genet 67:1611–1616, 2000

Nestadt G, Samuels J, Riddle MA, et al: The relationship between obsessive-compulsive disorder and anxiety and affective disorders: results from the Johns Hopkins OCD Family Study. Psychol Med 31:481–487, 2001

Pediatric OCD Treatment Study Team: Cognitive-behavior therapy, sertraline, and their combination for children and adolescents with obsessive-compulsive disorder: the Pediatric OCD Treatment Study (POTS) randomized controlled trial. JAMA 292:1969–1976, 2004

Perlmutter SJ, Leitman SF, Garvey MA, et al: Therapeutic plasma exchange and intravenous immunoglobulin for obsessive-compulsive disorder and tic disorders in childhood. Lancet 354:1153–1158, 1999

Piacentini J, Langley A: Cognitive behavior therapy for children with obsessive-compulsive disorder. J Clin Psychol 60:1181–1194, 2004

Piacentini J, Langley A, Roblek T: Overcoming Childhood OCD: A Therapist's Guide. New York, Oxford University Press, 2007a

Piacentini J, Peris T, Bergman RL, et al: Functional impairment in childhood OCD: development and psychometrics properties of the Child Obsessive-Compulsive Impact Scale—Revised (COIS-R). J Clin Child Adolesc Psychol 36:645–653, 2007b

Rapoport JL, Inoff-Germain G, Weissman MM, et al: Childhood obsessive-compulsive disorder in the NIMH MECA study: parent versus child identification of cases. J Anxiety Disord 14:535–548, 2000

Scahill L, Riddle MA, McSwiggin-Hardin M, et al: Children's Yale-Brown Obsessive Compulsive Scale: reliability and validity. J Am Acad Child Adolesc Psychiatry 36:844–852, 1997

Silverman WK, Albano AM: The Anxiety Disorders Interview Schedule for DSM-IV, Child and Parent Versions. New York, Oxford University Press, 1996

Swedo SE, Leonard HL, Garvey M, et al: Pediatric autoimmune neuropsychiatric disorders associated with streptococcal infections: clinical description of the first 50 cases. Am J Psychiatry 155:264–271, 1998

Swedo SE, Leonard HL, Rapoport JL: The pediatric autoimmune neuropsychiatric disorders associated with streptococcal infection (PANDAS) subgroup: separating fact from fiction. Pediatrics 113:907–911, 2004

Towbin KE, Riddle MA: Obsessive-compulsive disorder, in Lewis's Child and Adolescent Psychiatry: A Comprehensive Textbook, 4th Edition. Edited by Martin A, Volkmar FR. Baltimore, MD, Lippincott Williams & Wilkins, 2007, pp 548–566

▪ P a r t I I ▪

COMORBID COMPLEXITY

Introduction to Comorbid Complexity

Peter S. Jensen, M.D.
Cathryn A. Galanter, M.D.

In Part II, we present cases that are complicated because of multiple comorbidities. In such cases, careful attention to all of the precipitating and participating factors becomes essential. More often than not, effective treatment of a child with multiple comorbidities also means stabilizing key aspects of the child's environment. In addition, identifying how environmental factors precipitate and participate in maintaining the child's symptoms becomes especially critical.

In the first case, "Stealing the Car: Disruptive Behavior in an Adolescent" (Chapter 13), the commentators all note the importance of the environmental factors but recommend somewhat different approaches to assessment and diagnosis, including eschewing diagnosis altogether in multisystemic therapy. All three commentators, however, come to the same treatment conclusions.

In the second case, "Zero Tolerance: Threats to Harm a Teacher in Elementary School" (Chapter 14), differences are seen among the experts' attention-deficit/hyperactivity disorder (ADHD) diagnoses. In actual cases of ADHD, such distinctions will make a major difference (e.g., in deciding whether to use a stimulant), and these determinations may have a major impact on individuals' eventual outcomes and the likelihood of treatment success. Also in this case, the experts' Global Assessment of Functioning (GAF) scores have non-trivial differences. Again, this is not to say that one expert is right and another is wrong. The contributors are presented with only snippets of a case. The presentation of an actual patient with comorbid complexities may yield fewer or more differences across experts, depending on therapeutic approach, disciplinary background, and etiological inferences. In our view, for complicated cases, the need for multidisciplinary input and multiple interventions increases; thus, the integration of medication, psychotherapeutic, and environmental supports becomes increasingly essential. Often, because a single individual may lack expertise in all areas, optimal treatment approaches require multidisciplinary teams or close collaborations across disciplines.

In the case of "Anxious Adolescent in the Emergency Room: Possible Abuse of Prescription Medications" (Chapter 15), the experts differ in diagnosing anxiety. Presumably, many persons presenting with anxiety disorders also have histories of substance use. Similarly, many persons presenting with substance use may have histories of anxiety or related problems. Commonly, one or the other of the diagnoses is missed, depending on the clinical door the patient enters (i.e., based on the diagnostic beliefs and habits of a particular clinician). This case also demonstrates that comorbidity arises not only within psychiatric disorders (as in combined substance use disorder and anxiety disorder) but also with medical conditions, again illustrating the complexity of the information-integration task that the clinician faces.

In "The Worried Child: A Child With Multiple Anxiety Disorders" (Chapter 16), the experts differ in their patient impairment ratings (GAF scores) and in their determination of single versus multiple anxiety disorders. Although children with anxiety disorders often meet criteria for multiple anxiety disorders, our understanding of these distinctions and their possible importance remains rudimentary at this point. In this case, however, the extent to which the child has a specific phobia and/or a generalized anxiety disorder may be important. Although both of these anxiety disorders generally are thought to respond to cognitive-behavioral therapy, specific phobia per se has not been systematically investigated in terms of the benefits of medication. Evidence from a multisite study, however, has demonstrated the potential benefits of medication in treating other anxiety disorders (Research Unit on Pediatric Psychopharmacology Anxiety Study Group 2001). This case also illustrates—potentially dramatically—the differences in kinds of treatments that might be offered, depending on a clinician's disciplinary background and type of training. Those trained principally in medication may too quickly offer medication treatment for the presumed generalized anxiety disorder, whereas those trained in cognitive-behavioral therapy or exposure methods may tend to focus on the specific phobia and miss other aspects of the child's anxiety presentation that may in fact benefit from and require medication.

"Affective Storms: A Careful Assessment of Rage Attacks" (Chapter 17) exemplifies one of the problems that currently perplexes the field of child and adolescent psychiatry. The commentators were faced with deciding among an array of possible diagnoses, and they listed a variety. In fact, one commentator listed seven disorders to consider for this complex case. Notably, however, the commentators were more unified in the child's impairment ratings (GAF scores ranged from 45 to 50). Given the current confusion about discriminating among bipolar disorder not otherwise specified, oppositional defiant disorder, conduct disorder, ADHD, and related syndromes, this case demarcates questions of exceptional importance for further study within the field: For children with complex rages or "storms," to what extent are these disorders part and parcel of more commonplace disorders such as comorbid ADHD and oppositional defiant disorder? To what extent do they overlap with other disorders, such as bipolar I disorder, and to what extent do they make up discrete new syndromes altogether that need to be studied in their own right? While we in the field continue to debate about these problems depending on our various disciplinary backgrounds and theoretical persuasions, this group of children remains severely impaired and in need of effective treatments as determined through high-quality research—research that remains to be done.

The case of "Failing Out of School: Language and Reading Weaknesses" (Chapter 18) illustrates a much needed area of research: the overlap between ADHD and learning disabilities. In terms of federal research, ADHD historically has been studied almost exclusively by the National Institute of Mental Health. In contrast, learning disabilities have been studied most commonly by the National Institute of Child Health and Human Development and the Department of Education. Rarely have these two conditions—ADHD and learning disabilities—been studied explicitly together in treatment studies. Again, the diagnosis of learning disabilities or ADHD will likely depend on the clinical door the family enters. Also, the case presentation includes a long list of sophisticated psychoeducational tests. Most child and adolescent psychiatrists are not fully trained in the use or interpretation of these tests. Interestingly, one case commentator is a developmental-behavioral pediatrician who pursued and obtained substantial training in this area, allowing her to more accurately identify and delimit the learning conditions when they occur.

The last case in this section, "Functional Abdominal Pain in Child With Inflammatory Bowel Disease" (Chapter 19), aptly illustrates the complexity of working with children with medical illnesses and the difficulties in differentiating psychiatric illnesses from co-occurring or underlying medical morbidity. Despite these challenges, the commentators agree on the current functional nature of the child's pain syndrome; the stable nature of the Crohn's disease; and the importance of assisting the child in the context of the parent-child relationship, including addressing the potential role of family members in maintaining the child's difficulties. This case also illustrates that complex cases often require a multidisciplinary team, skilled not only in treating medical illnesses and understanding the biological factors related to those diseases, but also in using the necessary range of psychiatric medications and evidence-based psychotherapies in addressing such complex problems. Importantly, in the case of functional abdominal pain, we see that much of what we know is not based on studies of functional abdominal pain per se, but rather on inferences drawn from other areas of research and the accumulated evidence for effective treatments in related literatures, either with adults or in other studies of different child and adolescent populations. This represents yet another call for more research.

REFERENCE

Research Unit on Pediatric Psychopharmacology Anxiety Study Group: Fluvoxamine for the treatment of anxiety disorders in children and adolescents. N Engl J Med 344:1279–1285, 2001

■ CHAPTER 13 ■

Stealing the Car

Disruptive Behavior in an Adolescent

Peter S. Jensen, M.D.

CASE PRESENTATION

IDENTIFYING INFORMATION

Trey is a 17-year-old tenth grader who lives with his mother, a 12-year-old brother, and the mother's boyfriend.

CHIEF COMPLAINT

Trey was referred by a probation officer for an "urgent" mental health evaluation after he was arrested for "stealing" his family's car. He was accompanied to the evaluation by his mother and her boyfriend.

HISTORY OF PRESENT ILLNESS

Over the past 6 months, Trey has had increasing conflict with his mother and, more recently, arguments with his mother's boyfriend. Although Trey has always been "hard to handle" (his mother's words), the situation worsened after Trey turned 16 and earned his driver's license. At about the same time, the mother found a new boyfriend, who spends a lot of time in the home and recently started interceding when Trey and his mother argue. Arguments have principally turned on whether Trey is allowed to take the car out in the after-

Peter S. Jensen, M.D., is President and Chief Executive Officer of the REACH Institute (Resource for Advancing Children's Health) in New York, New York (for complete biographical information, see "About the Contributors," p. 613).

noons after school to "go places." Although he claims that he just goes to visit friends, in fact Trey had a recent accident 8 miles from where he said he would be, and the mother's coworkers have sighted Trey driving toward a seedy, drug-infested area of town where he is not supposed to go. For the accident, he received a ticket for being at fault (failing to yield, turning into an oncoming vehicle). His mother is reluctant to let him take the car, in part because she feels he is not telling her where he is really going and also because his driving "scares me," as he is often distracted. Although he has had only one accident, he seems to have had several "near misses" with his mother in the car.

One day, Trey and the mother's boyfriend got into a heated verbal argument when Trey wanted to take the car while his mother was away at work; the boyfriend said "no," and the two got into a shoving match. The boyfriend then grounded Trey and sent him to his room. Trey snuck out the window and drove the car over to a friend's house. The mother's boyfriend alerted the police, who found the car and arrested Trey.

PAST PSYCHIATRIC HISTORY

Trey had a history of behavior problems and learning difficulties beginning in first grade, just about a year after his father was killed in a trucking accident. Trey idolized his father, who often worked away from home as a long-distance trucker. Trey's difficulties in preschool and kindergarten had not aroused especial concerns, although his kindergarten teacher described him as "the Energizer Rabbit—he keeps on going." Toward the end of first grade, after the teacher expressed increasing concerns about Trey's difficulties staying seated, unwillingness to follow directions on the playground, aggression toward peers, and problems completing seat assignments, the mother took him for a medical evaluation with a pediatrician, who diagnosed attention-deficit/hyperactivity disorder (ADHD) and prescribed methylphenidate, 5 mg three times a day, with some benefit. Trey's mother discontinued his medication over the summer but restarted it in second grade. He continued taking the medication on and off for most of elementary school, but began to complain about taking it. In fifth grade, because of Trey's complaints, the pediatrician changed the prescription to osmotic-release methylphenidate (OROS-MPH), 18 mg/day, which Trey took for much of sixth and seventh grades but then stopped taking at the end of seventh grade.

Trey has had a long history of getting into heated arguments and conflicts, both at home and at his middle and high schools. He was suspended for fighting several times, and then expelled after hitting with his fist a teacher who was trying to break up a hallway fight in which Trey was involved. Trey claims it was "an accident." Because of these problems, as well as academic difficulties in most subjects, he was held back in ninth grade. After this incident, Trey seemed remorseful and sorry, but was also overheard bragging about it to a friend on the phone.

Trey has also had heated arguments with his mother and, on at least one occasion, has physically shoved her after she grounded him. In one incident, she fell and hit her head, needing stitches. Similarly, he is often physically aggressive toward his younger brother, including punching him and leaving bruises on his arm.

His mother notes that Trey has had long-standing problems with not minding her and staying out later than curfew. In ninth grade, he got caught skipping classes with another ninth grader, who has a history of drug abuse problems.

SUBSTANCE ABUSE HISTORY

Trey's mother says that she knows Trey is drinking, because "he sometimes smells like a brewery" after being out with friends on weekends. This has happened four or five times, and once when she confronted him about his drinking, he told his mother, "It's no big deal; everyone does it." His mother wonders if Trey has tried marijuana, noting that he keeps on display above his bed some paraphernalia, which he says are "for show," and that on two instances she wondered if he was "on drugs" as he came home with watery red eyes and a musky smell.

MEDICAL HISTORY

Trey had a tonsillectomy at age 9 after repeated bouts of strep throat. He has mild seasonal allergies and gets hives from eating shellfish.

DEVELOPMENTAL HISTORY

Trey was born at 38 weeks gestational age, with Apgar scores of 7 and 8 at 1 and 5 minutes, respectively. He had mildly elevated bilirubin and jaundice, for which he stayed an extra week in the hospital. Developmental milestones were normal or a bit precocious. His mother noted that he was "very active" beginning at about age 2, but this never worried her until teachers raised concerns in kindergarten and first grade.

SOCIAL HISTORY

Trey was raised by his mother and father until his father's death when Trey was in kindergarten. His mother was pregnant with the younger brother at the time of the father's death. She went back to work as a waitress to support the family. Trey has done fairly well in school, but his grades began a gradual decline in middle school, and he was held back in ninth grade for problems described above. His mother is concerned about his choice of friends, who tend to be "rockers" and bad students, and one of whom has known drug problems. Trey has several hobbies; he particularly likes playing guitar. He has been "jamming" with two friends after school for the past 2 years and wants to be in a band.

FAMILY HISTORY

Trey's father had a history of childhood and teenage problems in school, not doing homework, not getting along with others, and eventually dropping out. The father also had had alcohol and drug abuse problems until he joined Alcoholics Anonymous at age 25. Trey's mother and maternal grandmother have a history of depressive episodes, for which the mother has been treated with psychotherapy and a selective serotonin reuptake inhibitor.

MENTAL STATUS EXAMINATION

Trey presented dressed in jeans, sandals, a ball cap, and a KISS T-shirt. In the presence of the mother and boyfriend, he was sullen and angry about the interview, and particularly resentful about the mother's boyfriend and the subsequent arrest. His eye contact was poor, and his attitude was uncooperative. Upon interview without his mother and her boyfriend present, he appeared to warm up and to show more affect when talking about his future plans and interests in rock music. Trey denied suicidal or homicidal ideation. He said that his mother's boyfriend has "no right" to tell him what to do, because "he's not my dad." He stated that school does not interest him. Although he admitted that he has trouble concentrating, he claimed not to like medication because it "takes away my personality…I get nerdy." He admitted to some alcohol use with friends but stated, "It's not really a big problem. I know when to stop." Although he noted that one of his music friends has "drug problems," he stated, "I don't because it's not my style."

COMMENTARIES

Psychotherapeutic Perspective

Scott W. Henggeler, Ph.D.

DIAGNOSTIC FORMULATION

This commentary is written from the perspective of multisystemic therapy (MST; Henggeler et al. 1998), an evidence-based treatment typically used with adolescents referred from the juvenile justice system for serious antisocial behavior that places these youths at high risk for out-of-home placement. MST does not emphasize formal diagnostics, but rather focuses on identifying characteristics of the individual youth and the social systems in which he or she is embedded (i.e., family, peers, school, and neighborhood) that might be linked with the identified problems. Importantly, youth and social system strengths are also identified, because these are used as levers for change in the subsequent design of interventions. A multifaceted approach is taken to the assessment of problems, risk factors, and strengths; this approach includes interviews with family members (i.e., youth, caregivers, siblings, extended family as appropriate), teachers, peers, juvenile justice authorities, and others, as well as therapist observations of transactions within and between these systems. The MST therapist, in collaboration with other members of the MST treatment team, then synthesizes the assessment information into a coherent framework that will be used to guide and prioritize the design and implementation of interventions.

In the case of Trey, the likely consensus-identified problems include 1) physical aggression, 2) noncompliance, 3) substance abuse, and 4) lack of effort at school. These are serious and interrelated problems that place Trey at risk for incarceration (e.g., his physical confrontations with adults could readily lead to arrest and incarceration as an adult offender) as well as deleterious long-term outcomes (e.g., substance abuse and poor school/vocational performance are predictors of difficulties during adulthood). In delineating the risk factors linked with these problems, MST gives priority to proximal versus distal (e.g., early childhood experiences) factors. For purposes of illustration, hypothesized risk

Scott W. Henggeler, Ph.D., is Professor of Psychiatry and Behavioral Sciences and Director of the Family Services Research Center at the Medical University of South Carolina in Charleston, South Carolina (for complete biographical information, see "About the Contributors," p. 613).

factors for Trey's interpersonal aggression likely include genetic (i.e., from father) and biological (i.e., ADHD, substance abuse) predispositions for interpersonal aggression; weak parental monitoring and supervision at the family level;
extensive association with deviant friends at the peer level; and poor academic
and social performance at the school level. These risk factors likely combine
and interplay to support the development and maintenance of Trey's antisocial
behavior. On the other hand, as noted previously, the identification of systemic
strengths is also a critical emphasis of MST. For determining strengths, information provided in the case summary is less helpful, but several strengths can
be inferred. Trey's mother cares about him, the mother's boyfriend cares about
Trey's behavior, Trey is still in school (i.e., many 17-year-olds with his problems
would have dropped out by now), and Trey enjoys playing music.

DSM-IV-TR DIAGNOSIS

MST does not emphasize formal diagnostics, but rather focuses on identifying
characteristics that are described above in the diagnostic formulation. Thus, with
the case of Trey, this MST commentary does not include a DSM-IV-TR diagnosis.

TREATMENT RECOMMENDATIONS

The design of MST interventions is based on nine treatment principles
(Henggeler et al. 1998), and these interventions are developed and implemented in an iterative process: 1) the key risk factors for the identified problem
are specified, as noted above; 2) these factors are prioritized on the basis of
likelihood, if they are modified, to effect change in the identified problem;
3) interventions, derived primarily from evidence-based treatment protocols,
are developed for specific risk factors; 4) the interventions are implemented,
leveraging identified systemic strengths; 5) the outcomes of the interventions
are evaluated; and, assuming that success has not been complete, 6) the process is repeated, capitalizing on the knowledge gained from the relative success
or failure of the preceding interventions.

The development of MST interventions for Trey's physical aggression would
likely be multifaceted and sequential. Before these interventions can be developed,
however, a better understanding of the mother's lack of parenting competence is
needed, because improved parenting is often the key driver of youth clinical
change within MST. Even though Trey is 17, he is only in the tenth grade and will
likely be living in his mother's home for at least another 3 years. Common causes
of ineffective parenting include parental substance abuse or mental health problems, lack of social support, high stress, low knowledge, skill deficits, and having
"given up." The pertinent drivers of his mother's parenting difficulties would
need to be identified and resolved before interventions could be delivered optimally to Trey. Assuming that the barriers to effective parenting were addressed

effectively, the therapist would rely on the mother's love of her son and the boyfriend's caring for Trey's mother to develop a set of interventions that would be implemented by the mother. The boyfriend would not implement the interventions directly but would act as the mother's support system in her implementation.

In essence, interventions would be designed to change Trey's attitudes and the social environment that are currently supporting his physical aggression to counterparts that favor prosocial and responsible behavior. For example, Trey's substance use would be targeted with contingency management, which is an evidence-based treatment of substance abuse that has been successfully integrated into MST protocols for juvenile offenders (Henggeler et al. 2006). The parent monitors the youth's substance use through frequent drug screens and implements rewards (e.g., privileges, desired items) and sanctions (e.g., restrictions, loss of car privileges) based on the results of the screens. Similarly, cognitive-behavioral interventions, including both the youth and his mother, would be used to develop self-management strategies for dealing with high-risk substance use situations. Because impulsivity related to Trey's ADHD is also a likely contributor to his interpersonal aggression, psychiatric consultation would be obtained regarding the possibility of resuming evidence-based psychopharmacology. More challenging but critical interventions would also be designed (see Henggeler et al. 1998) to help the mother disengage Trey from his deviant peer group, connect him with more prosocial peer activities (e.g., leveraging his interest in guitar), and enhance his school and/or vocational functioning. These latter interventions are essential in promoting long-term behavioral change. Finally, throughout the course of treatment, the therapist would help the mother build an indigenous support system that could be accessed when problems inevitably reemerge.

Psychopharmacologic Perspective

Richard P. Malone, M.D.

DIAGNOSTIC FORMULATION

The assessment of conduct problems is accomplished by obtaining a detailed history that incorporates input from multiple sources, including the patient,

Richard P. Malone, M.D., is Professor of Psychiatry at the Drexel University College of Medicine in Philadelphia. Pennsylvania (for complete biographical information, see "About the Contributors," p. 613).

the family, and other community settings, especially the educational system. The history should focus on the development of symptoms over time and their impact on the patient, family, and educational performance, plus the history of past interventions and their effect.

In this case, Trey presents for evaluation after "stealing" the family car, a possible demonstration of conduct disorder. Review of the history reveals that he has a number of other conduct problems, including bullying, fighting, lying, skipping classes, school suspensions, and breaking curfew. Additionally, his history includes a number of features often associated with conduct disorder, such as poor frustration tolerance; temper outbursts; recklessness; a lack of empathy; and a family history of conduct problems, substance use, and mood disorders. As is common in conduct disorder, Trey has other comorbid conditions, including ADHD, learning problems, and drug and alcohol use.

Trey also has a history of persistent and significant aggression. Aggression can be a symptom of a number of psychiatric disorders and can also be a behavior that is independent of any psychiatric disorder. Regardless, aggression often becomes the focus of treatment and should be carefully assessed. A number of measures are available for assessing aggressive behavior, both for subtype (e.g., the Aggression Questionnaire; Vitiello et al. 1990) and for frequency and severity (e.g., the Overt Aggression Scale—Modified for Outpatients; Coccaro et al. 1991). Severe aggression in adolescents is usually preceded by a history of early childhood aggression, hyperactivity, and oppositionality (Loeber and Stouthamer-Loeber 1998).

DSM-IV-TR DIAGNOSIS

Axis I   312.81 Conduct disorder, childhood-onset type

314.01 ADHD, combined type

315.9 Learning disorder not otherwise specified

305.00 Alcohol abuse

Rule out marijuana abuse

Axis II   None

Axis III   Shellfish allergy

Axis IV   Psychosocial and environmental problems, including with primary support group, educational system, and legal system

Axis V   Global Assessment of Functioning=55 (current)

TREATMENT RECOMMENDATIONS

The treatment of disruptive behavior disorders such as conduct disorder requires a multimodal approach that incorporates behavioral, family, educational, and pharmacologic approaches. Comorbid conditions that are present and will shape the treatment plan in Trey's case are ADHD, learning problems, and substance abuse. Also, Trey's social problems at home and school and with teachers and peers will require psychosocial intervention. The family discord involving both his relationship with his mother and with her boyfriend has to be addressed. Furthermore, his decline in academic performance should be assessed, and further educational testing may be needed to assess the appropriateness of his school placement.

Psychopharmacologic treatment may be of benefit. Over the past year, Trey's problems with anger and aggression have increasingly interfered with his everyday functioning. Decreasing his aggression becomes a clinically important goal. However, the effectiveness of any treatment, including medication, can be difficult to assess. Environmental changes can have strong effects on the demonstration of aggressive behavior (Malone et al. 1997), but such changes are difficult to control and institute in a clinical setting. Also, many nonpharmacologic effects, including the expectations of caretakers and the use of placebos, influence the assessment of treatment success (Molling et al. 1962).

Double-blind, placebo-controlled trials of antipsychotic agents and mood stabilizers have demonstrated efficacy and safety for reducing aggression in conduct disorder. However, strategies developed by experts for using psychopharmacologic treatments to reduce aggression have emphasized the approach of treating the underlying psychiatric disorder and/or comorbid disorder before targeting aggression (Pappadopulos et al. 2003). Aggression itself may be reduced when comorbid conditions are treated. In the case of conduct disorder, drug treatments have been shown to be of benefit for reducing aggression but not for treating other symptoms, such as stealing, lying, and truancy.

In line with the notion of treating any comorbid disorders, the first approach pharmacologically might be to administer stimulant medication to treat comorbid ADHD. Stimulants are among the best-studied treatments in medicine and have been shown to be highly effective for reducing symptoms of ADHD. Results from large studies of children with ADHD suggest that stimulants also can reduce oppositional and aggressive behavior (Jensen et al. 2001). The history indicates that Trey has responded to stimulant medication in the past but discontinued usage because of a concern about perceived effects, a sign that discussions about adherence to medication usage will be a key part of his treatment.

Should Trey continue to have aggression despite optimal stimulant dosage, other medications as indicated above should be considered. For example, evidence indicates that antipsychotic drugs, both first- and second-generation agents, are effective for reducing aggression in disruptive disorders (Malone and Delaney 2003). Mood-stabilizing agents, such as lithium, have also been shown to be effective in reducing aggression in conduct disorder, but only in the inpatient setting (Malone et al. 2000). Although most experts agree that polypharmacy should be avoided, no guideline has been established regarding whether a stimulant should be continued or discontinued when another agent is being considered. Clearly, if another drug is added to a stimulant, the effect of later stopping the stimulant can be easily assessed, given the short-term activity of the stimulant drugs.

In summary, treatment of conduct disorder must be comprehensive and address not only the symptoms of the disorder but also comorbid disorders and environmental stressors. Medication can have a place in reducing aggression in conduct disorder. However, medication can first be used to treat comorbid conditions such as ADHD before medication to specifically reduce aggression is initiated.

Integrative Perspective

Peter S. Jensen, M.D.

DIAGNOSTIC FORMULATION

Trey, a 17-year-old living with his mother, his younger brother, and the mother's boyfriend, has a long history of troubled and troubling behaviors. Even prior to beginning kindergarten, he was a high-energy, hard-to-handle child. After the death of his father (the two reportedly had been quite close), he had increasing difficulties minding adults, aggression toward peers, and related troubles at school. In the last several years, his difficulties have increased, as demonstrated by his declining school grades, hanging out with other youths with known substance abuse problems, skipping school, breaking curfew, not minding adults, and in at least three instances becoming physically aggressive with adults. The most recent incident precipitating his referral was taking the family car without permission after an argument with the mother's boyfriend.

Trey has a number of risk factors that should be noted: elevated bilirubin levels at birth (known to be associated with ADHD), early childhood onset of aggression and hyperactive behaviors, the death of a father, and a single parent with likely difficulties in monitoring child behavior and multiple boyfriends. Trey has been treated for ADHD with some apparent benefit, but he has been noncompliant with medications since the end of seventh grade, after which he experienced drops in school grades and increased associations with problematic peers.

Trey's current difficulties appear to be greater than he and his family are willing to admit. The episodes of aggression appear to be impulsive, and the distinction between premeditated aggression and impulsive aggression is important in Trey's evaluation to determine whether his behavior difficulties are ego-syntonic or ego-dystonic. The clinician should find out whether Trey felt regret about injuring his mother or teacher. Simple cursory questions about these incidents are likely to provoke defensive responses; however, after establishing a therapeutic alliance, if the clinician can better determine the extent to which Trey felt remorse about the consequences of his behavior, both for himself and for others, this determination can be critical to determining Trey's prognosis and in guiding subsequent treatment. Similarly, developing a good therapeutic alliance would be helpful in better assessing the impact of Trey's mood on his symptoms, the role that inattention may play in activities that matter to him (such as playing guitar), and the full extent of his substance use.

Trey meets the criteria for oppositional defiant disorder (ODD). The clinician should consider whether to render the ODD diagnosis because, under DSM-IV-TR criteria, a conduct disorder diagnosis preempts the diagnosis of ODD. However, many of the difficulties related to his current problems—arguments with parents and adults, the refusal to mind adult requests, blaming of others (although this may have been defensive and not what he truly felt), an angry and resentful attitude, and often losing his temper—are related to his ODD symptoms.

The question of whether to render the conduct disorder diagnosis is based, in part, on whether Trey initiates the fights or whether they are initiated by others who tease him and possibly start a shoving or hitting match. He has no history of cruelty to persons or animals per se, and his several bouts of aggression toward peers and parents cannot be construed as cruelty per se, just as the history of taking the car cannot be fully considered as stealing when he has a history of driving the same car with permission under other circumstances. Also importantly, Trey does not appear to have the typical antisocial personality pattern of deceitfulness to obtain goods or back out of obligations. Trey's lies appear to serve the purpose of avoiding being caught. Likewise, regarding the conduct disorder diagnosis, Trey has no clear history of breaking curfew or truancy before age 13. Although he has a "long history" of staying out later than parental curfew, the case presentation is unclear whether this antedated the age of 13. Of note, because his aggression toward peers began shortly after his father's death, if the conduct disorder diagnosis were made, the criteria for childhood-onset type might be met. Although impulsive aggression is not a DSM-IV-TR diagnosis, discriminating impulsive from planned or predatory aggression is very important in Trey's case and needs to be considered as a part of the overall understanding of his prognosis and in constructing a treatment plan (Jensen et al. 2007; Vitiello et al. 1990).

In summary, Trey is a 17-year-old with a history of ADHD, significant oppositional and conduct problems, and substance use, yet he has an ability to engage with adults under the right conditions. He also has a history of significant instances of impulsive aggression when someone teases him about school, calls him names, makes fun of his music, or stops him from doing something that he feels he really "has to do." He shows affection, loyalty, and empathy toward his mother and friends, and he has the ability to relate in one-on-one interviews. Some capacity for insight and problem solving is apparent.

DSM-IV-TR DIAGNOSIS

Axis I   314.01 ADHD, combined type

313.81 Oppositional defiant disorder

Rule out conduct disorder

V61.20 Parent-child relational problem

V61.9 Relational problem related to a mental disorder

V62.3 Academic problem

Substance use disorder including marijuana, alcohol, and other substances

Axis II   Rule out emergent antisocial personality disorder

Axis III   None

Axis IV   Severity of psychosocial stressors

Family conflicts

Legal difficulties

Poor peer relationships

Blended family circumstances

Axis V   Global Assessment of Functioning=50

TREATMENT RECOMMENDATIONS

The most crucial aspect of Trey's treatment was first engaging him, his mother, and also the mother's boyfriend in the treatment process. In the case of Trey, motivational interviewing methods were used to help him recognize the problems that he was having and acknowledge that *he* wanted to improve how his life was going. Trey agreed to an overall plan, which included not using marijuana, intermittent urine drug tests for maintaining abstinence, a behavioral contract with car driving privileges tied to school attendance and homework completion, use of a long-acting stimulant medication, counseling to mother and boyfriend about their roles and appropriate noncoercive limit setting, weekly family communication sessions, and frequent weekly follow-up with therapist, at least initially.

Medication Treatment

Trey acknowledged his difficulties with sustained attention and completing activities, even with tasks that he liked doing, such as writing music. Because guitar practice was often tedious, he felt that he could be a better guitar player if he did not get bored so quickly during practice. In light of his early history of ADHD and present difficulties with sustained attention at school, at home, and in other settings, medication treatment with OROS-MPH was retried. Trey acknowledged that medication had helped him before but he did not want to feel different from other kids, which is why he stopped taking it. In light of his self-acknowledged difficulties with areas in which he himself now wanted to do better, including his music as well as school activities, Trey agreed to reexamine the benefits of a long-acting stimulant that had been beneficial during his earlier treatment plan. Although OROS-MPH, like any stimulant, can be diverted, it is relatively safe in that it cannot be crushed, ground, or snorted for abuse potential. Given the therapist's relationship with Trey, this approach was thought to be a reasonable first step. Should more concerns about diversion or abuse of medication develop, other approaches might be preferred (not done in Trey's case), including atomoxetine or lisdexamfetamine.

Trey's impulsive aggression and temper—arguably his most worrisome symptom—improved significantly after adequate titration of medication. Methylphenidate was titrated using a combination of ADHD rating scales from the homeroom teacher, his favorite music teacher, his mother, and himself. With Trey, rating scales were jointly inspected, and medication was adjusted so that the symptoms were as low as possible, thereby avoiding other side effects such as insomnia or extreme loss of appetite. Because Trey was slightly overweight, appetite issues were not a primary concern at the onset of treatment.

Trey's argumentativeness as well as his impulsivity and even the frequency of fights improved substantially (with a dosage of 72 mg/day of OROS-MPH, titrated over a 2-month period). In patients in whom impulsive aggression remains even after improvement of ADHD symptoms, other considerations (not employed in his case) include the use of a low-dose second-generation atypical antipsychotic, such as risperidone, or an α_2 agonist, such as clonidine or guanfacine. In the event of side effects or nonresponse, valproic acid might be considered (Pappadopulos et al. 2003). After 2 months of weekly psychotherapeutic engagement of Trey around the problems he felt he was experiencing, as well as close titration of his medication, Trey made significant progress on most fronts, except one weekend night when he admitted drinking at a party after being confronted by his mother. He did not drive the car on that occasion. He agreed to intermittent continued urine drug screens, applied for a summer job at a music store, and began to make arrangements to enroll in a community college to get his GED.

Because of the difficulties involving the role of the boyfriend in the home (this had been the mother's third boyfriend during Trey's growing-up years), Trey and his mother agreed to family therapy. Functional family therapy is an evidence-based treatment for youth with delinquent and antisocial behavior problems such as those experienced by Trey. In this context, behavioral contracting was done for critical changes in both Trey's behavior (attending school, controlling temper, avoiding drugs, and completing schoolwork) and his mother's behavior. The therapist, Trey, and his mother discussed the appropriate role that her boyfriend should have in Trey's discipline and those areas that needed to remain his mother's responsibilities. After several sessions, the boyfriend was invited to a session, and these arrangements were discussed and negotiated openly between Trey, the mother, and the boyfriend, with the therapist.

In cases such as Trey's, it is not uncommon that the youth careens further out of control, only to end up in juvenile justice, in an out-of-home placement, on the street, or in living arrangements with unseemly friends. In this instance, these outcomes were averted, at least for the time being, in part because of the engaging of Trey in the therapeutic process and the interruption of influences that were destructive in his life and leading him into further difficulties with substance use, problematic peers, and poor school performance. The therapeutic process involved reengaging Trey in working toward outcomes that he himself desired; the use of medication to address symptoms of ADHD, impulsivity, and aggression; the setting of appropriate boundaries in parenting relationships in a quasi-blended family; the use of behavioral and adolescent-relevant collaborative approaches toward problem solving; and the establishment of win-win behavioral contingencies. Although many similar cases have worse outcomes, due to less responsive family situations or different levels of motivation in the youngster, Trey's outcome was more favorable. Youth with similar difficulties and a similar trajectory but poor family circumstances and the inability or unwillingness to address increasing behavior problems may require more intensive forms of treatment, including multisystemic therapy (Henggeler et al. 1998), judicious use of an atypical antipsychotic for the aggressive symptoms (Pappadopulos et al. 2003), and substance use and rehabilitation programs.

REFERENCES

Coccaro EF, Harvey PD, Kupsaw-Lawrence E, et al: Development of neuropharmacologically based behavioral assessments of impulsive aggressive behavior. J Neuropsychiatry Clin Neurosci 3:S44–S51, 1991

Henggeler SW, Schoenwald SK, Borduin CM, et al: Multisystemic Treatment of Antisocial Behavior in Children and Adolescents. New York, Guilford, 1998

Henggeler SW, Halliday-Boykins CA, Cunningham PB, et al: Juvenile drug court: enhancing outcomes by integrating evidence-based treatments. J Consult Clin Psychol 74:42–54, 2006

Jensen PS, Hinshaw SP, Kraemer HC, et al: ADHD comorbidity findings from the MTA study: comparing comorbid subgroups. J Am Acad Child Adolesc Psychiatry 40:147–158, 2001

Jensen PS, Youngstrom E, Steiner H, et al: Consensus report: impulsive aggression as a symptom across diagnostic categories in child psychiatry: implications for medication studies. J Am Acad Child Adolesc Psychiatry 46:309–322, 2007

Loeber R, Stouthamer-Loeber M: Development of juvenile aggression and violence: some common misconceptions and controversies. Am Psychol 53:242–259, 1998

Malone RP, Delaney MA: Psychopharmacologic interventions in children with aggression: neuroleptics, lithium, and anticonvulsants, in Aggression: Assessment and Treatment. Edited by Coccaro EF. New York, Marcel Dekker, 2003, pp 331–349

Malone RP, Luebbert JF, Delaney MA, et al: Nonpharmacological response in hospitalized children with conduct disorder. J Am Acad Child Adolesc Psychiatry 36:242–247, 1997

Malone RP, Delaney MA, Luebbert JF, et al: A double-blind placebo-controlled study of lithium in hospitalized aggressive children and adolescents with conduct disorder. Arch Gen Psychiatry 57:649–654, 2000

Molling PA, Lockner AW Jr, Sauls RJ, et al: Committed delinquent boys: the impact of perphenazine and of placebo. Arch Gen Psychiatry 7:70–76, 1962

Pappadopulos E, Macintyre JC, Crismon ML, et al: Treatment recommendations for the use of antipsychotics for aggressive youth (TRAAY), part II: recommendations for clinicians. J Am Acad Child Adolesc Psychiatry 42:145–161, 2003

Vitiello B, Behar D, Hunt J, et al: Subtyping aggression in children and adolescents. J Neuropsychiatry Clin Neurosci 2:189–192, 1990

■ CHAPTER 14 ■

Zero Tolerance

Threats to Harm a Teacher in Elementary School

Karen C. Wells, Ph.D.

CASE PRESENTATION

IDENTIFYING INFORMATION

James is a 10-year-old who lives with his parents and two siblings, an 8-year-old sister and a newborn. He attends fifth grade.

CHIEF COMPLAINT

James was referred to the outpatient child psychiatry clinic by the emergency department of the local hospital, where he was taken for an emergency evaluation because of threatening to kill his teacher.

HISTORY OF PRESENT ILLNESS

On the day of evaluation, James had pulled a knife from his pocket at school and threatened to kill his teacher after she gave him an after-school detention and threatened to call his parents about his fighting on the playground. When James's parents could not be reached immediately, school security personnel

---

Karen C. Wells, Ph.D., is Associate Professor of Medical Psychology, Director of the Family Studies Program and Clinic, and Director of Psychology Internship in the Department of Psychiatry at Duke University Medical Center in Durham, North Carolina (for complete biographical information, see "About the Contributors," p. 613).

transported James to the emergency department because he continued to be combative and verbally defiant to the principal in the school office. Once at the emergency department, James became sullen and withdrawn and refused to speak to the medical personnel. When his parents arrived at the emergency department, they gave a history of James's disruptive behavior in school and oppositional and aggressive behavior from an early age, escalating to hitting his siblings and, more recently, hitting and kicking his parents when they attempted to discipline him and fighting at school. Although James had displayed disruptive behavior since an early age, his parents reported an increase in his anger and aggression since the recent birth of the sibling, as well as a corresponding increase in their anger and short-tempered reactions to James. In the emergency department, James denied suicidal or homicidal ideation or plans, and after several hours, he was released to the custody of his parents with an appointment scheduled the next day at the psychiatry clinic.

PAST PSYCHIATRIC HISTORY

Interview and history taken from James's parents at the psychiatry clinic indicated a child who from early infancy had had a difficult temperament, fussy irritability, and difficulty developing regular sleeping habits. His mother reported that James "never crawled or toddled but just seemed to get up and start running one day and has been running ever since." He was "into everything," seemingly fearless, and had to be constantly watched and monitored for dangerous behaviors, such as climbing bookcases. He did not respond when adults said "no," and when physically stopped or prevented from preferred or risky activities, he became very upset, screamed, cried, and threw tantrums. In kindergarten at age 5, James was aggressive toward other children, pinching and hitting them, and impulsively grabbed toys from other children. He threw tantrums when the teacher intervened to return the toy. He had difficulty making transitions from one activity to another and was unable to settle or rest at quiet time. The school administration suggested that he repeat kindergarten before going on to first grade.

In the early grades of elementary school, James continued to display disruptive behavior. He had difficulty sitting and paying attention in circle time and, later, at his desk, and he was frequently out of his seat walking around the room. He also continued to show aggression toward other children when frustrated, impulsively hitting them when he did not get his way. In the third and fourth grades, he continued to be aggressive toward classmates, had difficulty completing his assignments in class, and made disruptive noises in his seat that bothered other children. He seemed to be of average or higher intelligence but made poor grades, mainly due to not completing assignments or turning in homework. His teacher moved his desk to the front of the class by her desk. Over the years, as behavioral expectations in school increased and teacher tolerance decreased, his behavior elicited ever-increasing levels of corrective, negative feedback and criticism from teachers.

At home, his parents responded to James's behavior with increasing frustration, criticism, and hostility. The father spanked James frequently and, according to his mother, cursed at James when he was very angry, but this did not appear to reach the level of physical abuse. His mother admitted to yelling and scolding and calling James names, about which she later felt guilty. James first hit his mother in one of these disciplinary interactions. After this, his tantrums increased and would include hitting and kicking at both parents when he did not get his way. His parents admitted that these approaches did not seem to be working, but they did not know what would work. James appeared increasingly angry and out of control, and his parents were at a loss as to how to manage him.

SUBSTANCE ABUSE HISTORY

James and his parents deny that James has used alcohol, cigarettes, or recreational drugs.

MEDICAL HISTORY

James had a tonsillectomy at age 5 but no other significant medical history or procedures.

DEVELOPMENTAL HISTORY

James was the product of a normal, full-term pregnancy and delivery. His mother, a pack-a-day smoker prior to the pregnancy, reported that she tried to quit smoking while pregnant but succeeded only in cutting down from a pack a day to "several cigarettes a day." The remaining early developmental history was as described above.

SOCIAL HISTORY

James's mother worked full-time outside the home. His father was currently unemployed and had a work history of multiple job changes. Stressors included the father's unemployment, credit problems related to three automobile accidents that the father had had within the last 3 years, the new baby, an overburdened mother, and marital conflict related to all of the above.

FAMILY HISTORY

The father's brother had a history of attention-deficit/hyperactivity disorder (ADHD) and substance abuse, and several paternal cousins had ADHD. The father had never seen a psychiatrist or psychologist and had no formal diagnoses but reported having had significant difficulty in school despite a normal IQ. He reported being "bored" with his jobs and not finding an occupation that interested him, but his wife reported that he had been fired from several jobs due to "forgetfulness" and disorganization. According to his wife, he drank 6–12 beers per night. James's mother had a diagnosis of depression and was currently being treated with antidepressant medication.

MENTAL STATUS EXAMINATION

The interview revealed that James was a sullen boy who answered questions with one- or two-word responses. He stayed in his seat, shredding a tissue into tiny pieces, throughout the course of the interview. He stated that his mood was "fine" but that he got angry when people treated him unfairly. He denied that he had threatened his teacher with a knife, and said that the boys that he had been fighting with deserved to be punished, but that he did not. His reality testing was unimpaired, and he denied suicidal or homicidal ideation. He stated that he did not know why he was at the clinic and showed little insight about any contributions to his current difficulties.

COMMENTARIES

Psychotherapeutic Perspective

Caroline Lewczyk Boxmeyer, Ph.D.
Nicole Powell, Ph.D., M.P.H.
John E. Lochman, Ph.D., A.B.P.P.

DIAGNOSTIC FORMULATION

James's presentation suggests a history of disruptive behavior problems and family environmental stressors. A multimethod, multi-informant approach is recom-

Caroline Lewczyk Boxmeyer, Ph.D., is Research Scientist at the Center for the Prevention of Youth Behavior Problems, and Supervising Psychologist in the Psychology Clinic at The University of Alabama in Tuscaloosa, Alabama.

Nicole Powell, Ph.D, M.P.H., is Research Psychologist at the Center for the Prevention of Youth Behavior Problems at the The University of Alabama in Tuscaloosa, Alabama.

John E. Lochman, Ph.D., A.B.P.P., is Professor and Doddridge Saxon Chairholder in Clinical Psychology, and Director of the Center for Prevention of Youth Behavior Problems at the The University of Alabama in Tuscaloosa, Alabama.

For complete biographical information, see "About the Contributors," p. 613.

mended to assess the nature, onset, and severity of James's symptoms and to identify the specific biopsychosocial factors contributing to his current clinical
presentation. Specifically, information regarding James's current symptoms and
functioning, as well as his developmental, social, academic, and treatment history, should be obtained through 1) clinical interviews with James and his parents;
2) completion of behavioral checklists (e.g., Behavior Assessment System for Children, 2nd Edition; Reynolds and Kamphaus 2004) by James and his parents and
teacher; 3) school consultation; and 4) direct behavioral observation.

On the basis of the information provided, James is presenting with features of a
disruptive behavior disorder. He exhibits a number of symptoms of oppositional defiant disorder (ODD), and his history also indicates that he has symptoms of conduct disorder. According to DSM-IV-TR, because conduct disorder is felt to reflect
a more serious form of disruptive behavior, it takes precedence over the ODD diagnosis. The presenting incident in which James threatened to kill his teacher with
a knife meets the conduct disorder diagnostic criterion of using a weapon that can
cause serious physical harm to others. Reports of a number of other aggressive acts
toward children and adults, beginning at age 5, also indicate that James has been
exhibiting a repetitive and persistent pattern of behavior in which the basic rights of
others are violated. Although James's aggressive behavior reflects physical cruelty
toward others, given that the aggressive incidents described tended to be reactive in
nature, the clinician should determine whether James has also demonstrated more
proactive forms of aggressive, destructive, or deceitful behaviors, in an effort to further confirm that a conduct disorder diagnosis is most appropriate.

The descriptions of James's developmental and academic history also indicate that he has a number of symptoms of ADHD (e.g., impulsivity, hyperactivity, difficulty paying attention and completing assignments). Given the high
rate of co-occurrence of ADHD and ODD/conduct disorder (Jensen and
members of the MTA Cooperative Group 2002), as well as the paternal family
history of ADHD, the clinician should further assess James for ADHD and
consider how these symptoms may be affecting his behavior and academic performance. Research suggests that children with both conduct disorder and
ADHD have a poorer prognosis than children with only one of these disorders
(e.g., Waschbusch 2002) and that children with higher total numbers of conduct problems and ADHD symptoms are at risk for developing more severe
conduct disorder in adolescence (Whittinger et al. 2007), underscoring the
need to address both disorders if indicated.

Given James's difficult temperament in infancy, he was likely born with a
biological predisposition to social-emotional and/or behavior problems. However, a number of family environmental stressors appear to be exacerbating
James's behavior problems. His parents report an escalating cycle of harsh and
conflictual disciplinary interactions, which are reflective of the coercive family

process often seen in children with disruptive behavior disorders (Patterson 2002). Other key risk factors for conduct disorder are also reported, including maternal depression and paternal substance abuse, as well as situational stressors such as the father's unemployment, the birth of a new sibling, and financial concerns (Loeber and Farrington 1998).

DSM-IV-TR DIAGNOSIS

Axis I   312.81 Conduct disorder, childhood-onset type
            V61.20 Parent-child relational problem
            314.01 ADHD, combined type (provisional)
Axis II   None
Axis III   Intrauterine drug exposure (nicotine)
Axis IV   Adjustment to birth of new sibling, maternal depression, paternal unemployment and excessive alcohol use, family financial concerns, marital discord
Axis V   Global Assessment of Functioning=55

TREATMENT RECOMMENDATIONS

The information provided about James's current symptom presentation, psychosocial history, and family functioning indicates that a comprehensive treatment plan is needed to address his conduct problems. At a minimum, services should include individual and/or group therapy, parenting intervention, and collaboration with teachers. Should his disruptive behavior fail to improve or escalate while he is receiving these services, intervention might be intensified to include in-home therapy, day treatment, or placement in a residential facility.

As a first-line treatment, James and his parents should participate in an evidence-based program that addresses the characteristic skill deficits seen in children with conduct problems and their families (e.g., Lochman et al. 2008; Wells et al. 2008). Because James appears to have problems with anger management, he can benefit from improving his awareness of early cues to anger as well as from learning strategies such as positive self-statements (e.g., "I am not going to let this get to me") and relaxation. His reliance on aggression to resolve conflicts also is suggestive of a need for assistance in social problem solving. Therapeutic interventions in this area might include accurate recognition of others' intentions, appropriate problem identification, expanding his repertoire of problem-solving strategies (e.g., to include discussion and compromise), and improving his awareness of consequences for his choices. Aggressive children are likely to be rejected by their normative peer group, placing them at increased risk for association with deviant peers and escalating behavior problems (e.g., Coie et al. 1992). Improvement of James's social skills, addressed through in vivo practice during group therapy, increased parental supervision and monitoring, and involvement in well-supervised extracurricular activities, may decrease the risk of negative peer effects.

The main treatment goals with James's parents are to improve the parent-child relationship and establish effective behavioral management strategies. By spending one-on-one time each day engaging in enjoyable activities with James, and by increasing praise and attention to his positive behaviors, James's parents can work toward improving their interactions with him and increasing his prosocial behaviors. A therapist can also help them to broaden their range of discipline strategies to target minor disruptive behaviors (e.g., through selective ignoring) and more serious misbehavior (e.g., through privilege removal). Children with disruptive behaviors often respond well to structured behavioral programs that include clear expectations, rewards for appropriate behavior, and consequences for misdeeds, and a therapist can work with the family to develop a system for use in the home. To be maximally effective, the system should also encompass school behavior. This can be accomplished through establishing a written school-to-home report system, in which teachers indicate daily progress toward behavioral goals and parents provide rewards or consequences as indicated. Other important components of intervention with James's parents include providing support related to their current family stressors (which include James's behavior problems), teaching them to use stress management techniques, and referral for additional individual or marital therapy services as needed.

If further assessment supports an ADHD diagnosis for James, referrals for a medication evaluation and school accommodations would also be warranted.

Psychopharmacologic Perspective

Robert L. Findling, M.D.

DIAGNOSTIC FORMULATION

A thorough and thoughtful diagnostic assessment is the first step in a psychopharmacologic approach to a youngster with aggressive behavior (Pappadopulos

Robert L. Findling, M.D., is Rocco L. Motto, M.D., is Chair of Child and Adolescent Psychiatry at the Case Western Reserve University School of Medicine, and Director of the Division of Child and Adolescent Psychiatry at University Hospitals Case Medical Center in Cleveland, Ohio (for complete biographical information, see "About the Contributors," p. 613).

et al. 2003). Because James has a history of chronic restlessness and impulsivity, and his father has a history of academic and vocational underachievement, a diagnosis of ADHD seems to be a reasonable consideration for James.

The young man also has a chronic history of difficulties with oppositionality and impulsive aggressive behavior. Therefore, this youngster may also have a disruptive behavior disorder such as ODD or conduct disorder.

However, the case presentation suggests that other diagnoses might be considered as well. Based on the history of potentially excessive corporal punishment and possibly overly harsh verbal reprimands, the clinician should consider in the differential diagnosis whether James might also be suffering from posttraumatic stress disorder or a related anxiety disorder.

The patient's history also indicates multiple stressors within the home, all of which might be substantively impacting this youngster's behavior and emotional state. For this reason, these issues should also be thoughtfully evaluated and considered as part of a biopsychosocial evaluation. Once the evaluation is completed, a treatment plan can be formulated.

In James's age group, ADHD is frequently associated with comorbid disruptive behavior disorders (Pliszka and AACAP Work Group on Quality Issues 2007). Thus, although James may in fact be suffering from other psychiatric syndromes and likely has substantive psychosocial determinants for his behaviors, I will presume for heuristic purposes that he suffers from ADHD and comorbid conduct disorder.

DSM-IV-TR DIAGNOSIS

Axis I   314.01 ADHD, combined type
            312.81 Conduct disorder, childhood-onset type
Axis II   No diagnosis
Axis III   None
Axis IV   Problem with primary support group, birth of a sibling
            Educational problems, difficulty with teachers
Axis V   Global Assessment of Functioning=55

TREATMENT RECOMMENDATIONS

Pharmacotherapy alone might not be optimal for this patient, considering the multiple psychosocial stressors in his life and the psychological distress he is experiencing. Thus, medication therapy might be most effective for this child as part of a multimodal treatment plan.

A rational pharmacologic treatment approach, based on published recommendations, to treating such a youngster generally begins with pharmacotherapy of ADHD (Kutcher et al. 2004). Psychostimulants and atomoxetine have

U.S. Food and Drug Administration (FDA) approval for use in children with ADHD. A psychostimulant might be more reasonable for James, because extensive data suggest that treatment with psychostimulants is associated with both ADHD symptom amelioration and reductions in aggressive behavior in children with ADHD and aggression (Connor et al. 2002).

For youngsters like James, a long-acting stimulant (rather than a short-acting formulation) may be a rational starting point for ADHD pharmacotherapy, because a long-acting preparation may more readily afford a child the opportunity to have sustained symptom amelioration over the course of a day. However, for families that are particularly concerned about potential stimulant-related side effects, initial treatment with a short-acting stimulant may be a reasonable initial choice. Beginning therapy with a short-acting stimulant formulation may allow the family to become more comfortable with a more modest degree of medication exposure. This latter approach, therefore, can provide an opportunity to assuage the parents' concerns about psychostimulant treatment early in the course of drug therapy.

However, the extant evidence suggests that comorbidity with conduct disorder reduces psychostimulants' effectiveness in the treatment of aggression (Connor et al. 2002). Therefore, at the start of psychostimulant therapy, I would review with James's family the possibility that although James might have substantive reductions in ADHD symptomatology with optimized psychostimulant pharmacotherapy, he may not receive adequate reductions in his pathological aggression (Jensen et al. 2007).

Following FDA-approved dosing strategies for ADHD is recommended, because these dosing approaches are derived from scientific data. As mentioned above, although James might have good ADHD symptom amelioration with the first psychostimulant he is prescribed, satisfactory reductions in aggressive behavior may not occur. For a patient with residual and problematic aggression, I generally review two treatment options with the patient and family: 1) try another first-line treatment for ADHD (e.g., another psychostimulant or atomoxetine) to see if better overall response is seen or 2) consider an adjunctive agent specifically selected to address the aggression. Unfortunately, no methodologically stringent data are available to indicate whether option 1 or option 2 is best. However, my colleagues and I have the impression that replacing the psychostimulant with either another stimulant or atomoxetine is often not as successful as opting for a treatment course in which an adjunctive medication is initiated.

For some youths whose families are particularly concerned about the safety profile of possible adjunctive drugs, trying treatment with another psychostimulant (e.g., replacing a methylphenidate-based stimulant with an amphetamine, or vice versa) or atomoxetine may be reasonable. Should the family choose an adjunctive medication to address James's residual aggression despite effective treatment of his ADHD, risperidone (Pandina et al. 2006) and clonidine (Hazell and Stuart 2003) are commonly prescribed drugs with placebo-controlled evidence to support their being used in combination with psychostimulants in such children. However, of these two medications, risperidone has been studied more extensively in this patient population.

Presuming that the family would select risperidone because it has more data than clonidine to support its use, I would review the risks associated with this drug with the patient and his family. In addition, I would obtain baseline assessments so James could be monitored for weight gain and potential metabolic effects (Correll and Carlson 2006). Unfortunately, the presence of a psychostimulant does not appear to reduce the weight gain that is common during risperidone treatment (Aman et al. 2004). Dosing of risperidone should be gradually titrated upward and generally adhere to the maximum doses used in published studies of risperidone in this patient population. During the course of pharmacotherapy, the goal is to address both the youngster's ADHD with a stimulant and residual aggressive behavior with risperidone, while carefully monitoring for treatment-related side effects. To facilitate the monitoring of symptom severity, the use of rating scales that track these symptom domains may be quite useful (Kutcher et al. 2004; Pappadopulos et al. 2003).

Youth with ADHD and a comorbid disruptive behavior disorder diagnosis are at risk for poor outcomes (Connor et al. 2006). As a result, an appreciation of the poor outcomes that often befall these aggressive children needs to be incorporated into any risk/benefit consideration of combined pharmacotherapy—both at the outset and during ongoing pharmacotherapy.

Integrative Perspective

Karen C. Wells, Ph.D.

DIAGNOSTIC FORMULATION

James's case is a fairly typical example of a child whose disruptive, primarily aggressive and oppositional, behavior is the immediate presenting problem that brings him to the attention of the mental health system. However, this case illustrates the importance of taking a careful history, not only of the early onset and developmental course of symptoms, but also of the complex systems factors in the boy's surrounding psychosocial context. Review of the early history combined with the present symptom display reveals a boy who had a difficult early temperament and then began showing symptoms of impulsivity and hyperactivity at an early age, certainly prior to the age of 7, with symptoms persisting and escalating over the years to the present time. Of the primary symptom areas associated with ADHD, he displays at least four symptoms of inattention, at least five symptoms of hyperactivity, and at least two symptoms of impulsivity. This combination of symptoms qualifies him for a diagnosis of ADHD, predominantly hyperactive-impulsive type. However, given that he displays four of the six symptoms associated with inattention, the clinician should further inquire of the parents and/or teacher regarding behaviors reflecting disorganized behavior at home or in the classroom, forgetfulness, and distractibility. (In this regard, scales such as the Conners' Parent and Teacher Rating Scales [Conners 1997; Conners et al. 1998] would be useful for efficiently gathering the relevant information.) Display of two more of these symptoms would reach the threshold for diagnosing ADHD, combined type.

In general, children who meet criteria for a diagnosis of one disruptive behavior disorder are likely to show evidence of other disruptive disorders as well, and this seems to be the case with James. His immediate presenting problem primarily involves aggression, both at home and at school, both verbal and physical. He clearly meets two of the DSM-IV-TR criteria for a diagnosis of conduct disorder (initiating fights, using a weapon), and if further history taking shows any evidence of just one additional disruptive behavior, such as stealing, truanting, or lying, within the last 6 months, he would meet full criteria for a conduct disorder diagnosis. Given his relatively young age and the fact that he displays subthreshold conduct disorder currently, with a long-standing developmental history of aggressive behavior, if James goes without intervention, he will most likely reach full criteria for conduct disorder at some time in the future. This is important given the relatively poor long-term prognosis associated with a diagnosis of conduct disorder. Finally, James also displays at least four symptoms of ODD (i.e., losing temper, active defiance, blaming others, angry and resentful), so he presently meets criteria for a diagnosis of ODD as well. These comorbid diagnoses frequently occur together, with a large percentage of children (45% in community samples and 96% in clinical samples) showing these patterns of co-occurrence (Hinshaw et al. 1993).

In addition to the diagnostic issues, the clinician needs to consider psychosocial factors in James's surrounding context that are also important with regard to multiaxial diagnoses and treatment planning. Both of James's parents seem to have current psychiatric disorders that have implications for their ability to provide appropriate and responsive parenting to James. His mother has been diagnosed with depression and is overburdened with psychosocial stressors. His father seems to have many characteristics (both symptoms and functional impairments) of adult attention-deficit disorder (ADD). His father also uses/abuses alcohol excessively and daily. Each of these possible parent conditions (i.e., depression, adult ADD, substance abuse) bears a relationship to poor parenting and to the parents' ability to profit maximally from parent management training (e.g., Murray and Johnston 2006). In addition, marital discord is present and may contribute to the mother's depression as well as erode the ability of the spouses to work together effectively as parents. The recent birth of a new sibling may function as a psychosocial stressor and affect the parents' ability to pay positive attention to James and his needs, contributing to the increasing levels of anger that James has displayed most recently.

Both parents and James's teachers engage in what appears to be an escalating cycle of negative, hostile, and coercive interactions with James. In addition, the father engages in angry corporal punishment of James. Each of these processes 1) has the unintended effect of increasing and maintaining the very oppositional and aggressive behaviors that they are meant to diminish and 2) results in an increasingly angry child and frustrated and hostile parents and teachers (Patterson et al. 1992). The index event, in which James was reported to pull a knife on his teacher at school, was probably the end result of lengthy, escalating, coercive, interpersonal processes involving an impulsive and dysregulated child, frustrated teachers, and impaired, overstressed parents.

DSM-IV-TR DIAGNOSIS

Axis I   314.01 ADHD, predominantly hyperactive-impulsive type
            313.81 Oppositional defiant disorder
            312.9 Disruptive behavior disorder not otherwise specified
Axis II   None
Axis III   None
Axis IV   Problems with primary support group
Axis V   Global Assessment of Functioning=55

TREATMENT RECOMMENDATIONS

Treatment should follow from what is known about best, evidence-based practices for children displaying the multiple comorbidities and associated parent and social factors that are present in James's case. Each of the diagnostic components in the child and the parents, as well as the other parent, family, and interactional features, results in current functional impairment and also operates as a risk factor for continued and escalating disruptive disorders and poor prognostic outcome as this child ages. Thus, a multicomponent treatment plan that would include both medication treatment and psychosocial treatments for the child and the parents is indicated.

Multimodal treatment is recommended based on the current status of the treatment outcome research, which suggests that 1) stimulant medication is an effective short-term treatment approach for primary and some secondary symptoms of ADHD; 2) behavior therapy, including parent and teacher management training approaches, is an effective treatment for ODD alone, a useful treatment component for conduct disorder, and an effective, but not maximally effective, treatment for ADHD; 3) the combination of stimulant medication and comprehensive behavior therapy has (in some studies and on some measures) been shown to be more effective than either treatment alone for ADHD; 4) the combination of medication and behavioral treatment can result in equivalent behavioral improvements at lower doses of medication than when medication is used alone; and 5) combination treatment is most likely to result in full normalization of ADHD symptoms for some children than either treatment alone (see Wells 2004).

A review of all the relevant medications and discussion of medication choice are beyond the scope of this chapter. Suffice it to say that medication treatment would likely start with one of the stimulant medications, with ongoing evaluation of treatment response and side effects. Brief parent and teacher rating scales, such as the Conners' 10-item scales (Conners 1997; Conners et al. 1998), can be used to track treatment response. Increased dosage and/or medication switches would occur as needed until a stable treatment response with limited side effects is obtained.

Regarding psychosocial treatment, a comprehensive clinical behavioral therapy approach is recommended. This approach would involve structured interventions with the parents and teachers directed toward James and, given his subthreshold conduct disorder, individual cognitive therapy with James. Comprehensive clinical behavioral therapy for ADHD would involve structured parent management training sessions that include teaching parents how to implement the home component of home-school reinforcement systems, also known as daily report cards; how to use positive attention and reinforcement skills with their child; how to give appropriate instructions and set age-appropriate rules and expectations with their child; how to implement nonphysical punishment in an effective, consistent fashion; how to advocate for their child with the teacher and school personnel; and how to extend treatment effects to other community settings (Wells et al. 2000). A detailed parent training manual describes all of these parent interventions (Wells et al. 1996). Teachers receive consultation in areas such as setting up classroom or individual rules and expectations, classroom reward systems, and implementing the school component of the daily report card system (Wells et al. 2000). Finally, although individual cognitive therapy has been shown to be ineffective with children with ADHD, some evidence supports the effectiveness of these approaches in reducing the aggressive and antisocial behavior of children with conduct disorder. Two specific examples of effective programs are problem-solving skills training (Kazdin et al. 1987) and anger coping, utilizing the Coping Power program (Lochman and Wells 2002). Given James's noted outbursts of anger and his difficulty in solving peer problems in a nonaggressive manner, individual sessions involving problem-solving and anger-coping skills training might also be useful.

Wells (2005) suggested treating ADHD as a "family illness" for children such as James, whose parents suffer from their own possible psychiatric and substance use disorders, and marital and other stressors. In such cases, comprehensive, contextual treatment would involve evaluation and treatment of conditions that have an impact on the child's ADHD, on the adults' ability to parent their child effectively, on the parents' ability to cooperate with treatment, and on the parents' ability to cooperate with each other. Thus, James's parents should be offered treatment or referred for their own ADHD, depression, and marital conflict/dysfunction, and possibly assistance with substance use/abuse and life skills such as job/occupational skills. Some evidence in the literature suggests that treating parent psychopathology while also providing treatment for a child's disruptive behavior will result in better immediate and/or long-term outcomes for the child than when parent psychopathology goes untreated (e.g., Sanders and McFarland 2000). Finally, marital therapy should be recommended when marital conflict interferes obviously and significantly with co-parenting role functions and the ability to participate in parent management training. Wells (2005) described an integrated approach to family therapy for ADHD that incorporates all of the previously mentioned elements, including marital intervention, into a comprehensive, multicomponent psychosocial treatment approach that would be useful with James and his family.

REFERENCES

Aman MG, Binder C, Turgay A: Risperidone effects in the presence/absence of psychostimulant medicine in children with ADHD, other disruptive behavior disorders, and subaverage IQ. J Child Adolesc Psychopharmacol 14:243–254, 2004

Coie JD, Lochman JE, Terry R, et al: Predicting early adolescent disorder from childhood aggression and peer rejection. J Consult Clin Psychol 60:783–792, 1992

Conners CK: Conners' Rating Scales—Revised: Technical Manual. New York, Multi-Health Systems, 1997

Conners CK, Sitarenios G, Parker JD, et al: Revision and restandardization of the Conners' Teacher Rating Scale (CTRS-R): factor structure, reliability, and criterion validity. J Abnorm Child Psychol 26:279–291, 1998

Connor DF, Glatt SJ, Lopez ID, et al: Psychopharmacology and aggression, I: a meta-analysis of stimulant effects on overt/covert aggression-related behaviors in ADHD. J Am Acad Child Adolesc Psychiatry 41:253–261, 2002

Connor DF, Carlson GA, Chang KD, et al; Stanford/Howard/AACAP Workgroup on Juvenile Impulsivity and Aggression: Juvenile maladaptive aggression: a review of prevention, treatment, and service configuration and a proposed research agenda. J Clin Psychiatry 67:808–820, 2006

Correll CU, Carlson HE: Endocrine and metabolic adverse effects of psychotropic medications in children and adolescents. J Am Acad Child Adolesc Psychiatry 45:771–791, 2006

Hazell PL, Stuart JE: A randomized controlled trial of clonidine added to psychostimulant medication for hyperactive and aggressive children. J Am Acad Child Adolesc Psychiatry 42:886–894, 2003

Hinshaw SP, Lahey BB, Hart EL: Issues of taxonomy and comorbidity in the development of conduct disorder. Dev Psychopathol 5:31–49, 1993

Jensen PS and members of the MTA Cooperative Group: ADHD comorbidity findings from the MTA Study: new diagnostic subtypes and their optimal treatments, in Defining Psychopathology in the 21st Century: DSM-V and Beyond. Edited by Helzer JE, Hudziak JJ. Washington, DC, American Psychiatric Publishing, 2002, pp 169–192

Jensen PS, Youngstrom EA, Steiner H, et al: Consensus report on impulsive aggression as a symptom across diagnostic categories in child psychiatry: implications for medication studies. J Am Acad Child Adolesc Psychiatry 46:309–322, 2007

Kazdin AE, Esveldt-Dawson K, French NH, et al: Problem-solving skills training and relationship therapy in the treatment of antisocial child behavior. J Consult Clin Psychol 55:76–85, 1987

Kutcher S, Aman M, Brooks SJ, et al: International consensus statement on attention deficit/hyperactivity disorder (ADHD) and disruptive behavior disorders (DBDs): clinical implications and treatment practice suggestions. Eur Neuropsychopharmacol 14:11–28, 2004

Lochman JE, Wells KC: The Coping Power program at the middle-school transition: universal and indicated prevention effects. Psychol Addict Behav 16:540–554, 2002

Lochman JE, Wells KC, Lenhart L: Coping Power Child Component. New York, Oxford University Press, 2008

Loeber R, Farrington DP: Serious and Violent Juvenile Offenders: Risk Factors and Successful Interventions. Thousand Oaks, CA, Sage, 1998

Murray C, Johnston C: Parenting in mothers with and without attention-deficit/hyperactivity disorder. J Abnorm Psychol 115:52–61, 2006

Pandina GJ, Aman MG, Findling RL: Risperidone in the management of disruptive behavior disorders. J Child Adolesc Psychopharmacol 16:379–392, 2006

Pappadopulos E, Macintyre JC, Crismon ML, et al: Treatment recommendations for the use of antipsychotics for aggressive youth (TRAAY), part II. J Am Acad Child Adolesc Psychiatry 42:145–161, 2003

Patterson GR: The early development of coercive family process, in Antisocial Behavior in Children and Adolescents: A Developmental Analysis and Model for Intervention. Edited by Reid JB, Patterson GR, Snyder J. Washington DC, American Psychological Association, 2002, pp 25–44

Patterson GR, Reid JB, Dishion TJ: Antisocial Boys. Eugene, OR, Castalia, 1992

Pliszka S; AACAP Work Group on Quality Issues: Practice parameter for the assessment and treatment of children and adolescents with attention-deficit/hyperactivity disorder. J Am Acad Child Adolesc Psychiatry 46:894–921, 2007

Reynolds CR, Kamphaus RW: Behavior Assessment System for Children, 2nd Edition. Bloomington, MN, Pearson Assessments, 2004

Sanders MR, McFarland M: Treatment of depressed mothers with disruptive children: a controlled evaluation of cognitive behavioral family intervention. Behav Ther 31:89–112, 2000

Waschbusch DA: A meta-analytic examination of comorbid hyperactive-impulsive-attention problems and conduct problems. Psychol Bull 128:118–150, 2002

Wells KC: Treatment of ADHD in children and adolescents, in Handbook of Interventions That Work With Children and Adolescents: Prevention and Treatment. Edited by Barrett PM, Ollendick TH. West Sussex, UK, Wiley, 2004

Wells KC: Family therapy for attention-deficit/hyperactivity disorder (ADHD), in Handbook of Clinical Family Therapy. Edited by Lebow JL. Hoboken, NJ, Wiley, 2005

Wells KC, Abramowitz A, Courtney M, et al: Parent training for attention-deficit/hyperactivity disorder: MTA study. Unpublished manuscript, 1996

Wells KC, Pelham WE, Kotkin RA, et al: Psychosocial treatment strategies in the MTA study: rationale, methods, and critical issues in design and implementation. J Abnorm Child Psychol 28:483–505, 2000

Wells KC, Lochman JE, Lenhart L: Coping Power Parent Component. New York, Oxford University Press, 2008

Whittinger NS, Langley K, Fowler TA, et al: Clinical precursors of conduct disorder in children with attention-deficit/hyperactivity disorder. J Am Acad Child Adolesc Psychiatry 46:179–187, 2007

■ CHAPTER 15 ■

Anxious Adolescent in the Emergency Room

Possible Abuse of Prescription Medications

Jeffrey J. Wilson, M.D.

CASE PRESENTATION

IDENTIFYING INFORMATION

Chloe is a 15-year-old sophomore in high school with a history of superior academic performance until the middle of her freshman year, when her grades dropped to average and her participation in sports ceased.

CHIEF COMPLAINT

Chloe was referred to psychiatric treatment because of a 1-week history of panic attacks, resulting in three emergency room visits in the previous 2 days.

HISTORY OF PRESENT ILLNESS

Chloe's mother brought Chloe to her first outpatient psychiatry visit. The daughter complained of incessant anxiety, with periods of uncontrollable anxiety relieved only with benzodiazepines. She also felt that 1 mg of clonazepam was not able to calm her nerves, as evidenced by her last visit to the emergency room. At the emergency room, she presented with symptoms of anxiety and fear that she would lash

Jeffrey J. Wilson, M.D., is Assistant Professor of Clinical Psychiatry at Columbia University/New York State Psychiatric Institute in New York, New York (for complete biographical information, see "About the Contributors," p. 613).

out and hurt somebody. She feared she was going crazy, was short of breath, and had severe tremors. The record indicated that each time she was in the hospital, she escalated more until she received the medication. She reported that at home, 2 mg of clonazepam twice daily was helpful and had kept her out of the emergency room the past 3 days, but she was running out and would like a prescription as soon as possible, before her pharmacy closed. During her anxiety attacks, she experienced shortness of breath, headaches, nausea, vomiting, diarrhea, palpitations, diaphoresis, chest pains, abdominal pain, and a feeling that she was going crazy. At times, she seemed to endorse every symptom in the differential. Chloe's mother, exasperated, agreed with Chloe's assessment that so far the only thing that has helped with these recent episodes of anxiety is clonazepam, although sometimes only intramuscular lorazepam seemed to help. Chloe also thought that Vicodin would help, but her mother disagreed. Her mother seemed annoyed that Chloe had mentioned the Vicodin, which she had given Chloe at times for pain.

Past Psychiatric History

Although Chloe obtained multiple prescriptions for benzodiazepines in the past, she was never been seen by a mental health professional.

Substance Abuse History

Chloe admitted to using alcohol and marijuana, once or twice a week. She reported that she last smoked marijuana 3 or 4 days ago and she last used alcohol about a month ago. She also said that she generally drank alcohol two or three times a month. She denied the use of any prescription medicines except lorazepam (from the emergency room and sometimes a pediatrician) and, as needed, hydrocodone/acetaminophen (for chronic abdominal pain) and clonazepam (her mother's). She was at first evasive about her most recent use of hydrocodone/acetaminophen (Vicodin): "I never abuse it; in fact, Mom hasn't got it for me in a long time. I only take it for pain." When interviewed further, she stated that the first time she took it, a friend whose molars had been removed shared pills from her Vicodin prescription. She said, "After my appendicitis, it really helps my stomach pain. Nothing else seems to work." She denied ever using heroin, cocaine, lysergic acid diethylamide (LSD), Ecstasy, methamphetamine, ketamine, gamma-hydroxybutyric acid, or cough medicine "to get high." She denied every drinking or using drugs more than she intended to, and she denied "blackouts." Chloe reported that she first drank alcohol at age 12, and she first tried cigarettes at age 12 as well. She first tried smoking marijuana last year. Her mom permits drinking and smoking (cigarettes) at home at certain times; however, her father does not permit substance use.

Chloe denied any impairment due to alcohol or marijuana use, including any adverse impact on her responsibilities or functioning at home or at school, or on her social or interpersonal life. She denied any substance-related legal problems, or using in situations that could be physically hazardous. Chloe reported that she initially smoked more marijuana and drank more alcohol than she intended, but that was last year; she had "cut down" since then. She reported that last summer she developed a tolerance for alcohol. Several times in the past 2 months, she drank to alleviate panic attacks, and she reported that many of these times, she drank to excess (i.e., more than she intended). She also reported that she used pills to get rid of pain and anxiety, as described above. She reported that she cannot cut down any further on her drinking until somebody gives her something to alleviate her anxiety.

MEDICAL HISTORY

Chloe had an appendectomy, following which Chloe had chronic abdominal pain about a year before her initial presentation. She had a history of frequent ear infections as an infant, but her hearing was normal.

DEVELOPMENTAL HISTORY

At birth, Chloe weighed 7 lbs 14 oz, and her mother had had no difficulties with the pregnancy or delivery. She was an easy child and met all developmental milestones at the appropriate time. However, she has been behaviorally inhibited since preschool. She had separation anxiety until age 6. Chloe had a best friend until fourth grade, when her friend joined a group of highly competitive girls who did not like Chloe. Chloe refused to talk further about elementary school, as it appeared to upset her. Her mother reported that she became more withdrawn in middle school, around the time of her parents' separation and subsequent divorce. During middle school, she had only one friend, who went to a different school. She had many friends in high school, although she did next to no structured or school-sponsored activities, contrary to her interest in sports in the past.

SOCIAL HISTORY

Chloe is the younger of two children. Her older sister, age 23, is living on her own. Sometimes, Chloe goes to parties with her sister, volunteering, "I never drink or smoke with her though." Her parents have joint custody of Chloe, and she spends alternate weeks at each parent's house. Her parents seldom communicate except through her. Chloe has a group of friends, but their interests do not include athletic or other extracurricular activities.

FAMILY HISTORY

Chloe reported that her only problem was her mother and that everything was "fine" when she was with her father. Chloe reported that her mother drank too much and often argued with Chloe when intoxicated. When Chloe becomes really upset with her mother, she goes to her father's house. Although her father prohibits substances of abuse in his home, he has seldom confronted Chloe and does not seem as aware of her activities as her mother is.

Chloe's mother reported no history of substance abuse or of anxiety or mood disorders. She denied any family history of suicide or psychiatric hospitalization. She denied any familial medical disorders except her own hypothyroidism. Chloe's mother denied any alcohol or drug problems but reported that her ex-husband abused drugs in the past. She felt that Chloe exaggerated the mother's drinking to take the focus off Chloe's own use of alcohol and marijuana. Still, she did not feel that Chloe had a problem with either substance. Chloe's mother denied that Chloe had ever taken her prescription clonazepam prior to these recent episodes, and she was not aware of any other prescription drug use, except the Vicodin that Chloe sometimes took for abdominal pain. Chloe's mother claimed that Chloe had not fully recovered from surgery and at times asked for renewals of Vicodin. Her mother obtained these prescriptions from her neighbor, a cardiologist, but she and Chloe "didn't want to keep troubling the surgeon."

Chloe's father admitted to a history of cocaine dependence, in remission since Chloe was in seventh grade. Her father thought that his own father was possibly depressed and an alcoholic, and that his sister might have a problem with marijuana abuse. He denied any history of anxiety or mood disorders. He denied any family history of suicide or psychiatric hospitalization, except his own detoxification and rehabilitation when Chloe was in seventh grade.

MENTAL STATUS EXAMINATION

Chloe was dressed casually, if slightly provocatively, when she arrived at her first appointment. She was cooperative and talkative, but she spoke slowly. She closed her eyes often during the evaluation, but said that she was still listening. Her mood was "fine" and her affect full range. She laughed easily and appeared at ease, even when discussing her anxiety symptoms; her affect was not congruent with her mood. She said that she felt anxious "all the time" but that there were periods when the anxiety worsened acutely, as in the last emergency room visit. She said that "it's like I'm going crazy" and that she was "ready to jump out of her skin." She acknowledged every accompanying symptom possible (from palpitations to paresthesias), although her affect seemed considerably less concerned than what one would expect. She seemed invested in convincing the examiner about the severity of her attacks and the need for clonazepam. She denied that anything in the past had helped as much. She stated she was taking the clonazepam regularly and that she had smoked marijuana a few days before her emergency room visit. She could not explain why her urine drug screens were negative for marijuana and benzodiazepines when gently confronted. "I don't know—you're the doctor. You tell me....Those urine tests are always wrong, anyway." Chloe did talk about the importance of "partying" in her life, even though she felt that she "had it under control." She did not understand why people made such a "big deal" about marijuana. "Alcohol seems so much worse; I don't understand why marijuana's not legal." She denied any physical or sexual abuse and she denied any neglect. She thought she drank less than her mother, so she was OK. About her mother, she said, "She's the one who should be here, you know—I mean being evaluated." She denied any self-injurious behavior. She denied any current suicidal or homicidal ideation, plans, or intent. Her cognitive examination was unremarkable.

PHYSICAL EXAMINATION AND TOXICOLOGY DURING EMERGENCY ROOM VISITS

At her initial emergency room presentation, Chloe had a heart rate of 110, blood pressure of 125/95, respiratory rate of 18, and temperature of 98.4°F. Her weight was 130 lbs and her height was 5 ft 5 in. Her physical examination appeared normative except that she had pupillary dilatation, rhinorrhea, excessive lacrimation, and diffuse abdominal tenderness. Laboratory tests revealed normal electrolytes, complete blood count, serum glucose, and liver and thyroid function. At each visit, her urine toxicology was negative for cocaine, opiates, tetrahydrocannabinol (THC), and benzodiazepines. Alcohol Breathalyzer testing was negative at each visit. Following the first visit, she was prescribed 7 days of lorazepam, 0.5 mg twice daily as needed.

COMMENTARIES

Psychotherapeutic Perspective

Christianne Esposito-Smythers, Ph.D.
Robert Miranda, Jr., Ph.D.

DIAGNOSTIC FORMULATION

Chloe's assessment data are particularly notable for a recent 1-year history of opiate use, reportedly to manage chronic pain following an appendectomy. Although Chloe's symptom presentation includes features of panic attacks, her opiate use and drug-seeking behavior suggest that opiate withdrawal may better account for her anxiety and physiological symptoms. Opiate withdrawal is characterized by dysphoric mood, nausea or vomiting, muscle aches, lacrimation or rhinorrhea, pupillary dilatation, piloerection, sweating, diarrhea, yawning, fever, and insomnia. Notably, vomiting, pupillary dilatation, and diarrhea are characteristic of opiate withdrawal but are not typical of a panic attack. Although Chloe's presentation suggests that she abuses prescription medication, and potentially alcohol and marijuana, the diagnostic formulation for this case is complicated by discrepancies in the information obtained through clinical interviews and the repeated negative toxicology screens despite self-reported recent substance use. Consequently, differential diagnosis requires additional clinical evaluations with Chloe, her mother, and other knowledgeable informants.

To improve diagnostic accuracy, an additional evaluation should be conducted using a structured clinical interview specifically developed to assess substance use disorders in adolescents. Examples include the Schedule for Affective Disorders and Schizophrenia for School-Age Children—Present and Lifetime Version (Kaufman et al. 1997) and the Customary Drinking and

Christianne Esposito-Smythers, Ph.D., is Assistant Professor (Research) in the Department of Psychiatry and Human Behavior at Brown University, and on the training faculty of the Brown University Center for Alcohol and Addiction Studies in Providence, Rhode Island.

Robert Miranda, Jr., Ph.D., is Assistant Professor (Research) in the Department of Psychiatry and Human Behavior at Brown University in Providence, Rhode Island.

For complete biographical information, see "About the Contributors," p. 613.

Drug Use Record (Brown et al. 1998). Whichever instrument is used, it is important to collect specific information regarding the patterns (i.e., frequency, duration, contexts) and function (e.g., positive and/or negative reinforcement) of use as well as substance use disorder criteria. Moreover, Chloe and her parent(s) should be interviewed separately to improve the accuracy of reporting. Obtaining information from Chloe's father, school-based professionals (e.g., teachers, guidance counselor), and other knowledgeable parties may also prove useful. The clinician should also obtain another toxicology screen using a blood sample or other reliable method (e.g., observation of urine sample collection) to ensure the integrity of the test. Results will allow the evaluator to substantiate the diagnostic formulation. Finally, Chloe needs to be evaluated for the presence of co-occurring mental health disorders.

DSM-IV-TR DIAGNOSIS

Axis I   292.0 Opioid withdrawal

Axis II   No diagnosis

Axis III   Deferred (possible chronic pain following appendectomy)

Axis IV   Parent-child conflict

           Disruption of family by divorce

Axis V   Global Assessment of Functioning=60 (current)

TREATMENT RECOMMENDATIONS

Although the present diagnostic formulation includes opiate withdrawal, Chloe likely has more extensive substance involvement. A more thorough diagnostic evaluation, as recommended above, would likely yield a diagnosis of opioid dependence and possibly even a cannabis and/or alcohol use disorder. Under such conditions, we offer the following recommendations for psychosocial treatment. Depending on the severity of her withdrawal symptoms, inpatient hospitalization for purposes of detoxification may initially be required. After detoxification, a combination of individual skills-based treatment, such as cognitive-behavioral therapy (CBT), and family therapy may best address Chloe's treatment needs.

A number of randomized controlled clinical trials have examined the efficacy of CBT and family therapy for adolescent substance abuse (for reviews, see Waldron and Kaminer 2004; Williams and Chang 2000). Results of these trials suggest that CBT and family therapy, particularly when used in combination (e.g., Waldron et al. 2001), yield significant and clinically meaningful reductions in substance use. Because Chloe does not acknowledge problems associated with her regular use of substances, her CBT regimen may be best received if it is preceded by a motivational interview. Motivational interviewing is designed to heighten motivation for treatment and enhance self-efficacy for change through the use of personalized feedback and education in combination with nondirective therapeutic techniques. It has been used successfully in combination with CBT for adolescent substance abuse (Dennis et al. 2004). Moreover, if additional assessment reveals that Chloe also has one or more co-occurring mental health disorders, CBT techniques that directly address each disorder should be integrated into her treatment plan.

Equally important to Chloe's treatment plan is the involvement of her family. Chloe and her mother appear to have a conflictual relationship. Moreover, Chloe's mother has a permissive attitude toward her daughter's substance use, and apparently neither parent engages in parental monitoring or disciplinary practices to discourage use. These issues are further complicated by the possibility that Chloe's mother has an active alcohol use disorder. Notably, Chloe's mother has a prescription for clonazepam but denies a history of an anxiety disorder or a medical disorder other than hypothyroidism.

Because family conflict, insufficient parental monitoring, absent or ineffective discipline, and parental substance abuse are associated with the onset and maintenance of adolescent substance abuse (Hawkins et al. 1992), Chloe's chances of improvement would be greatly enhanced with family involvement. Examples of efficacious family therapies for adolescent substance abuse include brief strategic family therapy (Szapocznik and Williams 2000) and multidimensional family therapy (Liddle et al. 2001). Chloe's parents would benefit from psychoeducation on alcohol and drug use, as well as instruction in parental monitoring and effective disciplinary strategies. Chloe's parents will have to put aside their differences and work together as a team to effectively parent Chloe. This effort will involve direct communication between parents (not through Chloe), as well as consistent rules and disciplinary strategies across homes. Through family therapy, Chloe and her family will also need to work on improving their communication and relationships. The clinician also needs to gently engage Chloe's mother in a discussion about her own drinking. Chloe's mother should be encouraged to obtain an assessment and potential treatment for an alcohol use disorder. Finally, communication with Chloe's school about her drop in grades should be encouraged.

As suggested above, the most effective treatment plan will include an integrated intervention. Adolescent substance abuse interventions that concurrently address co-occurring mental health disorders, family functioning, peer and interpersonal functioning, and academic/vocational functioning may yield the greatest treatment gains (Bukstein 1997). Empirically based CBT and family therapy manuals for adolescent substance abuse are available for free online at the Chestnut Health Systems' Web site (http://www.chestnut.org/LI/bookstore) and may serve as the springboard for an effective treatment plan.

Integrative Perspective

Jeffrey J. Wilson, M.D.

DIAGNOSTIC FORMULATION

Chloe is a 15-year-old girl who is primarily complaining of the recent onset of severe anxiety, requiring three visits to the emergency room in the past 48 hours. During these visits, she complained of feeling like she would hurt somebody, but denied specific homicidal or otherwise aggressive ideation. She also complained of multiple symptoms commonly associated with anxiety, including fear of losing control, diaphoresis, palpitations, chills, nausea, paresthesia, and tremor. These symptoms are almost constant, with periods of further exacerbation resulting in her recent emergency room visits—a somewhat uncharacteristic history of panic disorder with or without agoraphobia (American Psychiatric Association 2000).

Prior to making a diagnosis of any anxiety disorder, the clinician should rule out medical or substance-related causes of the anxiety symptoms. Based on differential diagnosis (American Psychiatric Association 2000), common causes of medical illness related to anxiety appear unlikely given Chloe's normal vital signs, physical examination, and laboratories. Urine toxicology is negative for common drugs of abuse, and her alcohol Breathalyzer test results are negative. However, Chloe's symptoms of medication seeking (asking for benzodiazepines specifically), changing of prescriptions (taking the lorazepam and her mother's clonazepam), and obtaining prescriptions in inappropriate ways (getting hydrocodone from a physician friend of the family) raise suspicion for substance abuse. Although she admits to recent marijuana and alcohol use, if the quantities and frequencies are correct, this would not be terribly deviant from norms for her age. She denies all symptoms of alcohol or other substance abuse, yet she does admit to two symptoms of alcohol dependence: prior attempts to cut down on her alcohol use and a tolerance to alcohol. Negative drug screens for THC and benzodiazepines suggest the possibility of tampering; the lack of reported urinary creatinine makes it difficult to determine the concentration of the urine. Diluting urine is a common means of tampering with drug screens. Although both tests may have been false negatives, this is highly unlikely given their high sensitivity for drug metabolites. Interestingly, a negative urine screen for synthetic or semisynthetic opioids such as hydrocodone may be an exception, since the sensitivity of immunoassays for these compounds is variable and some labs have a restrictive definition of opioids. Pain clinics often use gas chromatography/mass spectrometry to confirm adherence to pain regimens because of the relatively low sensitivity of immunoassays to these opioid compounds (Heit and Gourlay 2004).

Several other factors place Chloe at high risk for some life course–persistent substance use disorder, including her father's history of narcotic addiction, a possible diagnosis of alcohol abuse in her mother, her mother's permissiveness toward Chloe's drug use, a family situation that makes monitoring inconsistent, a chronic pain disorder, and the early age at onset of Chloe's substance-related problems (Bukstein 1997; Kleber et al. 2007). She does not meet criteria for alcohol or substance abuse at the time of this evaluation, although she does endorse two symptoms of alcohol dependence. Pollock and Martin (1999) reported that these "diagnostic orphans" who do not meet criteria for substance abuse yet meet criteria for one or two symptoms of substance dependence have a similar prognosis to that of youths diagnosed with substance abuse per se. Based on the results of a 1993 study, girls ages 12–17 are at higher risk than boys are of both receiving prescriptions for abusable drugs and abusing these drugs (National Institute on Drug Abuse 2008). Prescription drugs were among the most commonly abused drugs by youths in 1994, with 4.0% of youths ages 12–17 reporting nonmedical use of these medications. Nearly twice as many individuals ages 12–13 reported nonmedical use of prescription drugs (1.8%) as reported using marijuana (1.0%) (National Institute on Drug Abuse 2008). Often during the initial assessment of substance abuse, more questions arise than there are answers, and the clinician needs to record possible clues for abuse or dependence as they arise during treatment.

Developmentally, Chloe may have some predisposition to anxiety attacks, given her early behavioral inhibition and separation anxiety. Moreover, her withdrawal during late childhood and early adolescence may have been related to some element of social phobia. Unfortunately, she was not ready to speak about this during the evaluation. Any comorbid anxiety disorder would further increase her risk of developing drug or alcohol dependence (Gorman et al. 1998). Genetic and familial risk factors coupled with a developmental lag in socialization may have placed her at high risk for developing a substance use disorder (Cicchetti and Rogosch 1999). Her drug and alcohol use appeared to become a problem about 1 year prior to her presenting for psychiatric treatment, around the same time she was hospitalized for appendicitis with a complication of persistent abdominal pain following the appendectomy. Her reportedly sporadic use of hydrocodone/ acetaminophen over the past year may have further contributed to the development of substance-related problems; alternatively, her substance-related problems may also have been an attempt to self-medicate pain, anxiety, or both.

Perhaps the most likely explanation for her symptoms during her presentation is opioid and/or sedative/hypnotic withdrawal. Her symptoms that are consistent with opioid withdrawal include pupillary dilatation, diaphoresis, rhinorrhea, diarrhea, chills, and anxiety. Although her anxiety, as the predominant symptom, may suggest an additional diagnosis of anxiety disorder, this diagnosis should not be made in the presence of a known intoxication or withdrawal syndrome, unless the anxiety is clearly in excess of that expected. Because the history of her hydrocodone use is suspect given her clinical presentation (i.e., she likely used more than she stated), the expected level of anxiety is difficult to determine. The clinician also needs to rule out alcohol and benzodiazepine dependence as a possible etiology because of the potential morbidity and mortality associated with withdrawal from these substances. Symptoms of tremor and elevated heart rate and blood pressure are also consistent with sedative/hypnotic withdrawal. The limited duration of Chloe's response to benzodiazepine injections would argue against this, although if she were dependent on benzodiazepines and/or alcohol, this might still be possible (Kleber et al. 2007).

DSM-IV-TR DIAGNOSIS

Axis I   292.0 Opioid withdrawal

300.00 Anxiety disorder not otherwise specified

Rule out pain disorder not otherwise specified

Rule out benzodiazepine and/or alcohol withdrawal

Rule out anxiety disorder due to benzodiazepine, opioid, alcohol, or polysubstance dependence

Rule out panic disorder

Rule out benzodiazepine abuse or dependence

Rule out opioid abuse or dependence

Rule out alcohol abuse or dependence

Rule out cannabis abuse or dependence

Axis II   Deferred

Axis III Chronic abdominal pain of unknown etiology

Axis IV Moderate psychosocial stressors related to her mother's alleged alcohol abuse

Consider additional stressors related to possible personal substance abuse

Axis V   Global Assessment of Functioning=75

TREATMENT RECOMMENDATIONS

History is arguably the most critical aspect of an assessment of prescription drug abuse, because a drug screen does not necessarily screen for all of the many possible drugs a person might take. In treating substance abuse, multiple assessments are often needed over time, as discussed above in "Psychotherapeutic Perspective." Oddly enough, as people recover, they often become more honest with themselves and their treatment providers. As a result, an important aspect of the treatment of a substance-abusing person, especially an adolescent, is continued unraveling of the person's substance abuse. In this case, a better history would be important to definitively confirm the diagnosis of opioid withdrawal. Additionally, tests to clarify how the urine tests were tampered with would be informative. Most simply, a urine creatinine can be added to the toxicology. Alternatively, urine tests for commonly used adulterants are available at some labs.

A critical first step is to obtain an accurate assessment of the patient's drug and alcohol use. Apprising the parents and the patient of the potential risks of detoxification given an inaccurate history may improve the validity of the history; risks of detoxification include severe symptoms, even death, depending on the substance. Confidentiality is essential to this process, because many young patients fear disclosing the precise nature of their drug use to their parents. All efforts should be used to maintain confidentiality except in cases where not revealing a risk could result in danger to the patient's safety. Most states have laws that restrict the provision to other parties of information that an adolescent provides, without the adolescent's consent. At times, an adolescent may agree to provide other parties with some general information, such as treatment recommendations. The clinician should clarify this right to privacy at the beginning of an evaluation. Both legally and ethically, an adolescent's right to privacy should be maximally respected (Bukstein 1997).

If opioid dependence is confirmed, several compounds are effective for opioid detoxification. Effective detoxification is critical to promoting completion of substance abuse treatment, in both outpatient and inpatient settings (Collins et al. 2007). Both methadone and Suboxone can be used for opioid detoxification, although Suboxone may be more effective and can be prescribed for opioid detoxification in an outpatient setting (Blondell et al. 2007). In cases where the dose of opioid is relatively low, clonidine may also be a reasonable choice; however, breakthrough symptoms, such as diarrhea and muscle aches, may require treatment with standard remedies. Both clonidine and Suboxone can be used for opioid detoxification in most outpatient settings (Ling et al. 2005).

The level of care (inpatient vs. outpatient) should be determined by the safety of the environment (relative risk of relapse), ability of the environment to support the patient's recovery, and the patient's and family's wishes. Emotional support, separation from actively drug-using peers, existence of drug-free alternative behaviors, and parent monitoring to minimize drug availability are generally thought to be key components of recovery. Another important consideration is the adolescent's motivation or readiness to change. Furthermore, any treatment plan requires consideration of the factors that have contributed to or may maintain the dependent state, including both positive reinforcers (euphoria, socialization, etc.) and negative reinforcers (preventing withdrawal or self-medication of pain or anxiety). In any case, understanding the role of pain is critical to preventing attrition and relapse following treatment.

In Chloe's case, because of a precontemplative state (Prochaska and Di-Clemente 1983), an environment unlikely to be able to support and/or maintain change, an unexplained pain syndrome, and signs of opiate withdrawal, inpatient detoxification and rehabilitation are indicated. In brief, detoxification from synthetic opioids such as hydrocodone generally involves substitution of the drug of abuse with a longer-acting medication, such as methadone or buprenorphine, followed by gradual tapering of the substituted medication. In this case, residential treatment would be highly recommended following detoxification. The most effective rehabilitation programs would include family therapy and CBT, as discussed above in "Psychotherapeutic Perspective." Reduction of anxiety and pain is also necessary to minimize the risk of relapse and should be emphasized as part of a comprehensive treatment plan. For pain patients, relief of pain through non-narcotic means, such as physical therapy, nonsteroidal anti-inflammatory drugs, and meditation, is an important part of a comprehensive treatment plan. Finally, continued anxiety during the rehabilitation process should be treated with evidence-based treatments such as CBT or selective serotonin reuptake inhibitors.

REFERENCES

American Psychiatric Association: Diagnostic and Statistical Manual of Mental Disorders, 4th Edition, Text Revision. Washington, DC, American Psychiatric Association, 2000

Blondell RD, Smith SJ, Servoss TJ, et al: Buprenorphine and methadone: a comparison of patient completion rates during inpatient detoxification. J Addict Dis 26(2):3–11, 2007

Brown SA, Myers MG, Lippke L, et al: Psychometric evaluation of the Customary Drinking and Drug Use Record (CDDR): a measure of adolescent alcohol and drug involvement. J Stud Alcohol 59:427–438, 1998

Bukstein O: Practice parameters for the assessment and treatment of children and adolescents with substance use disorders. J Am Acad Child Adolesc Psychiatry 36 (suppl 10):140–156, 1997

Cicchetti D, Rogosch FA: Psychopathology as risk for adolescent substance use disorders: a developmental psychopathology perspective. J Clin Child Psychol 28:355–365, 1999

Collins ED, Horton T, Reinke K, et al: Using buprenorphine to facilitate entry into resi-
    dential therapeutic community rehabilitation. J Subst Abuse Treat 32:167–175,
    2007
Dennis N, Godley SH, Diamond G, et al: The Cannabis Youth Treatment (CYT) Study:
    main findings from two randomized trials. J Subst Abuse Treat 27:197–213, 2004
Gorman J, Shear K, Cowley D, et al: Practice Guideline for the Treatment of Patients
    With Panic Disorder. Washington, DC, American Psychiatric Association, 1998
Hawkins JD, Catalano RF, Miller JY: Risk and protective factors for alcohol and other
    drug problems in adolescence and early adulthood: implications for substance
    abuse prevention. Psychol Bull 112:64–105, 1992
Heit HA, Gourlay DL: Urine drug testing in pain medicine. J Pain Symptom Manage
    27:260–267, 2004
Kaufman J, Birmaher B, Brent D, et al: Schedule for Affective Disorders and Schizo-
    phrenia for School-Age Children—Present and Lifetime Version (K-SADS-PL): Ini-
    tial reliability and validity data. J Am Acad Child Adolesc Psychiatry 36:980–988,
    1997
Kleber HD, Weiss RD, Anton RF Jr, et al; Work Group on Substance Use Disorders;
    American Psychiatric Association; Steering Committee on Practice Guidelines:
    Treatment of patients with substance use disorders, second edition. Am J Psychiatry
    164 (4 suppl):5–123, 2007
Liddle HA, Dakof GA, Diamond GS, et al: Multidimensional family therapy for ado-
    lescent substance abuse: results of a randomized clinical trial. Am J Drug Alcohol
    Abuse 27:651–687, 2001
Ling W, Amass L, Shoptaw S, et al: A multicenter randomized trial of buprenorphine-
    naloxone versus clonidine for opioid detoxification: findings from the National In-
    stitute on Drug Abuse Clinical Trials Network. Addiction 100:1090–1100, 2005
National Institute on Drug Abuse: Trends in prescription drug abuse. July 15,
    2008. Available at: http://www.drugabuse.gov/ResearchReports/Prescription/
    prescription5.html. Accessed July 16, 2008.
Pollock NK, Martin CS: Diagnostic orphans: adolescents with alcohol symptoms who
    do not qualify for DSM-IV abuse or dependence diagnoses. Am J Psychiatry 156:897–
    901, 1999
Prochaska JO, DiClemente CC: Stages and processes of self-change of smoking: toward
    an integrative model of change. J Consult Clin Psychol 51:390–395, 1983
Szapocznik J, Williams RA: Brief strategic family therapy: twenty-five years of interplay
    among theory, research and practice in adolescent behavior problems and drug
    abuse. Clin Child Fam Psychol Rev 3:117–134, 2000
Waldron HB, Kaminer Y: On the learning curve: the emerging evidence supporting
    cognitive-behavioral therapies for adolescent substance abuse. Addiction 99:93–
    105, 2004
Waldron HB, Slesnick N, Brody JL, et al: Treatment outcomes for adolescent substance
    abuse at 4- and 7-month assessments. J Consult Clin Psychol 69:802–813, 2001
Williams RJ, Chang SY; Addiction Centre Adolescent Research Group: A comprehen-
    sive and comparative review of adolescent substance abuse treatment outcome.
    Clinical Psychology: Science and Practice 7:138–166, 2000

■ CHAPTER 16 ■

The Worried Child

A Child With Multiple Anxiety Disorders

Wendy K. Silverman, Ph.D., A.B.P.P.
Carla E. Marin, M.S.

CASE PRESENTATION

IDENTIFYING INFORMATION

Miguel, a 12-year-old Hispanic boy, was referred to a childhood anxiety disorders specialty research clinic by his pediatrician. He lives with his biological parents, 14-year-old brother, and maternal grandmother.

CHIEF COMPLAINT

Miguel's mother called the clinic because she was increasingly concerned about her son's weight loss of 10 lbs over the past 2 months, stemming from Miguel's refusal to eat any solid foods.

Wendy K. Silverman, Ph.D., A.B.P.P., is Professor of Psychology at Florida International University in Miami, Florida.

Carla E. Marin, M.S., is a doctoral candidate in life span developmental science at Florida International University in Miami, Florida.

For complete biographical information, see "About the Contributors," p. 613.

This case presentation and the integrative commentary were written with support from National Institute of Mental Health grant K24 MH073696 awarded to Wendy K. Silverman.

HISTORY OF PRESENT ILLNESS

Miguel's mother attributed her son's refusal to eat solid foods to an extreme fear of choking. To ensure that Miguel had some food intake, in the last 3 weeks she began allowing her son to limit his food intake to soft foods, such as yogurt, gelatin snacks, and ice cream. She also allowed him to drink two large glasses of juice and/or water with his meals to soften the food, which was something Miguel wanted to be allowed to do.

According to his mother, Miguel also voiced frequent concerns regarding his safety and security. Both Miguel and his mother reported that he demanded constant reassurance regarding safety and security that was unrelated to his primary diagnosis of specific phobia. At night, he needed to make sure the doors and windows were locked; he also checked his room to make sure "no one could get in"; and he needed to check under his bed, inside his closet, and behind the curtains.

Miguel and his mother both indicated during the initial evaluation that Miguel's main difficulties with eating began about 6 months prior to their clinic presentation, when he choked on a banana while riding in the car with his mother. Although he was able to cough up the piece of fruit, he became frightened about eating anything shortly thereafter. To alleviate these fears, not only would Miguel drink large amounts of liquid with his meals, as described above, but he also would take up to an hour to finish meals. Specifically, Miguel stated that he did not want to eat as much as he did before because he was afraid he would choke again and die. He explained that he preferred to eat slowly, sometimes taking up to an hour to finish a meal, because he needed to chew several times and needed to drink at least two full, large glasses of water or juice to avoid any chances of choking again. Miguel also avoided going to restaurants with his family because it had turned into an unpleasant experience.

PAST PSYCHIATRIC HISTORY

Miguel has no history of mental illness or substance abuse.

MEDICAL HISTORY

Miguel has no current medical illnesses and takes no medications. As an infant and toddler, however, he suffered from recurrent ear infections. Miguel's mother reported that her son had no history of any kind of medical condition, such as hypoglycemia, hyperthyroidism, cardiac arrhythmias, seizure disorders, or migraines. The pediatrician was concerned about Miguel's limited food intake and recommended that Miguel's mother take him to the anxiety disorders clinic.

DEVELOPMENTAL HISTORY

Miguel learned to walk at age 11 months and was potty trained by the time he was age 3 years. His speech development was unremarkable, with no significant delays.

Miguel was reported by his mother as always being timid and shy. She further reported that Miguel was fearful and usually withdrawn in unknown situations.

SOCIAL HISTORY

According to Miguel and his mother, he has no history of abuse or neglect. As an infant, he was described as "hard to warm up" in that he was unusually fearful, shy, and quiet, as previously noted. As a toddler, and even in the early elementary school years, he displayed marked physiological arousal when placed in a new setting. Kagan et al. (1987) would describe this temperament as behaviorally inhibited. Specifically, Miguel would stay away from unfamiliar people and would become distressed when his mother left him alone with his grandmother while the mother ran errands. His mother also reported that he was not happy to see her return, but was instead upset and withdrawn from her. Upon further probing, his mother stated that she was unsure why her son responded to her return in this way. She speculated, however, that maybe Miguel was "mad" at her for having "left him." After a few minutes upon her return, though, Miguel usually warmed up to her again.

Miguel is currently in seventh grade at a large middle school. Although he has only a few close friends, he has no difficulties making or keeping friends. He has a 14-year-old brother with whom he is very close. His mother reports that each considers the other his best friend. Miguel is not involved in any extracurricular activities.

FAMILY HISTORY

The immediate and extended family have no history of mental illness. Notably, his father has returned to work as a mechanic after 3 months of being unemployed.

MENTAL STATUS EXAMINATION

Using the guidelines suggested by Folstein et al. (1975), the clinician obtained information about Miguel's mental status. Overall, Miguel had no obvious delusions, hallucinations, or thought disorders. He showed appropriate insight and good judgment, as ascertained by the introductory sections of the child interview schedule (Anxiety Disorders Interview Schedule for DSM-IV—Child and Parent Versions [ADIS-C/P]; Silverman and Albano 1996), which asks the client to report his or her name, age, and home address; the name of his or her school; and his or her reasons for presenting to the clinic. Miguel also showed socially appropriate appearance and behavior.

During the assessment interview, Miguel made appropriate eye contact and displayed proper posture and coordination. Although he appeared nervous and shy, his mood was otherwise suitable. Miguel acknowledged that he was "nervous" about coming to the clinic because he had "never been to a psychologist before."

COMMENTARIES

Psychotherapeutic Perspective

Bruce F. Chorpita, Ph.D.

DIAGNOSTIC FORMULATION

Miguel appears to have a primary diagnosis of specific phobia, other type. The onset of this disorder appears to have been triggered by a combination of his temperamentally heightened inhibition and an aversive conditioning experience related to his choking on a banana 6 months prior to the interview. Some children may choke on food and not develop the extreme fear and avoidance demonstrated by Miguel, and such differences in conditioning thresholds may involve overall differences in temperament (Vasey and Dadds 2001).

Miguel also may have additional anxiety problems, which could involve a diagnosis of generalized anxiety disorder (GAD) or separation anxiety disorder (SAD), both of which can be associated with nighttime fears and safety concerns and which commonly co-occur with specific phobias. To assist in the determination of possible additional diagnoses, the clinician should arrange for administration of a structured diagnostic interview (e.g., the Anxiety Disorders Interview Schedule for DSM-IV—Child and Parent Versions [ADIS-C/P]; Silverman and Albano 1996) and a self-report measure with scales corresponding to relevant DSM syndromes such as worry and separation anxiety (e.g., the Revised Child Anxiety and Depression Scales; Chorpita et al. 2000). Furthermore, the clinician should determine whether Miguel's nighttime fears are in fact excessive and unrealistic before considering any diagnosis. For example, Miguel might live in a neighborhood in which break-ins are common (although his repeated checking of the closet and under the bed is not likely to be an adaptive behavior in all but the most dangerous contexts).

Given the high level of interference caused by Miguel's specific phobia, most notably the extreme weight loss, this diagnosis would likely be primary on Axis I.

DSM-IV-TR DIAGNOSIS

Axis I   300.29 Specific phobia, other type
Axis II   No diagnosis

Bruce F. Chorpita, Ph.D., is Professor of Psychology at University of California, Los Angeles (for complete biographical information, see "About the Contributors," p. 613).

Axis III None

Axis IV None

Axis V   Global Assessment of Functioning=60 (current)

TREATMENT RECOMMENDATIONS

As suggested by the substantial literature on the treatment of specific phobia (Chorpita and Southam-Gerow 2006) and the demonstrations of successful behavioral treatments of choking phobia (Zelikovsky et al. 2001), the primary treatment plan for Miguel would involve a cognitive-behavioral intervention (Chorpita 2007) with a focus on those treatment strategies most commonly associated with successful treatments of phobias (see Chorpita et al. 2005). The centerpiece of these strategies would be exposure, which would involve having Miguel practice eating foods that are safe but anxiety provoking. Miguel would be asked to provide ratings of fear before, during, and after each eating task that he performs with the clinician. These ratings would be used to guide the pace and intensity of exposure (see Chorpita 2007).

Practice exercises would be supported by several other techniques, each with a separate rationale. First, a period of relationship building or getting acquainted would be important before the clinician begins exposure. Because the clinician will later ask Miguel to participate in relatively distressing exercises, a positive relationship would likely reduce the probability of refusal or dropout. Given that the child is at risk due to weight loss and nutritional problems, this period of relationship building would need to happen quickly—perhaps in a single session involving some conversation and games. Next, a list of feared items would be developed to facilitate both measurement of progress, using weekly distress ratings for each item targeted, and selection of new items to practice in each meeting. If motivation were to become an issue, a reward program could be added whereby Miguel earns points for each practice session and redeems them for rewards. Finally, to increase the probability of Miguel's engaging in exposure exercises, the clinician could model eating feared foods to the extent possible, such that the clinician would eat some of a banana just prior to asking Miguel to eat some banana.

Successful treatment would conclude with a review of skills and some planning and preparation for how to handle future difficulties should they arise. If the treatment is not making sufficient progress despite intensive troubleshooting and adjusting of the outpatient treatment program, one might consider very brief inpatient treatment (Burklow and Linscheid 2004) or medication (Banerjee et al. 2005), given some evidence of their success in the literature. Following successful treatment, one would need to evaluate whether Miguel's remaining anxiety concerns continue to warrant attention, and to develop a new plan accordingly.

Psychopharmacologic Perspective

Daniel Pine, M.D.

DIAGNOSTIC FORMULATION

The assessment of anxiety in children and adolescents involves elicitation of history from both the child and a series of parallel informants, including parents and teachers. Although this assessment can be facilitated by the use of various standardized rating forms or structured interviews, the core aspect of an evaluation involves direct elicitation of the relevant information by a competent mental health professional. Complications in the assessment of pediatric anxiety often arise due to the relatively low rate of agreement among informants, and clinical expertise provides particularly useful guidance in these situations. The assessment typically focuses on delineation of events and scenarios that elicit fear and distress in the child, while paying particularly close attention to situations that are avoided due to fear. Impairment due to pediatric anxiety disorders frequently follows from high levels of avoidance.

Some aspects of Miguel's presentation illustrate key clinical features of pediatric anxiety disorders, as they often appear on clinical assessment. Most children and adolescents presenting for treatment of an anxiety disorder exhibit signs and symptoms of multiple anxiety disorders (Research Unit on Pediatric Psychopharmacology [RUPP] Anxiety Study Group 2001; Pine and Klein 2008). In Miguel's case, he shows features of a specific phobia, manifest as marked and persistent fear of a discernible, circumscribed situation. This fear is accompanied by high levels of distress and avoidance, with clear interference in function. Moreover, Miguel also shows features of other anxiety disorders beyond specific phobia. He demonstrates concerns about safety and fear of harm that might represent manifestations of SAD, although full diagnostic criteria are not clearly met. As a result, these symptoms could be considered nonspecific aspects of an emerging anxiety disorder, probably reasonably classified using the "not otherwise specified" designation. Similarly, he shows some signs

Daniel Pine, M.D., is Chief of the Section on Development and Affective Neuroscience; Chief of the Emotion and Development Branch; and Chief of Child and Adolescent Research in the Mood and Anxiety Disorders Program at the National Institute of Mental Health Intramural Research Program in Bethesda, Maryland (for complete biographical information, see "About the Contributors," p. 613).

of social anxiety disorder or of having had a known developmental precursor, behavioral inhibition, which refers to a temperamental profile of excessive timidity within the first years of life (Pérez-Edgar and Fox 2005). Finally, some of Miguel's anxieties represent extreme variants of fears manifest in healthy children at earlier stages of development. For example, although fear of harm at night or in the dark frequently manifests in typically developing toddlers or young children free of an anxiety disorder, identical symptoms in an adolescent represent signs of pathology (Pine and Klein 2008).

Other aspects of Miguel's clinical picture are relatively atypical. For example, virtually all anxiety disorders, including specific phobia, occur at higher rates among girls than boys, and, unlike Miguel, children presenting for treatment rarely manifest specific phobia as the most prominent feature of their anxiety disorder (Pine and Klein 2008). Moreover, Miguel's presentation is somewhat unusual because a phobia specified as "other type" is seen less commonly in the clinic than are "situational" or "natural environment" types. The 6-month duration of the phobia also just passes the minimal duration criterion and raises questions on the role of acute stress in the presentation. Along these same lines, the association between Miguel's fear of choking and a traumatic exposure, during which he choked on a banana, calls to mind the considerable controversy relating phobias to fear conditioning (Lissek et al. 2005). The juxtaposition between trauma and anxiety also raises questions on presentations of pediatric posttraumatic stress disorder, which can differ in children and adults (Scheeringa et al. 2006). Although many theories attribute phobias to traumatic conditioning, the weight of the evidence does not support this view, based on a review of fear conditioning research and prospective investigations following traumatic exposures (Lissek et al. 2005).

DSM-IV-TR DIAGNOSIS

Axis I   300.29 Specific phobia, other type
            300.00 Anxiety disorder not otherwise specified
Axis II   None
Axis III   None
Axis IV   None
Axis V   Global Assessment of Functioning=55
            Currently experiencing moderate difficulty

TREATMENT RECOMMENDATIONS

The first step in appropriate treatment for pediatric anxiety disorders is to collect more information to arrive at a more definitive diagnosis, including all relevant target disorders. As noted above, Miguel may manifest symptoms of many possible anxiety disorders, in addition to specific phobia. Moreover, given the strong cross-sectional and longitudinal association between pediatric anxiety and depression (Pine et al. 1998), Miguel may have a current mood disorder or the risk for a future mood disorder. The presence of any of these complicating factors dramatically influences choices about treatment. After the target disorders have been determined, treatment of the specific conditions can be considered.

Relatively few randomized controlled trials have considered treatment options for specific phobias in pediatric populations, a fact that probably relates to the low frequency with which patients present to the pediatric clinic with specific phobia as an isolated condition. Cognitive-behavioral therapy (CBT) represents the only treatment examined in any detail using a randomized controlled trial, and some evidence supports the efficacy of this treatment (Silverman et al. 1999). In Miguel's case, a few features of the clinical presentation illustrate principles important for implementing CBT. For example, the focus of Miguel's anxiety on a relatively narrow set of scenarios provides an excellent opportunity to create a hierarchy of feared objects and situations, each associated with risk for choking. In CBT, graded exposure can be used to gradually assist children as they confront items on this hierarchy while using newly learned cognitive techniques designed to facilitate exposure. Virtually no research has examined the efficacy of non-CBT treatments, including psychotherapies or medications, for specific phobia.

More data are available concerning the treatment of anxiety disorders other than specific phobia. These data are relevant to the treatment of specific phobia, because children included in studies of other anxiety disorders often suffer from specific phobia as well. In particular, considerable data exist for treatments of patients with social anxiety disorder, SAD, and GAD, conditions frequently complicated by specific phobia. For these disorders, CBT has been shown to be effective, as have a range of selective serotonin reuptake inhibitor (SSRI) antidepressants (RUPP Anxiety Study Group 2001; Pine and Klein 2008). For most cases, CBT represents a reasonable first-line treatment, given concerns about adverse behavioral reactions, such as suicidal thoughts, that can occur with the SSRIs. Nevertheless, not all children with extreme anxiety can tolerate the distressing aspects of exposures involved in many forms of CBT. For these children, SSRIs also represent a reasonable first-line treatment. For children failing these two therapeutic options, virtually no data exist to inform subsequent interventions.

Integrative Perspective

Wendy K. Silverman, Ph.D., A.B.P.P.
Carla E. Marin, M.S.

DIAGNOSTIC FORMULATION

To derive diagnoses, the clinician administered Miguel and his mother the respective forms of the Anxiety Disorders Interview Schedule for DSM-IV—Child and Parent Versions (Silverman and Albano 1996). The ADIS-C/P is a semistructured diagnostic interview schedule designed to derive primary anxiety disorder diagnoses in youth. The ADIS-C/P and its previous versions (Silverman 1991) have been used most frequently in the youth anxiety disorders research literature relative to other interview schedules. Studies have confirmed the reliability and validity of diagnoses using the ADIS-C/P, with several studies confirming interrater (Grills and Ollendick 2003; Rapee et al. 1994; Silverman and Nelles 1988) and test-retest reliability for specific diagnoses (Silverman and Eisen 1992; Silverman et al. 2001) and symptom patterns (Silverman and Rabian 1995). With regard to validity, concurrent validity of ADIS-C/P diagnoses of SAD, GAD, social phobia, and panic disorder also has been confirmed (Wood et al. 2002).

Miguel's behavior of refusing to eat solid foods met DSM-IV-TR criteria for a primary diagnosis of specific phobia of choking under the subtype of "other," according to the ADIS-C/P. According to DSM-IV-TR, subtypes may be specified to indicate the focus of fear or avoidance in cases of specific phobia. The subtype "other" was specified in Miguel's case because his fear was cued by stimuli other than animals, the natural environment, blood, injection, or injury. Miguel's need for constant reassurance and excessive worry also were found to meet criteria for a secondary diagnosis of GAD.

DIFFERENTIAL DIAGNOSIS

Individuals with specific phobia, unlike those with other anxiety disorders such as panic disorder or GAD, do not present with pervasive anxiety, because the fear is limited to a specific object or event (American Psychiatric Association 2000). A diagnosis of panic disorder was not warranted in Miguel's case because he was only avoiding specific objects (i.e., food) and situations (i.e., restaurants) and did not report panic attacks. Also, a diagnosis of anorexia nervosa or bulimia nervosa was not warranted because the nature of Miguel's fear was not related to body image, but rather to an irrational fear of choking after experiencing a conditioning event.

As noted, Miguel also presented with GAD and reported that his main worries were regarding thieves breaking into his house. However, both Miguel and his mother indicated in discussion and in interference ratings of his specific phobia and GAD worries (using a 0–8 scale) that the problems relating to specific phobia were interfering more with Miguel's functioning at school, with his friends, and with his family than were his GAD worries. Indeed, the specific phobia could result in serious health and medical complications if left untreated. Taking all these factors together, the clinician felt that a primary diagnosis of specific phobia of choking and a secondary diagnosis of GAD were warranted, and that specific phobia should be targeted in treatment.

Individuals diagnosed with specific phobia often have comorbid anxiety disorders, as well as other internalizing and externalizing behavior problems (e.g., Anderson et al. 1987; Last et al. 1987; Strauss et al. 1988). Although estimates of comorbidity among anxiety disorders vary across studies, the rate may be as high as 50% (Beidel and Turner 1988). In fact, rates of comorbidity may be underestimated in studies due to the use of pooled diagnostic groups (e.g., a group of "anxious" children that includes children who present with multiple anxiety disorders, such as SAD, overanxious disorder, and phobic disorder). Last et al. (1992) reported that of 80 children with diagnoses of simple phobia, 75% had a lifetime history of additional, specific anxiety disorders; 32.5% had a lifetime history of any depressive disorder; and 22.5% had a lifetime history of any behavior disorder.

DSM-IV-TR DIAGNOSIS

Axis I   300.29 Specific phobia, other type
            300.02 Generalized anxiety disorder
Axis II   None
Axis III   Recurrent ear infections until age 3
Axis IV   Financial difficulties
            Father recently started work after 3 months of unemployment
Axis V   Global Assessment of Functioning=54

TREATMENT RECOMMENDATIONS

INITIAL TREATMENT PLAN AND RATIONALE FOR CHOICE

Miguel and his mother participated in a 14-week CBT program. CBT is the primary choice of treatment for anxiety disorders and phobias because of its efficacious outcome (Silverman and Kurtines 2005; Silverman et al. 2008). The main components of CBT are graduated exposure to the feared object or event, contingency management, and cognitive restructuring. The aim of the graduated exposure approach was to gradually increase Miguel's food intake to solid foods. The contingency management component of CBT entails teaching the parent specific learning principles and procedures, such as positive reinforcement, shaping, extinction, and contingency contracting. Contingency management also involves teaching the parent to ignore the child's fear-based behaviors, such as avoidance or reassurance seeking, and to limit the child's avoidance of feared activities or environments. In Miguel's case, his mother was asked to limit her son's eating in his room and to limit the amount of liquids he drank during meals.

Cognitive restructuring, the last component of CBT, was used to facilitate Miguel's graduated exposure to the feared or avoided situations. Specifically, Miguel was taught to challenge his irrational beliefs by facing the situation and obtaining the "evidence" that there "really" is nothing to be afraid of. Through the use of cognitive restructuring, Miguel learned to modify his maladaptive and irrational thoughts to more adaptive and rational ones.

IMPLEMENTING THE TREATMENT PLAN

The treatment plan was implemented by devising a fear hierarchy to which both Miguel and his mother agreed. They concurred that they wanted Miguel to eat a variety of foods, not just soft foods, but also foods such as chicken, rice, and fruit. His mother further stated that she wanted her son to eat like "he did before," not to take so long to eat, and not to drink large amounts of juice or water with his meals. Miguel, his mother, and the clinician devised the fear hierarchy together in the third treatment session, and Miguel and his mother were asked to devise a "rewards list" for the following session. The rewards list is part of the contingency management component of the therapy, described above. After the three agreed on an exposure task for the week, the clinician drew up a contract that stated explicitly what the exposure task was and what reward Miguel would receive if he completed the task. For instance, if Miguel were to complete a specific exposure task (e.g., finishing breakfast in 20 minutes; drinking only one glass of water with his meals; eating a small piece of fruit), then his mother would provide him with a reward (e.g., chocolate bar; taking him to the movies; allowing him to stay up to watch his favorite show).

Based on the fear hierarchy, the types of food Miguel ate, the amount of time he spent eating, and the amount of liquids he drank during meals were targeted for exposure. After Miguel had successfully completed several exposures (e.g., eat cereal [or waffles or pancakes] in 20 minutes; eat cereal [or waffles or pancakes] in 20 minutes with one glass of milk or juice), the clinician introduced the cognitive restructuring component of the treatment. Miguel was asked a series of questions that pertained to reality checking ("What is the chance of choking again?") and decatastrophizing ("If I start to choke on a piece of fruit/food, will I surely die?"). Miguel was helped to understand that although it is possible to die from choking on food, the probability is low. Specifically, through responding to the series of questions, Miguel came to understand that if one eats one's food at a reasonable pace (i.e., not too fast but also not too slowly), chews the food appropriately, swallows, refrains from talking while eating, and so on, then the probability of choking is relatively low. Thus, the questioning helped Miguel to realize there are more constructive and adaptive ways of thinking about the situation rather than jumping to the worst conclusion.

Although the focus of the cognitive strategies was on Miguel's fears relating to choking, the clinician explained to him that he could apply similar strategies to help manage his worries about his safety and security, as part of his difficulties with GAD. He practiced utilizing these strategies in the office. The clinician further emphasized to Miguel's mother that whenever he approached her for reassurance, she should respond by saying, "You remember what you are learning? Use what you are learning." In this way, Miguel needed to seek out solutions on his own, rather than seeking reassurance and solutions from his mother, as in the past.

MONITORING THE PATIENT'S RESPONSE

Miguel and his mother responded well to the treatment, as evidenced by the monitoring form that Miguel completed each week prior to the session. Specifically, at the beginning of each session, Miguel was asked to complete a brief questionnaire, on which he indicated what the specific exposure task was for that week and whether he completed the task, and then rated on a scale of 0–8 the level of fear he experienced both before and after the completion of the exposure task. By completing this brief questionnaire, Miguel confirmed that he was completing each assigned task. Most importantly, he generally reported decreased fear from the beginning to the end of each exposure task.

SUMMARY AND OUTCOME

By the end of the tenth treatment session, Miguel was able to eat a whole banana, something he had not done in over 8 months. He also began to join his family at dinnertime, and the family was again able to enjoy a pleasant meal at restaurants. He reported that "every now and then" he worried about choking, but he now understood that the chances of this happening were very small. He also reported that he no longer needed to check his room for robbers; he said he felt safe and stated that the STOP technique (an acronym representing "scared," "thoughts," "other thoughts," and "praise"), which he learned during the cognitive restructuring phase of treatment, helped him to realize that his fears of someone breaking into the house would probably never come to fruition.

To prevent relapse, the clinician discussed two main concepts with Miguel and his mother during the last two treatment sessions. The first concept was the importance of practice and continued exposure. Essentially, Miguel would continue to eat as usual and not avoid restaurants, and his mother could not make special meals (mashed potatoes, smoothies, etc.) for Miguel. The other concept was that at some point a "slip" was likely to occur. Specifically, one day Miguel might feel nervous again about choking. The clinician emphasized that if this were to occur, Miguel needed to interpret the event as a one-time occasion and not feel that everything he had learned was lost or ruined. The importance of continued practice was again emphasized as being useful to help prevent "slipping." Miguel's prognosis was positive in light of his successful exposure tasks, his high level of compliance, and his mother's high level of motivation.

REFERENCES

American Psychiatric Association: Diagnostic and Statistical Manual of Mental Disorders, 4th Edition, Text Revision. Washington, DC, American Psychiatric Association, 2000

Anderson JC, Williams SM, McGee R, et al: DSM-III disorders in preadolescent children: prevalence in a large sample from the general population. Arch Gen Psychiatry 44:69–76, 1987

Banerjee S, Bhandari R, Rosenberg D: Use of low-dose selective serotonin reuptake inhibitors for severe, refractory choking phobia in childhood. J Dev Behav Pediatr 26:123–127, 2005

Beidel DC, Turner SM: Comorbidity of test anxiety and other anxiety disorders in children. J Abnorm Child Psychol 16:275–287, 1988

Burklow K, Linscheid T: Rapid inpatient behavioral treatment for choking phobia in children. Child Health Care 33:93–107, 2004

Chorpita BF: Modular Cognitive-Behavioral Therapy for Childhood Anxiety Disorders. New York, Guilford, 2007

Chorpita BF, Southam-Gerow M: Fears and anxieties, in Treatment of Child Disorders, 3rd Edition. Edited by Mash EJ, Barkley RA. New York, Guilford, 2006, pp 271–335

Chorpita BF, Yim LM, Moffitt CE, et al: Assessment of symptoms of DSM-IV anxiety and depression in children: a revised child anxiety and depression scale. Behav Res Ther 38:835–855, 2000

Chorpita BF, Daleiden E, Weisz JR: Identifying and selecting the common elements of evidence based interventions: a distillation and matching model. Ment Health Serv Res 7:5–20, 2005

Folstein MF, Folstein SE, McHugh PR: "Mini-mental state": a practical method for grading the cognitive state of patients for the clinician. J Psychiatr Res 12:189–198, 1975

Grills AE, Ollendick TH: Multiple informant agreement and the Anxiety Disorders Interview Schedule for Parents and Children. J Am Acad Child Adolesc Psychiatry 42:30–40, 2003

Kagan J, Reznick JS, Snidman N: The physiology and psychology of behavioral inhibition in children. Child Dev 58:1459–1473, 1987

Last CG, Strauss CC, Francis G: Comorbidity among childhood anxiety disorders. J Nerv
Ment Dis 175:726–730, 1987

Last CG, Perrin S, Hersen M, et al: DSM-III-R anxiety disorders in children: socio-
demographic and clinical characteristics. J Clin Child Adolesc Psychol 31:1070–
1076, 1992

Lissek S, Powers AS, McClure EB, et al: Classical fear conditioning in the anxiety disorders: a meta-analysis. Behav Res Ther 43:1391–1424, 2005

Pérez-Edgar K, Fox NA: Temperament and anxiety disorders. Child Adolesc Psychiatr
Clin N Am 14:681–706, viii, 2005

Pine DS, Klein RG: Anxiety disorders, in Rutter's Child and Adolescent Psychiatry, 5th
Edition. Edited by Rutter M, Bishop D, Pine DS, et al. Oxford, UK, Blackwell, 2008,
pp 628–647

Pine DS, Cohen P, Gurley D, et al: The risk for early adulthood anxiety and depressive
disorders in adolescents with anxiety and depressive disorders. Arch Gen Psychiatry
55:56–64, 1998

Rapee RM, Barrett PM, Dadds MR, et al: Reliability of the DSM-III-R childhood anxiety disorders using structured interview: interrater and parent-child agreement. J Am
Acad Child Adolesc Psychiatry 33:984–992, 1994

Research Unit on Pediatric Psychopharmacology Anxiety Study Group: Fluvoxamine
for the treatment of anxiety disorders in children and adolescents. N Engl J Med
344:1279–1285, 2001

Scheeringa MS, Wright MJ, Hunt JP, et al: Factors affecting the diagnosis and prediction of PTSD symptomatology in children and adolescents. Am J Psychiatry
163:644–651, 2006

Silverman WK, Albano AM: Anxiety Disorders Interview Schedule for DSM-IV. San
Antonio, TX, Psychological Corporation/Graywind, 1996

Silverman WK, Eisen A: Age differences in the reliability of parent and child reports
of child anxious symptomatology using a structured interview. J Am Acad Child Adolesc Psychiatry 31:117–124, 1992

Silverman WK, Kurtines WM: Progress in developing an exposure-based transfer-of-
control approach to treating internalizing disorders in youth, in Psychosocial
Treatments for Child and Adolescent Disorders: Empirically Based Strategies for
Clinical Practice, 2nd Edition. Edited by Hibbs ED, Jensen PS. Washington, DC,
American Psychological Association, 2005, pp 97–119

Silverman WK, Nelles WB: The Anxiety Disorders Interview Schedule for Children. J Am
Acad Child Adolesc Psychiatry 27:772–778, 1988

Silverman WK, Rabian B: Test-retest reliability of the DSM-III-R childhood anxiety
disorders symptoms using the Anxiety Disorders Interview Schedule for Children.
J Anxiety Disord 9:1–12, 1995

Silverman WK, Kurtines WM, Ginsburg GS, et al: Contingency management, self-
control, and education support in the treatment of childhood phobic disorders: a
randomized clinical trial. J Consult Clin Psychol 67:675–687, 1999

Silverman WK, Saavedra LM, Pina AA: Test-retest reliability of anxiety symptoms and diagnoses using the Anxiety Disorders Interview Schedule for DSM-IV: Child and Parent Versions. J Am Acad Child Adolesc Psychiatry 40:937–944, 2001

Silverman WK, Pina AA, Visweswaran C: Evidence-based psychosocial treatments for phobic and anxiety disorders in children and adolescents. J Clin Child Adolesc Psychol 37:105–130, 2008

Strauss CC, Last CG, Hersen M, et al: Association between anxiety and depression in children and adolescents with anxiety disorders. J Abnorm Child Psychol 16:57–68, 1988

Vasey MW, Dadds MR: The Developmental Psychopathology of Anxiety. New York, Oxford University Press, 2001

Wood J, Piacentini JC, Bergman RL, et al: Concurrent validity of the anxiety disorders section of the Anxiety Disorders Interview Schedule for DSM-IV: Child and Parent Versions. J Clin Child Adolesc Psychol 31:335–342, 2002

Zelikovsky N, MacNaughton K, Geffken G: A review of choking phobia in children: diagnosis, assessment, and treatment. Journal of Psychological Practice 7:23–32, 2001

■ CHAPTER 17 ■

Affective Storms

A Careful Assessment of Rage Attacks

Gabrielle A. Carlson, M.D.

CASE PRESENTATION

IDENTIFYING INFORMATION

Brad is a 10-year-old boy who has just finished fifth grade in an inclusion class. He has been classified as having multiple disabilities since kindergarten. He lives with both parents.

CHIEF COMPLAINT

Brad's mom wanted a second opinion regarding the diagnosis of bipolar disorder her son had received. She is concerned because 1) bipolar disorder runs in her husband's family and 2) she is aware of the popular media descriptions equating rages with bipolar disorder. The family was referred by the Child and Adolescent Bipolar Foundation.

HISTORY OF PRESENT ILLNESS

Brad has difficulties in several domains. His mother describes "rages" or outbursts during which he throws valuable objects at her or says he wants to kill

Gabrielle A. Carlson, M.D., is Professor of Psychiatry and Pediatrics and Director of the Division of Child and Adolescent Psychiatry at State University of New York at Stony Brook (for complete biographical information, see "About the Contributors," p. 613).

himself, and he has threatened both himself and his mom with a kitchen knife. Brad's rages occur when he does not get something he wants, feels criticized, does not have demands met instantly, misunderstands what others are saying, or is asked to comply with requests; his rages last up to 2 hours. After that point, Brad is often still irritable but can be distracted from a rage.

At the time of referral, even though Brad has been taking divalproex, atomoxetine, and risperidone, his mother reports that he is extremely distractible, disorganized, and forgetful, but not especially hyperactive. With regard to conduct/oppositional symptoms, his mother says that Brad lies, intimidates, starts fights, has stolen things, and has been deliberately destructive, although these are infrequent problems. He can be extremely oppositional, at least at home.

Brad is anxious. He asks questions almost for the sake of asking questions and, according to his mom, does not care about the answers. He has difficulty with change, although this has improved with age, and, when excited, has hand mannerisms (stretches his fingers a certain way) that sound like stereotypies. He sometimes head bangs when he is writing, although writing is a frustrating task for Brad.

Brad's mother describes him as generally cheerful, without any sustained depressed mood. He does cry easily. If something does not go his way, he decompensates. For instance, if he wants to play with someone and that person is not available (which usually happens), he gets very agitated and angry. He tries to get other children to like him by acting silly. His mother is not sure whether this behavior is euphoria or a misguided attempt at socialization. He has low self-esteem. Brad denies sustained feelings of excessive happiness, sadness, or irritability. He does not endorse any psychotic symptoms in a convincing way.

The family attends church regularly. Brad often asks if he will go to Hell if he is bad, and he is afraid that God will be mad at him. He also asks lots of questions about sex but, although he is curious about the subject, has not acted out inappropriately. Brad does not have sleep problems when he is off medication.

The teacher in Brad's inclusion class has observed that he has symptoms of inattentiveness and disorganization but not much hyperactivity. The teacher also observed symptoms of oppositionality, anxiety (Brad often goes to the school nurse with physical complaints), low self-esteem, sometimes trouble relating to other children, and getting upset with change.

Brad really has no friends, although he does not acknowledge this and has described himself as popular (this statement was considered grandiose by one of his doctors). He does enjoy playing with much younger children and loves babies. He has had serious learning issues (see cognitive summary below).

Medications being taken at the time of referral consisted of divalproex 500 mg/day (blood level is 97 µg/mL), risperidone 0.75 mg/day, and atomoxetine 60 mg/day.

Past Psychiatric History

Brad's tantrums began when he was around age 4. Behaviorally, he was very hyperactive. He climbed out of windows, would not stay in the supermarket carriage, and would not stick to play activities in preschool or at home. At age 5, he was referred for an evaluation for attention-deficit/hyperactivity disorder (ADHD) and was started on stimulant medication. His rages had not occurred frequently and had not been a problem in school. Brad's psychiatrist treated him with venlafaxine at age 9 years for his prominent anxious behavior, including his unusual fears. For instance, Brad got agitated seeing cars pass the car he was riding in. He could not explain why. While taking venlafaxine, Brad began talking in his sleep and, when he woke up, thought he saw a face when nothing was there. He went to bed at 10:00–11:00 P.M. and woke up at 6:00 A.M. Also, while taking this medication, he perseverated more on the subject of God and wanted to go to confession all the time. Recalling his feelings while taking venlafaxine, Brad said he could not sit still. Additionally, his rages increased in frequency, occurring at least daily. When his mom complained that he was getting more irritable, his doctor raised the dosage to a maximum of 225 mg/day. Finally, after several trips to the emergency room because Brad was out of control, the emergency room doctor suggested that his mother stop giving Brad the drug. When Brad was no longer taking venlafaxine, his rages returned to their previous frequency. Other medications that Brad took in the past included stimulants, which appeared to cause tics and compulsions, and gabapentin, which was stopped for unknown reasons.

Medical History

Brad has had no significant medical problems.

Developmental History

Brad was born vaginally, 2 weeks after his due date, and there was no amniotic fluid when he was born. He was a demanding baby, never slept through the night, and needed predigested formula. His speech was late (he did not speak sentences until age 3 years), and he was evaluated at a special education preschool. His mother also noted that Brad repeated other people's words when he was learning to speak, and he fought with peers because he did not understand sharing or turn-taking. Rather than using toys for imaginative play, Brad lined up toys in intricate ways and then was done with them.

Brad was always clumsy and accident-prone and had a high pain threshold, so he would end up with lumps and bruises that did not seem to bother him. He had no other symptoms of sensory defensiveness, however.

In addition to speech services, Brad received occupational therapy for visual-motor difficulties.

SOCIAL HISTORY

Brad's mother is a high school graduate who works as a lab technician. Brad's father is a construction worker who dropped out of school at age 16.

FAMILY HISTORY

Brad's mother had separation anxiety as a child but was a reasonable student. Other relatives have obsessive-compulsive disorder, panic disorder, and a gambling problem. Brad's father had learning disabilities and temper problems, and as an adult is recovering from alcoholism. The father's sister was identified as "bipolar"; based on further questioning, if she has bipolar disorder, it is bipolar II disorder because of her serious depressions. The father has other siblings who have alcohol abuse.

COGNITIVE TESTING

On the Wechsler Intelligence Scale for Children, 3rd Edition (Wechsler 1991), Brad achieved a Verbal IQ of 88 (Arithmetic 5; Comprehension 8; Information 10), Performance IQ of 81 (Picture Completion 3; Block Design/Picture Arrangement 9), and Full Scale IQ of 83. His performance on the Bender Visual Motor Gestalt Test (Brannigan and Decker 2003) was within normal limits. Language testing was done in preschool when he was referred for early intervention, but subsequent testing no longer qualified him for services. Table 17–1 shows the results of Brad's achievement tests.

TABLE 17–1. Brad's achievement test results[a]

| | Grade | | | | |
Test	1	2	3	4	5
Math	k.4 (1st %ile)	—	1.2	1.7	2.3
Reading					
Comprehension	k.8 (9th %ile)	—	1.8	1.7	2.0
Vocabulary	k.5 (8th %ile)	—	2.0	1.1	2.7
Scanning	—	—	2.5	3.3	3.6

Note.   k=kindergarten.
[a]Results are given as year (before decimal) and month (after decimal) of school. (No test results are available for second grade.)

MENTAL STATUS EXAMINATION

Brad is a cute youngster who both looks and relates like a much younger child. He has an odd gait and body posture, and his general appearance is that of a child with neurological dysfunction. Contributing to his immature behavior is his "Tigger-like" friskiness, which one associates with preschool children. He is disinhibited and overly friendly, and he frequently interrupted the psychiatrist's interview with his mother (although he could be distracted and would leave). During the one-to-one interview with Brad, while he had the examiner's complete attention, his behavior was more appropriate.

Brad's language expression was like that of a younger child in its simplicity; however, he had content in his head. If prompted and asked to elaborate further, he would give more complex answers to the questions. For instance, Brad had been watching the movie *Mighty Joe Young* in the waiting room, and in an effort to get him to talk, the clinician asked him what the movie was about. Brad could not summarize it, but he was able to provide more of a summary when asked specific questions, such as "Who was in it?" "What did he do?" "What happened next?"

Brad also did poorly summarizing in a "listening to paragraphs" task, although he had the drift of the stories. He was nonverbally and verbally quite expressive when he spoke. Not one of his comments was off topic. Brad was able to read a first grade–level story for the examiner, reading "Leo the Late Bloomer" with very dramatic expression. When he was told what *blooming* meant in the context of the book, he said, "I hope that's me."

Brad was weak in math. He said 5+3 was 7, and he could not subtract without making marks on a sheet of paper and then crossing them out.

Brad said he gets angry when kids in school make fun of him and when people tell him "no." When asked what he does when he gets angry, he showed the examiner by banging his head repeatedly into his hands. When asked what makes him sad, Brad responded, "Movies," although this response hearkened to what happened to Mighty Joe Young. After discussion with the examiner, Brad decided that it is sad if the animal dies, so when he was asked what makes him sad, "movies" made sense as a response. Brad replied that what makes him happy is "parties" and what makes him scared is "when my parents fight." He also worries about God because he knows that he himself is often bad and in trouble.

SCREENING INSTRUMENTS

Social problems and somatic symptoms got the highest endorsements (>99th percentile) on the Teacher Report Form (Achenbach 1991). On a language screen, the teacher reported that Brad misses the point of a conversation, makes comments that are off topic, confuses sequences of events, and does not always seem to care that others do not understand him. Other than irritability, no manic symptoms were observed in school. On the Parent Version of the Child Mania Rating Scale (Pavuluri et al. 2006), he scored 31, but his mother later told the clinician that she had completed the form based on Brad's behavior while he was taking venlafaxine.

COMMENTARIES

Psychotherapeutic Perspective

Penelope Knapp, M.D.

DIAGNOSTIC FORMULATION

The differential diagnosis of stormy affective behavior includes 1) bipolar disorder, 2) ADHD, and 3) developmental regulatory disorders, as well as 4) intellectual disabilities impairing adaptive response to ordinary stresses. Brad has a history of tantrums, and his current symptoms include irritability, attention-deficit constellation (without hyperactivity), anxiety, rages when he is thwarted, and inability to communicate his needs or have them met instantly.

Brad's initial evaluation included, appropriately, family history, developmental history, and collateral information from school. The initial list of symptoms might lead to any of several diagnoses. Indeed, many such children would receive two or more diagnoses and, like Brad, receive prescriptions for multiple psychotropic medications. What else does the clinician need to know for diagnostic clarity and treatment planning for Brad?

1. The presenting complaint is possible bipolar disorder; however, Brad's mood symptoms do not appear to be due to bipolar disorder. He does not have a strong family history or a clear pattern of alternating elevated and depressed mood. His baseline mood is cheerful, but he is labile and becomes agitated when events turn in directions he finds unpredictable or unacceptable. An extended evaluation should pursue more detail about those situations to explore for a pattern of triggering stressors.

Penelope Knapp, M.D., is Professor Emeritus of Psychiatry and Pediatrics at University of California Davis, and Medical Director of the California Department of Mental Health in Sacramento, California (for complete biographical information, see "About the Contributors," p. 613).

2. Brad has previously received a diagnosis of ADHD, based on his hyperactivity, impulsivity, and tantrums, leading to the prescription of stimulant medications since he was age 5. It will be important to clarify what effect if any this class of medications had, especially as his teacher notes continuing disorganization and inattention. Brad continues to have difficulty managing his attention at an age-appropriate level. Attention, however, is not a unitary function, and neuropsychological testing would clarify whether Brad's difficulties are with deploying, sustaining, or shifting his attention, in relation to other executive functions.

3. Developmental regulatory disorders may arise from inborn child characteristics or from a child's reaction to early experiences with caregiving, including disordered attachments or traumatic experiences (Knapp 2006). The developmental history suggests regulatory problems since infancy. Following a late delivery with oligohydramnios, Brad was a demanding baby, did not sleep through the night, and "needed predigested formula." DSM-IV-TR does not specifically characterize developmental regulatory disorders, although the Diagnostic Classification of Mental Health and Developmental Disorders of Infancy and Early Childhood (DC:0-3) does (Zero to Three 1994); many children older than age 36 months who meet diagnostic criteria for various DSM-IV-TR diagnoses can be found by history to have also met DC:0-3 diagnostic criteria for a regulatory disorder. This diagnosis requires both a distinct behavioral pattern and a sensory, sensory-motor, or organizational processing difficulty. Several types of regulatory disorder have been identified; Brad might most closely fit type III, motorically disorganized, impulsive. However, self-regulation also describes whether the infant or toddler has been able to establish a rhythm of hunger, arousal, and sleep, and whether the child can self-soothe or modulate his or her feelings to an age-appropriate degree, and Brad's history of feeding problems and "demandingness" may be indicative of earlier roots to his present problems.

   Anxiety is a nonspecific symptom. Brad's unusual fears and somatic complaints, with frequent visits to the school nurse, indicate that he struggles with anxiety. An attempt was made to treat this with a serotonin-norepinephrine reuptake inhibitor (venlafaxine), leading to reduced sleep, increased rages, and perseverative religious thoughts. This reaction suggests that Brad does not suffer from a simple anxiety disorder per se, but rather that anxiety may be a feature of his difficulty with self-regulation as well as a reaction to continuing stresses related to his handicaps in school and in interpersonal communication, as evidenced by head banging when frustrated and rages when he misunderstands others.

4. Intellectual disability is part of Brad's picture. Testing shows that Brad has a Full Scale IQ of 83, with scatter, but that his academic achievement

progresses at a level below what his IQ would predict in all areas. Not only does Brad have low normal intellectual functioning, but a developmental language disorder is strongly indicated. He had late language acquisition, possibly had echolalia (repeated other people's words), and currently has significant difficulty with pragmatic aspects of language, such as understanding sharing or turn-taking. The history indicates that language testing was done in preschool and that subsequent testing no longer qualified him for services. Further diagnostic clarity should be pursued, beginning with obtaining the report of the earlier testing results to see if testing focused on achievement of language milestones with respect to expressive and receptive language or if it also included language pragmatics.

Currently, Brad expresses himself as would a first-grade child, with congruent affect. He has trouble reporting about a series of sentences but could make use of therapist armature to organize his responses. A crucial component of diagnostic assessment is the clinician's self-observation of the means he or she must use to establish verbal and nonverbal communication and the level at which this communication occurs; this will inform which therapeutic modality might best succeed, an important step to treatment planning.

Autistic spectrum disorder is an important diagnostic category to consider. Brad demonstrates several symptoms that might lead to consideration of an autistic spectrum disorder. He has difficulty with change, possible stereotypies, and no imaginative play; he lines up toys in "intricate ways"; he has no friends. Less specifically, he is motorically clumsy and has a high pain threshold.

Finally, the family history—anxiety, obsessive-compulsive disorder, learning disabilities, alcohol abuse, and depression—is rudimentary, and the current family relationships are not described. Brad's troubling preoccupations with religiosity need to be understood in the context of the family's religious beliefs, to determine if his views are congruent (learned) with those of his family's culture or if they represent his own constructions. Also, although a history of previous alcoholism in the father was reported, the clinician needs to inquire about the mother's alcohol use during pregnancy, because fetal alcohol syndrome may present with impairments in attention, impulsivity, and cognition.

DIAGNOSIS

Having determined that Brad's affective storms are not due to bipolar disorder, the clinician might peruse DSM-IV-TR and find that Brad has sufficient symptoms to meet criteria for the following diagnoses:

315.9   Learning disorder not otherwise specified (NOS)
315.4   Developmental coordination disorder

315.32   Mixed receptive-expressive language disorder

299.80   Pervasive developmental disorder NOS (PDD-NOS) (including atypical autism)

314.9   ADHD NOS

The clinician might choose one or more of these or diagnose the following:

313.9   Disorder of infancy, childhood, or adolescence NOS

However, if a diagnosis is to inform treatment planning, none of these diagnoses offers a particularly useful map to guide the next steps. Assigning a diagnosis to children with impaired reciprocal social interaction may be difficult because several developmental pathways to this problem are possible (Knapp and Jensen 2006).

The first diagnosis to consider is PDD-NOS, although Brad's odd gait, posture, and movements might indicate a less specific neuropsychiatric condition, and his disinhibited, overly friendly demeanor with a benign therapist, as well as his implied capacity for joint attention in a structured one-to-one setting, might lead some to discard this diagnostic option.

In addition to PDD-NOS, the clinician might consider several non-DSM diagnoses that have been described for children with disordered interpersonal relatedness. These include multisystem (or multiplex) developmental disorder, nonverbal learning disability syndrome, semantic-pragmatic language disorder (SPLD), attachment disorders (besides reactive attachment disorder, referencing theories of developmental limbic system damage), and schizoid personality disorder (Scheeringa 2001).

Multiplex developmental disorder (Zalsman and Cohen 1998), or multiple complex developmental disorder (van der Gaag et al. 2005), is being considered as a separate subcategory for DSM-V. This disorder transcends "comorbidity" in that it describes a developmental disorder that spans several developmental strands. Children with this disorder have the severe, early-appearing social and communicative deficits characteristic of autism, as well as some of the emotional instability and disordered thought processes that resemble schizophrenic symptoms. Brad has symptoms in the three categories for this disorder: 1) impaired social behavior/sensitivity, similar to that seen in autism, such as impaired peer relations, and possibly limited capacity for empathy or understanding what others are thinking or feeling; 2) affective symptoms, including impaired regulation of feelings, intense and inappropriate anxiety, recurrent panic, and possibly emotional lability without obvious cause; and 3) thought disorder symptoms, such as possible sudden, irrational intrusions on normal thoughts, or magical thinking as manifested by his religious fears.

Children with SPLD have disordered semantic processing and pragmatics of language use. Some authorities classify SPLD in the autism spectrum of disorders, whereas others consider it a language disorder. SPLD may occur in combination with a non–autistic spectrum disorder such as ADHD. The accurate diagnosis of SPLD may involve a speech-language pathologist, clinical psychologist, or occupational therapist.

If a DSM-IV-TR diagnosis must be chosen, the best Axis I option is probably PDD-NOS. Mixed receptive-expressive language disorder might be an alternative diagnosis, but as yet no testing has been done to confirm to what extent this is present, whereas there is significant history to suggest a pragmatic language handicap.

DSM-IV-TR DIAGNOSIS

Axis I   299.80 Pervasive developmental disorder not otherwise specified

Axis II   None

Axis III   None

Axis IV   Educational problems: continuing stress due to difficulty succeeding in school placement

Other problems: inability to make friends

Axis V   Global Assessment of Functioning=50

Serious impairment in school functioning and social functioning

TREATMENT RECOMMENDATIONS

The initial treatment plan would be to work with Brad, together with his family, through the course of a more extended evaluation, to understand how the family perceives his function level and how they assist him, and to guide them through the fuller diagnostic assessment necessary for treatment planning and for executing a new educational approach.

Because Brad's achievement is below age level and also below that to be predicted from his IQ testing, and because his teacher reports low self-esteem and anxiety, the latter propelling him to the nurse's office with somatic complaints, the clinician needs to obtain testing that informs an individualized education program that will allow Brad to enjoy success in learning.

One advantage of a PDD-NOS diagnosis is that it might open the door to a broader array of services for Brad. This diagnosis may be necessary, because Brad needs help with interpersonal communication and with the basic skills underlying academic achievement. To confirm the diagnosis, the evaluator might employ the Social Communication Questionnaire (for children ages 4 years and older), Autism Spectrum Screening Questionnaire (Berument et al. 1999), or Childhood Autism Rating Scale (Ehlers et al. 1999).

Regardless of the DSM-IV-TR diagnosis, further assessment of Brad's language function is necessary for planning an educational and remedial approach, and will also be strategically useful for his therapist. The Clinical Evaluation of Language Fundamentals, 3rd Edition (Semel et al. 1995), the Test of Language Development—Primary, 3rd Edition (Newcomer and Hammill 1997), and the Test of Language Development—Intermediate, 3rd Edition (Hammill and Newcomer 1997) meet standards for reliability, validity, and the availability of representative normative data.

Brad's difficulties with language pragmatics and expression are functionally impairing him, although he has not reportedly tested at a level that qualifies him for services supporting academic progress. Brad's impulsivity might be reduced if he understands and attends better; Bishop and Norbury (2005) found that inhibitory deficits are neither specific to autism nor linked to particular aspects of autistic symptomatology, but rather appear to be associated with poor verbal skills and inattention. Therapy for a pragmatic language disorder would include scripting language for various social situations and question formats.

Being informed that their child has an intellectual or learning disability can be a severe blow to parents. However, a foundation for building a treatment plan with the parents is laid by having them understand the information gained by the evaluation, including not only Brad's areas of delay or deficiency, but also his strengths. Because the family is a tactical resource for his learning and growing, the family members' capacities and areas of difficulty will also have to be understood. In family sessions, the therapist can identify how Brad can and could learn, not just what he has not learned. Improved language and communication skills would enable the child to construct a coherent sense of himself (Paul et al. 1999). Recognizing how PDD-NOS or multiplex developmental disorder affects both language and self-regulation and how these affect the child's internal sense of himself has implications for treating the child for whom several aspects of development are atypical. Also, a social communication skills group would allow Brad to gain experience and competence at successfully communicating to other children his age.

The purpose of this commentary is not to address pharmacologic intervention. However, I would like to note that currently Brad's symptoms of affective dysregulation are being targeted by a mood-stabilizing anticonvulsant (divalproex), his symptoms of ADHD by a selective norepinephrine reuptake inhibitor (atomoxetine), and his general difficulty with emotional regulation and/or his odd/psychotic thinking by a seond-generation antipsychotic (risperidone). Fuller characterization of all of Brad's symptom patterns is necessary, as is specification of target symptoms for any medication prescribed, to allow tracking of the treatment effect. Moreover, coordination between nonpharmacologic and pharmacologic treatment is necessary to understand treatment response and adjust doses. A detailed medication evaluation would organize such information. If medication is part of Brad's treatment, his parents should receive psychoeducation about each medication and should actively participate in observing its effects on their child.

Psychopharmacologic Perspective

Jon McClellan, M.D.

DIAGNOSTIC FORMULATION

Brad presents with a complicated set of behavioral and emotional challenges, including aggression, impulsivity, volatility, conduct problems, anxiety, cognitive rigidity, and demoralization. Many of his symptoms are reactive, are context specific, and represent ineffective coping strategies in response to conflict or stress. Such clinical presentations often arise in youth with difficult reactive temperaments coupled with poor impulse control, developmental lags, negativity, and disinhibition. These difficulties may lead to maladaptive interpersonal negotiation or problem-solving strategies that are inadvertently reinforced by well-meaning adults (including therapists) who struggle to address behavioral escalations and emotional torment. As these interactive patterns evolve, negative behavioral and emotional repertoires can become fixed and may escalate over time.

Brad's symptoms cross over several DSM-IV-TR diagnostic categories, including mood disorders, disruptive behavior disorders, anxiety disorders, and learning/developmental disorders. No single defined syndrome characterizes his clinical picture in toto. He does not present with well-demarcated mood states that meet full criteria for either major depression or mania. His symptoms of irritability, excessive silliness, anger outbursts, reckless behaviors, and mood swings can arguably be classified as bipolar disorder NOS. However, the specificity of this characterization is debatable and may have no relationship to

Jon McClellan, M.D., is Professor in the Department of Psychiatry and Behavioral Sciences at the University of Washington in Seattle; and Medical Director of the Child Study and Treatment Center in the Division of Mental Health, Washington State (for complete biographical information, see "About the Contributors," p. 613).

what has classically been characterized as bipolar disorder in adults (McClellan et al. 2007).

Brad's symptoms best fit the descriptor "severe mood dysregulation," coined by Leibenluft and colleagues (Brotman et al. 2006). Severe mood dysregulation is defined by a persistently abnormal baseline mood (i.e., irritability, anger, and/or sadness), hyperarousal (e.g., physical restlessness, distractibility, rapid speech, intrusiveness), and increased reactivity to negative emotional stimuli (e.g., temper outbursts). Severe mood dysregulation is not a DSM-IV-TR diagnosis, although the concept is being considered for DSM-V.

DSM-IV-TR DIAGNOSIS

Axis I   296.80 Bipolar disorder NOS

314.00 ADHD, predominantly inattentive type

312.81 Conduct disorder, which subsumes oppositional defiant disorder

300.00 Anxiety disorder NOS

299.80 Pervasive developmental disorder NOS

Axis II   None

Axis III   None

Axis IV   Family conflicts, difficulties at school, and poor peer relationships

Axis V   Global Assessment of Functioning=45

Currently experiencing moderate impairment at school, at home, and with peers, with frequent aggression, oppositionality, and anxiety

TREATMENT RECOMMENDATIONS

Prior to initiating new treatments, the clinician needs to review past therapies. Brad has previously taken stimulants, gabapentin, and venlafaxine. The venlafaxine appears to have caused significant activation that exacerbated his irritability and rage outbursts. He may be at risk for activation with other antidepressants as well. Stimulants were associated with tics and increased compulsiveness and do not appear to be an option. The indications for gabapentin were not noted. Presumably, it was used for anxiety because it has not been found to be helpful for bipolar disorder, at least in adults (Sachs and Gardner-Schuster 2007).

Brad is currently taking divalproex 500 mg/day (blood level=97 µg/mL), risperidone 0.75 mg/day, and atomoxetine 60 mg/day. This combination appears to have been designed to target problems with inattention, impulsivity, and explosive outbursts. The history does not indicate whether Brad has had a significant therapeutic response or developed toxicities to any of these agents, why he is on three different agents, and whether ongoing treatment with each or all is indicated. His ongoing behavioral and emotional struggles suggest that dosage adjustments and/or modifications in the regimen should be considered.

When considering pharmacologic options, the clinician needs to review the extant literature supporting the use of different agents for specific indications. Pediatric psychopharmacology trials have not typically addressed mood and behavioral dysregulation; however, the treatment literature addressing ADHD, bipolar disorder, and aggression in youth arguably applies.

For youth, atomoxetine and risperidone have the best empirical support. Atomoxetine has been approved by the U.S. Food and Drug Administration for treating ADHD in youth and is recommended for children with ADHD who cannot tolerate stimulants or for those who have comorbid anxiety (Pliszka and AACAP Work Group on Quality Issues 2007). However, this agent may increase activation, which could be contributing to Brad's current problems. Furthermore, atomoxetine does not appear to have as large a clinical effect size as stimulants (Pliszka and AACAP Work Group on Quality Issues 2007), thus raising questions as to its utility for youth with more serious impairments.

Risperidone has been found to be beneficial for youth with explosive behaviors and those with bipolar disorder (Findling et al. 2005). In general, the atypical antipsychotics appear helpful for aggression and impulsiveness (Findling et al. 2005). Although anticonvulsants are presumed to be helpful as well, negative randomized controlled trials of divalproex (Wagner et al. 2007) and oxcarbazepine (Wagner et al. 2006) for pediatric bipolar disorder raise questions as to whether second-generation antipsychotic agents are a better first choice.

Assessing whether Brad needs to be taking three different agents is important. The goal is to use the fewest possible medications to adequately address symptoms across different diagnostic groupings. Polypharmacy is a growing concern in pediatric psychopharmacology, especially for youth diagnosed with bipolar disorder (Duffy et al. 2005). Multiple agents are often added over a relatively short period of time given clinical acuity. Pressures within systems of care, such as efforts to shorten lengths of hospital stay, also add to the rapidity with which medications are added.

For Brad, risperidone is perhaps the best single option to better control his aggression, poor impulse control, and reactivity. The current dosage, 0.75 mg/day, may not be adequate to address his symptoms. Slowly increasing the risperidone as tolerated, up to a target dosage of about 3 mg/day, may improve his current functioning. As he stabilizes, the next step would be to reassess the need for divalproex and/or atomoxetine, with consideration of a stepwise taper of one or the other, while closely monitoring for an exacerbation of symptoms. Preferably each medication step will be undertaken in sequence, not concurrently, with sufficient time to adequately gauge the response. Potential side effects need to be systematically monitored, including the risk for weight gain and other metabolic complications.

Finally, medications alone are not likely to resolve Brad's emotional and behavioral challenges. Medication therapy should be considered adjunctive to psychoeducational and cognitive-behavioral interventions designed to improve problem-solving strategies, coping skills, and parenting effectiveness. The goal with use of medications for Brad is to stabilize his aggression and volatility, thus increasing the likelihood that psychotherapeutic strategies can be implemented. As these strategies are effective, Brad's need for medications hopefully will be reduced.

Integrative Perspective

Gabrielle A. Carlson, M.D.

DIAGNOSTIC FORMULATION

Brad has had a little bit of many things. He met criteria for ADHD, combined type, as a younger child. Although his hyperactivity is in partial remission, he is left with problems of executive function that atomoxetine did not adequately address. He had a number of motor tics that seemed to worsen when he was treated with stimulants. His mother and teachers feel he is touchy, easily annoyed, and often defiant and argumentative—features that meet the criteria for oppositional defiant disorder, although his behavior is characterized by low frustration tolerance rather than deliberate flaunting of authority.

Brad has serious social delays, more so than the "typical" child with ADHD. He experienced language delay and brief echolalia, and he continues to have some expressive language difficulties. Ironically, his speech therapy was discontinued in first grade when he tested out of services. He has not been tested or treated since. In Sweden, Brad's motor clumsiness and learning disabilities along with the attention problems would be considered DAMP, which stands for deficits in attention, motor control, and perception (Gillberg 2003). In DSM-IV-TR terms, however, although he had some symptoms of PDD as a preschool child, his social behavior and language are now immature rather than instrumental. The current understanding in the field is that autism and its component parts are on a continuum (Constantino and Todd 2003). Nevertheless, as demonstrated in follow-up studies of youngsters with language impairment (Clegg et al. 2005; Howlin et al. 2000) and children with PDD-NOS

(Michelotti et al. 2002), significant social and behavioral impairments continue, as is the case with Brad.

Although Brad does not have mental retardation, his learning trajectory is in the mentally retarded range. The achievement test results listed in Table 17–1, which appeared earlier in this chapter, indicate that Brad gains half a grade level every year, giving him a developmental quotient of about 50. In other words, at this rate, when he is in twelfth grade, he will have sixth-grade skills, assuming he continues to learn (which can be expected if he does not have mental retardation). Clearly, Brad has significant learning disabilities, possibly based on his language disorder.

Brad's mother wanted to know if her son had bipolar disorder. Although this diagnosis is increasingly given to children who have serious tantrums, this behavior is not what constitutes the disorder. Although Brad can be silly and disinhibited, these behaviors may not stem from euphoria. Because his social awareness is poor, his calling himself popular may not be inflated self-esteem. Brad certainly appeared to have manic symptoms on venlafaxine; all of his behaviors were exaggerated, including his activity level, irritability/aggression, and religious concerns. These returned to baseline when the drug was stopped. Adults with bipolar depression have developed mania when treated with venlafaxine (Post et al. 2006), and antidepressant-induced mania in adults with bipolar disorder has been the subject of considerable discussion (Ghaemi et al. 2003). Whether the toxic response to a drug represents the same phenomenon in a prepubertal child who was not depressed is not clear. Prepubertal children appear to be more sensitive to activation produced by selective serotonin reuptake inhibitors (Martin et al. 2004; Safer and Zito 2006) than are adolescents and adults. Children with PDDs appear to be especially sensitive to psychotropic medication (Posey et al. 2006). Another important consideration is that had the diagnostic assessment been restricted to the interview usually used for mood and behavior disorders (Schedule for Affective Disorders and Schizophrenia for School-Age Children—Present and Lifetime Version; Kaufman et al. 1997), there would have been no reference to Brad's learning, language, or autism spectrum disorder problems.

Brad is very stressed at school. He denies worry per se, and his anxiety is not generalized, but his academic and social failures are probably behind the somatic complaints that he experiences. Spending time in the nurse's office serves as an avoidance mechanism.

Although Brad also meets official criteria for oppositional defiant disorder and learning disabilities, these conditions do not do justice to the level of social, language, and mood/anxiety symptoms he manifests. One could argue that he has PDD-NOS, in partial remission, and substance-induced mania. If he is diagnosed with PDD, then his executive function symptoms will be attributed to this condition and not diagnosed as ADHD.

DSM-IV-TR DIAGNOSIS

Brad is diagnostically homeless. In the current health care system, clinicians are forced to choose a diagnosis for purposes of reimbursement. The following are the closest for Brad:

Axis I   314.01 ADHD, combined type

300.00 Anxiety disorder NOS

Possible pervasive developmental disorder NOS, in partial remission

Substance-induced mood disorder with manic features, onset during venlafaxine treatment

315.1 Mathematics disorder

315.00 Reading disorder

315.32 Mixed receptive-expressive language disorder

Axis II   None

Axis III None

Axis IV   School placement

Limited social contact

Axis V   Global Assessment of Functioning=45

TREATMENT RECOMMENDATIONS

The clinician recommended to the school that Brad's language function be retested. His percentile ranks were <3 for both expressive and receptive language functioning. As a result, he was placed in a self-contained class for his academic classes and given speech-language interventions twice a week.

Brad's mother was coached in collaborative problem-solving approaches (Greene and Ablon 2006) and learned to anticipate Brad's meltdowns, which actually decreased in frequency after his classroom change. Although he had not had rages in school, his family bore the brunt of the anxiety he experienced there. The more appropriate classroom placement reduced his anxiety.

Divalproex was discontinued, and Brad was treated with a small dose of methylphenidate during the day, which also improved his focus and decreased his silly behavior. Ironically, he appeared to respond better to two doses of short-acting medication than to longer-acting preparations, which increased his irritability. Risperidone was continued because his mother was afraid to stop it.

REFERENCES

Achenbach TM: Manual for the Teacher Report Form. Burlington, University of Vermont, Department of Psychology, 1991

Berument SK, Rutter M, Lord C, et al: Autism Screening Questionnaire: diagnostic validity. Br J Psychiatry 175:444–451, 1999

Bishop DV, Norbury CF: Executive functions in children with communication impairments, in relation to autistic symptomatology, 2: response inhibition. Autism 9:29–43, 2005

Brannigan GG, Decker SL: Bender Visual-Motor Gestalt Test, 2nd Edition. Itasca, IL, Riverside Publishing, 2003

Brotman MA, Schmajuk M, Rich BA, et al: Prevalence, clinical correlates, and longitudinal course of severe mood dysregulation in children. Biol Psychiatry 60:991–997, 2006

Clegg J, Hollis C, Mawhood L, et al: Developmental language disorders—a follow-up in later adult life: cognitive, language and psychosocial outcomes. J Child Psychol Psychiatry 46:128–149, 2005

Constantino JN, Todd RD: Autistic traits in the general population: a twin study. Arch Gen Psychiatry 60:524–530, 2003

Duffy FF, Narrow WE, Rae DS, et al: Concomitant pharmacotherapy among youths treated in routine psychiatric practice. J Child Adolesc Psychopharmacol 15:12–25, 2005

Ehlers S, Gillberg C, Wing L: A screening questionnaire for Asperger syndrome and other high-functioning autism spectrum disorders in school age children. J Autism Dev Disord 29:129–141, 1999

Findling RL, Steiner H, Weller EB: Use of antipsychotics in children and adolescents. J Clin Psychiatry 66 (suppl 7):29–40, 2005

Ghaemi SN, Hsu DJ, Soldani F, et al: Antidepressants in bipolar disorder: the case for caution. Bipolar Disord 5:421–433, 2003

Gillberg C: Deficits in attention, motor control, and perception: a brief review. Arch Dis Child 88:904–910, 2003

Greene RW, Ablon JS: Treating Explosive Kids: The Collaborative Problem-Solving Approach. New York, Guilford, 2006

Hammill DD, Newcomer PL: Test of Language Development—Intermediate, 3rd Edition. Austin, TX, PRO-ED, 1997

Howlin P, Mawhood L, Rutter M: Autism and developmental receptive language disorder—a follow-up comparison in early adult life, II: social, behavioural, and psychiatric outcomes. J Child Psychol Psychiatry 41:561–578, 2000

Kaufman J, Birmaher B, Brent D, et al: Schedule for Affective Disorders and Schizophrenia for School-Age Children—Present and Lifetime Version (K-SADS-PL): initial reliability and validity data. J Am Acad Child Adolesc Psychiatry 36:980–988, 1997

Knapp P: Understanding early development and temperament from the vantage point of evolutionary theory, in Toward a New Diagnostic System for Child Psychopathology: Moving Beyond the DSM. Edited by Jensen PS, Knapp P, Mrazek DA. New York, Guilford, 2006, pp 38–57

Knapp P, Jensen PS: Recommendations for DSM-V, in Toward a New Diagnostic System for Child Psychopathology: Moving Beyond the DSM. Edited by Jensen PS, Knapp P, Mrazek DA. New York, Guilford, 2006, pp 162–182

Martin A, Young C, Leckman JF, et al: Age effects on antidepressant-induced manic conversion. Arch Pediatr Adolesc Med 158:773–780, 2004

McClellan J, Kowatch R, Findling RL; Work Group on Quality Issues: Practice parameter for the assessment and treatment of children and adolescents with bipolar disorder. J Am Acad Child Adolesc Psychiatry 46:107–125, 2007

Michelotti J, Charman T, Slonims V, et al: Follow-up of children with language delay and features of autism from preschool years to middle childhood. Dev Med Child Neurol 44:812–819, 2002

Newcomer PL, Hammill DD: Test of Language Development—Primary, 3rd Edition. Austin, TX, PRO-ED, 1997

Paul R, Cohen D, Klin A, et al: Multiplex developmental disorders: the role of communication in the construction of a self. Child Adolesc Psychiatr Clin N Am 8:189–202, 1999

Pavuluri MN, Henry D, Devineni B, et al: Child Mania Rating Scale: development, reliability, and validity. J Am Acad Child Adolesc Psychiatry 45:550–560, 2006

Pliszka S; AACAP Work Group on Quality Issues: Practice parameter for the assessment and treatment of children and adolescents with attention-deficit/hyperactivity disorder. J Am Acad Child Adolesc Psychiatry 46:894–921, 2007

Posey DJ, Erickson CA, Stigler KA, et al: The use of selective serotonin reuptake inhibitors in autism and related disorders. J Child Adolesc Psychopharmacol 16:181–186, 2006

Post RM, Altshuler LL, Leverich GS, et al: Mood switch in bipolar depression: comparison of adjunctive venlafaxine, bupropion and sertraline. Br J Psychiatry 189:124–131, 2006

Sachs GS, Gardner-Schuster EE: Adjunctive treatment of acute mania: a clinical overview. Acta Psychiatr Scand Suppl 434:27–34, 2007

Safer DJ, Zito JM: Treatment emergent adverse events from selective serotonin reuptake inhibitors by age group: children versus adolescents. J Child Adolesc Psychopharmacol 16:159–169, 2006

Scheeringa MS: The differential diagnosis of impaired reciprocal social interaction in children: a review of disorders. Child Psychiatry Hum Dev 32:71–89, 2001

Semel E, Wiig EH, Secord WA: Clinical Evaluation of Language Fundamentals, 3rd Edition. San Antonio, TX, Psychological Corporation, 1995

van der Gaag RJ, Caplan R, van Engeland H, et al: A controlled study of formal thought disorder in children with autism and multiple complex developmental disorders. J Child Adolesc Psychopharmacol 15:465–476, 2005

Wagner KD, Kowatch RA, Emslie GJ, et al: A double-blind, randomized, placebo-controlled trial of oxcarbazepine in the treatment of bipolar disorder in children and adolescents. Am J Psychiatry 163:1179–1186, 2006

Wagner KD, Redden L, Kowatch R, et al: Safety and efficacy of divalproex extended release (ER) in youth with mania. Paper presented at the annual meeting of the American Academy of Child and Adolescent Psychiatry, Boston, MA, October 2007

Wechsler D: Wechsler Intelligence Scale for Children, 3rd Edition. San Antonio, TX, Psychological Corporation, 1991

Zalsman G, Cohen DJ: Multiplex developmental disorder. Isr J Psychiatry Relat Sci 35:300–306, 1998

Zero to Three: National Center for Infants, Toddlers and Families. Diagnostic Classification of Mental Health and Developmental Disorders of Infancy and Early Childhood (DC:0-3). Arlington, VA, Zero to Three, 1994

■ CHAPTER 18 ■

Failing Out of School

Language and Reading Weaknesses

Lynn M. Wegner, M.D., F.A.A.P.

CASE PRESENTATION

IDENTIFYING INFORMATION

Michael is a 12-year-old sixth grader who attends an inner-city public middle school. He lives with his widowed father and 16-year-old sister. His father is employed as a security guard at a local chemical research facility, and his sister is enrolled in her junior year of a college-preparatory public high school program.

CHIEF COMPLAINT

Michael is failing his language arts, science, and social studies classes. Retention for sixth grade is being discussed.

HISTORY OF PRESENT ILLNESS

Michael is enrolled in regular sixth-grade classes and receives no supplemental services from school personnel or formal supplemental tutoring. When asked to read aloud in any of his classes, he reads slowly and with mistakes and many pauses. His social studies and earth science teachers report that he seems very interested in the content in their classes when demonstrations or slide lec-

Lynn M. Wegner, M.D., F.A.A.P., is Associate Clinical Professor and Director of the Developmental/Behavioral Pediatrics Division in the Department of Pediatrics at University of North Carolina at Chapel Hill School of Medicine in Chapel Hill, North Carolina (for complete biographical information, see "About the Contributors," p. 613).

tures are given. When he has to read independently, however, he quickly seems to lose interest and stares vacantly away from the text. He does not interfere with other students; however, he is not engaged at all in the classroom activities when no "visual presentation" accompanies the discussions or readings. Michael also was a strong math student in previous grades. He was on the accelerated math track, but his prealgebra instructor is puzzled; although Michael did very well in previous classes in which he studied geometry and elaborate fractionation and multiplication/division, he is currently struggling with word problems.

Michael's father reports that no changes have occurred in the home. His teachers have not seen any altered interactions with peers. He has been perceived as a "quiet boy" by all teachers and administrative staff at his middle school.

PAST PSYCHIATRIC HISTORY

Michael had difficulty separating from his parents when he first began attending day care at age 3 years. He never had significant temper tantrums, but when his mother died during a car accident when he was age 4, he seemed to be more "clingy" to his father.

During the middle of Michael's fifth-grade year, the student support team met to discuss referring Michael for evaluation for attention-deficit disorder, although they acknowledged that he never exhibited behavior problems at school. "At times I forget he is in the classroom," his teacher commented. "He never raises his hand to ask questions, and when I call on him, he stares at me as though he hasn't heard what I said." The other students seemed to like him, although they rarely talked to him at recess or lunchtime.

During his sixth-grade year he has shown no improvement, although the school guidance counselor has assigned a mentor to help him after school with his homework and to make sure he catches the late school bus home. The mentor thinks Michael enjoys working with him, but he admitted, "It's hard to know what he thinks or feels. He doesn't talk much."

DEVELOPMENTAL HISTORY

Michael was the second pregnancy for his 28-year-old mother. The pregnancy was uncomplicated by hypertension, vaginal bleeding, maternal cigarette smoking, or iron deficiency. He was born at term, weighed over 5½ lbs, and had no perinatal problems. He quickly established a regular schedule of sleeping and eating. He did not cry excessively.

His social, motor, and language skills were attained at "usual" times. His father did not remember temper tantrums between 12 and 24 months of age, but he noted that his son "did not talk a lot."

Throughout preschool, his caregivers commented that he spoke little but seemed to know what was going on. He often seemed "a million miles away" during circle time and did not sit quietly when books were read aloud by his teachers. However, his ability to assemble puzzles was consistently perceived to be a strength, and his ability to assemble LEGO bricks into sophisticated structures seemed very advanced for his age.

Although no "real" problems were reported in day care or preschool, Michael did not pass the kindergarten entry screening for language skills. Subsequent formal language testing showed a mixed pattern of expressive and receptive skills "more than two standard deviations below the mean value for his age (i.e., standard score [SS]<70.)" Michael was referred for language therapy, provided in twice-weekly small group sessions at his school. He received Title I reading support in first and second grades, but all supplemental services, including the speech and language therapy, were terminated at the end of second grade when he "exited" on the basis of having met the criteria of "average" receptive and expressive skills on standardized testing administered by the speech-language pathologist. Michael had no additional developmental evaluations or therapeutic interventions.

Michael passed the third-grade end-of-grade standardized examinations; however, his fourth-grade teacher made numerous notations on interim grading reports that he seemed inattentive and poorly focused on classroom discussions. His reading comprehension progressively deteriorated through fourth and fifth grades, although he was able to earn "low passing" grades. His written assignments, brief as they were, showed many spelling errors.

MEDICAL HISTORY

Michael has never had a seizure, head trauma resulting in loss of consciousness, or central nervous system infection. He has had no sensory impairments, chronic illnesses, past hospitalizations, or surgeries. He has no history of iron deficiency or lead exposure. He takes no medications on a daily basis.

FAMILY HISTORY

Michael's only sibling is an honors student in the eleventh grade. His mother was a registered nurse, with no need for supplemental services at any point in her education or mental health consultations. His father graduated from high school but admitted he does not like to read and "barely" passed the twelfth grade. He noted he has always been a "quiet" person and wonders if he talked with Michael enough after his wife died. Michael's father has two brothers, neither of whom completed the ninth grade, and he acknowledged that his father "couldn't even read the Bible."

MENTAL STATUS EXAMINATION

Michael slowly entered the interview room and did not make immediate eye contact with the interviewer. He made no spontaneous comments, and he frequently nodded assent or shook his head in disagreement rather than reply to the examiner's questions. He remained seated throughout the interview, but his body was oriented away from the interviewer and he frequently rubbed his face. He denied any problems with his mood, rejecting any thoughts of hurting himself or others. At one point he answered the question "Are you sad?" by replying, "Doesn't everyone get mad sometimes?" His reality testing was unimpaired.

The following lists include the record reviews, interviews, and testing that were done so the clinician could fully consider Michael's case.

Clinical Assessment, Observations, and Nonstandardized Scales

- Review of medical and school records
- Clinical interview with father and Michael
- Review of nonstandardized summary questionnaire from all five sixth-grade teachers
- School ANSER Form (Levine 1996)

Standardized Questionnaires

- Behavior Assessment for Children—Second Edition (BASC-2): Parent Version, Teacher Version, and Self-Report Profile (Reynolds and Kamphaus 2004)
- Behavior Rating Inventory of Executive Function (BRIEF): Parent Version, Teacher Version, and Self-Report Version (Guy et al. 2005)

Standardized Testing

- Clinical Evaluation of Language Fundamentals—Fourth Edition (CELF-4; Semel et al. 2003)
- Comprehensive Test of Phonological Processing (CTOPP; Wagner et al. 1999)
- Leiter International Performance Scale—Revised (Leiter-R; Roid and Miller 1995)
- Peabody Picture Vocabulary Test—Fourth Edition (PPVT-4; Dunn and Dunn 2007)
- Test of Language Competence—Expanded Edition (Wiig and Secord 1989)

- Wechsler Intelligence Scale for Children—Fourth Edition (WISC-IV; Wechsler 2004)
- Woodcock-Johnson Tests of Achievement—Third Edition (WJ-III; Woodcock et al. 2001)

Evaluation Results

The BASC-2 and BRIEF rating scales administered to Michael's father and teacher yielded a few consistencies and several discrepant endorsements. His teacher noted clinically significant concerns for attention, atypicality, and withdrawal, whereas his father endorsed responses reflecting significant concerns only for withdrawal. Both Michael's father and teacher endorsed several areas of weakness in executive function: planning, initiation of actions and comments, mental energy, and working memory. Michael's self-report on BASC-2 was significant for anxiety, depression, attitude to school, self-esteem, and sense of inadequacy. He endorsed significant areas of concern for working memory and task completion.

All Michael's current teachers completed the School ANSER questionnaire. All noted "significantly delayed more than 1 year" for all reading, language, and writing skills. His math teacher noted delays of more than 1 year in Michael's "understanding word problems." In all classes, Michael's teachers observed that his "mental energy" was weak and he did not interact with peers at age level.

Formal standardized testing was administered in three morning sessions. During each session, the examiner noted that Michael seemed willing to participate but progressively became cognitively fatigued, often rubbing his face and hair. He stretched his arms several times and yawned. When asked if he had slept well the night before the session, he nodded each time. Notably, the examiner observed that Michael answered questions with one word or two- to three-word phrases. Michael's testing yielded the results listed in Table 18–1.

TABLE 18–1.   Michael's standardized test results

Test	Standard score	%ile
Clinical Evaluation of Language Fundamentals—Fourth Edition		
Core Language Composite	70	2
Receptive Language	61	0.5
Expressive Language Composite	80	9
Language Memory Composite	66	1
Comprehensive Test of Phonological Processing		
Phonological Awareness Composite	76	5
Phonological Memory Composite	67	1
Rapid Naming Composite	79	8
Alternate Phonological Composite	70	2
Alternate Rapid Naming Composite	76	5
Leiter International Performance Scale—Revised		
Fluid Reasoning	102	55
Full Scale IQ	110	75
Peabody Picture Vocabulary Test—Fourth Edition	80	9
Test of Language Competence—Expanded Edition		
Composite	65	1
Wechsler Intelligence Scale for Children—Fourth Edition		
Verbal Comprehension Index	73	4
Perceptual Reasoning Index	94	34
Working Memory Index	86	18
Processing Speed Index	88	21
Full Scale IQ	81	10
Woodcock-Johnson Tests of Achievement—Third Edition		
Broad Reading Composite	77	6
Broad Math Composite	95	37
Broad Written Language	72	3

Note.   All standardized results were based on a mean value of 100 with a standard deviation of 15.

COMMENTARIES

Psychotherapeutic Perspective

Joshua M. Langberg, Ph.D.
Jeffery N. Epstein, Ph.D.

DIAGNOSTIC FORMULATION

Mixed receptive-expressive language disorder is characterized by impairment in both receptive and expressive language development compared to a child's nonverbal intellectual capacity. Furthermore, DSM-IV-TR criteria require evidence that the language problems are interfering with functioning. Michael's receptive and expressive language scores across a range of measures (e.g., CELF-4, PPVT-4) are below the 10th percentile for children his age and are more than one standard deviation below his Full Scale IQ as measured by the Leiter-R. It is interesting to note that Michael's Full Scale IQ (110) on the Leiter-R, a nonverbal test of IQ, is considerably higher than his Full Scale IQ (81) on WISC-IV, which relies heavily on language comprehension. This presentation is typical of children with language disorders. Because Michael is failing the majority of his classes and is in danger of being retained, the DSM-IV-TR impairment criterion is clearly met.

Michael's achievement scores and impairment in the school setting also suggest that he meets DSM-IV-TR criteria for a reading disorder. His reading scores are well below average and are highly discrepant from his Full Scale IQ on the Leiter-R. Furthermore, his WJ-III Broad Reading Composite score (SS=77, 6th percentile) is considerably lower than his Broad Math Composite score (SS=95, 37th percentile). This finding is replicated in the school setting, where Michael achieved at grade level in math and began struggling when the

Joshua M. Langberg, Ph.D., is Assistant Professor in the Center for Attention Deficit Hyperactivity Disorder at Cincinnati Children's Hospital Medical Center in Cincinnati, Ohio.

Jeffery N. Epstein, Ph.D., is Associate Professor of Pediatrics in the Division of Behavioral Medicine and Clinical Psychology at Cincinnati Children's Hospital Medical Center and in the Department of Psychology at University of Cincinnati; and Director of the Center for Attention Deficit Hyperactivity Disorder at Cincinnati Children's Hospital Medical Center in Cincinnati, Ohio.

For complete biographical information, see "About the Contributors," p. 613.

curriculum progressed to include word problems, which require reading comprehension. Finally, all of Michael's scores on the CTOPP lend support to the reading disorder diagnosis (i.e., all subscale scores are below the 10th percentile) and suggest that delays in phonological processing may be contributing to his reading difficulties.

Additional evaluation of Michael's attention, anxiety, and mood also appears warranted. Michael's case presentation does not contain sufficient information to determine if he meets DSM-IV-TR criteria for attention-deficit/hyperactivity disorder (ADHD). The determination of whether he may have comorbid ADHD is complicated by the fact that children with mixed receptive-expressive language disorders often appear confused, seem to have difficulties with attention, and provide off-topic responses (American Psychiatric Association 2000). Parent and teacher rating scales that focus on screening for specific DSM ADHD symptoms, such as the Vanderbilt ADHD Rating Scales (Wolraich et al. 1998, 2003) or the ADHD Rating Scale—IV (DuPaul et al. 1998), should be administered to determine the number and severity of ADHD symptoms Michael is displaying across home and school environments. Also, a caregiver interview should be added that includes assessment of the specific ADHD symptoms listed in DSM-IV-TR, including their frequency, age at onset, duration, and associated impairment. Determining whether symptoms of inattention are present in all settings or only in settings that involve language and/or reading requirements is imperative.

Michael's father and teacher both endorsed responses on BASC-2 reflecting concern with withdrawal, and Michael endorsed problems with anxiety, depression, self-esteem, and a sense of inadequacy. Some of these internalizing symptoms may be sequelae related to the early loss of his mother. Again, the presence of a language disorder complicates establishing whether a comorbid mood or anxiety disorder is present. Children with language disorders often present as exceptionally quiet and withdrawn (American Psychiatric Association 2000). To more carefully evaluate Michael's symptoms of anxiety and mood, the clinician could administer the Multidimensional Anxiety Scale for Children (March 1997) and the Children's Depression Inventory (Kovacs 1992), self-report measures that assess anxiety and depressive behaviors, respectively.

DSM-IV-TR DIAGNOSIS

Axis I   315.32 Mixed receptive-expressive language disorder
           315.00 Reading disorder
           Rule out ADHD
Axis II   None
Axis III   None
Axis IV   Educational problems

Axis V   Global Assessment of Functioning=55
          Currently failing multiple core classes and in danger of failing sixth
          grade

TREATMENT RECOMMENDATIONS

The evaluation results should be shared with Michael's school, with the goal of resuming the speech, language, and reading support services that he received in early elementary school. The fact that Michael's language and reading deficits have persisted despite this early intervention is not surprising. Recent research clearly demonstrates the chronic nature of both language and reading impairments and supports the need for ongoing intervention (Glogowska et al. 2006; Shaywitz et al. 1999). Currently, no published, evidence-based guidelines for the treatment of language disorders are available. Nevertheless, compelling evidence indicates that speech and language therapy is effective in improving expressive language delays, although receptive language delays are more resistant to treatment (Boyle et al. 2007).

In addition to speech and language therapy, Michael should receive some form of reading intervention that directly teaches reading skills. Although reading problems tend to be more difficult to treat in older children and adolescents, explicit and systematic reading interventions do result in improved reading comprehension and fluency (Lyon et al. 2006). Evidence supports the efficacy of multiple types of reading intervention. The selected reading intervention should target Michael's specific areas of reading deficit. For example, addressing Michael's phonological awareness deficits by teaching phonological awareness with parallel instruction in other reading skills (e.g., reading fluency or reading comprehension) would likely be productive. Regardless of intervention type, intervention efforts should include explicit and systematic direct instruction in deficient skills and also provide continued cumulative review of mastered content (Lyon et al. 2006). This instruction could be provided on an individual basis (e.g., tutoring) or within the context of school-based special education instruction.

If further evaluation suggests that Michael has comorbid ADHD or if Michael continues to demonstrate attentional difficulties after his language and reading problems have been addressed, his ADHD symptoms and related impairments will need intervention. If Michael meets criteria for ADHD, he will likely meet criteria for predominantly inattentive type. The best treatment approach for children with ADHD is a multimodal intervention including pharmacologic and psychosocial treatments (MTA Cooperative Group 1999). A trial with psychostimulants might be considered. Concordantly, psychosocial interventions should be initiated. Unfortunately, the majority of psychosocial interventions for children with ADHD (e.g., behavioral parent training) are geared toward children with hyperactive/impulsive and disruptive behaviors. However, some evidence supports the effectiveness of skills training (e.g., organizational, study, daily living) combined with typical behavioral intervention (e.g., token economy) for children with ADHD, predominantly inattentive type (Pfiffner et al. 2007).

Psychopharmacologic Perspective

Lacramioara Spetie, M.D.
L. Eugene Arnold, M.D., M.Ed.

DIAGNOSTIC FORMULATION

Michael is a 12-year-old referred for a psychiatric evaluation because his poor reading skills, inattention, and lack of participation in class are impairing his academic functioning despite his obvious willingness and efforts to learn.

Michael's mother had an uncomplicated full-term pregnancy with no perinatal complications, and Michael had no history of medical conditions that might account for his difficulties. As an infant, Michael had a regular schedule for sleeping and eating and he did not cry excessively. Michael's father, both paternal uncles, and his paternal grandfather had significant reading difficulties that impaired their ability to complete their schooling. Michael's father also described himself as rather "quiet," suggesting a genetic predisposition toward dyslexia and possibly an easy, regular temperament.

Michael was diagnosed with a mixed receptive-expressive language disorder in preschool and continued to present with limited speech volume and only limited verbal communication in general.

Michael's long-standing history of reading difficulties supports the diagnosis of dyslexia. Dyslexia is "a specific learning disability characterized by difficulties with accurate and/or fluent word recognition and poor spelling and

Lacramioara Spetie, M.D., is Assistant Professor of Psychiatry at The Ohio State University in Columbus, Ohio.

L. Eugene Arnold, M.D., M.Ed., is Professor Emeritus of Psychiatry; Former Director of the Division of Child and Adolescent Psychiatry; Former Vice Chair of Psychiatry; and Interim Director of the Nisonger Center of Excellence in Developmental Disabilities at The Ohio State University in Columbus, Ohio.

For complete biographical information, see "About the Contributors," p. 613.

decoding abilities" (Shaywitz et al. 2008). The main deficit is in the ability to identify and manipulate phoneme-level units of language (i.e., phonological awareness). Michael's scores on all tests measuring phonological processing pointed to a severe deficit. His impairment had been overlooked in school, leading to severe deficits in academic achievement together with symptoms of anxiety and depression. His efforts at reading and writing had consistently been exhausting, leading to a great deal of mental fatigue, followed by daydreaming and lack of participation in classroom activities.

Dyslexia is highly comorbid with ADHD (Martin and Volkmar 2007). A diagnosis of ADHD is supported by Michael's history of having difficulties sitting still, as early as preschool, together with an ongoing history of daydreaming, poor focus, poor concentration, difficulties staying on task, and so forth.

Unresolved grief following his mother's death is also worth exploring. Children perceive death differently than do adults. At the time of his mother's sudden death, Michael was 4 years old, an age when children see death as temporary and reversible, and they may provide magical explanations or blame themselves for the death (Himebauch et al. 2008). Michael did not receive mental health intervention at the time. His father already had difficulties expressing himself, possibly due to his own language disorder issues, therefore impairing his ability to help Michael with the grieving process. Diagnoses to be considered include dysthymic disorder and major depressive disorder, chronic, mild to moderate, without psychotic features. The symptoms of anxiety and depression may have added further to Michael's social withdrawal, poor attention, poor concentration, lack of motivation, worrying, low self-esteem, mental fatigue, and so on.

Several clinical instruments are helpful in Michael's case: the Child Depression Inventory (Kovacs 1985; see also Fristad 1997; Merrell 2003) to help clarify a diagnosis of depression, and SNAP-IV Teacher and Parent ADHD Rating Scale (Swanson 1992) or Conners' Rating Scales—Revised for parents and teachers (Conners 1997) to further clarify the diagnosis of ADHD.

DSM-IV-TR DIAGNOSIS

Axis I   315.00 Reading disorder (dyslexia)

         315.32 Mixed receptive-expressive language disorder

         Rule out ADHD

         Rule out dysthymic disorder

         Rule out major depressive disorder, mild to moderate, without psychotic features

Axis II   Borderline intellectual functioning

Axis III   Noncontributory

Axis IV   Unresolved grief
          Academic failure
          Limited social support
          One-parent household
Axis V   Global Assessment of Functioning=50–60

TREATMENT RECOMMENDATIONS

Dyslexia is a disorder with various degrees of severity, in which phonological processing has been found to play a critical role. Recent neuroimaging studies have shown that early reading intervention facilitates the development of those neural systems that underlie normal reading (left anterolateral occipitotemporal region). Such interventions are most effective when implemented at the earliest possible age, when the brain responds best. Close monitoring of the progress children make in learning how to read, starting in kindergarten or first grade, will help teachers identify the children who struggle and provide reading interventions at an early age, rather than waiting until the children repeatedly fail and are then found to meet the criteria for a reading disorder of more than two standard deviations below the value expected. The interventions for young children in earlier grades focus on phonemic awareness, phonics, fluency, vocabulary, and comprehension, and aim to help children improve their phonological awareness and word identification skills (Lonigan 2003). Children in third grade or higher receive various remedial interventions (Lovett and Barron 2003).

Speech therapy may further help Michael improve his phonological awareness and communication skills.

Stimulants (methylphenidate-based and amphetamine-based drugs) are usually considered the first line of treatment for ADHD (MTA Cooperative Group 1999; "Moderators and Mediators of Treatment Response" 1999). Although not currently the standard of practice, obtaining a baseline electrocardiogram may be advisable in case cardiovascular side effects occur. Serial electrocardiograms may be indicated in some cases, especially if a cardiovascular indicator changes. In any event, vital signs (heart rate, blood pressure), weight, and height should be closely monitored while a patient is taking a stimulant. Extended-release products are generally preferred to avoid the need for midday dosing at school (Arnold 2006). Titration should start with the lowest dose of the chosen extended-release product, with weekly increases based on clinical benefit and side effects. Some patients may benefit from a booster dose of an immediate-release product in the afternoon for homework or organized high-performance activities.

Another first-line drug is atomoxetine (Cheng et al. 2007), which may also mildly benefit comorbid internalizing symptoms. This drug should be titrated weekly, starting with 0.5 mg/kg. Most patients respond to about 1.0–1.2 mg/kg, but the safety of doses up to 1.8 mg/kg was demonstrated in premarketing studies. Although many of its side effects are similar to those of stimulants, atomoxetine differs by not interfering with sleep and even sometimes inducing drowsiness or fatigue. For this reason and because of its long pharmacodynamic half-life, it can be given at bedtime to make a virtue of the sedative side effect.

Given Michael's reports of depression and anxiety, atomoxetine might be the best choice to try first. Another option might be a tricyclic antidepressant or bupropion, which might help depression and anxiety and have documented efficacy for ADHD symptoms. However, they are not considered first-line drugs, and the tricyclics present their own cardiovascular risk. If Michael's depression or anxiety persists after attempts to treat both ADHD and internalizing symptoms with one drug, cognitive-behavioral therapy should be added if not already implemented. If treatment still is not sufficient, the clinician might consider fluoxetine, which has been more effective than placebo in treating depression in children and adolescents. Michael and his father should be educated about the potential for an increased suicide risk during treatment with antidepressants and instructed about how to monitor for such risk and what to do in case of an emergency.

In addition to cognitive-behavioral therapy for depression and anxiety, psychoeducational and other individual, group, or family therapy may help Michael address unresolved grief, understand his learning disorder, and address self-esteem issues.

Speech and Language Pathology Perspective

Helen Nelson Willard, M.Ed., CCC-SLP

DIAGNOSTIC FORMULATION

Michael is a 12-year-old boy in sixth grade. He has failing grades in language arts, science, and social studies. He is a well-behaved, quiet child who does not initiate communication often or express his feelings to others. A review of evaluation re-

Helen Nelson Willard, M.Ed., CCC-SLP, is in private practice in Cary, North Carolina (for complete biographical information, see "About the Contributors," p. 613).

sults and school records suggests that no accommodations, modifications, or strategies are in place to address Michael's current academic and communication deficits, other than an assigned mentor to assist with homework after school.

Michael's academic and language difficulties began in kindergarten. Language evaluation results identified significant receptive and expressive deficits, which were addressed through language therapy twice a week until therapy was terminated at the end of second grade. After 4 years of no apparent academic support, Michael is experiencing increased difficulty with written and spoken language in all areas of the sixth-grade curriculum. He has difficulty attending to and focusing on assigned tasks, and he exhibits feelings of anxiety, inadequacy, and withdrawal.

A thorough assessment requires consideration of Michael's strengths and weaknesses, which follow.

Strengths: Global nonverbal intelligence
              Pleasant, quiet behavior and liked by his peers
              Apparent good health with no sensory impairments
Weaknesses: Ability to initiate requests for assistance and/or clarification
              Ability to talk freely and to share feelings with others
              Feelings of anxiety, inadequacy, and withdrawal
              Executive functions: planning, initiation of actions and
                  comments, mental energy, and working memory
              Phonological processing
              Receptive vocabulary
              General language skills
              Metalinguistic abilities/language use
              Significant delays in reading, language, writing, and math
              Reading fluency and comprehension

Michael should be assessed further to find out if the following behaviors are concerns for him.

Unknown: Behaviors that may be contributing to auditory processing
                  weakness
              Auditory processing and central auditory processing abilities
              Phonemic awareness
              Specific strengths/weaknesses in phonological awareness
              Specific spelling error patterns
              Behaviors symptomatic of pragmatic language weakness

The following tools are recommended to assess these behaviors:

- The Listening Inventory (Geffner and Ross-Swain 2006): Quantifies behaviors to determine the need for further evaluation of auditory processing abilities.
- Differential Screening Test for Processing (Richard and Ferre 2006): Differentiates among the various levels of the processing hierarchy to identify deficit areas for referral or further evaluation.
- Lindamood Auditory Conceptualization Test—Third Edition (Lindamood and Lindamood 2004): Measures phonemic awareness.
- Phonological Awareness Test—Second Edition (Robertson and Salter 2007): Identifies specific strengths and weaknesses in phonological awareness knowledge. Although administering this test to a student who is older than age 9 may be appropriate and provide useful information for planning an instructional program to meet the student's specific needs, normative data should not be applied to testing results (Robertson and Salter 1997).
- Spelling Performance Evaluation for Language and Literacy (Masterson et al. 2006): Identifies error patterns and provides specific recommendations for spelling intervention.
- Clinical Evaluation of Language Fundamentals—Fourth Edition (Semel et al. 2003): The Pragmatic Profile identifies strengths and weaknesses in the understanding or use of speech intentions that are expected for social and school interactions in mainstream U.S. classrooms. The Observational Rating Scale measures the ability to meet school curriculum objectives for following teacher instructions and self-managing classroom behavior and interactions.

DIAGNOSIS

In this section, I use *International Classification of Diseases*, 9th Revision, Clinical Modification (ICD-9-CM) codes (World Health Organization 1978) to describe the diagnoses that a speech-language pathologist will treat, as opposed to the DSM-IV-TR codes, which are used mainly by health care providers working with mental health conditions. The diagnoses made by the speech-language pathologist play an important role in the overall diagnostic process in that language is the foundation from which all communication originates and the knowledge of Michael's existing language deficits can impact the clinical perspective when profiling disorders and conditions using the DSM-IV-TR multiaxial system. The speech-language pathologist offers a unique perspective when analyzing the evaluation results and may initiate referrals to other professionals to pursue the assessment of areas that may be impacting Michael's ability to navigate the demands of communication in different contexts.

A diagnosis of a mixed receptive-expressive language disorder (ICD-9-CM 315.32) is supported by the available standardized testing; however, as I discuss in "Diagnostic Formulation" above, the list of evaluation tools should be used to assess the "unknown" behaviors. Michael's severe to profound deficits in phonological processing, his standardized test results, and the documentation of dyslexia in the family history also support the diagnosis of dyslexia (ICD-9-CM 784.61).

On the basis of ICD-9-CM diagnoses, the multidisciplinary team treating Michael should consider his language and phonological processing deficits as possible sources for his feelings of anxiety and withdrawal from communication with others. These same deficits may also contribute to his inability to attend to and focus on the curriculum.

According to Shaywitz and Shaywitz (2007), "Results from large and well-studied populations confirm that a deficit in phonology represents the most robust and specific correlate of dyslexia and form the basis for the most successful and evidence-based interventions designed to improve reading" (p. 20). For Michael, a treatment program targeting the strengthening of phonological processing and language is recommended. Michael's emotional status should be monitored during treatment to determine if further evaluation or treatment in this area is warranted.

TREATMENT RECOMMENDATIONS

Michael presents a complex profile of language and literacy skills that must be strengthened so he can access the curriculum. At Michael's age, traditional language therapy designed to fill in the gaps is not appropriate or practical. Treatment must focus on the development and/or strengthening of phonemic awareness, phonological awareness, and orthographic knowledge, while at the same time enhancing development of the language skills necessary for Michael to survive in his present setting. Such a treatment program must address these language and literacy skills in a functional way; therefore, language therapy should be based on strategy acquisition rather than memorization of specific information about the content areas. This learning strategy model will allow Michael to generalize basic skills across situations, settings, and curricula (McKinley and Lord-Larson 1985).

The most effective strategy for developing knowledge and use of phonemic awareness, phonological awareness, and orthographic rules for children who have not responded to traditional phonics instruction is the Lindamood Phoneme Sequencing Program for Reading, Spelling, and Speech (LiPS; Lindamood and Lindamood 1998). The LiPS Program provides explicit, systematic, highly organized linguistic instruction that will target Michael's identified literacy weaknesses with an emphasis on how the sounds *feel* rather than how they *sound*. This unique approach of using the sensory system will allow Michael to learn a different way to understand and monitor what he reads, hears, and writes, and the highly organized presentation of the material will enhance working memory and long-term memory. Socratic questioning and the participatory format of this program will allow Michael's other language deficits to be addressed in tandem. The nature of the LiPS Program will require Michael to summarize, paraphrase, analyze, predict, and infer while developing phonemic awareness, the basis of all literacy skills. As his phonological and language skills are used and strengthened, his comprehension skills will begin to improve. This type of treatment plan will provide Michael with the opportunity to practice his language in a functional manner, which will equip him with the tools needed to interact successfully in the classroom setting. Although other phonics programs are available, these programs use the same avenue of learning—listening to the sound system—that has not been successful with Michael in the past. Also, these other phonics programs do not allow for the development of language skills, including critical thinking skills, to the degree that the LiPS Program provides.

As treatment progresses, three other interventions should be integrated into Michael's therapy: Seeing Stars: Symbol Imagery for Phonemic Awareness, Sight Words and Spelling (Bell 1997); Visualizing and Verbalizing for Language Comprehension and Thinking (Bell 1991); and SPELL-Links to Reading and Writing: A Word Study Curriculum (Wasowicz et al. 2004).

At the outset of treatment, the speech-language pathologist must carefully analyze the language expectations of the curriculum and the teacher, and problematic behaviors noted on the Pragmatic Profile of CELF-4 must be examined, to determine appropriate modifications, interventions, and/or strategies. The management of any auditory processing needs that are identified by additional testing should be a priority. Finally, the delivery of treatment should be a collaborative effort involving all members of the multidisciplinary team.

Integrative Perspective

Lynn M. Wegner, M.D., F.A.A.P.

DIAGNOSTIC FORMULATION

Michael is a young adolescent with persistently disordered expressive and receptive language skills. He meets the diagnostic criteria for specific language impairment because he has normal hearing thresholds, his language test scores are >1.25 standard deviations below the mean, and his nonverbal IQ is in the average or better (SS≥85) range. Although as a young child, he was correctly identified as having a language delay and offered formal intervention for several years, his performance on language reevaluation at the end of second grade apparently yielded a composite score in the average range. Because public school systems are mandated to offer therapy only to those children whose scores are "below average," Michael's assistance was withdrawn. During the intervening 6½ years, he has not acquired language skills commensurate with those of his peers, and his language development has plateaued. Results of his current formal testing on CELF-4 and PPVT-4 substantiate this. Michael expresses himself at a very low average to borderline level, but his understanding and memory for aural information are significantly weaker. His receptive skills now are weaker than those of 99 of 100 same-age peers, and his overall language abilities, his Core Language Composite on CELF-4, would surpass those of only 2 of 100 of his peers.

The impact of Michael's language weakness can be seen in his educational achievement, as supported by scores on WJ-III, and his formally assessed language-dependent cognitive abilities, as supported by scores on WISC-IV. Michael's reading is significantly weak for his grade. He is a slow reader, with many mispronunciations and substitutions. He forgets what he has read by the end of a passage and has to reread. The CTOPP results clearly document his weak phonological skills, which are needed for word decoding. Moreover, he is not cognitively "wired" for adept recognition of sight words (e.g., *eight; height*), because his rapid automatic naming skills are not strong. His auditory working memory, as assessed on WISC-IV (SS=86, 18th percentile), is not strong either. Michael does not have the requisite abilities to be even an average sixth-grade reader; therefore, he understands little of what he reads in school. Even his ability to apply math concepts in word problems is impacted, because he misunderstands the description of the problems.

Dyslexia is a language learning disorder that is not reflective of hearing impairment or weak nonverbal intelligence, and that is characterized by significant difficulties in reading, spelling, and written expression (Sawyer 2006). A primary weakness is phonological processing, which includes the ability to segment speech into smaller units and the ability to associate sounds with letters. Individuals with dyslexia also have problems with rapid label naming, and therefore experience slow and inaccurate lexical access (Siegel 2008). Michael shows weaknesses in both phonological processing and rapid label naming. For Michael, reading weaknesses are accompanied by weak language skills (Snowling and Hayiou-Thomas 2006). His dual disabilities likely reflect both genetic and environmental elements, because both specific language impairment and reading disorders have genetic contributions (Olson and Byrne 2005).

Michael may not have been referred for formal evaluation until this point because no one expected him to perform any better than he has been doing. His expressive language skills fall in the "very low average/borderline" range, and adults working with him have probably thought that was his overall cognitive level. Certainly, that is what the WISC-IV results indicated (Full Scale IQ=81, 10th percentile). When Michael was offered cognitive testing devoid of language understanding or expression, however, his "upper average" nonverbal problem-solving and conceptualization abilities were seen (Leiter-R Full Scale IQ=110, 75th percentile). Michael clearly has areas of unidentified strength.

What has life been like for Michael as he has struggled to understand what was being said to him and tried to learn in school? This is a boy who understands the world at an "upper average" level in nonverbal domains but is trapped by his problems with understanding what he hears and with expressing his thoughts, ideas, and feelings. It should not be surprising that he seems detached and withdrawn, lost in his own world. His teachers have noted his vacant stares but have interpreted this as possibly representing inattentive attention-deficit disorder. Although children and adolescents with language impairment certainly may demonstrate comorbid attention-deficit disorder with or without hyperactivity (Damico et al. 1999), efforts to differentiate possible inattention from weak aural understanding are important. On BASC-2, Michael clearly reported what he is experiencing: problems with anxiety, depression, attitude to school, self-esteem, and a sense of inadequacy. His language struggles and associated poor academic achievement are likely linked with the anxious feelings he has when he attempts to understand and explain using language skills he does not possess. Recurrent negative responses from both adults and even peers might engender feelings of inadequacy and even hopelessness. Leonard (1998) reported that children with normal language skills direct fewer comments to peers with language impairment and seek them out less frequently for play.

DSM-IV-TR DIAGNOSIS

Axis I   315.32 Mixed receptive-expressive language disorder

315.02 Developmental dyslexia

315.2 Disorder of written expression

Axis II   None

Axis III None

Axis IV   None

Axis V   Global Assessment of Functioning=60

TREATMENT RECOMMENDATIONS

IMMEDIATE CONFERENCE WITH MICHAEL AND HIS FATHER

Both Michael and his father need to hear the results of the evaluation explained by a professional who can describe the meaning of the scores in real terms. Accompanying the explanation with a drawing of a normal curve will allow both Michael and his father to visually understand Michael's nonverbal cognitive strength. The professional should allow more time than usually scheduled for this discussion, pausing frequently to permit Michael (and maybe his father) to process the information.

CONFERENCE WITH ALL SCHOOL PERSONNEL WORKING WITH MICHAEL

Michael's language abilities, as they impact his daily performance and behavior, should be fully explained to all teachers, guidance counselors, mentors, and tutors. His "upper average" nonverbal cognitive abilities should be emphasized several times during the discussion so the school personnel will understand the significance of his weak receptive and overall language abilities.

DEVELOPMENT OF AN INDIVIDUALIZED EDUCATION PROGRAM

A team of professionals should develop an Individualized Education Program for Michael under the following specific language impairment identifications: receptive-expressive language disorder; learning disorder in reading; and learning disorder in written expression. In addition to direct special education services addressing his weak academic skills, Michael should also be offered language therapy services in school. This therapy should include instruction in pragmatics, as well as vocabulary, syntax, organization, and fluency.

SOCIAL-EMOTIONAL ASSESSMENT

Michael should be formally assessed for significant anxiety and/or depression by a professional who understands assessment of a young adolescent with language impairment.

LANGUAGE THERAPY DURING SUMMER VACATION

Michael's medical provider should refer him for private services during prolonged school vacations. The school speech-language pathologist and the private therapist should exchange information at the beginning and end of the vacations.

FAMILY ASSESSMENT

Michael's father is a single parent who related a family history that suggests language weakness. His reading skills may be weak. Careful and tactful inquiry might identify a desire to improve his personal literacy level. Assessment of family functioning might also identify stress in the older sister, who may have been put in the parental role because she appears to be bright and her mother is deceased.

REFERENCES

American Psychiatric Association: Diagnostic and Statistical Manual of Mental Disorders, 4th Edition, Text Revision. Washington, DC, American Psychiatric Association, 2000

Arnold LE: New ADHD medication options: advances in long-term treatment for a chronically impairing condition. Advances in ADHD 1:23–29, 2006

Bell N: Visualizing and Verbalizing for Language Comprehension and Thinking, Revised Edition. Paso Robles, CA, Academy of Reading Publications, 1991

Bell N: Seeing Stars: Symbol Imagery for Phonemic Awareness, Sight Words and Spelling. San Luis Obispo, CA, Gander, 1997

Boyle J, McCartney E, Forbes J, et al: A randomised controlled trial and economic evaluation of direct versus indirect and individual versus group modes of speech and language therapy for children with primary language impairment. Health Technol Assess 11:iii–iv, xi–xiii, 1–139, 2007

Cheng JY, Chen RY, Ko JS, et al: Efficacy and safety of atomoxetine for attention-deficit/hyperactivity disorder in children and adolescents—meta-analysis and meta-regression analysis. Psychopharmacology (Berl) 194:197–209, 2007

Conners CK: Conners' Rating Scales—Revised. North Tonawanda, NY, Multi-Health Systems, 1997

Damico JS, Damico SK, Armstrong MB: Attention-deficit hyperactivity disorder and communication disorders, in Child and Adolescent Clinics of North America: Language Disorders. Edited by Paul R. Philadelphia, PA, WB Saunders, 1999, pp 37–60

Dunn LM, Dunn DM: Peabody Picture Vocabulary Test, 4th Edition. San Antonio, TX, Pearson, 2007

DuPaul GJ, Power TJ, Anastopoulos AD, et al: The ADHD Rating Scale—IV: checklists, norms, and clinical interpretation. New York, Guilford, 1998

Fristad MA, Emery BL, Beck SJ: Use and abuse of the Children's Depression Inventory. J Consult Clin Psychol 65:699–702, 1997

Geffner D, Ross-Swain D: The Listening Inventory. Novato, CA, Academic Therapy Publications, 2006

Glogowska M, Roulstone S, Peters TJ, et al: Early speech- and language-impaired children: linguistic, literacy, and social outcomes. Dev Med Child Neurol 48:489–494, 2006

Guy SC, Isquith PK, Gioia GA: Behavior Rating Inventory of Executive Function. Lutz, FL, Psychological Assessment Resources, 2005

Himebauch A, Arnold R, May C: Grief in children and developmental concepts of death #138. J Palliat Med 11:242–243, 2008

Kovacs M: Children's Depression Inventory (CDI). Psychopharmacol Bull 21:995–998, 1985

Kovacs M: Children's Depression Inventory. North Tonawanda, NY, Multi-Health Systems, 1992

Leonard L: Children With Specific Language Impairment. Cambridge, MA, MIT Press, 1998

Levine MD: ANSER System. Cambridge, MA, Educators Publishing Services, 1996

Lindamood P, Lindamood P: The Lindamood Phoneme Sequencing Program for Reading, Spelling, and Speech. Austin, TX, PRO-ED, 1998

Lindamood PC, Lindamood P: Lindamood Auditory Conceptualization Test, 3rd Edition. Austin, TX, PRO-ED, 2004

Lonigan C: Development and Promotion of Emergent Literacy Skills in Children at Risk of Reading Difficulties. Baltimore, MD, York, 2003

Lovett M, Barron BN: Effective Remediation of Word Identification and Decoding Difficulties in School Age Children With Reading Difficulties. New York, Guilford, 2003

Lyon GR, Fletcher JM, Fuchs LS, et al: Learning disabilities, in Treatment of Childhood Disorders, 3rd Edition. Edited by Mash EJ, Barkley RA. New York, Guilford, 2006, pp 512–591

March JS: Multidimensional Anxiety Scale for Children. North Tonawanda, NY, Multi-Health Systems, 1997

Martin A, Volkmar FR: Lewis's Child and Adolescent Psychiatry—A Comprehensive Textbook, 4th Edition. Baltimore, MD, Lippincott, Williams & Wilkins, 2007

Masterson JJ, Apel K, Wasowicz J: Spelling Performance Evaluation for Language and Literacy. Evanston, IL, Learning By Design, 2006

McKinley N, Lord-Larson V: Neglected language-disordered adolescent: a delivery model. Lang Speech Hear Serv Sch 16:1–4, 1985

Merrell KW: Behavioral, Social, and Emotional Assessment of Children and Adolescents. Mahwah, NJ, Erlbaum, 2003

Moderators and mediators of treatment response for children with attention-deficit/hyperactivity disorder: the Multimodal Treatment Study of children with attention-deficit/hyperactivity disorder. Arch Gen Psychiatry 56:1088–1096, 1999

MTA Cooperative Group: A 14-month randomized clinical trial of treatment strategies for attention-deficit/hyperactivity disorder. Multimodal Treatment Study of Children With ADHD. Arch Gen Psychiatry 56:1073–1086, 1999

Olson RK, Byrne B: Genetic and environmental influences on reading and language ability and disability, in The Connections Between Language and Reading Disabilities. Edited by Catts H, Kahmi A. Mahwah, NJ, Erlbaum, 2005, pp 173–200

Pfiffner LJ, Mikami AY, Huang-Pollack C, et al: A randomized, controlled trial of integrated home-school behavioral treatment for ADHD, predominantly inattentive type. J Am Acad Child Adolesc Psychiatry 46:1041–1050, 2007

Reynolds CR, Kamphaus RW: Behavior Assessment for Children, 2nd Edition. Bloomington, MN, Pearson Assessments, 2004

Richard GJ, Ferre JM: Differential Screening Test for Processing. East Moline, IL, LinguiSystems, 2006

Robertson C, Salter W: The Phonological Awareness Test. East Moline, IL, LinguiSystems, 1997

Robertson C, Salter W: The Phonological Awareness Test, 2nd Edition. East Moline,
    IL, LinguiSystems, 2007

Roid GH, Miller LJ: Leiter International Performance Scale—Revised (Leiter-R). Lutz,
    FL, Psychological Assessment Resources, 1995

Sawyer DJ: Dyslexia: a generation of inquiry. Topics in Language Disorders 26:1–5,
    2006

Semel E, Wiig EH, Secord WA: Clinical Evaluation of Language Fundamentals, 4th
    Edition. San Antonio, TX, Psychological Corporation, 2003

Shaywitz SE, Shaywitz BA: The neurobiology of reading and dyslexia. ASHA Leader
    12:20–21, 2007

Shaywitz SE, Fletcher JM, Holahan JM, et al: Persistence of dyslexia: the Connecticut
    Longitudinal Study at adolescence. Pediatrics 104:1351–1359, 1999

Shaywitz SE, Morris R, Shaywitz BA: The education of dyslexic children from child-
    hood to young adulthood. Annu Rev Psychol 59:451–475, 2008

Siegel LS (ed): Understanding the linguistic aspects of dyslexia: beyond phonological
    processing. Topics in Language Disorders 28:1–5, 2008

Snowling MJ, Hayiou-Thomas ME: The dyslexia spectrum: continuities between read-
    ing, speech and language impairments. Topics in Language Disorders 26:110–126,
    2006

Swanson JM: The SNAP-IV Teacher and Parent Rating Scale. 1992. Available at: http://
    www.adhd.net/. Accessed July 21, 2008.

Wagner R, Torgesen J, Rashotte C: Comprehensive Test of Phonological Processing.
    Austin, TX, PRO-ED, 1999

Wasowicz J, Apel K, Masterson JJ, et al: SPELL-Links to Reading and Writing: A Word
    Study Curriculum. Evanston, IL, Learning by Design, 2004

Wechsler D: Wechsler Intelligence Scale for Children, 4th Edition. San Antonio, TX,
    Pearson, 2004

Wiig EH, Secord W: Test of Language Competence, Expanded Edition. San Antonio,
    TX, Pearson, 1989

Wolraich ML, Feurer ID, Hannah JN, et al: Obtaining systematic teacher reports of dis-
    ruptive behavior disorders utilizing DSM-IV. J Abnorm Child Psychol 26:141–152,
    1998

Wolraich ML, Lambert EW, Baumgaertel A, et al: Teachers' screening for attention def-
    icit/hyperactivity disorder: comparing multinational samples on teacher ratings of
    ADHD. J Abnorm Child Psychol 31:445–455, 2003

Woodcock RW, McGrew KS, Mather N: Woodcock-Johnson Tests of Achievement, 3rd
    Edition. Itasca, IL, Riverside, 2001

World Health Organization: International Classification of Diseases, 9th Revision,
    Clinical Modification. Ann Arbor, MI, Commission on Professional and Hospital
    Activities, 1978

■ CHAPTER 19 ■

Functional Abdominal Pain in a Child With Inflammatory Bowel Disease

Eva M. Szigethy, M.D., Ph.D.

CASE PRESENTATION

IDENTIFYING INFORMATION

Ryan is a 13-year-old who was diagnosed with Crohn's disease, a common inflammatory bowel disease (IBD), 4 years ago. He lives at home with his parents and attends eighth grade in a regular education classroom. He was referred for a behavioral health evaluation by his gastroenterologist.

CHIEF COMPLAINT

Ryan reports that he would be fine "if this stupid pain was not ruining my life."

HISTORY OF PRESENT ILLNESS

Over the past month, Ryan developed persistent abdominal pain that was interfering with his school performance. The pain was worse in the morning and was not accompanied by the symptoms (e.g., bloody diarrhea and weight loss) that usually accompany a flare-up of his IBD. The pain did not seem to be triggered by food or eating. Ryan went to his pediatric gastroenterologist 1 month after the pain began, but neither his physical examination nor laboratory tests were consistent with IBD activity or any other physical illness–related cause for his pain.

According to Ryan's mother, he was doing well until approximately 6 months prior, when he began to seem sad, become easily frustrated, com-

Eva M. Szigethy, M.D., Ph.D., is Assistant Professor of Psychiatry and Pediatrics at the University of Pittsburgh School of Medicine, and Director of Medical Coping Clinic in the Department of Gastroenterology at Children's Hospital of Pittsburgh in Pittsburgh, Pennsylvania (for full biographical information, see "About the Contributors," p. 613).

plain of fatigue in spite of sleeping more than 10 hours per night, have difficulty concentrating, and have decreased appetite but with little weight loss.
She also noted that he was making more negative self-comments ("I am stupid") and at times endorsed "wishing I was dead" but had no active suicidal intent. He missed more than 40 days of eighth grade at a public school during
this period, resulting in a downward drift in his usually above average grades.
His mother was also concerned about his increased isolation from his friends;
he often spent hours alone in his room listening to music and watching TV.

Ryan denied feeling depressed but did endorse that the pain was making
him very tired and making it too hard to concentrate in school, so he stopped
trying. Ryan also felt stressed by the constant tension between his parents, who
were arguing a lot and talking about getting a divorce. Ryan felt that the pain
also helped him get more attention from his father. He denied any other symptoms of depression. In terms of anxiety, he endorsed worrying that he would
have a flare-up of his IBD but denied any other anxiety symptoms. He denied
that the anxiety interfered with sleep or caused muscle tension or restlessness.

PAST PSYCHIATRIC HISTORY

Ryan and his mother denied that Ryan had any previous problems with depression. He reported that he remembers feeling more "down" when he was getting intermittent high-dose steroid treatments for his IBD flare-ups but did not
have lengthy school absences. He has had no previous psychiatric treatment.
He has no history of attention-deficit/hyperactivity disorder or a learning disability to account for his declining grades.

MEDICAL HISTORY

Ryan and his mother denied that Ryan has had previous problems with persistent abdominal pain. He did endorse having stomach pains during his two previous flare-ups of his Crohn's disease. He was medically hospitalized at age 9 at
the time of his IBD diagnosis but did not find this experience to be particularly
traumatic. His current medications for his IBD include mercaptopurine, an
immunosuppressant, and omeprazole (Prilosec) for possible gastric reflux.
There have been no recent changes in medications or dosages.

DEVELOPMENTAL HISTORY

Ryan is on target for meeting developmental milestones.

SOCIAL HISTORY

Ryan's father is a Vietnam War veteran who is unemployed. His mother works
as a high school teacher and often buries herself in her work to escape conflict
at home. Ryan is an only child.

FAMILY HISTORY

The family history is significant for possible colitis, depression, and alcoholism in his father.

MENTAL STATUS EXAMINATION

Ryan appeared small for his age (25th percentile for age-appropriate height). He was slightly unkempt, with hair in his eyes and loose-fitting T-shirt and jeans. He was not happy to be at the evaluation and stated, "It was my mother's idea." He was shy and reserved for the majority of the interview. He endorsed an abdominal pain level of 7 out of 10 but did not appear in any acute distress. He had poor eye contact through much of the interview, often looking at the floor. Ryan tended to give short, monotonic answers in a soft voice. He was occasionally fidgety in a nervous manner, cracking his knuckles and shaking his leg, but otherwise no motor abnormalities were noted.

Ryan's affect was constricted in the depressed range. He also appeared anxious, particularly on topics such as returning to school or getting along with friends. His thought process was organized. Ryan denied current suicidality or psychosis. Ryan was alert and oriented. His insight and judgment were developmentally appropriate in most realms but impaired regarding how he is coping with abdominal pain.

COMMENTARIES

Psychotherapeutic Perspective

David R. DeMaso, M.D.

DIAGNOSTIC FORMULATION

Ryan, an early adolescent with Crohn's disease, has had persistent abdominal pain over the last month. His subjective pain complaints, physical examination, and laboratory testing are inconsistent with an acute gastrointestinal illness flare-up, suggesting that his IBD is currently under good medical control

David R. DeMaso, M.D., is Professor of Psychiatry and Pediatrics at Harvard Medical School, and Psychiatrist-in-Chief at Children's Hospital Boston in Boston, Massachusetts (for complete biographical information, see "About the Contributors," p. 613).

with mercaptopurine and omeprazole. Although there is not enough evidence that he has an active general medical condition (e.g., Crohn's disease, gastric reflux, and/or side effects from their treatment) contributing to his current pain, the possibility that one or more physical conditions may be contributing at some physiological level to his gastrointestinal symptom production cannot be completely ruled out. Even if a medical condition is contributing to his symptoms, the condition is unlikely to fully account for the severity of his pain complaints or the degree of his functional disability.

Emotionally, Ryan appears to be experiencing a major depressive disorder (MDD), single episode, as evidenced by nearly 6 months of disabling depressed mood, diminished interests, hypersomnia, fatigue, feelings of worthlessness, diminished ability to concentrate, and recurrent thoughts of dying, in the context of a biological vulnerability to depression (e.g., paternal illness). These symptoms cannot be attributed to steroid-induced or steroid-exacerbated depressive symptoms because he is not currently being treated with steroids.

The clinically significant distress and impairment in his social and academic functioning, combined with his pain symptoms following the onset of a mood disturbance and no evidence for an etiological general medical condition, suggest that Ryan has a co-occurring pain disorder associated with psychological factors. He has no apparent disabling anxiety, temperament issues, or substance abuse, all of which are commonly involved in somatic presentations of this nature. Although his parents are likely caring and supportive, they clearly have significant relational problems, as evidenced by his father's unemployment and alleged alcohol problems, as well as his mother's avoidance of conflict. The degree of marital discord that Ryan has witnessed in the home in unknown, but this discord does represent a major stress for a young adolescent.

DSM-IV-TR DIAGNOSIS

Axis I   296.20 Major depressive disorder, single episode, unspecified

307.80 Pain disorder associated with psychological factors (acute)

Rule out pain disorder associated with both psychological factors and general medical condition

V61.20 Parent-child relational problem

Axis II   Diagnosis deferred

Axis III   Crohn's disease (treated with mercaptopurine)

Reflux, esophageal (treated with omeprazole)

Axis IV   Problems with primary support group (parental discord)

Axis V   Global Assessment of Functioning=55

TREATMENT RECOMMENDATIONS

Communication of the diagnostic formulation is the critical first step in responding to Ryan (Shaw and DeMaso 2006). He and his family likely believe that Ryan's month-long pain is due to a general medical condition. This view of the problem needs to be reframed to a biopsychosocial understanding, which should be communicated by the psychiatrist first to the gastroenterologist. Then an "informing conference" should be scheduled, which includes the gastroenterologist and family (Shaw and DeMaso 2006). It can be helpful for the psychiatrist to join this meeting depending on the gastroenterologist's expertise and comfort in communicating the biopsychosocial findings.

In this meeting, Ryan and his family are presented with the diagnostic formulation, generally by the gastroenterologist, in a supportive and nonjudgmental manner (Shaw and DeMaso 2006). The family should be told that many important things have been discovered—for example, "We have good news. We have ruled out a number of serious physical illnesses, and this is not a flare-up of your Crohn's disease." Statements that should be avoided include "We couldn't find anything," "It's in your mind," and "The symptoms are not real." Statements can focus on describing the common co-occurrence of mood and pain symptoms. Close attention and careful response to the family's words allows the family to be integrated into a more biopsychosocial formulation, thereby facilitating family acceptance (Shaw and DeMaso 2006).

Following the family's acceptance of a new formulation, the psychiatrist can facilitate the formation of a medical-psychiatric team, with the goal being an integrated medical and psychiatric approach (Shaw and DeMaso 2006). This team supports simultaneously the gastroenterologist's ongoing monitoring and treatment and the psychiatrist's interventions. The gastroenterologist should provide ongoing follow-up while avoiding unnecessary medical investigations and procedures. Clinical experience suggests that Ryan's co-occurring mood and pain disorders will respond to psychotherapy and medications (Fritz et al. 1997).

Nonpharmacologic intervention recommendations would include individual psychotherapy and family therapy, with treatment of Ryan's depression being a primary focus. Supportive, narrative, interpersonal, cognitive-behavioral, and/or behavioral modification therapies can be used to help change Ryan's erroneous cognitions about his ability to resume functioning and to encourage more adaptive coping mechanisms (Shaw and DeMaso 2006). Family therapy can explore ways in which Ryan's symptoms may serve to stabilize the family (i.e., the family's focus on the symptoms allows for avoidance of conflict) (Shaw and DeMaso 2006). Parent guidance can discourage reinforcement of the symptoms and promote positive reinforcement for improvement of functioning. The use of physical therapy, biofeedback, and/or relaxation techniques, along with a graduated return to his usual activities, may be additional interventions. Szigethy et al. (2007b) described a controlled trial with adolescents with IBD and depression; results suggest a positive response to cognitive-behavioral therapy (CBT) with family and narrative therapy modifications.

Although the literature contains little information pertaining to pharmacologic treatment of comorbid psychiatric disorders in the pediatric population (Berde and Sethna 2002), Ryan would benefit from a trial of an antidepressant medication targeting his depression. The impact of antidepressant medications on his pain symptoms is not clear because data are significantly limited regarding the use of these medications in pediatric patients with pain disorders. Clinical experience would suggest that the psychiatrist and gastroenterologist must be careful not to undertreat Ryan's pain, given that he may have both psychological and physical contributing factors at different points in his treatment (DeMaso and Beasley 2005). It is important to consider the use of analgesics to treat pain due to any subsequent flare-up of his IBD. Undertreated physical pain will only exacerbate any associated depressive symptoms and maintain his functional disability (DeMaso and Beasley 2005).

Should Ryan's pain symptoms persist and/or become more disabling, a rehabilitation model may need to be adopted in which his pain is accepted as a symptom that may not go away (Shaw and DeMaso 2006). The focus becomes one of improving independent functioning and skill building to improve coping. Ryan's progress is measured by changes in adaptive functioning, including school attendance and resuming normal social and recreational activities. This approach can be a hard shift for patients and their families, because acknowledging the pain without continuing to make medical inquiry into the etiological causes requires a large paradigm shift on their part (Shaw and DeMaso 2006).

Although the described treatment approach is successful in many cases, some families remain resistant to psychiatric intervention (DeMaso and Beasley 2005). If Ryan's family becomes resistant, the psychiatrist should remain a consultant to the gastroenterologist to advise alternative ways in which the gastroenterologist can decrease reinforcement for the sick role while encouraging Ryan's mobilization and responding to his depressive illness.

Psychopharmacologic Perspective

John V. Campo, M.D.

DIAGNOSTIC FORMULATION

Ryan, a 13-year-old with a history of Crohn's disease, presents with 1 month of persistent abdominal pain and 6 months of dysphoric mood, fatigue, poor concentration, hypersomnia, decreased appetite, negative self-image, passive death wish, social isolation, and declining school performance and attendance. In addition to the boy's chronic physical illness, significant psychosocial stressors include parental marital conflict and threatened separation, and paternal alcoholism and unemployment. Although no clear evidence for an anxiety disorder has been given, the details of the history provide reason to suspect anxiety. Therefore, the patient and parent(s) should be questioned further, and consideration should be given to offering a questionnaire focused on anxiety symptoms.

Any credible differential diagnosis must include unrecognized physical disease as a potential cause of Ryan's abdominal pain. The boy's history, physical evaluation, and lack of discernible pathology or tissue damage suggest that his Crohn's disease remains in remission, and little information is provided to suggest the presence of other explanatory physical disease in the traditional sense. Additional medical tests and procedures are probably unnecessary in the absence of new information, because relentless testing to rule out physical disease can inadvertently cause physical harm to the patient and/or create the false conviction for patients and families that a serious physical disease has been "missed." Abdominal pain and depressive symptoms are common in patients with Crohn's disease who appear to be in remission and thus show no evidence of active gut pathology (Farrokhyar et al. 2006). A growing body of evidence suggests that prior gut inflammation increases the risk of subsequent "medically unexplained" abdominal pain, perhaps by generating heightened gut sensitivity (i.e., visceral hypersensitivity) and lowering the threshold for particular sensations to be experienced as painful or distressing, with the mechanism likely involving serotonin (Spiller 2007).

John V. Campo, M.D., is Chief of the Division of Child and Adolescent Psychiatry; Medical Director of Pediatric Behavioral Health; and Professor of Clinical Psychiatry at The Ohio State University and Nationwide Children's Hospital in Columbus, Ohio (for complete biographical information, see "About the Contributors," p. 613).

Patients with pain in the absence of demonstrable disease create a nosological conundrum in Western medicine and are typically described as suffering from a functional somatic syndrome or disorder. Ryan would thus be considered to be suffering from functional abdominal pain (FAP) by his gastroenterologist and be diagnosed with a functional gastrointestinal disorder. In current psychiatric nosology, the diagnostic category of somatoform disorder is defined by the presence of somatic symptoms that suggest a physical disorder but are not fully explained by an associated general medical condition, the direct effects of a substance, or another mental disorder; the symptoms must cause distress or functional impairment and should not appear to be voluntarily or intentionally produced. Nothing in the case description suggests that Ryan's pain is feigned, fabricated, or intentionally produced, as one might find in factitious disorder, where the presumed incentive for the symptom is internal (i.e., a psychological wish or need to assume the sick role), or in malingering, where the incentive is considered to be external (i.e., a wish to obtain some reward or avoid unpleasant duties or obligations). Pain disorder is the specific somatoform disorder diagnosed when pain in one or more anatomical sites is of sufficient severity to warrant clinical attention and to cause significant distress or functional impairment, with the stipulation being that the pain is not better accounted for by a mood, anxiety, or psychotic disorder. The three subtypes are pain disorder associated with psychological factors, in which psychological factors are judged to play the predominant role in the causation or persistence of the pain; pain disorder associated with both psychological factors and a general medical condition, in which psychological factors and a general medical condition are judged to interact significantly in the development or maintenance of pain; and pain disorder associated with a general medical condition, in which psychological factors appear to play no more than a minimal role. The third subtype is not considered a mental disorder and is coded only on Axis III. The disorder is considered *acute* if less than 6 months in duration and *chronic* when lasting 6 months or more.

Youth with Crohn's disease appear to be at increased risk of experiencing depressive symptoms and disorders compared to healthy children (Mackner and Crandall 2007), and evidence is accumulating that depression can negatively influence the course of disease, making the identification and treatment of depression in youth with Crohn's disease particularly important. FAP is also commonly associated with high rates of anxiety and depressive disorders relative to those in healthy children (Campo et al. 2004a). Other than some hints of anxiety in Ryan that would suggest a more focused evaluation, perhaps including offering the child and a parent an anxiety-focused questionnaire, no clear evidence indicates that a specific anxiety disorder is present. Because Ryan meets criteria for MDD, the clinician must decide whether to classify the boy's abdominal pain as representative of a somatoform disorder or to consider the pain as being fully attributable to MDD. The requirement that the clinician decide whether the pain is better accounted for by mood, anxiety, or psychotic disorder introduces considerable diagnostic subjectivity and is likely to decrease diagnostic reliability. Several experts in the field have suggested that the somatoform disorder category be eliminated in future iterations of DSM and that functional somatic symptoms be coded on Axis III, in keeping with the diagnostic practices of our colleagues in general medicine (Mayou et al. 2005). For this patient, the decision to be made is whether the pain is a distinct problem that should be coded as pain disorder or whether it should be considered subordinate to the patient's MDD. Given the predominance of the pain, the patient's subjective focus on pain as the primary complaint, and the premorbid Crohn's disease, the following diagnostic formulation is offered.

DSM-IV-TR DIAGNOSIS

Axis I   307.89 Pain disorder associated with both psychological factors and a general medical condition, acute

296.22 Major depressive disorder, single episode, moderate

Rule out anxiety disorder not otherwise specified

Axis II   Deferred

Axis III   Functional abdominal pain

Crohn's disease, in remission

Axis IV   Parental marital conflict and threatened separation

Paternal alcoholism

Paternal unemployment

Axis V   Global Assessment of Functioning=45

TREATMENT RECOMMENDATIONS

A treatment approach that restores the patient to normal functioning and provides relief for his abdominal pain and depressive symptoms would be ideal. Treatment begins after the clinician, patient, and family reach diagnostic consensus and appropriate education is provided to allow for true informed consent. The clinician should provide reassurance that Ryan's Crohn's disease appears to remain in remission and that his abdominal pain is not a signal of ongoing tissue damage or a life-threatening and progressive physical disease. While emphasizing that the Crohn's disease is in remission, the clinician should also help the patient and family to understand that a history of Crohn's disease is likely a risk factor for both FAP and MDD, that both disorders tend to be chronic and potentially impairing in their own right, and that untreated depression may negatively impact the course of the Crohn's disease and increase the likelihood of relapse. Patient, family, and professional roles and responsibilities should be clarified, and the importance of good communication and collaboration must be emphasized. The psychiatric consultant and referring physician should communicate regularly and coordinate planning to maintain the physician-patient alliance and prevent unnecessary "doctor shopping" by the family.

Existing treatment options for FAP and MDD should be reviewed comprehensively, with a focus on what is known and not known and on facilitating informed treatment choices for the patient and family. The evidence base available to guide the management of youth with FAP is limited, and although evidence is growing that psychotherapy and/or antidepressant medications are effective for depressed adolescents, youth with chronic physical illness have typically been excluded from clinical trials, leaving clinicians to rely on studies of youth without documented physical disease or to extrapolate from experience with adults. The clinician should review with the patient and family the available clinical research specific to youth with Crohn's disease and depression, most notably the encouraging work of Szigethy and colleagues in the application of cognitive-behavioral psychotherapy to depressed youth with Crohn's disease (Szigethy et al. 2006). Cognitive-behavioral psychotherapy (Sanders et al. 1989, 1994) and interventions such as relaxation training, guided imagery, and hypnosis also have shown some promise in the treatment of FAP in youth.

Psychopharmacologic treatment is worthy of consideration, particularly if the patient and family favor pharmacologic management or the combination of medication with psychotherapy treatment, or if psychotherapeutic interventions fail. Unfortunately, no large randomized controlled trials of psychoactive medications have been done for the treatment of pediatric FAP or depression in youth with Crohn's disease. Nevertheless, the demonstrated efficacy of selective serotonin reuptake inhibitor (SSRI) antidepressant medications for MDD in adolescents (Bridge et al. 2007) makes the use of an SSRI the most reasonable initial consideration, because there is little reason to suspect that the presence of Crohn's disease would obviate its use. A recent case report describes the successful treatment of chronic pain and MDD in two adolescent girls with Crohn's disease, using the selective serotonin-norepinephrine reuptake inhibitor duloxetine (Meighen 2007). Although Ryan's Crohn's disease appears to be quiescent, it is worth noting that a handful of case reports have associated Crohn's disease remission with the initiation of the antidepressants bupropion (Kane et al. 2003) and phenelzine, a monoamine oxidase inhibitor (Kast 1998). Bupropion has been reported to lower levels of tumor necrosis factor–alpha (TNF-α), a circulating proinflammatory cytokine that has been associated with gut mucosal erosions in Crohn's disease (Brustolim et al. 2006). Although clinical studies are lacking, a report that mirtazapine may increase levels of TNF-α led some to presumptively recommend that the use of mirtazapine be avoided in patients with Crohn's disease (Kast 2003).

Although research on the pharmacologic treatment of pediatric FAP has been judged inconclusive to date (Campo 2005), adults with FAP have reportedly benefited from treatment with antidepressant medications (Drossman et al. 2003; Jailwala et al. 2000), including the SSRI citalopram (Tack et al. 2006). An open trial of citalopram for pediatric FAP found that 21 of 25 treated youth (84%) responded positively as judged by clinician ratings of "much improved" or "very much improved," and child and parent ratings of abdominal pain, anxiety, depression, other somatic symptoms, and functional impairment all improved significantly over the course of the study as well (Campo et al. 2004b). Although pediatric gastroenterologists have often favored the use of tricyclic antidepressants in youth with FAP, based in part on adult experience, it is difficult to advocate their use in this case given their lack of proven efficacy in the treatment of pediatric depressive disorders, as well as their toxicity in overdose and a handful of reports of sudden death in pediatric patients (Geller et al. 1999).

Based on the intersection of evidence supporting the use of SSRIs for depression in adolescents and at least one open trial suggesting that SSRIs may be of benefit in treating FAP, the most prudent choice of a pharmacologic agent in Ryan's case would likely be an SSRI such as fluoxetine or citalopram. This choice would be especially apt should further assessment demonstrate the presence of significant anxiety, because other potential antidepressant choices such as bupropion would be unlikely to prove beneficial in an anxious patient. Also, no reports have indicated that bupropion or other antidepressants are of use in pediatric FAP, save a single case report of duloxetine (Meighen 2007). Because both of Ryan's current medications (i.e., mercaptopurine and omeprazole) are metabolized by cytochrome P450 2D6, the clinician may wish to minimize pharmacokinetic concerns by using citalopram or escitalopram, because fluoxetine is a reasonably potent inhibitor of 2D6. My clinical approach has been to initiate SSRI treatment at a low dosage (e.g., citalopram 10 mg/day), increase to a potentially therapeutic dosage (e.g., 20 mg/day) over the next week, and then advance to higher dosages (e.g., 40 mg/day) at approximately week 4 in the absence of full improvement. The clinician should understand and communicate that antidepressant treatment in Ryan represents off-label use, and would be obligated to discuss potential risks and benefits in detail, including the recent black box warning that antidepressant use can be associated with suicidal thinking and/or behavior and the need for careful follow-up and safety monitoring.

Regardless of whether the specific treatment chosen is psychotherapeutic, pharmacologic, or a combination, the clinician needs to instill realistic hope and positive expectations for the patient and family. Care is likely best framed by a *rehabilitative approach*, which directs the patient and family away from finding a "cure" to instead coping with and overcoming the illness by returning to usual activities and responsibilities. Health-promoting patient behaviors and a return to normal functioning should be encouraged and rewarded, and any familial or social reinforcement of the illness or its symptoms (i.e., secondary gain) should be minimized or extinguished (see Campo and Fritz 2007). The rehabilitative approach challenges existing misperceptions about the child's health, communicates that healthy activity is safe and desirable, and emphasizes the child's fundamental strength and adaptability. School attendance and performance should be emphasized as critical indicators of developmentally appropriate functioning, and full school attendance should be a goal to be achieved either immediately or incrementally. Homebound instruction should be avoided. Respect for the importance of school should be communicated by attempting to schedule follow-up visits outside of regular school hours whenever possible. Ideally, coordination of the child's medical care should be consolidated with a single physician or clinician, and regularly scheduled visits can prove useful in reassuring the patient and family that their concerns have not been dismissed and that the patient need not be ill to see the doctor (Campo and Fritz 2007). Other potential treatment targets in Ryan's case include parental marital conflict, the father's alcoholism, and associated psychiatric disorders in either parent, particularly depression and/or posttraumatic stress disorder in the father. Also, additional assessment should explore whether there is need to be concerned about domestic violence or maltreatment in the home.

Integrative Perspective

Eva M. Szigethy, M.D., Ph.D.

DIAGNOSTIC FORMULATION

Ryan is a 13-year-old male who presents with a 6-month history of new-onset abdominal pain accompanied by persistent depressive symptoms, which collectively were resulting in functional impairment both at school and socially. He has several biological predisposing factors for his depression. IBD has been associated with increased rates of depression (Engstrom 1992), and although these depressive symptoms have been linked with cytokine-mediated inflammation and medications used to treat IBD, they can occur during periods of relative IBD remission (Szigethy et al. 2004b). The symptom of abdominal pain could also represent somatization, described as a tendency to express emotional distress through physical symptoms in the absence of pathophysiologic findings, and is often seen in depressed youth (Campo et al. 1999). In children with IBD, the perceived pain can be secondary to cytokine-related visceral hyperalgesia (Kelley et al. 2003). Ryan's paternal history of depression could also be a predisposing factor, coupled with the increased risk of Ryan's emerging adolescence. From a psychological perspective, his pain may provide secondary gain in helping him avoid conflict situations, gain attention from his parents, or avoid school-related shame of possible failure, particularly given his low self-esteem. Ryan may also be modeling the sick-role behavior or learned helplessness exhibited by his father, particularly given his mother's relative withdrawal. Parental conflict and social isolation from friends also have been shown to be predisposing factors for pediatric depression (Engstrom 1999; Mackner et al. 2004).

Diagnostically, if both self-report and maternal reports are taken into consideration, Ryan meets DSM-IV-TR criteria for MDD. Although he has a medical condition and is on medication, no temporal relationship is apparent between onset of depressive symptoms and either active IBD or medication change. If the abdominal pain occurred in the absence of depressive symptoms, he would be diagnosed with undifferentiated somatoform disorder or pain disorder. Generalized anxiety disorder needs to be considered because although Ryan only endorses worrying about his physical illness and not other realms of his life, he does have fatigue, decreased concentration, and irritability. Given his shy temperament (a risk factor for future anxiety disorder) and the high rates of anxiety disorders reported in youth with IBD (Szigethy et al. 2004a), anxiety needs to be tracked longitudinally to determine if it resolves as part of Ryan's mood disorder.

DSM-IV-TR DIAGNOSIS

Axis I   296.23 Major depressive disorder
            Rule out generalized anxiety disorder
Axis II   None
Axis III   Crohn's disease
Axis IV   Problems with primary support group
            Educational problems
Axis V   Global Assessment of Functioning=55 (current)

TREATMENT RECOMMENDATIONS

With the help of Ryan's gastroenterologist, medical causes for depression and abdominal pain were ruled out. Ryan was started on an 11-week course of CBT aimed at addressing skill deficits (e.g., difficulty self-soothing, withdrawal from peers, difficulty negotiating conflicts) and maladaptive cognitive habits (e.g., lack of perceived control and resulting helplessness, low self-esteem) that were likely causing and/or maintaining his depression (Szigethy et al. 2004a, 2007a). Ryan was taught more active problem-solving techniques; relaxation and distraction techniques for his pain, including forcing himself to become more active; and cognitive restructuring techniques for his negative attributions. Part of the work also involved parent sessions, during which the behavior of both parents was addressed and their help elicited in better supporting Ryan's return to health. The school was also contacted to set up a Section 504 educational plan designed to help Ryan receive the help he needed after missing school due to his chronic physical illness.

Over the following 3 months, Ryan's depressive symptoms improved, and he was able to return to school on a more regular basis. His parents decided to get a divorce during this time, and his father moved out, but Ryan was able to maintain contact with him and was relieved that the tension at home had significantly improved.

Even with remission of his depressive symptoms, Ryan's abdominal pain had not completely resolved, although it had diminished. Because Ryan had experienced a strong positive response to relaxation techniques for pain, the clinician decided to try a course of weekly hypnosis to help further reduce the pain. Hypnosis has shown promise in adults with irritable bowel disorder (Tan et al. 2005). Further relaxation and visual imagery, coupled with hypnotic suggestions to let the pain go, resulted in a complete resolution of Ryan's abdominal pain over the next several months.

Ryan's abdominal pain and depressive symptoms stayed in remission for approximately 1 year with maintenance CBT sessions every few months. Then Ryan had an exacerbation of his IBD, with bloody diarrhea, fatigue, and a 10-lb weight loss over 1 month. He was placed on high-dose prednisone and within the first week developed a significant major depression, with the presence of both neurovegetative and cognitive symptoms. His CBT sessions were again intensified to weekly; however, because his depressive symptoms persisted, he was started on citalopram, titrated to 20 mg/day, as an adjunct to his therapy. Within the next several weeks, his depressive symptoms improved significantly, as did his symptoms of IBD, and he was continued on citalopram and intermittent booster sessions of CBT over the next year, with sustained remission of both his IBD and depression. Citalopram has been shown to have promise in youth with FAP (Campo et al. 2004b), and SSRIs have been shown to have positive effects for certain cytokine-mediated depressive symptoms in adults treated with interferon, an exogenous cytokine (Capuron et al. 2003). Interestingly, several case reports indicate that antidepressants are associated with improvement in depression and IBD course in adults (Mikocka-Walus et al. 2006). Ryan's course and his response to a combination of CBT and antidepressant for sustained remission are consistent with the longitudinal treatment course and response observed in other adolescents with IBD (Szigethy et al. 2006).

SUMMARY

Ryan's presentation is typical of youth with functional abdominal pain. As the case illustrates, such pain—defined as at least 6 months of abdominal pain in the absence of clear organic etiology—can be seen in children and adolescents with IBD in remission, as well as in youth without any identified physical illness. In addition, children with comorbid depressive and anxiety symptoms are at higher risk for persistent abdominal pain and related impairment. Thus, it is particularly important that they are aggressively treated (Mulvaney et al. 2006). Even with this complex etiology, the treatment of pain appears to be similar across different etiologies: 1) identify comorbid depression and anxiety; 2) consider psychosocial issues; 3) if there is an underlying physical illness, collaborate with the medical team to make sure it is adequately treated; and 4) begin CBT, including family involvement in a developmentally appropriate manner, as first-line treatment, with careful addition of an antidepressant if clinically warranted. Youth who are encouraged to return to their usual peer activities and academics, with the assistance of an educated and empathic educational staff, appear to improve more quickly than children and adolescents who remain inactive in the sick role.

REFERENCES

Berde CB, Sethna NF: Analgesics for the treatment of pain in children. N Engl J Med 347:1094–1103, 2002

Bridge JA, Iyengar S, Salary CB, et al: Clinical response and risk for reported suicidal ideation and suicide attempts in pediatric antidepressant treatment: a meta-analysis of randomized controlled trials. JAMA 297:1683–1696, 2007

Brustolim D, Ribeiro-dos-Santos R, Kast RE, et al: A new chapter opens in anti-inflammatory treatments: the antidepressant bupropion lowers production of tumor necrosis factor-alpha and interferon-gamma in mice. Int Immunopharmacol 6:903–907, 2006

Campo JV: Coping with ignorance: exploring pharmacologic management of pediatric functional abdominal pain. J Pediatr Gastroenterol Nutr 41:569–574, 2005

Campo JV, Fritz GK: Somatoform disorders, in Lewis's Child and Adolescent Psychiatry: A Comprehensive Textbook, 4th Edition. Edited by Martin A, Volkmar F. Baltimore, MD, Lippincott Williams & Wilkins, 2007, pp 633–647

Campo JV, Jansen-McWilliams L, Comer DM, et al: Somatization in pediatric primary care: association with psychopathology, functional impairment, and use of services. J Am Acad Child Adolesc Psychiatry 38:1093–1101, 1999

Campo JV, Bridge J, Ehmann M, et al: Recurrent abdominal pain, anxiety, and depression in primary care. Pediatrics 113:817–824, 2004a

Campo JV, Perel J, Lucase A, et al: Citalopram treatment of pediatric recurrent abdominal pain and comorbid internalizing disorders: an exploratory study. J Am Acad Child Adolesc Psychiatry 43:1234–1242, 2004b

Capuron L, Neurauter G, Musselman DL, et al: Interferon-alpha-induced changes in tryptophan metabolism: relationship to depression and paroxetine treatment. Biol Psychiatry 54:906–914, 2003

DeMaso DR, Beasley PJ: The somatoform disorders, in Clinical Child Psychiatry, 2nd Edition. Edited by Klykylo WM, Kay JL. West Sussex, UK, Wiley, 2005

Drossman DA, Toner BB, Whitehead WE, et al: Cognitive-behavioral therapy versus education and desipramine versus placebo for moderate to severe functional bowel disorders. Gastroenterology 125:19–31, 2003

Engstrom I: Mental health and psychological functioning in children and adolescents with inflammatory bowel disease. J Child Psychol Psychiatry 33:563–582, 1992

Engstrom I: Inflammatory bowel disease in children and adolescents: mental health and family functioning. J Pediatr Gastroenterol Nutr 28:S28–S33, 1999

Farrokhyar F, Marshall JK, Easterbrook B, et al: Functional gastrointestinal disorders and mood disorders in patients with inactive inflammatory bowel disease: prevalence and impact on health. Inflamm Bowel Dis 12:38–46, 2006

Fritz GK, Fritsch S, Hagino O: Somatoform disorders in children and adolescents: a review of the past 10 years. J Am Acad Child Adolesc Psychiatry 36:1329–1338, 1997

Geller B, Reising D, Leonard HL, et al: Critical review of tricyclic antidepressant use in children and adolescents. J Am Acad Child Adolesc Psychiatry 38:513–516, 1999

Jailwala J, Imperiale T, Kroenke K: Pharmacologic treatment of the irritable bowel syndrome: a systematic review of randomized, controlled trials. Ann Intern Med 133:136–147, 2000

Kane S, Altschuler EL, Kast RE: Crohn's disease remission on bupropion (letter). Gastroenterology 125:1290, 2003

Kast RE: Crohn's disease remission with phenelzine treatment. Gastroenterology 115:1034–1035, 1998

Kast RE: Anti- and pro-inflammatory considerations in antidepressant use during medical illness: bupropion lowers and mirtazapine increases circulating tumor necrosis factor–alpha levels. Gen Hosp Psychiatry 25:495–496, 2003

Kelley KW, Bluthe RM, Dantzer R, et al: Cytokine-induced sickness behavior. Brain Behav Immun 17:S112–S118, 2003

Mackner L, Crandall WV: Psychological factors affecting pediatric inflammatory bowel disease. Curr Opin Pediatr 19:548–552, 2007

Mackner LM, Sisson DP, Crandall WV: Review: psychosocial issues in pediatric inflammatory bowel disease. J Pediatr Psychol 29:243–257, 2004

Mayou R, Kirmayer L, Simon G, et al: Somatoform disorders: time for a new approach in DSM-V. Am J Psychiatry 162:847–855, 2005

Meighen KG: Duloxetine treatment of pediatric chronic pain and co-morbid major depressive disorder. J Child Adolesc Psychopharmacol 17:121–127, 2007

Mikocka-Walus AA, Turnbull DA, Moulding NT, et al: Antidepressants and inflammatory bowel disease: a systematic review. Clin Pract Epidemol Ment Health 2:24–33, 2006

Mulvaney S, Lambert EW, Garber J, et al: Trajectories of symptoms and impairment for pediatric patients with functional abdominal pain: a 5-year longitudinal study. J Am Acad Child Adolesc Psychiatry 45:737–744, 2006

Sanders MR, Rebgetz M, Morrison M, et al: Cognitive-behavioral treatment of recurrent nonspecific abdominal pain in children: an analysis of generalization, maintenance, and side effects. J Consult Clin Psychol 57:294–300, 1989

Sanders MR, Shepherd RW, Cleghorn G, et al: The treatment of recurrent abdominal pain in children: a controlled comparison of cognitive-behavioral family intervention and standard pediatric care. J Consult Clin Psychol 62:306–314, 1994

Shaw RJ, DeMaso DR: Clinical Manual of Pediatric Psychosomatic Medicine: Mental Health Consultation With Physically Ill Children and Adolescents. Washington, DC, American Psychiatric Publishing, 2006

Spiller RC: Irritable bowel syndrome: bacteria and inflammation—clinical relevance now. Curr Treat Options Gastroenterol 10:312–321, 2007

Szigethy EM, Levy-Warren A, Whitton S, et al: Cognitive-behavioral therapy for depression in adolescents with inflammatory bowel disease: a pilot study. J Am Acad Child Adolesc Psychiatry 43:1469–1477, 2004a

Szigethy EM, Whitton S, Levy-Warren A, et al: Depressive symptoms and inflammatory bowel disease in children and adolescents: a cross-sectional study. J Pediatr Gastroenterol Nutr 39:395–403, 2004b

Szigethy E, Carpenter J, Baum E, et al: Case study: longitudinal treatment of adolescents with depression and inflammatory bowel disease. J Am Acad Child Adolesc Psychiatry 45:396–400, 2006

Szigethy E, Kenney E, Carpenter J, et al: Cognitive-behavioral therapy for adolescents with inflammatory bowel disease and sybsyndromal depression. J Am Acad Child Adolesc Psychiatry 46:1290–1298, 2007a

Szigethy ES, Kenney E, Carpenter J, et al: A randomized efficacy trial of cognitive behavioral therapy for adolescents with inflammatory bowel disease and mild to moderate depression: two-site study. J Am Acad Child Adolesc Psychiatry 10:1290–1298, 2007b

Tack J, Broekaert D, Fischler B, et al: A controlled crossover study of the selective serotonin reuptake inhibitor citalopram in irritable bowel syndrome. Gut 55:1095–1103, 2006

Tan G, Hammond DC, Gurrala J: Hypnosis and irritable bowel syndrome: a review of efficacy and mechanism of action. Am J Clin Hypn 47:161–178, 2005

▪Part III▪

TOUGHEST CASES
Diagnostic and
Treatment Dilemmas

Introduction to Toughest Cases

Peter S. Jensen, M.D.
Cathryn A. Galanter, M.D.

In Part III, we present cases that pose diagnostic and therapeutic challenges to clinicians. In some instances, these difficulties are simply due to the absence of critical research to discriminate various syndromes. In other cases, clinicians may encounter difficulties in deciding which subtle diagnostic distinctions are possible and important. In still other instances, clinicians may face a dilemma as to which component of the patient's overall presentation to treat first.

In "Frequent Tantrums: Oppositional Behavior in a Young Child" (Chapter 20), our expert commentators vary in the differential diagnosis of tantrum behavior in a 6-year-old child. In essence, the case presents difficulties in distinguishing between oppositional defiant disorder and bipolar disorder not otherwise specified. The commentators also differ in assigning the child Global Assessment of Functioning scores and in invoking the presumed etiological models. They vary in the extent to which they invoke primarily parenting and psychosocial factors; a combination of factors; and biological factors that require a whole array of biological, pharmacologic, supportive, and psychotherapeutic approaches. In our view, this case could easily exemplify the use of any of the three approaches as most correct.

The challenge for our field — and one that still lies ahead of us — is ferreting out how to distinguish among these cases, and to do it reliably in research settings and clinical practice. The goal is to better understand those family, constitutional, and environmental factors that predispose children in different directions and then to use that information to provide optimal prevention and treatment interventions. Thus, perhaps the child in this case has four or five different disorders, using the Robins and Guze (1970) and Cantwell-modified (Cantwell 1995) disorder validation criteria — disorders that could be ferreted out once we know where to look in the brain, the genes, the family, and the developmental and environmental factors. More research is needed before this child's story can be completed.

In "Toddler With Temper Tantrums: A Careful Assessment of a Dysregulated Preschool Child" (Chapter 21), a 4½-year-old boy illustrates some of the difficulties in making diagnoses with very young children, as well as the differences among experts with different persuasions as to etiological factors and preferred approaches to treatment. For one of the commentators, oppositional defiant disorder symptoms seemed central, whereas for other commentators, issues of anxiety, separation and attachment difficulties, and sleep problems take center stage.

Although all of the commentators invoke various approaches to parent support and treatment using behavioral methods, they differ in the extent to which anxiety and attachment issues are approached in the course of that parent-directed treatment. For various reasons, parent-directed treatment requires the clinician to carefully assess the environment, including the nature of the parent-child relationship. The following are all necessary for success: reliance on multiple informants (including other caretakers); a separate determination of the child's affective state apart from his or her behavior; generous use of rigorous rating scales; speech and language testing; and psychoeducational, intelligence, and environmental assessments.

"Won't Leave His Room: Clinical High Risk for Developing Psychosis" (Chapter 22) presents the case of a 15-year-old who shows progressive deterioration in functioning over time. The commentators all agree that the youth's impairment is substantial, yet they proffer different diagnoses with likely different prognoses. Of interest in this case is the youth's response to nonmedical intervention after medications were refused. This case illustrates a typical clinician bias (Cohen and Cohen 1984): because a clinician often sees long-term chronic patients, the clinician might assume that all patients presenting with a particular syndrome or disorder must be similarly chronic, but in fact many psychotic episodes may remit without further evidence of relapse, as was the general outcome for this youth. Thus, this case presents an argument for clinical humility and more clinical research.

In "I Just Want to Die: Double Depression" (Chapter 23), the case is presented of a youth with an apparent long-standing history of depression. Various therapeutic approaches are outlined by commentators, and they cite the importance of the Treatment for Adolescents with Depression Study and its relevance to offering both medication and cognitive-behavioral therapy (CBT) interventions when possible. Particularly in complex and/or unremitting cases, multiple treatments have become de rigueur, even in the absence of evidence.

This case also illustrates the difficulties in determining which disorder appeared first. In this case, not only did the dysthymia precede the major depression, but also the inattentive attention-deficit/hyperactivity disorder symptoms may have preceded the dysthymia and depression. Interestingly, the commentators suggest three forms of treatments: CBT; CBT and medication; and CBT, a selective serotonin reuptake inhibitor, and a stimulant medication. In this instance, these differences are best understood as a function of the experts' responses to an incomplete vignette rather than what they would do with a real patient. However, in the real world, similar differences in approach are likely, depending on the clinical door into which each patient walks, providing yet another argument for humility and the need for clinicians to continue learning from each other.

Similar differences in therapeutic approach are also seen in the case of "Cutting Helps Me Feel Better: Nonsuicidal Self-Injury" (Chapter 24). Although some commentators inferred the diagnosis of major depression, others did not. Yet all tended to consider various forms of psychotherapy, CBT, or dialectical behavior therapy. Also demonstrated in this case is the important role of diaries in helping experts better understand the unique precipitants and consequences of the youth's suicidal behavior. This type of intermittent behavior, like many clinical phenomena, can be difficult to understand through the use of rating scales alone, and clinicians often must work with the patient and family to do careful detective work to tease out possible precipitants, motives, and reinforcing consequences of a specific behavior.

"From Foster Care to the State Hospital: Psychotic Symptoms in a Child Who Is the Victim of Neglect" (Chapter 25) demonstrates some of the most daunting challenges faced in treating children and youth with the most severe impairments. Often, no single treatment is satisfactory, and even multiple treatments leave something to be desired. Multiple medications—often in combinations whose risks and benefits are unknown—end up being used. Sometimes, it is only through the diagnostic course, in hindsight, that a clinician learns about the true nature of a child's disorder. This case also aptly illustrates the aphorism "the secret of patient care is caring for patients"; for many patients, what clinicians are seeking is care and not necessarily a cure, and the goal of treatment (and the ultimate measure of treatment success) is the ongoing maintenance of a relationship, continued problem solving, and finding what "works" for a given patient and family.

REFERENCES

Cantwell DP: Child psychiatry: introduction and overview, in Comprehensive Textbook of Psychiatry, 6th Edition. Edited by Kaplan HI, Sadock BJ. Baltimore, MD, Williams & Wilkins, 1995, pp 2151–2154

Cohen P, Cohen J: The clinician's illusion. Arch Gen Psychiatry 41:1178–1182, 1984

Robins E, Guze SB: Establishment of diagnostic validity in psychiatric illness: its application to schizophrenia. Am J Psychiatry 126:983–987, 1970

■ CHAPTER 20 ■

Frequent Tantrums

Oppositional Behavior in a Young Child

Ross W. Greene, Ph.D.
J. Stuart Ablon, Ph.D.

CASE PRESENTATION

IDENTIFYING INFORMATION

Sam is a 6-year-old boy who lives with his parents and 3-year-old sister. He is in kindergarten at a local public school. Sam's mother was 5 months pregnant with the couple's third child at the time of referral.

CHIEF COMPLAINT

Sam and his family were referred to an outpatient psychiatrist's office for Sam's significant oppositional behavior and aggressive outbursts.

Ross W. Greene, Ph.D., is Associate Clinical Professor in the Department of Psychiatry at Harvard Medical School, and Cofounder of the Collaborative Problem Solving Institute in the Department of Psychiatry of Massachusetts General Hospital in Boston, Massachusetts.

J. Stuart Ablon, Ph.D., is Associate Clinical Professor of Psychiatry at Harvard Medical School, and Associate Director and Cofounder of the Collaborative Problem Solving Institute in the Department of Psychiatry of Massachusetts General Hospital in Boston, Massachusetts.

For complete biographical information, see "About the Contributors," p. 613.

History of Present Illness

Sam's pediatrician recommended Sam for psychiatric evaluation because prior intervention had not improved his challenging behavior. Sam's parents reported that Sam had always had difficulty managing his emotions, and they described Sam as extremely "willful," as "wanting to control everyone in the family," and as "refusing to take no for an answer." His oppositional behaviors include screaming, throwing or destroying property, and sometimes hitting. Although he does not use profanity, he does make disrespectful comments directed at his mother, such as "I hate you" and "I wish you weren't my mommy." The parents indicate that Sam is "fine" as long as things are "going his way." The tantrums at home began before Sam was 2 years old. The father reported that his wife was too lenient and inconsistent in her discipline, whereas Sam's mother felt that her husband had little appreciation for all that was involved in getting Sam through a typical day at home.

When Sam was age 5, his parents sought the guidance of a mental health professional for the first time. The mental health professional recommended some adjustments to the existing home-based contingency management program, suggested that Sam spend more special time with his father, and saw the parents briefly for marital counseling. The mental health professional suggested that Sam's difficulties with transitions and poor impulse control when angered might be a sign of looming attention-deficit/hyperactivity disorder (ADHD). At the time, the parents were becoming increasingly concerned about the effect that Sam's behavior was having on his sister and on their marriage; these concerns linger.

Recently, Sam's mother began searching the Internet for anything she could find regarding her son's difficulties. She felt that Sam did not really meet criteria for ADHD, because he was not especially hyperactive and he did not seem to have trouble focusing. She came across information on sensory hypersensitivities, which also did not seem to fit Sam. When she read about pediatric bipolar disorder, she thought this seemed closer to the mark because of Sam's temper outbursts; additionally, Sam seemed to fit some criteria for some definitions of grandiosity, in that he always wanted his own way and sometimes told his parents, "You're not my boss." However, Sam did not seem "manic," and his mood only appeared to be "rapidly cycling" when he was upset. The mother also read about Asperger's disorder and felt that some features described her son—he was pretty inflexible and was bossy and controlling with his friends— but a lot of the criteria for Asperger's disorder did not seem to fit at all.

Past Psychiatric History

Sam's parents reported that he was a fussy infant and somewhat demanding as a toddler. However, once Sam entered preschool, greater difficulties began to emerge. Sam's preschool teachers reported that he had more difficulty sharing than his peers, was somewhat bossy, and always wanted his own way (and would lash out when things did not go his way). These reports caused Sam's mother to wonder if she had catered too much to his every whim when he was a toddler (this possibility was also suggested by one of the preschool teachers), if her mild postpartum depression after Sam's birth was having lingering effects, or if Sam was still reacting badly to the addition of his younger sister to the family.

At the time, the mother had a brief discussion about her concerns with Sam's pediatrician and was relieved when the pediatrician suggested that Sam was "just a boy," would probably "grow out of it," and would just have to adapt to the presence of his sister and the parents' divided affections. The pediatrician recommended a few parenting books. Based on what they read, and with additional prodding from the preschool teacher, the parents implemented a contingency management program and began using a time-out procedure. Over the first few months of implementation, Sam's parents and teachers noted the heightened severity of Sam's temper outbursts, especially when he was placed in time-out. During the worst episodes, Sam's screaming and crying could last as long as 45 minutes and could be touched off by triggers such as being told to get out of the bathtub, being asked to turn off the TV and come to dinner, and having to shift from one activity to another at school. Sam's parents were reassured by what they read: that Sam's temper outbursts would diminish once he realized that he could not always have things his way.

SUBSTANCE ABUSE HISTORY

Sam has no history of substance abuse.

MEDICAL HISTORY

Sam does not have any medical illnesses.

DEVELOPMENTAL HISTORY

Sam achieved developmental milestones within expectations.

SOCIAL HISTORY

Sam has one close friend who lives next door (and who seems to enjoy Sam's creative ideas for play and is willing to go along for the ride), but his parents report that Sam rarely receives invitations for playdates from his friends at school.

FAMILY HISTORY

Sam's mother had a mild postpartum depression after Sam was born. A distant paternal uncle abused alcohol.

MENTAL STATUS EXAMINATION

Sam was a neatly dressed boy who appeared his stated age. He did not have any atypical facial features. Sam was friendly and generally cooperative with the interview and interviewer, but he became increasingly active as the interview progressed, moving from his chair to the toy table and making crashing motions and noises with the cars. This behavior made it increasingly difficult for him to focus on the interviewer's questions. Sam's mood appeared to be cheerful; he volunteered that he sometimes gets "really mad." His thought process was fairly linear. He denied psychotic symptoms. He also denied thoughts of wanting to harm himself. He first denied any wish to harm others but, with some gentle prodding, admitted that sometimes he gets angry and hits his sister but is sorry afterward. Sam appeared to be of average or above average intelligence, with a good fund of knowledge (e.g., he could name the president), and he was able to repeat three words and recall them several minutes later. Sam's speech was of regular tone and volume. At the end of the interview, Sam demanded that his mother buy him candy from the vending machine. The interviewer heard this discussion continue outside his office. After Sam whined and raised his voice, his mother said she would buy him candy "just this once."

COMMENTARIES

Psychotherapeutic Perspective

Alison Zisser, M.S.
Sheila M. Eyberg, Ph.D., A.B.P.P.

DIAGNOSTIC FORMULATION

Sam was referred for diagnosis and treatment of significant oppositional behavior and aggressive outbursts. Background information from the clinical interview and mental status examination will be supplemented with additional interview

Alison Zisser, M.S., is a graduate student in the Department of Clinical and Health Psychology at the University of Florida in Gainesville, Florida.

Sheila M. Eyberg, Ph.D., A.B.P.P., is Distinguished Professor in the Department of Clinical and Health Psychology at the University of Florida in Gainesville, Florida.

For complete biographical information, see "About the Contributors," p. 613.

and assessment procedures required for differential diagnosis and treatment planning. Specific modules of the Diagnostic Interview Schedule for Children (Shaffer et al. 2000) will be administered to obtain further information on symptom presence, duration, and functional impairment related to oppositional defiant disorder (ODD), conduct disorder, ADHD, and major depressive disorder.

Sam's behavior meets DSM-IV-TR diagnostic criteria for ODD: He has demonstrated a pattern of hostile or defiant behavior toward authority figures for at least 6 months, resulting in significant impairment in social or academic functioning. Sam's parents described him as defiant, willful, and controlling at home and school, and noted that simple parent or teacher commands set off temper tantrums that include screaming, throwing things, destroying property, and sometimes hitting others. They indicated that Sam's behavior has negatively affected his peer relationships and school learning and has contributed to stress in their marriage.

DSM-IV-TR diagnostic criteria for ODD stipulate that the disruptive behaviors occur outside an episode of mood or psychotic disorder and require that criteria for conduct disorder are not met. Although Sam's behavior was described as grandiose at times, his parents did not report other manic symptoms or rapid cycling beyond times when Sam is upset. Sam's linear thought processes and denial of psychotic symptoms during the mental status examination suggest that he does not have a psychotic disorder. Conduct disorder may be dismissed because Sam does not meet full diagnostic criteria for behaviors that violate the rights of others or break age-appropriate social norms.

The rule-out of comorbid ADHD is the most difficult diagnostic decision in Sam's case. ADHD is a common comorbid condition in young children with ODD. Although Sam's mother described him as "not especially hyperactive" or inattentive, she also described him as a fussy baby, and Sam demonstrated increasingly active and inattentive behavior during the mental status examination. Sam's kindergarten teacher reported his difficulty sharing with peers but did not comment on inattentiveness or hyperactivity. A teacher rating scale such as the SNAP-IV (Swanson 1992) would provide a better understanding of Sam's symptom expression at school. Information available at this point does not provide sufficient evidence for an ADHD diagnosis.

DSM–IV–TR DIAGNOSIS

Axis I   313.81 Oppositional defiant disorder
Axis II   None
Axis III   None
Axis IV   Parents experiencing strain in marriage
Axis V   Global Assessment of Functioning=60

TREATMENT RECOMMENDATIONS

Child factors, such as difficult temperament (Rubin et al. 2003) and impaired social information processing (Crick and Dodge 1994), as well as familial factors, such as maternal depression (Webster-Stratton and Hammond 1990) and parent conflict regarding child rearing (Bearss and Eyberg 1998), contribute to the development of disruptive behaviors. The behaviors described by Sam's parents, their description of their own parenting and discipline, and observations by the examiner reveal a parent-child interaction pattern in which parent behaviors reinforce child behavior problems. The association between parenting style and child behavior problems (Campbell 1997) suggests that treatment focused on the parent-child interaction will benefit Sam by changing the coercive interactions into a healthy parent-child relationship.

Parent-child interaction therapy (PCIT; Brinkmeyer and Eyberg 2003) is an evidence-based treatment for families with children ages 2–6 years with disruptive behavior disorders. Families attend weekly 1-hour sessions for an average of 12–16 weeks. Treatment is not time limited and is completed when parents have mastered the PCIT skills and rate their child's behavior within normal limits.

In addition to establishing a diagnosis, the pretreatment assessment is used to gather information to inform treatment planning and provide baseline measures against which progress is assessed. The clinical interview addresses past discipline strategies. With Sam's parents, a behavioral analysis of their implementation of the time-out procedure will be important for identifying errors that can be clarified when time-out is introduced in the second phase of PCIT.

The pretreatment assessment will also include behavioral observations of Sam interacting with each parent in three structured play situations that vary in the degree of parental control. Frequencies of child and parent behaviors will be recorded using the Dyadic Parent-Child Interaction Coding System (Eyberg et al. 2005). Sam's parents will also complete the Eyberg Child Behavior Inventory (Eyberg and Pincus 1999) to assess the frequency of Sam's disruptive behaviors at home. Given the mother's history of depression and marital stress, screening for current depressive symptomatology with the Beck Depression Inventory (Beck et al. 1996) will also be included.

In the first phase of PCIT, the child-directed interaction, parents learn play therapy skills designed to strengthen the parent-child relationship. The parent and child develop a cooperative, positive, reciprocal interaction, which increases enjoyment of their relationship and the child's inclination to obey. Parents must meet preset child-directed interaction skill levels before progressing to the second phase of treatment, the parent-directed interaction.

During parent-directed interaction, parents learn to use clear, positively worded direct commands and to implement consistent consequences following child compliance and noncompliance. Parents are taught a precise, step-by-step time-out procedure to begin whenever their child disobeys a direct command. Parents learn to apply the skills first at home and then in public settings, and to sibling interactions. During treatment, therapists actively coach the parents, providing prompts and feedback as the parents practice the skills with their child. Between sessions, parents spend 5–10 minutes each day practicing the skills at home.

Sam's behavior is expected to improve steadily each week during treatment. Once the family meets criteria for treatment completion, the posttreatment assessment will be scheduled. If Sam's behavior does not show regular improvement each week, the therapist will address family stressors that may be interfering with the parents' adherence to home practice. If Sam's parents report practicing the PCIT skills regularly without expected effect, other treatment options, such as referral for mood disorder medication, will be considered.

Psychopharmacologic Perspective

Mani Pavuluri, M.D., Ph.D.

DIAGNOSTIC FORMULATION

Sam is a 6-year-old boy presenting with chronic oppositional behavior and explosive outbursts. On the biological front, Sam has a difficult temperament and has a family history of affective illness (i.e., his mother had postpartum depression). He also has executive function difficulties, with potential cognitive problems. On the psychological front, his bossy, intrusive behavior is leading to conflicted interpersonal relationships, which in turn may feed low self-esteem. It is possible that Sam's feelings of competence at home and school are severely compromised by his executive function difficulties, as well as the family conflict that surrounds him, which essentially appears to be secondary to his difficult behavior. On the social front, Sam's mother has two young children and will soon have a third child. In a matter of 4 months, she will have three children age 6 and under, which is a burden.

Mani Pavuluri, M.D., Ph.D., is the Founding Director of the Pediatric Mood Program in the Center for Cognitive Medicine at the University of Illinois, Chicago (for complete biographical information, see "About the Contributors," p. 613).

DSM-IV-TR DIAGNOSIS

Axis I   296.80 Bipolar disorder not otherwise specified (NOS)

Consider oppositional defiant disorder (cannot be diagnosed in the presence of bipolar diathesis)

Rule out ADHD (This diagnosis is considered if Sam had clear impulsivity, inattention, or hyperactivity preceding bipolar diathesis; however, given that his problems started since he was 2 years old, it is likely that his emotional problems were present chronically for a long period, and it is difficult to ascertain an ADHD diagnosis with this current clinical picture.)

Axis II   Learning disorder (may be a possible outcome once Sam is challenged academically in higher classes)

Axis III Deferred

Axis IV   Moderate, given the difficulties at home and school and the interpersonal conflicts encroaching on his function

Axis V   Global Assessment of Functioning=48

THE ISSUE OF BIPOLAR DISORDER NOS DIAGNOSIS AND COMORBID CONDITIONS

Given that Sam does not have a clear episodic history of illness—the case presentation does not include a clear description of elated mood, grandiosity, hypersexuality, rapid flow of speech, or sleep difficulties—ascertaining whether he has a typical or narrow phenotype of bipolar disorder is difficult. The clinical picture seems to be an exacerbated state of affective dysregulation layered on top of a difficult temperament. Sam may have explosive rages when one says "no" to his requests. This reactivity starts as oppositional behavior but escalates to greater heights due to severe affect dysregulation. His parents would need psychoeducation to understand that this is not a simple case of oppositionality that could be tied to a "no" answer. The clinician should not automatically consider Sam's behavior to be a result of parental inconsistency (although it might be), because parents often have to "give in" to children's requests intuitively to avoid severe explosive outbursts in children with poor emotional regulation. This behavior in children is often misconstrued as being secondary to parental mismanagement. Also, parents often disagree on discipline, especially because mothers tend to be the main target of strong-willed oppositional behavior in emotionally dysregulated children. Additional examples of grandiosity might clarify whether Sam in fact has bipolar disorder symptoms. The descriptions of his general bossiness and overbearing behavior are not sufficient examples of grandiosity to diagnose bipolar disorder. Assuming that Sam's aggressive rages are not essentially resulting from parental management (although this possibility needs to be clarified) and because Sam does not have all the symptoms of mania or fit the DSM-IV-TR timeline criteria for bipolar disorder, a diagnosis of bipolar disorder NOS may do justice at the current time. This diagnostic approach is especially important for the parsimonious reasons of giving the right treatment.

The Child Mania Rating Scale (Pavuluri et al. 2006) and the parent report portion of the General Behavior Inventory (Youngstrom et al. 2001) might be two good scales to use for screening in Sam's case. However, given the intensity of his explosive rages and the limited number of symptoms, Sam may fall short of meeting the criteria on any rating scale. In this case, a thorough diagnostic interview may be more effective than simply getting more information through rating scales.

TREATMENT RECOMMENDATIONS

Considering the case presentation described earlier, the clinician needs to obtain a clear history of manic symptoms as well as depressive symptoms in a systematic manner. Answers to the following questions about Sam's mood cycles are important: How long do they last? What are the symptoms and signs? What situations trigger them? Is a depressive episode couched between the manic episodes? Does Sam have a mixed episode (which is common rather than pure manic or depressive episodes in children)? Does he have interepisodic inattention or impulsivity, suggesting a comorbid diagnosis of ADHD?

A referral for neuropsychological assessment should be made by the pediatrician (better for insurance purposes than referral by a psychiatrist). That assessment makes more apparent any potential cognitive difficulties, such as executive function problems, attention difficulties, verbal memory problems, visual-spatial perception problems, and working memory deficits. Then the neuropsychologist and clinician can meet with the school personnel, either through a teleconference or in person, to offer their recommendations.

COMMUNICATION WITH PARENTS

The clinician needs to educate Sam's parents in a detailed manner, maintaining an optimistic tone that this is an issue of strong temperament. Although one cannot know when the psychopathology ends and bipolar diathesis begins, the tendency is to diagnose bipolar spectrum disorder if the functional disturbance is severe enough to be encroaching on the well-being of the child and the family. Children should not be overdiagnosed. After the formal diagnosis is made, the family must decide whether they would like to use the label "bipolar disorder" or refer to Sam as having emotional dysregulation. If Sam were my patient, I would check the comfort level of the family regarding using the diagnosis, using medications, and communicating with the school about these matters. Medications, while essential in severe situations, are not necessary in a case such as Sam's. I would encourage the family to visit the Child and Adolescent Bipolar Foundation Web site (http://www.bpkids.org) to learn more about bipolar spectrum disorders. I would also tell the parents that as Sam grows up, he may gain more emotional control, which typically occurs if a child is intelligent and the parents offer good support in a manner that is conducive to the child's emotional growth.

PHARMACOTHERAPY

If no clear-cut depression is associated with Sam's extreme irritability and explosive outbursts, the clinician might consider a second-generation antipsychotic medication in small doses, such as risperidone 0.5–1 mg/day. Parents need to be educated about possible extrapyramidal side effects, weight gain, and prolactin increase with risperidone. The second choice would be aripiprazole in very small doses, such as 0.5 mg/day. Quetiapine (Seroquel) is another alternative, starting with 25 mg/day (pharmacotherapy algorithm: Pavuluri et al. 2004b; treatment guidelines: Kowatch et al. 2005).

PSYCHOTHERAPY

The child- and family-focused cognitive-behavioral therapy, or RAINBOW, approach appears to be extremely successful in children such as Sam (Pavuluri et al. 2004a). The acronym RAINBOW is easy to remember and introduce: routine; affective/regulation anger control; "I can do it"; no negative thoughts; "be a good friend"/balanced lifestyle with parents; "Oh, how can I solve this problem?" (using collaborative problem-solving methods); and ways to get support. Essentially, these principles are based on building the child's self-esteem, regulating daily routines, establishing open communication, and dealing with the child in an extremely compassionate way. Community practitioners, especially psychotherapists, need to be educated not to use contingency management invariably because it goes against the management of intense children. Consistency is important, but instituting negative consequences can work against negotiating effectively with a child who rapidly swings into a negative cycle.

If initial pharmacotherapy with antipsychotics does not work, alternatives may be considered. The clinician can either add a mood stabilizer, such as lithium, divalproex sodium, or lamotrigine, to the existing antipsychotic or prescribe a different antipsychotic. A patient may need one or more additional medications, such as a treatment for comorbid ADHD or an antidepressant to treat severe anxiety or depression. Stabilizing the symptom complex, as well as addressing side effects and associated autonomic hyperarousal, will pose challenges. West et al. (2007) provide a systematic medication algorithm and a plan for troubleshooting psychological issues through a maintenance model of psychotherapy.

Integrative Perspective

Ross W. Greene, Ph.D.
J. Stuart Ablon, Ph.D.

DIAGNOSTIC FORMULATION

Sam's psychiatrist felt that Sam met diagnostic criteria for ODD and that there was some (but not compelling) evidence for a possible diagnosis of ADHD. However, she was also clear that neither diagnosis would provide much specific guidance to the family to help them reduce the likelihood of explosive outbursts at home. She noted that the various procedures Sam's parents had implemented thus far had not seemed to reduce Sam's difficulties, and questioned whether locking him in his room would ever do the trick.

She conducted a situational analysis for the purpose of exploring factors that seemed to "trigger" Sam's worst moments at home. The parents responded that Sam's worst triggers were "the word 'no'" and "his sister." In an attempt to achieve greater specificity, the psychiatrist asked the parents to describe scenarios in which Sam was most frequently being told "no" and in which he and his sister had the greatest difficulties together. The parents indicated that Sam was frequently told "no" when he wanted to eat certain foods; when he wanted to play alone, away from his sister; when he hit or screamed at his sister, especially when he wanted her to be quiet; and when he asked to watch more than his allotment of cartoons. They further indicated that Sam's difficulties with his sister were fairly constant but were particularly acute when his sister wanted to play with Sam's toys, when she would not follow his directives, and when she played her *Sesame Street* CD. The psychiatrist also met with Sam to determine if he could shed further light on triggers and to get a feel for any developmental issues. When asked what made him upset most often, Sam replied, "My sister…she's annoying." When asked for clarification, Sam said, "She makes too much noise…She plays that stupid *Sesame Street* CD…She always wants to play with the toys I'm playing with…and she won't leave me alone."

The psychiatrist pointed out to Sam's parents that Sam's outbursts actually seemed fairly predictable and therefore permitted proactive interventions that could be used before Sam became so upset that he lost his capacity for rational thought. Based on what she had heard about and observed of Sam, the psychiatrist also suggested that Sam might be lacking important cognitive skills for handling frustration, being flexible, and solving problems. Using a model originated by Greene (Greene 2005; Greene 2008), she inquired more specifically about a host of skills crucial for handling demands for flexibility, frustration tolerance, and problem solving and subsequently surmised that Sam was beginning to sound like a very black-and-white thinker who had tremendous difficulty shifting from one cognitive configuration to another, seemed to have difficulty appreciating the impact of his behavior on others, and seemed to have trouble separating his emotional response to a problem or frustration from the thinking required for resolving the problem. The psychiatrist described these difficulties as a "developmental delay" of sorts, in many ways similar to other recognized delays "in reading, writing, and arithmetic." The parents inquired about what diagnosis applied to these lagging skills; the psychiatrist responded that no diagnoses really seemed to apply neatly to this constellation of skill deficits. The parents asked if a medication might be helpful; the psychiatrist responded that although medications exist that might "lengthen Sam's fuse," no medication would solve the problems setting the stage for Sam's outbursts or teach him the cognitive skills he lacked. The psychiatrist opined that in Sam's case, medication should be an option of "last resort."

DSM-IV-TR DIAGNOSIS

Axis I   313.81 Oppositional defiant disorder

Axis II   None

Axis III None

Axis IV None

Axis V   Global Assessment of Functioning=65

TREATMENT RECOMMENDATIONS

The psychiatrist refuted the notion that Sam simply required more firm or consistent discipline. She noted that the skills she described Sam as lacking would not be taught via reward and punishment procedures. She also noted that Sam had remarked that he, too, was unhappy with how things were going in the family and was already quite motivated to work on making things better. She recommended that the family begin using the Collaborative Problem-Solving approach (described in Greene 2005, 2008; Greene and Ablon 2005; Greene et al. 2003a, 2003b, 2004). She explained to the parents that this treatment model was aimed at helping them pursue their expectations for Sam, reduce the likelihood of explosive outbursts, and simultaneously teach him the cognitive skills he seemed to be lacking. The psychiatrist began to help Sam's parents prioritize the problems they would be trying to resolve collaboratively with Sam and helped the parents recognize that imposition of adult will was, in fact, a very reliable precipitant to Sam's worst moments. She then began to teach the parents the nuts and bolts of solving problems collaboratively with Sam.

The father, in particular, expressed skepticism about the message being sent to Sam by this new way of doing things.

> **Father:** Isn't Sam going to get the idea that he's always going to get his way?
>
> **Psychiatrist:** No, when you're solving problems collaboratively, the solutions are mutually satisfactory, so your concerns will still be addressed…It's just that Sam's concerns will be addressed as well.
>
> **Father:** He never wants to try to resolve anything when he's upset.
>
> **Psychiatrist:** That's why we're going to resolve the problems causing his outbursts *before* he's upset—*proactively*—rather than waiting for him to get upset before we start trying to solve the problem.
>
> **Father:** This is not the way I was raised.
>
> **Psychiatrist:** Yes, so this is a new way of doing things for all of you. Thankfully, you apparently didn't have the challenges with frustration tolerance, flexibility, and problem solving that Sam has. Sam seems to need a different approach.

In early sessions, the psychiatrist guided the parents and Sam in trying to resolve one problem at a time by proactively working toward mutually satisfactory solutions together. The psychiatrist ensured that all perspectives and concerns related to a particular problem were identified and then invited collaboration aimed at reconciling the concerns. Each week, the parents tried to use the model independently; in early sessions, the psychiatrist began sessions by hearing about these attempts and would then troubleshoot ways in which the process went awry. Slowly, the parents' comfort level with this new way of interacting with their son increased. Problems that had been plaguing their interactions with their son for years began showing signs of resolution. Solutions for sharing toys, eating "treats," allowing Sam his time alone and away from his sister, and the amount of time allotted for television were agreed upon, implemented, and revised as needed.

Each time the psychiatrist heard new stories of the parents' attempts to use the Collaborative Problem-Solving approach, additional information about Sam's difficulties became apparent. Other lagging skills, especially related to pragmatic language, became evident. Together with Sam and his parents, the psychiatrist created a list of four verbalizations Sam could use when he became frustrated with his sister. The parents would provide Sam with reminders of these verbalizations. His parents initially grew frustrated with the lack of immediate results, but the psychiatrist reminded them that as with other developmental delays, this skill would not be trained overnight. Several weeks later, the parents reported that after repeated reminders and practice (and with some revisions to the phrases recommended by Sam), Sam had begun to use the verbalizations (although not every time just yet) and that, correspondingly, the frequency of his aggressive outbursts toward his sister had decreased significantly.

Over the course of eight sessions, progress had been made on resolving many of the problems that had been precipitating a significant percentage of Sam's episodes. The parents had begun solving problems with Sam independent of the psychiatrist. Along the way, the parents stopped using many of the procedures that had been exacerbating Sam's outbursts over the years. Sam became more skilled not only at articulating his concerns but also at generating solutions. Treatment continued for a few more weeks until Sam and his parents felt they were ready to go it alone. They were encouraged to return to treatment as needed at any time in the future.

REFERENCES

Bearss K, Eyberg SM: A test of the parenting alliance theory. Early Educ Dev 9:179–185, 1998

Beck AT, Steer RA, Brown GK: Manual for the Beck Depression Inventory, 2nd Edition. San Antonio, TX, Psychological Corporation, 1996

Brinkmeyer M, Eyberg SM: Parent-child interaction therapy for oppositional children, in Evidence-Based Psychotherapies for Children and Adolescents. Edited by Kazdin AE, Weisz JR. New York, Guilford, 2003, pp 204–223

Campbell S: Behavior problems in preschool children: developmental and family issues. Advances in Clinical Child Psychology 19:1–26, 1997

Crick NR, Dodge KA: A review and reformulation of social information-processing mechanisms in children's social adjustment. Psychol Bull 115:74–101, 1994

Eyberg SM, Pincus D: Eyberg Child Behavior Inventory and Sutter-Eyberg Student Behavior Inventory: Professional Manual. Odessa, FL, Psychological Assessment Resources, 1999

Eyberg SM, Nelson MM, Duke M, et al: Manual for the Dyadic Parent-Child Interaction Coding System, 3rd Edition. 2005. Available at: http://www.phhp.ufl.edu/~eyberg/PCITWEB2004/DPICSfiles/DPICS%20Draft%203.03.pdf. Accessed November 5, 2008.

Greene RW: The Explosive Child: A New Approach for Understanding and Parenting Easily Frustrated, Chronically Inflexible Children, 3rd Edition. New York, HarperCollins, 2005

Greene RW: Lost at School: Why Our Kids With Behavioral Challenges Are Falling Through the Cracks and How We Can Help Them. New York, Scribner, 2008

Greene RW, Ablon JS: Treating Explosive Kids: The Collaborative Problem Solving Approach. New York, Guilford, 2005

Greene RW, Ablon SA, Goring JC: A transactional model of oppositional behavior: underpinnings of the Collaborative Problem Solving approach. J Psychosom Res 55:67–75, 2003a

Greene RW, Ablon SA, Goring JC, et al: Treatment of oppositional defiant disorder in children and adolescents, in Handbook of Interventions That Work With Children and Adolescents: Prevention and Treatment. Edited by Barrett P, Ollendick TH. West Sussex, UK, Wiley, 2003b, pp 369–393

Greene RW, Ablon JS, Goring JC, et al: Effectiveness of Collaborative Problem Solving in affectively dysregulated children with oppositional-defiant disorder: initial findings. J Consult Clin Psychol 72:1157–1164, 2004

Kowatch RA, Fristad M, Birmaher B, et al; Child Psychiatric Workgroup on Bipolar Disorder: Treatment guidelines for children and adolescents with bipolar disorder. J Am Acad Child Adolesc Psychiatry 44:213–235, 2005

Pavuluri MN, Grayczyk P, Carbray J, et al: Child and family focused cognitive behavior therapy in pediatric bipolar disorder. J Am Acad Child Adolesc Psychiatry 43:528–537, 2004a

Pavuluri MN, Henry D, Naylor M, et al: A pharmacotherapy algorithm for stabilization and maintenance of pediatric bipolar disorder. J Am Acad Child Adolesc Psychiatry 43:859–867, 2004b

Pavuluri MN, Henry D, Devineni B, et al: Child Mania Rating Scale: development, reliability and validity. J Am Acad Child Adolesc Psychiatry 45:550–560, 2006

Rubin K, Burgess KB, Dwyer KM, et al: Predicting preschoolers' externalizing behaviors from toddler temperament, conflict, and maternal negativity. Dev Psychol 39:164–176, 2003

Shaffer D, Fisher P, Lucas CP, et al: NIMH Diagnostic Interview Schedule for Children Version IV (NIMH DISC-IV): description, differences from previous versions, and reliability of some common diagnoses. J Am Acad Child Adolesc Psychiatry 39:28–38, 2000

Swanson JM: School Based Assessments and Interventions for ADD Students. Irvine, CA, KC Publishing, 1992

Webster-Stratton C, Hammond M: Predictors of treatment outcome in parent training for families with conduct problem children. Behav Ther 21:319–337, 1990

West AE, Pavuluri MN: Maintenance model of integrated psychosocial treatment in pediatric bipolar disorder. J Am Acad Child Adolesc Psychiatry 46:205–212, 2007

Youngstrom EA, Findling RL, Danielson CK, et al: Discriminative validity of parent report of hypomanic and depressive symptoms on the General Behavior Inventory. Psychol Assess 13:267–276, 2001

■ CHAPTER 21 ■

Toddler With Temper Tantrums

A Careful Assessment of a Dysregulated Preschool Child

Helen Egger, M.D.

CASE PRESENTATION

IDENTIFYING INFORMATION

Jacob is a 4½-year-old boy with no prior psychiatric history. He is an only child who lives with his biological parents.

CHIEF COMPLAINT

Jacob is having difficulty with tantrums, defiance, sleep, and separation anxiety. His parents are concerned that he is "unable to control his emotions." When he is frustrated or things do not "go as he planned," he has a temper tantrum. They describe him as a "mama's boy" who does not like to be separated from his mother. His parents are also worried because he complains of fatigue during the day, despite adequate hours of sleep at night. Jacob's pediatrician referred him to the infant/preschool mental health clinic for a comprehensive mental health evaluation.

Helen Egger, M.D., is Assistant Professor at the Center for Developmental Epidemiology in the Department of Psychiatry and Behavioral Sciences at Duke University Medical Center, and Clinical Director of the Duke Preschool Psychiatric Clinic in Durham, North Carolina (for complete biographical information, see "About the Contributors," p. 613).

INFORMANTS AND STRUCTURE OF THE EVALUATION

Evaluation occurred over three sessions. Jacob's parents attended the first session. Jacob and his parents attended the second and third sessions. Jacob's parents completed several rating scales, which are listed at the end of this case presentation. Information was also obtained over the phone from Jacob's preschool teacher. Results of the assessment and recommendations for treatment were discussed with the parents (without Jacob) during a fourth session.

HISTORY OF PRESENT PROBLEMS

Tantrums and Other Behavioral Problems

Jacob's parents report that Jacob was a "hot-tempered," intense baby whose tantrums started when he was 6 months old. Jacob has frequent (4–10 tantrums each day), violent, and uncontrollable tantrums. According to his mother, on some days the tantrums seem to occur "all day." They can be triggered by frustration or a change in routine, or come "out of the blue." Examples of triggers include the fact that his sock does not fit on his foot the right way, or he wants a blue cup rather than a green cup. He can be happy one moment and then erupt in anger or tears the next moment. When he has a tantrum, Jacob yells, curses, hits his mother, kicks, writhes on the floor, throws objects, bangs his head, and bites himself. Tantrums last from a few minutes to half an hour. They occur primarily at home or when he is out with his parents. Recently, Jacob has been having tantrums with his grandparents and at school.

On certain days, "nothing seems right," and he is irritable, touchy, and easily annoyed by others. On these days, he is also oppositional and defiant, challenging his parents' requests in an angry and rigid manner. As long as "things go his way" and the daily routine remains the same, Jacob can appear happy. His parents often feel that they are "walking on eggshells" because they do not know what will change his mood. Jacob does seem to feel remorseful about his misbehavior and tantrums, particularly if he has been physically aggressive. At times, he will cry inconsolably for an hour or more, saying he is a "bad boy."

Neither his parents nor his teacher reports that Jacob has high levels of hyperactivity or inattention. He is able to sit in his seat at dinner. He does not have difficulty paying attention for sustained periods of time (e.g., doing crafts projects, reading with his parents). Although he interrupts his mother's conversations, intrudes into other children's games, and has trouble waiting his turn, this impulsive and intrusive behavior often seems secondary to anxiety or a lack of social skills.

Sleep Problems

Although Jacob goes to bed at 8 P.M. and wakes at 7 A.M., he is always sluggish and tired in the morning. "When he wakes up, he seems as tired as he did when he went to bed," says his mother. He is a restless sleeper. He complains of fatigue during the day and almost always falls asleep in his car seat when in the car for more than 15 minutes, although he no longer takes regular naps. To fall asleep at night, he needs to have his mother lying beside him in his bed. Every night, he goes into his parents' bed and sleeps the rest of the night next to his mother. Jacob does not have difficulty falling asleep, and he has no nightmares, night terrors, or sleepwalking. His teacher notes that he is often sleepy and complains of fatigue at school.

Anxiety

As noted above, Jacob has difficulty separating from his mother at night. At home, he follows his mother from room to room and becomes upset and begins yelling for her if he finds himself alone in a room. At school, he has difficulty separating from his mother, but after a month of daily crying and clinging, he now separates without as much difficulty. His parents "cannot remember" the last time they went out without Jacob, because he becomes so distressed when they attempt to leave him with a babysitter. He says that he is afraid that his parents will not come back. He also has significant anticipatory worry, repeatedly seeking reassurance from his mother about upcoming events. He is slow to warm up with unfamiliar adults and children, although he is outgoing and friendly when he gets to know others. His parents do not report obsessive thoughts or compulsions.

Mood Symptoms

Jacob's mood is often irritable. His parents describe him as "stressed out" but do not feel that he is a "sad kid." His parents do not report appetite or weight changes, anhedonia, fixated talk or play about death or dying, flights of ideas, pressured speech, racing thoughts, hypersexuality, grandiosity, or bizarre or disorganized behavior.

Past Psychiatric History

Jacob has no previous psychiatric history.

Medical History

Jacob has seasonal allergies and a history of ear infections but no history of hospitalizations, head injuries, accidents, or significant illnesses. He takes no medications and has no known history of drug allergies.

Developmental History

Jacob was born at 42 weeks by cesarean section and weighed 8 lbs 10 oz. He had no difficulties at birth. His mother describes the pregnancy as very stressful because she was on bed rest for the last trimester due to preterm labor. She also had difficulty with breast-feeding.

Jacob met all of his developmental milestones at expected times. His parents describe him as an intense baby who had difficulty with transitions. He has never been a good sleeper. During his first year, he began to bang his head or bite himself when angry or frustrated. No language, gross motor, or fine motor difficulties were noted.

The Peabody Picture Vocabulary Test—Third Edition (Dunn and Dunn 1997) was administered to assess Jacob's receptive vocabulary (i.e., what he understands), which is strongly associated with verbal intelligence. Jacob's standardized score of 121 was in the superior range, the age-equivalent of a child age 6 years 7 months.

SOCIAL HISTORY

Jacob is an only child, as are both parents. His parents (both in their mid-30s) have been married for 15 years. His father works 55–60 hours per week. His mother does not work outside the home. Both parents describe themselves as shy, socially isolated, and "stressed out." Jacob's maternal grandparents live nearby but have become annoyed with Jacob's behaviors and critical of their daughter's parenting. His parents deny a history of major traumas, including physical or sexual abuse.

Jacob attends preschool 5 mornings a week. He enjoys school, although he does not like to say good-bye to his mother in the morning. His teacher notes that Jacob has difficulty controlling his temper, often annoys other children, is often fearful in new situations or with new people, and becomes upset over small changes in routine. Jacob has never been suspended or expelled from school or day care.

His peer relationships are fair. He has very few playdates both because he is not invited to other children's houses and because his mother is concerned about how Jacob might behave if a friend were invited home. He tends to be controlling with peers and will hit or yell if he does not get his way.

FAMILY HISTORY

Jacob's mother has a history of major depression and generalized anxiety. She has been treated effectively in the past with the selective serotonin reuptake inhibitors (SSRIs) Prozac and Paxil. She is not currently taking medication or receiving treatment. The maternal family history is significant for the maternal grandmother's agoraphobia (which was never evaluated or treated). Jacob's father does not report a personal or family history of psychiatric symptoms or treatment. Results of the depression and anxiety screenings of both parents during Jacob's evaluation suggest that his mother currently has clinically significant levels of depressive and anxiety symptoms.

MENTAL STATUS EXAMINATION

Jacob was observed during two sessions. Jacob is a cute and articulate 4-year-old boy who was cooperative but initially wary when he met the interviewer. After this initial hesitancy, he had good eye contact with the interviewer. By the end of the session, he was smiling and engaged, although he preferred to remain physically close to his mother and repeatedly checked in with her visually. The interviewer observed Jacob's many strengths (i.e., intelligence, curiosity, enthusiasm, cooperativeness, warmth), as well as his mother's strengths as a parent (i.e., warm, supportive). Jacob's and his mother's interactions were mutually warm and close. Although he clearly enjoyed playing with her, he also seemed worried about doing things correctly. When putting together a puzzle with her, he repeatedly asked her if he had put the piece in the right place, despite her supportive reassurance. He was able to separate from his mother, but his affect became anxious and sad while she was gone, and he complained of feeling tired. He was visibly relieved when she returned. He said that he was a "happy kid" except that he is "sad" when he is "bad." He said that he is afraid of being alone in the house. He worries that something bad will happen to his mother. At the end of the session, he became physically exuberant, although not disruptive. He was able to leave the playroom without difficulty.

CLINICAL ASSESSMENT AND OBSERVATION

The following lists include the record reviews, interviews, and testing that were done so the clinician could fully consider Jacob's case. For reviews of measures for assessing preschool psychopathology, see Carter et al. (2004), DelCarmen-Wiggins and Carter (2004), Egger et al. (2006), Luby (2006), and Zeanah (2000).

RECORD REVIEWS AND INTERVIEWS

- Review of available records
- Clinical interview with parents
- Developmental and family history questionnaire
- Parent section of Disruptive Behavior Diagnostic Observation Schedule (Wakschlag et al. 2005, 2008a, 2008b)
- Clinician-child play
- Phone interview with teacher

PARENT QUESTIONNAIRES

- Child Behavior Checklist 1½–5 (Achenbach and Rescorla 2000)
- Early Childhood Symptom Inventory–4: Parent Checklist (Gadow and Sprafkin 1997; Gadow et al. 2001)

- Temperament and Atypical Behavior Scale (Neisworth et al. 1999)
- Parenting Stress Index—Short Form (Abidin 1995)
- Family Impact Survey (Ford and Barlow 1994)
- Beck Depression Inventory—Second Edition (Beck et al. 1996)
- Beck Anxiety Inventory (Beck and Steer 1993)

TEACHER QUESTIONNAIRE

- Early Childhood Symptom Inventory–4: Teacher Checklist (Sprafkin and Gadow 1996)
- Social Skills Rating System (Fantuzzo et al. 1998; Gresham and Elliott 1990)

TESTING

- Peabody Picture Vocabulary Test—Third Edition (Dunn and Dunn 1997)

COMMENTARIES

Psychotherapeutic Perspective

M. Jamila Reid, Ph.D.
Carolyn Webster-Stratton, Ph.D.

DIAGNOSTIC FORMULATION

The description of Jacob's history and his current behavior indicate both defiant-disruptive and anxious-fearful symptoms. It is not uncommon for young children to exhibit both externalizing and internalizing behaviors, and the cli-

M. Jamila Reid, Ph.D., is Affiliate Assistant Professor in the Department of Psychology and on the staff of the Parenting Clinic at the University of Washington in Seattle, Washington.

Carolyn Webster-Stratton, Ph.D., is Professor in the Department of Psychology and and Director of the Parenting Clinic at the University of Washington in Seattle, Washington.

For complete biographical information, see "About the Contributors," p. 613.

nician may have difficulty teasing apart the etiology of the two groups of behaviors. The most likely primary diagnosis for Jacob is oppositional defiant
disorder (ODD). Jacob's history of intense tantrums and reactive behavior at
an early age is consistent with the ODD diagnosis. His current oppositional,
defiant, and challenging behaviors at home and at school are also typical of
ODD.

Jacob's fears of separation from his mother at bedtime and at school, as well as
his anticipatory worries about upcoming separations, are somewhat consistent with
separation anxiety disorder. However, although Jacob's symptoms are in excess of
those exhibited by many 4-year-old children, they may not currently be severe
enough to warrant a diagnosis. Moreover, they are frequently part of the oppositional behavior problems and are likely to have been reinforced by his parents' responses. Many young children prefer to sleep with their parents and exhibit some
fear when faced with new settings, and if the parents are anxious, inconsistent, and
unpredictable, they can reinforce the children's sense of insecurity. Part of typical
development is experiencing the discomfort of separations and learning the predictability of reunions. If these normal separations and reunions occur frequently
and without excess parental distress and negativity, most children learn to accept
the separations with a minimum of discomfort. Prior to making a diagnosis of separation anxiety disorder, the clinician needs to examine the predictability of the
routines that have been established around separations at home (including bedtime) and at school. Jacob's fears and separation tantrums may be exacerbated by
his ODD behaviors and temperamental difficulties, because his extreme responses to change may have made it more likely that his parents will "give in,"
thereby reinforcing his desire to be with them at all times. For example, their willingness to let him sleep in their bed and their inability to go out for an evening indicate their difficulty with limit setting. The parents also report being shy and
socially isolated, so Jacob has likely had fewer early separation experiences than
other children his age. If, after treatment, Jacob continues to experience intense
separation difficulties and fears, then an anxiety diagnosis could be revisited.

Parent report, direct observation of the child, and teacher report are all important in assessing this family. Looking at Jacob's behavior across the home
and school settings provides information on how he reacts to different caregivers. His scores on standardized questionnaires would provide interesting information on how his behavior compares to that of other children his age, as well
as a baseline against which therapy progress can be measured.

Both Jacob and his parents report that he is fatigued during the day despite
apparently adequate hours of sleep. Therefore, the clinician needs to rule out
a sleep disorder, such as sleep apnea, because lack of sleep could contribute
significantly to irritability and behavioral difficulties.

DSM-IV-TR DIAGNOSIS

Axis I   313.81 Oppositional defiant disorder

Axis II   None

Axis III   Rule out sleep disorder (e.g., apnea)

Axis IV   Problems with primary support group
          Educational problems

Axis V   Global Assessment of Functioning=60 (current)

TREATMENT RECOMMENDATIONS

Parent management training is the recommended treatment for oppositional behavior in young children and would be appropriate in Jacob's case. Brestan and
Eyberg (1998) identified only two treatments as well established for children in
Jacob's age range; both are parent training programs. The first intervention is
based on Patterson and Gullion's (1968) manual *Living With Children*, and the
second is Webster-Stratton's Incredible Years Parent Training Series (e.g., Webster-Stratton and Hammond 1997; Webster-Stratton et al. 2004). These two treatments share a similar foundation in social learning principles, and either would
be appropriate for this family. Both programs have demonstrated outcomes, including changes in parent behavior (more positive and less coercive parenting)
and in child behavior (less aggressive and noncompliant behavior and more cooperative and prosocial behavior) in comparison to untreated controls. *Living
With Children* has primarily been researched and delivered in an individual format, whereas the Incredible Years program uses a group model. Because Jacob's
family is somewhat isolated and has little external support, the group format of the
Incredible Years program might provide community support for Jacob's parents,
as well as providing some normalizing frame of reference for their concerns.

The Incredible Years parent program content focuses on strengthening
parent competencies, fostering parents' involvement with school, decreasing
children's problem behaviors, and strengthening children's social, emotional,
and academic competencies. The treatment program is delivered in a 20-week
group format in which a trained leader facilitates discussions and collaborations among parents about parenting issues. Videotaped vignettes of parents in
a variety of common parenting situations serve as starting points for these discussions, and role-plays and homework assignments provide opportunities for
parents to practice new skills. Parents are also encouraged to provide support
and feedback to each other. Jacob's parents would each be assigned "buddies"
to call and check in with during the course of the therapy group. Frequently,
participating parents feel for the first time that they can be honest with other
parents about the difficulties they are facing with their children, and many establish close friendships that last beyond the group sessions. For Jacob's par-

ents, this relationship building might prove to be a valuable part of the group experience because it will decrease their sense of isolation.

The program begins by having parents identify their own individual goals for their children and themselves. Jacob's parents' goals would likely include learning ways to respond that would help Jacob to regulate his extreme emotional responses, to comply with their requests, to sleep in his own bed, to separate from them and feel confident about his ability to cope with new situations on his own, and to interact with peers in a prosocial way.

After parents set their goals, the therapists begin to work with the group in a collaborative way to introduce the program material and help parents apply each topic to their own situation. Program topics include child-directed play, social and emotional coaching, encouragement, praise, tangible reinforcement, monitoring, setting up predictable schedules and routines, ignoring, limit setting, natural and logical consequences, time-out, and problem solving. A therapist working with Jacob's parents would help them think about the way their interactions with Jacob could begin to meet their goals for him. For instance, Jacob's parents would be encouraged to apply "the attention principle" to their goals for helping Jacob to become less fearful of separations. During play sessions and other interactions with Jacob, they would be encouraged to use emotion coaching and to comment on times when he was calm, brave, confident, and independent. The therapists would also discuss with the parents the value of providing less attention around fearful and withdrawal behaviors. For instance, instead of providing extensive comfort at times when Jacob was upset at the thought of separation, they would be helped to provide a predictable separation routine including brief reassurance, then expression of confidence that Jacob will be fine in their absence, followed by ignoring of the protests and tantrums. In the group, the parents would practice a routine such as the following: "Jacob, I know you are sad that I am going to leave, but I'm sure that you're going to have a good time today. Remember how much fun you had yesterday building with the LEGO blocks? I love you, and I will see you this afternoon." At that point, his parents would be coached to leave, even if Jacob expressed continued distress or tantrums. The fact that Jacob seems to enjoy school after the initial separation seems promising for his eventual adjustment to separations. Jacob's teacher would also be encouraged to notice and comment on his ability to cope with his sad feelings. "Wow! I know that you were sad when your mom left, but you started making a really tall tower with the LEGO blocks, and it looks to me like you're feeling better and are happy now. That was a brave choice to make!"

A similar approach would be taken to help Jacob's parents think about his tantrums and noncompliant behavior. During the initial sessions on child-directed play, his parents would be encouraged to let Jacob take the lead during daily play sessions, thereby providing Jacob with consistent parental attention and control over one part of his interactions with his parents. During these play sessions, his parents would learn social and emotional coaching skills so that they would comment on times when Jacob was cooperative, friendly, and calm, and when he was using appropriate social skills such as sharing and helping. As the program progressed, they would think about what behaviors they wanted to praise (e.g., cooperation, accepting "no"), as well as what behaviors they wanted to ignore (e.g., tantrums, whining). They would learn how to set up an incentive system for specific target behaviors (e.g., compliance to their limit setting or requests) and, finally, to use selected consequences (time-out or privilege removal) for repeated noncompliance or aggressive behavior.

In addition to learning cognitive-behavioral principles, parents in the Incredible Years program are helped to understand and accept individual differences in their child's temperament, needs for attention, and ability to regulate emotions, as well as to learn how their child's unique "wiring" will determine particular parenting approaches. Jacob has a fairly long history of being emotionally volatile, irritable, and shy or anxious. Therapists would problem-solve with the group about how children with this kind of temperament require their parents to model patience and calm responses and to provide practice for their children in how to calm down (using puppets or stories) as well as learning trials in following parents' directions. Jacob's parents would spend time thinking about ways that they could be proactive in their parenting to meet Jacob's temperament needs. Perhaps Jacob needs a longer bedtime routine and more transition time before going to sleep on his own, or maybe the parents need to provide more predictable structure to his day and more positive play times so that he feels secure in his relationship with them.

The Incredible Years Advance parent program also covers material on adult and child anger management, adult mood regulation, working with schools and teachers, academic success, communication, problem solving with adults and children, and encouraging children's positive peer relationships. Because Jacob's social and behavioral difficulties extend to the school setting, the material on working with the school and his classroom teacher would be particularly relevant. In addition, because Jacob's mother has a history of depression, some of the mood regulation material in the program might help her to understand how her own mood responses both provide modeling for and impact her responses to Jacob's behavior. After getting to know Jacob's mother in the group format, therapists would also work with her to determine whether a referral for her own depressive and anxious symptoms is warranted. Occasionally, the support of the group and the assistance around parenting issues make this unnecessary, but for parents with serious depression and anxiety, individual therapy and/or medication would be recommended.

The Incredible Years series also has a child treatment program, called Dinosaur School, and a teacher classroom management program. Dinosaur School would provide direct training to Jacob in a group of five other children. Children learn appropriate ways to be in a group and to follow developmentally appropriate school rules and routines. Units on feelings, problem solving, anger management, friendship, and communication are individualized to address the needs of each child in the group. The teacher training program covers content similar to that delivered in the parent program, but specific to the school context. Webster-Stratton et al. (2004) found that children whose behavior was pervasive across home and school settings benefited from adding either the child or the teacher program to the parent program. If Jacob's behavior continues to be challenging after participation in the parent program, then adding either the child or the teacher program would be recommended.

Psychopharmacologic Perspective

Joan L. Luby, M.D.

DIAGNOSTIC FORMULATION

Jacob, a 4½-year-old boy, presents with prominent symptoms of anxiety associated with behavioral rigidity and oppositionality. Temper tantrums precipitated by Jacob's inability to adhere to rigid routines or minor frustrations and characterized by physical aggression directed at others occur multiple times daily. Separation and anticipatory anxieties are also daily occurrences. Of importance is the absence of symptoms indicative of a mood disorder, such as elated or sad mood, grandiosity, or hypersexuality. Daytime fatigue despite sufficient sleep is described. However, no other neurovegetative signs (e.g., change in appetite) are present, and Jacob does not appear anhedonic or preoccupied with negative or death themes in play.

In this case, the absence of key symptoms and the presence of symptoms are both informative to the diagnostic formulation. Although irritable mood and disruptive behavior are prominent, the absence of any evidence of grandi-

Joan L. Luby, M.D., is Associate Professor of Psychiatry (Child) and Founder and Director of the Early Emotional Development Program at the Washington University School of Medicine in St. Louis, Missouri (for complete biographical information, see "About the Contributors," p. 613).

osity, elation, decreased need for sleep, and racing thoughts suggests that bipolar disorder is an unlikely diagnosis. Although Jacob is described as oppositional and rigid, he is not described as having an inflated sense of powers and abilities. In addition, and central to a diagnosis of bipolar disorder, the case description does not indicate that Jacob demonstrates a sustained elated mood. Elated mood, as opposed to normative joyful moods highly typical of a preschool child, would be demonstrated by a sustained and intense elevated mood that arises without an apparent precipitant and cannot be alleviated.

Along these lines, despite Jacob's prominent anxiety, the absence of anhedonia, preoccupation with death (in thoughts or play), or persistent sad mood also suggests that the diagnosis of depression is unlikely. Although symptoms of depression are often seen in anxious children, this case is notable for the absence of specific symptoms of depression. Outside of irritability, a highly nonspecific symptom in young children, the only symptom that might suggest depression is Jacob's daytime fatigue despite adequate sleep at night. Neurovegetative signs and symptoms, such as changes in sleep and appetite patterns, have been shown to be specific to depression and are known to characterize a more severe melancholic subtype (Luby et al. 2004).

Another important diagnosis to rule out in this case is a pervasive developmental disorder. The presence of behavioral rigidity, anxiety that also has an obsessive component, and some suggestion of impairment in peer play raises some concern for this diagnosis. However, Jacob's social interest in peers and his ability for age-appropriate social interaction after becoming more comfortable in an unfamiliar situation, as well as his lack of other developmental delays, suggest that this diagnosis is also unlikely.

Anxiety appears to be the central and most impairing symptom for Jacob. Given the absence of key specific symptoms of a mood disorder, as described above, the most likely diagnosis is an anxiety disorder with comorbid ODD. Based on the symptoms described, he would appear to meet criteria for separation anxiety disorder as well as generalized anxiety disorder. Considering the prominence of anxiety, the likelihood that the oppositional and disruptive behaviors are related to the underlying anxiety and rigidity must be considered. That is, due to his high levels of anxiety, Jacob needs his environment to be controlled and predictable. When the environment deviates, he becomes overwhelmed with anxiety and acts out disruptively. The case represents an interesting example of a child with both internalizing and externalizing psychopathology who does not have a clinical picture suggestive of bipolar disorder.

DSM-IV-TR DIAGNOSIS

Axis I   309.21 Separation anxiety disorder
          300.02 Generalized anxiety disorder

313.81 Oppositional defiant disorder

Axis II   None

Axis III   Rule out medical etiology for daytime fatigue

Axis IV   Mild psychosocial stressors

Axis V   Global Assessment of Functioning=60

TREATMENT RECOMMENDATIONS

Before proceeding with treatment, the clinician should conduct a comprehensive evaluation that includes observation of dyadic play between the primary caregiver and Jacob. Ideally, the child should be observed on more than one occasion and with more than one caregiver so that state- and relationship-specific elements of his mental state can be considered. A number of standardized measures of early-onset psychopathology are now available for research use. Although some may be useful as an adjunct to a clinical evaluation, a detailed history and multisession observation are essential and have become the standard of care for the assessment of a preschool-age child (Thomas et al. 1997).

Psychotherapeutic treatment should be the primary intervention for anxiety disorders and ODD during the preschool period. Because insufficient empirical data are available to guide psychopharmacologic treatment for children in this age group, psychotherapeutic interventions, which have fewer inherent risks, are considered primary. Furthermore, the use of medications in preschoolers is, in almost all cases, off-label because controlled data on safety and efficacy remain unavailable. However, if Jacob's symptoms of anxiety and ODD remain impairing and unresponsive to a reasonable trial of psychotherapy, pharmacologic treatment would be a next step. Medications should be initiated only after a detailed discussion with parents about other treatment alternatives, the off-label use, and the unknown effects on growth and development, after which formal consent should be obtained.

In Jacob's case, symptoms of anxiety appear to be central to the clinical picture and may underlie temper tantrums and aggression. Therefore, an anxiolytic would be the medication class of first choice. Because paradoxical activation has been observed frequently with benzodiazepines in children, particularly in young children, this class of agents is not appropriate for treatment of preschoolers' anxiety disorders. Furthermore, sedation is a highly undesirable side effect in a preschooler, another reason why benzodiazepines are not a feasible treatment option. The SSRIs have been shown to be effective in the treatment of anxiety disorders in older children and would be the class of agents of first choice (Hammerness et al. 2006). However, some evidence suggests that paradoxical activation, a known side effect of the SSRIs in children, may occur even more frequently in younger children (Zuckerman et al. 2007). For this reason, as well as given the small size of preschool children, titration should be very slow, with careful monitoring for side effects. When preschool children are taking an SSRI, they should be monitored closely by parents and seen frequently in the clinic, especially as the dose is titrated upward.

The choice of a specific SSRI is based largely on the treating clinician's preferences, clinical experience, and comfort level. Because the largest database for children is available for fluoxetine, many clinicians prescribe this medication. This issue of which medications are more likely to produce activation remains unclear and anecdotal. In general, medications would not be indicated for the treatment of ODD per se, unless symptoms were unusually severe and unresponsive to behavioral management. In Jacob's case, the symptoms of ODD will likely subside as his anxiety is diminished.

Integrative Perspective

Helen Egger, M.D.

DIAGNOSTIC FORMULATION

Jacob is a very bright, appealing 4-year-old boy with clinically significant symptoms, including difficulty controlling his anger and frustration, aggressive tantrums, oppositional behavior, separation anxiety, and sleep difficulties. Jacob's symptoms occur most frequently with his parents, particularly his mother. He has similar symptoms at school, but they are much less frequent and intense. They are causing significant disturbances and distress at home and in his relationships with his parents, other adults, and peers. Recently, the symptoms have begun to increase at school and affect his school functioning.

Jacob meets criteria for separation anxiety disorder, based on his difficulty being physically separated from his mother, his fears of her not returning or of harm befalling her, his difficulty falling asleep or sleeping through the night alone, and his difficulty separating to attend school (Egger and Angold 2006a, 2006b). Jacob also meets criteria for ODD, based on his irritability, defiance, arguing, and severe and frequent tantrums. The intensity and frequency of these behaviors and his dysregulated anger are much greater than found in typically developing preschoolers (Egger and Angold 2006b). He has begun to demonstrate these behaviors with other adults, with peers, and outside of the home, and the behaviors are adversely affecting his relationships with his parents and other adults and children, suggesting that the behaviors are becoming more pervasive and uncontrollable. Studies have shown that preschoolers with anxiety or depression commonly also have tantrums and may meet criteria for ODD (Egger and Angold 2006b). Frequent tantrums that are aggressive (hitting, biting, kicking, or breaking objects) are strongly associated with both emotional disorders, particularly separation anxiety disorder and depression, and behavioral disorders such as ODD (Egger and Angold 2006b). Although Jacob presents with other symptoms of ODD, he may well be expressing his anxious distress through his irritability and tantrums. Treatment must address his anxiety symptoms and distress, not merely his dysregulated anger and aggressive and out-of-control tantrums (Egger and Angold 2006a).

Although Jacob does not meet criteria for a depressive disorder at this time, his irritability, intermittent sadness, guilt, tiredness, and sleep problems suggest that he might be at risk for a depressive disorder. Although his severe emotional dysregulation and tantrums could be described as mood swings, he does not have other symptoms of mania, such as excessive talking, pressured speech, grandiosity, hypersexuality, or decreased need for sleep.

A prominent symptom described by Jacob's parents and observed in the clinic assessment is Jacob's daytime fatigue. In the clinic, his fatigue seemed to be a response to anxiety. However, his parents describe a persistent pattern of restless, nonrestorative sleep, night waking, morning sleepiness, and persistent tiredness and fatigue. These may be symptoms of an anxiety disorder (e.g., generalized anxiety disorder) or depressive disorder but also may reflect a primary sleep disorder. Jacob's sleep difficulties may be contributing to or be one cause of his emotional and behavioral dysregulation (Bates et al. 2002; Lavigne et al. 1999).

The other clinically significant finding in this evaluation is that Jacob's mother is experiencing moderate to severe depression, moderate anxiety, and severe stress in her role as a parent. Jacob's father is experiencing stress at his job and seems detached and emotionally withdrawn from Jacob and his mother. The mother's depression and anxiety and the family stress may also be contributing to Jacob's own anxiety and difficulty managing his anger and aggression (Beardslee et al. 1993a, 1996; Carter et al. 2001; Kim-Cohen et al. 2005; Needlman et al. 1991; Webster-Stratton and Hammond 1988).

DSM-IV-TR DIAGNOSIS

Axis I   307.47 Dyssomnia not otherwise specified (NOS)

309.21 Separation anxiety disorder

313.81 Oppositional defiant disorder

Rule out generalized anxiety disorder

Rule out depressive disorder NOS

Axis II   None

Axis III   History of ear infections, seasonal allergies

Axis IV   Significant parental stress

Maternal depression and anxiety

Parental occupational stress

Possible marital stress due to child's behaviors

Family social isolation

Axis V   Jacob's Global Assessment of Functioning=70

Mother's Global Assessment of Functioning=60

TREATMENT RECOMMENDATIONS

PARENT SUPPORT AND PARENTING SKILLS

Jacob's parents are encouraged to work with the clinician to develop consistent and effective parenting strategies to help Jacob develop ways to manage his feelings and behaviors, to reduce the conflict and stress at home, and to increase Jacob's compliance and cooperation (Nixon 2002; Webster-Stratton and Hammond 1997).

COGNITIVE-BEHAVIORAL THERAPY

Jacob and his parents should participate in an 8- to 12-week course of cognitive-behavioral therapy (CBT) focused on helping him and his parents learn and practice strategies to reduce and manage his anxiety (Compton et al. 2002; Egger and Angold 2006a; Farmer et al. 2002; Ollendick and March 2004).

REFERRAL FOR A SLEEP EVALUATION

Because Jacob's sleep is nonrestorative and he is tired much of the day, Jacob should have a workup at a sleep disorders clinic to rule out a primary sleep disorder, such as sleep apnea, that might be effectively treated and could be one cause of, not simply a symptom of, his emotional and behavioral symptoms (Anders and Eiben 2000).

PSYCHIATRIC TREATMENT FOR JACOB'S MOTHER

Jacob's mother should seek treatment for her depression and anxiety. Recommended treatment might be a combination of medication for the depression and anxiety symptoms and then short-term CBT to provide effective coping tools. CBT might not only help Jacob's mother feel better about herself, as an individual and as a parent, but also provide a much needed source of support. These interventions would likely significantly reduce the stress that the family is experiencing (Beardslee et al. 1992, 1993b).

RESPITE

Jacob's parents also should consider obtaining some child care for Jacob, either in the afternoon, on weekends, or in the evening. The clinician's experience with Jacob during the examination suggests that he will be able to connect with and have fun with a friendly caregiver, such as a graduate student, for a few hours. Regular child care may reduce the mother's parenting stress, give her time to do some things for herself (e.g., take a walk, have coffee with a friend), and provide time for the parents to be together as a couple. Jacob's parents expressed anxiety and shyness about finding a babysitter. This anxiety might be addressed and practical solutions developed in CBT.

After these evaluations and interventions are completed, the preschool mental health team should reevaluate Jacob. If a significant reduction has not occurred in Jacob's symptoms and the impairment they are causing at home, other therapeutic interventions should be considered, including psychotherapy and medications (Gleason et al. 2007).

REFERENCES

Abidin RR: Parenting Stress Index, 3rd Edition: Professional Manual. Lutz, FL, Psychological Assessment Resources, 1995

Achenbach TM, Rescorla LA: Manual for the ASEBA Preschool Forms and Profiles: An Integrated System of Multi-Informant Assessment. Burlington, University of Vermont Department of Psychiatry, 2000

Anders T, Eiben L: Sleep disorders, in Handbook of Infant Mental Health. Edited by Zeanah CH Jr. New York, Guilford, 2000, pp 326–338

Angold A, Egger HL: Preschool psychopathology: lessons for the lifespan. J Child Psychol Psychiatry 48:961–966, 2007

Angold A, Egger H, Carter A: The measurement of psychopathology in children under the age of six, in Age and Gender Considerations in Psychiatric Diagnosis: A Research Agenda for DSM-V. Edited by Narrow W, First M, Sirovatka P, et al. Arlington, VA, American Psychiatric Association, 2007, pp 177–189

Bates J, Viken RJ, Alexander D, et al: Sleep and adjustment in preschool children: sleep diary reports by mothers relate to behavior reports by teachers. Child Dev 73:62–74, 2002

Beardslee WR, Hoke L, Wheelock I, et al: Initial findings on preventive intervention for families with parental affective disorders. Am J Psychiatry 149:1335–1340, 1992

Beardslee WR, Keller MB, Lavori PW, et al: The impact of parental affective disorder on depression in offspring: a longitudinal follow-up in a non-referred sample. J Am Acad Child Adolesc Psychiatry 32:723–730, 1993a

Beardslee WR, Salt P, Porterfield K, et al: Comparison of preventive interventions for families with parental affective disorder. J Am Acad Child Adolesc Psychiatry 32:254–263, 1993b

Beardslee WR, Keller MB, Seifer R, et al: Prediction of adolescent affective disorder: effects of prior parental affective disorders and child psychopathology. J Am Acad Child Adolesc Psychiatry 35:279–288, 1996

Beck AT, Steer RA: Beck Anxiety Inventory Manual. San Antonio, TX, Harcourt Assessment, 1993

Beck AT, Steer RA, Brown GK: Beck Depression Inventory Manual, 2nd Edition. San Antonio, TX, Harcourt Assessment, 1996

Brestan EV, Eyberg SM: Effective psychosocial treatments of conduct-disordered children and adolescents: 29 years, 82 studies, and 5,272 kids. J Clin Child Psychol 27:180–189, 1998

Carter AS, Garrity-Rokous FE, Chazan-Cohen R, et al: Maternal depression and comorbidity: predicting early parenting, attachment security, and toddler social-emotional problems and competencies. J Am Acad Child Adolesc Psychiatry 40:18–26, 2001

Carter AS, Briggs-Gowan MJ, Davis NO: Assessment of young children's social-emotional development and psychopathology: recent advances and recommendations for practice. J Child Psychol Psychiatry 45:109–134, 2004

Compton SN, Burns BJ, Egger HL, et al: Review of the evidence base for treatment of childhood psychopathology: internalizing disorders. J Consult Clin Psychol 70:1240–1266, 2002

DelCarmen-Wiggins R, Carter A (eds): Handbook of Infant, Toddler, and Preschool Mental Health Assessment. New York, Oxford University Press, 2004

Dunn LM, Dunn LM: Peabody Picture Vocabulary Test, 3rd Edition. Circle Pines, MN, American Guidance Service, 1997

Egger HL, Angold A: Anxiety disorders, in Handbook of Preschool Mental Health: Development, Disorders, and Treatment. Edited by Luby J. New York, Guilford, 2006a, pp 137–164

Egger HL, Angold A: Common emotional and behavioral disorders in preschool children: presentation, nosology, and epidemiology. J Child Psychol Psychiatry 47:313–337, 2006b

Egger HL, Erkanli A, Keeler G, et al: The test-retest reliability of the Preschool Age Psychiatric Assessment (PAPA). J Am Acad Child Adolesc Psychiatry 45:538–549, 2006

Fantuzzo JW, Manz PH, McDermott PA: Preschool version of the Social Skills Rating System: an empirical analysis of its use with low-income children. J Sch Psychol 36:199–214, 1998

Farmer EMZ, Compton SN, Burns JB, et al: Review of the evidence base for treatment of childhood psychopathology: externalizing disorders. J Consult Clin Psychol 70:1267–1302, 2002

Ford J, Barlow J: The Ru Rua Family Impact Survey. J Intellect Dev Disabil 19:121–138, 1994

Gadow KD, Sprafkin J: Early Childhood Symptom Inventory, 4th Edition, Norms Manual. Stony Brook, NY, Checkmate Plus, 1997

Gadow KD, Sprafkin J, Nolan EE: DSM-IV symptoms in community and clinic preschool children. J Am Acad Child Adolesc Psychiatry 40:1383–1392, 2001

Gleason MM, Egger HL, Emslie GJ, et al: Psychopharmacological treatment for very young children: contexts and guidelines. J Am Acad Child Adolesc Psychiatry 46:1532–1572, 2007

Gresham F, Elliott S: Social Skills Rating System Manual. Circle Pines, MN, American Guidance Service, 1990

Hammerness P, Vivas F, Geller D: Selective serotonin reuptake inhibitors in pediatric psychopharmacology: a review of the evidence. J Pediatr 148:158–165, 2006

Kim-Cohen J, Moffitt TE, Taylor A, et al: Maternal depression and children's antisocial behavior. Arch Gen Psychiatry 62:173–181, 2005

Lavigne JV, Arend R, Rosenbaum D, et al: Sleep and behavior problems among preschoolers. J Dev Behav Pediatr 20:164–169, 1999

Luby J (ed): Handbook of Preschool Mental Health: Development, Disorders, and Treatment. New York, Guilford, 2006

Luby JL, Mrakotsky CM, Heffelfinger A, et al: Characteristics of depressed preschoolers with and without anhedonia: evidence for a melancholic depressive subtype in young children. Am J Psychiatry 161:1998–2004, 2004

Needlman R, Stevenson J, Zuckerman B: Psychosocial correlates of severe temper tantrums. J Dev Behav Pediatr 12:77–83, 1991

Neisworth JT, Bagnato SJ, Salvia JJ, et al: Temperament and Atypical Behavior Scale (TABS): Early Childhood Indicators of Developmental Dysfunction. Baltimore, MD, Paul H Brookes, 1999

Nixon RDV: Treatment of behavior problems in preschoolers: a review of parent training programs. Clin Psychol Rev 22:525–546, 2002

Ollendick T, March JS: Phobic and Anxiety Disorders in Children and Adolescents: A Clinician's Guide to Effective Psychosocial and Pharmacological Interventions. New York, Oxford University Press, 2004

Patterson GR, Gullion ME: Living With Children: New Methods for Parents and Teachers. Champaign, IL, Research Press, 1968

Sprafkin J, Gadow KD: Early Childhood Inventories Manual. Stony Brook, NY, Checkmate Plus, 1996

Thomas JM, Benham AL, Gean M, et al: Practice parameters for the psychiatric assessment of infants and toddlers (0–36 months). J Am Acad Child Adolesc Psychiatry 36 (suppl 10):21S–36S, 1997

Wakschlag LS, Leventhal B, Briggs-Gowan MJ, et al: Defining the "disruptive" in preschool behavior: what diagnostic observation can teach us. Clin Child Fam Psychol Rev 8:183–201, 2005

Wakschlag LS, Briggs-Gowan MJ, Hill C, et al: Observational assessment of preschool disruptive behavior, part II: validity of the Disruptive Behavior Diagnostic Observation Schedule (DB-DOS). J Am Acad Child Adolesc Psychiatry 47:632–641, 2008a

Wakschlag LS, Hill C, Carter AS, et al: Observational assessment of preschool disruptive behavior, part I: reliability of the Disruptive Behavior Diagnostic Observation Schedule (DB-DOS). J Am Acad Child Adolesc Psychiatry 47:622–631, 2008b

Webster-Stratton C, Hammond M: Maternal depression and its relationship to life stress, perceptions of child behavior problems, parenting behaviors, and child conduct problems. J Abnorm Child Psychol 16:299–315, 1988

Webster-Stratton C, Hammond M: Treating children with early onset conduct problems: a comparison of child and parent training interventions. J Consult Clin Psychol 65:93–109, 1997

Webster-Stratton C, Reid MJ, Hammond M: Treating children with early onset conduct problems: intervention outcomes for parent, child, and teacher training. J Clin Child Adolesc Psychol 33:105–124, 2004

Zeanah CH Jr (ed): Handbook of Infant Mental Health, 2nd Edition. New York, Guilford, 2000

Zuckerman ML, Vaughan BL, Whitney J, et al: Tolerability of selective serotonin reuptake inhibitors in thirty-nine children under seven: a retrospective chart review. J Child Adolesc Psychopharmacol 17:165–174, 2007

■ CHAPTER 22 ■

Won't Leave His Room

Clinical High Risk for Developing Psychosis

Cheryl M. Corcoran, M.D.

CASE PRESENTATION

IDENTIFYING INFORMATION

James is a 15-year-old adolescent who was referred for social withdrawal, declining school function, some depressive symptoms, and school refusal. He lives with his mother and older brother. He was referred by his school counselor.

CHIEF COMPLAINT

"I don't know why my school wanted me to come here today."

HISTORY OF PRESENT ILLNESS

James has always been somewhat shy and awkward, although he has had some close friends and maintained an A to B average in school. His mother reports that during his recent summer vacation, he spent a few weeks in July visiting their extended family in South Carolina, where he spent time with his cousins, hanging out and playing basketball. When he returned, his local friends in New York City

Cheryl M. Corcoran, M.D., is Florence Irving Assistant Professor of Clinical Psychiatry and Director of the Center of Prevention and Evaluation at Columbia University/New York State Psychiatric Institute in New York, New York (for complete biographical information, see "About the Contributors," p. 613).

called to invite him to go to the movies, to play basketball, and so on. However, he usually declined, saying it was too hot to go outside. Instead, he stayed mostly in his room, up to 10 hours at a time, watching cartoon channel episodes and playing multiplayer online games. Instead of joining the family for dinner, he would grab a sandwich and go back to his room. James began to stay up most of the night and sleep during the day. His room became increasingly messy, he changed his clothes less often, and he began showering every other day, only with nagging by his mother. For his birthday, his mother offered to take him to his favorite restaurant, but he was very resistant to this. She coaxed him to go. In the car, he slumped in the backseat, covering his face with his hand. At the restaurant, he kept his menu throughout the meal, hiding his face by holding it upright. He ate all of the shrimp he ordered but without his usual delight.

With the beginning of the school year, James's mother was optimistic that he would do better. In the first few weeks of school, in September, he went to school daily and mostly did his homework. Upon coming home, he still went straight to his room, where he remained on his computer for hours. His room was still quite messy, and he showered and changed clothing only with repeated prodding.

By October, he had become somewhat irritable, especially with a younger niece, who wanted to spend time with him. His clear preference was to be alone. His friends had stopped calling him. His mother said it was like he had become a stranger, unlike himself, and she worried if maybe he was using drugs or if this was just adolescence. His first report card in the fall had mostly C's. His teachers reported that he was very quiet in class, typically looking out the window or doodling and drawing. His English teacher saw his drawings and was impressed by the nihilistic themes, with images of explosions and violence. Although James could complete other types of assignments, he had particular difficulty with writing assignments. He would write a first sentence and then stop, saying he was not sure what else to add. At school, the janitor found him sitting alone in the bathroom after hours; James could not or would not say why he was there.

By December, James refused to go to school, and again would not say why. Resorting to desperate measures, his mother locked him out of the apartment during the day so that he would go to school. When she returned from work, she found him just sitting quietly. At the school's urging, James's mother brought him in for a psychiatric evaluation.

Past Psychiatric History

In the past, he reportedly had "inattention without hyperactivity."

Medical History

James was the product of a full-term, normal vaginal delivery. He had mild asthma as a young boy, for which he was prescribed albuterol inhalers. He has not received steroids, required emergency room admission, or been intubated as a result of his asthma.

DEVELOPMENTAL HISTORY

As an infant and toddler, James was a much easier baby than his brother, who had been colicky. His mother reports that when she took him shopping, he would sit in the cart quietly. James began walking at 14 months. His mother thinks he may have started speaking a little later than his brother, but she is not sure. James responded well to cuddling and played with other children. He has always been a little clumsy and less athletic and outgoing than his brother.

When James went to preschool and then kindergarten, he separated easily, but his teachers noted he was a little shy and needed to be drawn out. He rarely initiated play with other children but joined in when invited. His mother describes him as being more compliant and less mischievous than his brother.

James was referred for evaluation in the second grade for inattention without hyperactivity. The reports have been lost, but his mother reports that he was briefly prescribed a stimulant of unclear dose, which was not particularly helpful. Of note, James was taller than the other boys in his class—like a "gentle giant"—and other children provoked and teased him to see if he would respond. His teachers all liked him immensely and tried to protect him, as they perceived him to be somewhat vulnerable.

James's school performance over several years was marked by A's and B's, compliance, and the development of friendships, although he was somewhat shy and awkward.

SOCIAL HISTORY

James lives in a one-bedroom apartment in northern Manhattan with his mother and older brother, with whom he shares a bedroom. James has never known his father. When he was age 3, he was in foster care for a few months with his brother when his mother was hospitalized (see below). He has no history of abuse or neglect. The family is supported by his mother's salary as a secretary and some income from his older brother.

FAMILY HISTORY

James's mother was hospitalized 25 years ago for an episode of psychosis, which has never recurred. James's mother said that she had thought she was hearing the voice of an older uncle, named Jimmy Carter, who had recently died. She said the doctors mistakenly thought she was having auditory hallucinations of the U.S. president. She was given chlorpromazine briefly and discharged within a few weeks. The symptoms have not recurred, and she has not taken any additional psychiatric medications or received any care since the hospitalization.

Mental Status Examination

James appeared younger than his stated age and was quite slender. He wore age-appropriate clothing, including a basketball jersey and jeans, and a baseball cap turned backward. He appeared awkward and shy and sat quietly while his mother described the course of events leading up to the evaluation.

When interviewed alone, James was compliant with the interview, answering all questions. He maintained fair eye contact and spoke softly, smiling occasionally while tapping his foot. He described his mood as "OK." His thought pattern was a little tangential and at times odd.

When asked about the past few months, James acknowledged that he did prefer to be by himself. He felt uncomfortable around others. He was not sure how to act with his friends and he did not think they liked him much anymore. In crowds, he felt like people looked at him and thought he was weird or menacing, especially as a young, tall black male. He was not sure whether he should make eye contact with others. His neighborhood felt increasingly dangerous, and he felt like he had to look over his shoulder. On the other hand, he did not feel like anyone had singled him out or was plotting against him in any way.

James also reported that he had been thinking a lot about politics, and he thought U.S. society as a whole was controlled by television and mass marketing. He thought George Bush was a "jerk" and wondered if George Bush had something to do with the 9/11 attacks so he could get a lot of power. James acknowledged a lot of fantasizing about blowing up the world—building a tube to the center of the earth and dropping a nuclear bomb—so that all the mistakes and problems would be erased. On the other hand, James has considered that a better approach would be to become a rap star and spread the message of God and love and peace instead.

James also described having feelings of déjà vu every few months, and also wondering if he had dreamed about things before they happened, such as a teacher's being absent from school. He also felt sometimes that if he saw a white car drive by, something bad might happen. He thought these were strange ideas that did not make much sense, and he was not sure why he thought them. He confirmed that his thoughts were clearly his own and he did not feel controlled by anyone or anything else.

When asked about sensory perceptions, James acknowledged that when he returned to New York City from South Carolina in the summer, the city seemed much louder and smellier and dirtier than before. Therefore, he preferred to stay in the apartment. Sometimes, he thought he heard his name in the wind. Late at night, when he was in his bedroom, he sometimes thought he saw a black object moving briefly in the periphery of his vision. However, he denied any voices or any other type of hallucination.

COMMENTARIES

Psychotherapeutic Perspective

Jean Addington, Ph.D.

DIAGNOSTIC FORMULATION

James does not appear to meet criteria for any DSM-IV-TR disorder, although the clinician should rule out depression and seriously consider that he may be developing a psychotic illness. The Structured Interview for Prodromal Syndromes (Miller et al. 2003) can be used to determine if James meets prodromal criteria or may actually have a psychotic illness. From the information presented, James most likely meets criteria for the attenuated psychotic symptom syndrome, which puts him at clinical high risk of developing psychosis. Most notable is his decline in functioning: isolation from friends and family, decline in school performance, and lack of self-care. He describes experiencing unusual thought content, ideas of reference, suspiciousness, grandiosity, and perceptual abnormalities. All of these symptoms are at the attenuated level, none meet psychotic intensity, some may be occurring infrequently, and all have begun or worsened in the past year. He may also have depression, which would be a comorbid diagnosis because these attenuated psychotic symptoms are unlikely to be explained by depression.

DSM-IV-TR DIAGNOSIS

Axis I   Rule out depressive disorder not otherwise specified (NOS)

Axis II   Deferred

Axis III None

Axis IV   None

Axis V   Global Assessment of Functioning=50

Jean Addington, Ph.D., is Professor of Psychiatry at the University of Toronto; Research Scientist and Director of Psychosocial Treatments in the First Episode Psychosis Program; and Director or the PRIME Research Clinic at the Centre for Addiction and Mental Health in Toronto, Ontario, Canada (for complete biographical information, see "About the Contributors," p. 613).

TREATMENT RECOMMENDATIONS

The initial treatment plan for James would include further evaluation, the development of a formulation of the presenting problems, and a cognitive-behavioral approach to treatment. It is necessary to assess all presenting problems that are seen as troubling to James, including those that could potentially increase the risk of developing psychosis, because he appears vulnerable to psychosis. This assessment would help not only to identify targets for treatment but also to develop an individualized case formulation. The recommended therapeutic approach for James is based on a range of assessment, engagement, formulation, and treatment options from authors and researchers around the world described in a treatment handbook for those at risk of developing psychosis (Addington et al. 2006) plus cognitive-behavioral therapy (CBT; French and Morrison 2004).

For James, a cognitive assessment would be useful to determine if there is any evidence of cognitive decline, so that appropriate expectations for school performance could be set. Further assessment would focus on symptoms, behavior, and beliefs about his symptoms. By conducting a comprehensive psychological assessment, the clinician is beginning to educate James about the nature and likely cause of his symptoms and to develop a rationale for treatment that will follow the assessment. The model that is used to explain the possible onset of psychosis is the stress-vulnerability model, which fits well for those at clinical high risk of psychosis.

In developing the formulation, the clinician would want to consider predisposing, precipitating, perpetuating, and protective factors. For James, predisposing factors or life experience would include being shy, awkward, and tall from an early age; the fact that James spent a brief time in foster care; and the family history of psychosis or at least a vulnerability to psychosis. Precipitating and/or perpetuating factors need further exploration but may include teasing in school. Protective factors could be a supportive family and schoolteachers. After gaining a good sense of James's life experiences, the clinician would focus on understanding the beliefs that James has about himself and others. These include his core beliefs about himself that have developed from his life experiences and may include beliefs that he is not a good person, or that people are out to get him, or that he is not likable. Through a brief exploration of his history, the clinician can begin to understand James's self-beliefs.

The next step would be to conceptualize his psychotic-like experiences in terms of events or intrusions. For James, these include people looking at him in a menacing way, but the clinician would also want to pursue the origin of James's political beliefs, as well as details about his seeing the white car and the black object or hearing his name called in the wind. An important goal is to clarify the events and intrusions that he experiences and separate them from the way he makes sense of them. First, the clinician must identify the perceptual anomalies (psychotic-like experiences) and then understand how James makes sense of them. For example, he *thinks* people are looking at him (the event or anomaly) and he *believes* they think he is weird or menacing (how he makes sense of it). The impact on James is that he isolates himself and keeps away from his friends. The connection is that James's core beliefs about himself and the world play a major role in how he interprets the perceptual anomalies that he experiences and the attributions that he makes about his these anomalies.

Therapeutically, work with James would follow several phases (French and Morrison 2004). The first step would focus on normalizing, where possible, some of James's experiences and dealing with the associated distress. Addressing the meaning of the perceptual anomalies and then generating and evaluating alternative explanations for these experiences are typical CBT strategies that would be used at this point. A next step is to address his safety behaviors, which are those responses to the intrusions that instead of helping, actually serve to maintain the dysfunctional interpretations of intrusions. For example, James sees people staring at him; he thinks they see him as "weird." His safety behavior is that he avoids their gaze, does not talk to people, and no longer goes out. The result is that they may indeed think he is "weird." A third step is to address and challenge his core beliefs. Strategies for these steps are well described in two texts (Addington et al. 2006; French and Morrison 2004). The clinician may also address James's social isolation, which may be a safety behavior or may indicate that he needs some help with his social interaction.

In summary, a psychological approach would be based on an individualized formulation for James, taking into account his life experiences, his beliefs about himself, the anomalies he experiences and his attributions about those anomalies, his safety behaviors, and his goals. The tasks of therapy have to be set in a context of support and consideration of how best to engage with this young person, recognizing the fear and panic that may be accompanying these early psychotic-like experiences.

Psychopharmacologic Perspective

Christoph U. Correll, M.D.
Andrea Auther, Ph.D.
Barbara A. Cornblatt, Ph.D., M.B.A.

DIAGNOSTIC FORMULATION

James is a 15-year-old male who presented for evaluation for social withdrawal, depressive symptoms, and school refusal. According to his history, James has undergone a several-month decline in functioning, including increased social withdrawal, problems with hygiene, day-night sleep reversal, anhedonia, some odd behavior (e.g., hiding his face in public places, hiding at school), and difficulties with attention and concentration. He also recently developed irritable mood, accompanied by an emergence of nihilistic and violent thoughts, although these thoughts do not seem to have influenced his behavior. James was sent for evaluation by the school counselor after his decline in school functioning worsened into total school refusal.

James had no known birth complications, and the only reported medical problem was mild asthma when he was younger. However, several nonspecific difficulties reported in his developmental history are consistent with characteristics found to be early precursors of adult schizophrenia (e.g., Cornblatt et al. 2003; Jones et al. 1994). Some examples are the suggested delays in James's verbal and motor development, his referral for evaluation for inattention (without hyperactivity) in the second grade, and his description as being "a little shy." In addition, there is a possible familial loading for a psychotic illness, although the details of his mother's hospitalization are unclear.

Christoph U. Correll, M.D., is Assistant Professor of Psychiatry and Behavioral Sciences at Albert Einstein College of Medicine in Bronx, New York, and Medical Director of the Recognition and Prevention Program at The Zucker Hillside Hospital in Glen Oaks, New York.

Andrea Auther, Ph.D., is Assistant Director of the Recognition and Prevention (RAP) Program at The Zucker Hillside Hospital in Glen Oaks, New York.

Barbara A. Cornblatt, Ph.D., M.B.A., is Professor of Psychiatry at the Albert Einstein College of Medicine in Bronx, New York; Investigator at the Feinstein Institute for Medical Research; and Director of the Recognition and Prevention Program at The Zucker Hillside Hospital in Glen Oaks, New York.

For complete biographical information, see "About the Contributors," p. 613.

Upon direct interview, James also reported a variety of symptoms and experiences that appear to fall in the prodromal range as specified by the widely used Scale of Prodromal Symptoms (McGlashan et al. 2001; Miller et al. 1999). This scale comprises 19 items that make up four subscales: positive, negative, disorganized, and general symptoms. Items are rated on a 7-point scale (0–6), with scores of 0–2 not considered clinically significant and a score of 6 representing "psychotic intensity." James had no symptoms that reached the level of psychosis.

To meet criteria for the schizophrenia prodrome, an individual must display a recent onset or worsening of at least one of five positive symptoms at an "attenuated" level (i.e., at a score of 3–5). James displayed several moderate attenuated positive symptoms. He reported unusual ideas such as conspiracy theories about 9/11 and destruction of the world. He also described déjà vu experiences and strange thoughts that perplexed him. In addition, he reported a high level of suspiciousness and indicated that he was uncomfortable around people. He stated that he thought people were looking at him and did not like (or feared) him. This symptom, though clinically significant, is nevertheless at an attenuated, or prodromal, level because James did not have any specific indication that others were plotting to harm him or single him out directly. Additionally, James reported perceptual abnormalities in the prodromal range, such as changes in his environment, hearing his name in the wind, and seeing things out of the corner of his eye. Lastly, his somewhat tangential and odd thought processes reached a prodromal level of disorganized communication. James's feeling that he could become a rap star and "spread the message of God and love and peace" is evidence of mild (below prodromal level) grandiosity.

Other attenuated symptoms (negative, disorganized, and general), although not required to meet prodromal criteria, are nevertheless essential components of the prodromal state. James demonstrated a range of additional symptoms, especially negative, which included decline in school functioning, social isolation, and a decline in goal-directed activities (anhedonia). Other potentially prodromal symptoms from the disorganized and general subscales of the Scale of Prodromal Symptoms include odd behavior, trouble with focus and attention, impairment in hygiene, sleep disturbance, dysphoric mood, and perhaps intolerance to stress (e.g., at school).

DIAGNOSTIC CONSIDERATIONS

As previously mentioned, James does not evidence any symptoms that are at a psychotic level of intensity. However, he is reporting putatively prodromal symptoms and symptoms that may be indicative of a mood or anxiety disorder. Thus, the following differential diagnoses would be considered: 1) depressive disorder NOS, as indicated by anhedonia, decreased concentration, irritability, and decreased functioning; and 2) anxiety disorder NOS, as indicated by social avoidance and persistent worrying. Although not currently included in DSM-IV-TR, the schizophrenia prodrome is suggested by the recent emergence of several moderate attenuated positive symptoms, including suspiciousness, unusual thought content, and perceptual abnormalities. If symptoms are persistent and no worsening occurs in the absence of antipsychotic treatment, then schizotypal and schizoid personality disorders should be considered. Finally, despite absence of any relevant subthreshold mania symptoms at the time of presentation, the possibility of a bipolar disorder prodrome cannot be ruled out, because depressive, anxious, and attenuated positive and negative symptoms have been observed in patients who ultimately developed bipolar disorder (Correll et al. 2007a, 2007b).

DSM-IV-TR DIAGNOSIS

Axis I   311 Depressive disorder NOS
           Rule out anxiety disorder NOS
Axis II   Rule out schizotypal and schizoid personality disorders
Axis III   Mild asthma
Axis IV   Educational problems
           Problems related to social environment
Axis V   Global Assessment of Functioning=45–50

TREATMENT RECOMMENDATIONS

Although James does not meet DSM-IV-TR criteria for a specific Axis I disorder, his decline in functioning and moderate to severe levels of attenuated positive and negative symptoms (with recent onset and worsening) warrant an intervention (Correll and Kane 2004). Pharmacologic treatment would be directed at current symptom amelioration as well as prevention of a full-blown Axis I disorder, particularly a psychotic illness. We recommend a symptom- or problem-based strategy, using the most benign treatment possible, and moving to higher-risk interventions if needed. For this case, five potential treatment targets are identified: 1) depressive and/or anxiety symptoms, 2) problems with attention and concentration, 3) social isolation, 4) academic dysfunction, and 5) attenuated positive symptoms. First-line interventions typically used in the Hillside Recognition and Prevention (RAP) program for all patients meeting criteria for prodromal schizophrenia include psychoeducation (involving the patient and family) and individual, group, and/or multifamily group therapy. If this line of intervention does not yield the desired improvement, then pharmacologic interventions targeted to specific problems are added. In this case, James's depressive and anxious symptoms could be treated with a selective serotonin reuptake inhibitor (SSRI). This medication may also improve the other deficit areas (e.g., school attendance, socializing) if they are, in fact, related to depression and/or anxiety. Moreover, as shown by a recent study, antidepressants may prevent worsening of positive symptoms and emergence of full psychosis (Cornblatt et al. 2007). Because of the remote possibility of a bipolar prodrome presentation, the family should be educated and the patient should be carefully monitored for emergence of antidepressant-induced mania or hypomania and/or suicidality. If irritability worsens and other potential symptoms of mania emerge during treatment, the antidepressant may need to be replaced by a mood stabilizer with some antidepressant activity, such as lamotrigine or lithium.

If school refusal persists, short-term home schooling may have to be considered until James can return to school or until a more suitable educational setting is located. If attention and concentration problems persist, cognitive remediation may be recommended. Because attention-deficit/hyperactivity disorder (ADHD) does not seem to be present and because stimulants may aggravate attenuated positive symptoms, stimulants are not currently indicated. In addition, or as an alternative to antidepressants, CBT could be used, as this treatment has been shown not only to reduce anxiety and depression, but also to reduce the likelihood of conversion to psychosis in high-risk patients (Morrison et al. 2004). With further worsening of attenuated symptoms despite adherence to the treatment plan, a switch to or augmentation with an atypical antipsychotic may be necessary; an agent with the least likelihood of sedation, extrapyramidal symptoms, and weight gain is our first choice.

As is standard in the RAP program, the clinician needs to follow this patient frequently to adjust treatment and to monitor symptom response, treatment side effects, and/or emergence of new symptoms as part of the transition to psychosis or mania (e.g., suicidality, substance abuse, overt aggression toward self or others).

Integrative Perspective

Cheryl M. Corcoran, M.D.

DIAGNOSTIC FORMULATION

James is a 15-year-old who has developed over the past few months a marked social withdrawal with concomitant school refusal and functional decline. He has some affective symptoms—questionably depressive symptoms, as well as irritability that is evident specifically in the context of social demands. Neuro-vegetative symptoms include sleep-wake reversal, decrease (or change) in interests, and poor concentration, but no evidence of guilt, low energy, change in appetite, or suicidal ideation. James also has some unusual thoughts and experiences. His previous history includes poor attention without hyperactivity, with alleged poor response to stimulants, as well as social awkwardness and clumsiness. James lives in a single-parent household of limited means and has a family history of psychosis, diagnoses unclear.

This young man has a wide range of symptoms that do not obviously fit any clear DSM-IV-TR diagnosis, except possibly social phobia. The different categories of diagnoses are addressed individually in the following subsections.

Disorders Usually First Diagnosed in Infancy, Childhood, or Adolescence

James does not have mental retardation or a learning disorder; until recently, he did well in school. Although somewhat clumsy, he plays basketball well, so motor skills disorder is unlikely. He has no impairment in communication, ruling out communication disorders and autism.

Although James is somewhat odd and currently has significant social impairment, the onset of this is recent, such that Asperger's disorder can be ruled out. Furthermore, he has not had repetitions or stereotypies.

James has had long-standing difficulties with attention and was prescribed stimulants without any apparent effect. No hyperactivity or impulsivity was noted. Therefore, he is given a provisional diagnosis of ADHD, predominantly inattentive type.

Mood Disorders

Although his mother describes James as having been depressed and at times irritable, he denies this and it is not evident on interview. He has had poor concentration, which appears unrelated to mood. Although he has experienced a shift in interests from peer-related to solitary activities, he does not have anhedonia and enjoys computer games and cartoons. Despite sleep-wake reversal, he has had neither insomnia nor hypersomnia. No fatigue, change in appetite, guilt, feelings of worthlessness, thoughts of death, or psychomotor abnormalities have been reported or observed. Hence, he cannot have major depression or dysthymia.

James's alleged irritability was context specific, and he displayed no irritability on interview. Although some grandiose themes were expressed by James in his nihilistic fantasies and his dreams about becoming a rap star, these are not persistent and may overlap with what is normal for adolescent boys. James does not have any other symptoms of mania and does not fulfill criteria for bipolar disorder.

In sum, no diagnosis of mood disorder could be made for James.

ANXIETY DISORDERS

James may meet the criteria for social phobia if it is determined that he has the capacity for age-appropriate social relationships with familiar people. It is questionable whether he does because he describes difficulty in knowing how to act with peers. His symptoms have lasted nearly 6 months and have impaired his function. However, his social anxiety may be atypical in that it does not involve fears about performance, and he additionally has some suspiciousness. Therefore, James may fulfill criteria for social phobia.

PSYCHOTIC DISORDERS

Because James does not have delusions, hallucinations, or disorganized speech and behavior, he does not fulfill any criteria for a DSM-IV-TR diagnosis of psychotic disorder. However, James does have a number of psychotic symptoms in attenuated or subthreshold form. Although he does not have any fixed, false ideas, he has a number of overvalued ideas with several themes. Although not paranoid, he is suspicious and somewhat referential, feeling that people consider him weird or menacing (but in fact he is a young black man in a neighborhood that others consider dangerous). His consideration that George Bush may have been involved with 9/11 is an idea that was widespread in his community. James also has had nihilistic fantasies and somewhat grandiose plans, as well as some sense of premonition. Overall, James lacks conviction or certainty about these various ideas and in fact considers them strange.

Also, although James has not had hallucinations, he did report perceptual disturbances, including altered and enhanced perception in olfactory, visual, and auditory modalities. He has had the illusions of hearing his name in the wind and seeing an object move briefly in his visual periphery.

Of note, none of these subthreshold or attenuated psychotic symptoms has appreciably affected his behavior or function.

MOVING BEYOND DSM-IV-TR

Of all the DSM-IV-TR psychotic disorders, schizophrenia is the only one that has a documented description of a prodrome, which precedes a first episode of frank psychosis and is characterized by negative symptoms and/or attenuated psychotic symptoms. Were James to go on to develop psychosis, his current clinical picture would retrospectively be characterized as prodromal. However, no DSM-IV-TR diagnosis exists for a putative prodromal or clinical high-risk state.

Many clinicians nonetheless would agree that James is at enhanced risk for a psychotic disorder, given both his own symptoms and the history of psychosis in his mother. When results of the Structured Interview for Prodromal Syndromes/Scale of Prodromal Symptoms (Miller et al. 2003) are considered,

James fulfills criteria for two prodromal syndromes: 1) attenuated positive symptom syndrome and 2) genetic risk and deterioration syndrome. Cornblatt (2002) noted that putative prodromal states are typically accompanied by cognitive, academic, and social impairments, which are also evident in James.

DSM-IV-TR DIAGNOSIS

Axis I   314.00 ADHD, predominantly inattentive type
          300.23 Social phobia
Axis II   None
Axis III Asthma
Axis IV   None
Axis V   Global Assessment of Functioning=43

TREATMENT RECOMMENDATIONS

James had a normal physical examination and blood work, and magnetic resonance imaging, obtained as he participated in a research protocol, demonstrated no abnormalities. His earlier records of diagnosis and treatment of putative ADHD were not obtainable.

NEUROPSYCHOLOGICAL TESTING

The clinician prioritized neuropsychological testing for a host of reasons, including James's attentional problems, his recent decline in academic performance, and new reports of difficulty in planning and organization, especially for less structured tasks such as writing an essay. James was given the Wechsler Intelligence Scale for Children—Third Edition (WISC-III; Wechsler 1991), as well as the Wechsler Memory Scale—Revised (WMS-R; Wechsler 1987). James was found to have a Verbal IQ of 110 and a Performance IQ of 90. He had significant spread in ability among cognitive domains. His reading ability was a strength, although he demonstrated impairment in explicit verbal memory and verbal working memory.

James's processing speed was below the 30th percentile. Attentional deficits were observed, and James was observed to often rush through tasks. Overall, across domains, his test performance was very dependent on the extent to which the task was structured. James refused to attempt many mathematical problems. Of interest, this pattern of performance is not atypical in adolescents putatively prodromal for psychosis (Keefe et al. 2006).

PHARMACOLOGIC TREATMENTS

Stimulants were considered as treatment for James's attentional difficulties, but they were not prescribed because of concerns that stimulants might exacerbate James's subthreshold psychotic symptoms.

SSRIs were considered because they have been shown to be effective for adolescents with social phobia (March et al. 2007). Also, preliminary data suggest that antidepressants may protect against attenuated psychotic symptoms reaching a threshold level (Cornblatt et al. 2007). If James were to take an SSRI, he would be monitored closely for any emergent suicidal thoughts or behaviors.

Antipsychotic medications were also considered as a means to treat his current attenuated psychotic symptoms and prevent their progression. Two randomized clinical trials have examined the effects of antipsychotics on arresting psychotic symptom progression in putatively prodromal young people. In one, olanzapine led to sizable weight gain and no clear efficacy compared to placebo (McGlashan et al. 2006). In the other, low-dose risperidone, when "bundled" with CBT, was efficacious when compared with "treatment as usual" (McGorry et al. 2002). Because CBT alone may be protective (Morrison et al. 2004), the role of antipsychotics for "prodromal" symptoms remains unclear.

In any event, James's mother refused the prescription of any medications to her son, given her own negative experience with chlorpromazine in the past.

PSYCHOLOGICAL TREATMENTS

Effective group therapies for adolescents with primary social phobia focus on improving social effectiveness and social skills (Albano 2003). However, James was reluctant to join any sort of group.

CBT was attempted, as this may be effective for prodromal symptoms (Morrison et al. 2004), but James could not identify any problems to work on.

OTHER INTERVENTIONS

Support and education were provided to James's mother. The clinician worked with her to obtain a home-based tutor, given James's school refusal. This enabled James to keep up with his work. Ultimately, mainly through his mother's advocacy with the board of education, James was placed in a residential school in rural upstate New York for children with emotional problems. There, he received supportive therapy, and class size was small. He flourished there, attending classes and receiving A's. He developed friendships with peers and even ran for and was elected the president of his small class. He reported being very happy to be out of his small apartment, out of New York City in general, and in "nature." In sum, his academic and social function improved, although his subthreshold psychotic symptoms remained.

CONCLUSIONS

Notably, the designation of a putatively prodromal state, reflecting a combination of cognitive, academic, and social dysfunction with subthreshold symptoms, has a yield of "conversion" to psychosis of less than 50%. The discovery of biological markers should improve the specificity of this syndrome. No clear evidence base exists for treatment of current morbidity and symptoms, or for prevention of progression to psychosis. Clearly, more research is needed on this putative prodrome to psychosis seen in adolescents (Lieberman and Corcoran 2007).

REFERENCES

Addington J, Francey SM, Morrison AP: Working With People at High Risk of Developing Psychosis: A Treatment Handbook. Chichester, UK, Wiley, 2006

Albano AM: Treatment of social anxiety in adolescents, in Casebook of Cognitive-Behavioral Therapy With Children and Adolescents, 2nd Edition. Edited by Reinecke M, Dattilio F, Freeman A. New York, Guilford, 2003, pp 128–161

Cornblatt BA: The New York High Risk Project to the Hillside Recognition and Prevention (RAP) program. Am J Med Genet 114:956–966, 2002

Cornblatt BA, Lencz T, Smith CW, et al: The schizophrenia prodrome revisited: a neurodevelopmental perspective. Schizophr Bull 29:633–651, 2003

Cornblatt BA, Lencz T, Smith CW, et al: Can antidepressants be used to treat the schizophrenia prodrome? Results of a prospective, naturalistic treatment study of adolescents. J Clin Psychiatry 68:546–557, 2007

Correll CU, Kane JM: The psychotic prodrome: how effective are early interventions? Advances in Schizophrenia and Clinical Psychiatry 1:2–10, 2004

Correll CU, Penzner JB, Frederickson AM, et al: Differentiation in the preonset phases of schizophrenia and mood disorders: evidence in support of a bipolar mania prodrome. Schizophr Bull 33:703–714, 2007a

Correll CU, Penzner JB, Lencz T, et al: Early identification and high risk strategies for bipolar disorder. Bipolar Disord 9:324–338, 2007b

French P, Morrison AP: Early Detection and Cognitive Therapy for People at High Risk of Developing Psychosis. Chichester, UK, Wiley, 2004

Jones P, Rodgers B, Murray R, et al: Child developmental risk factors for adult schizophrenia in the British 1946 birth cohort. Lancet 344:1398–1402, 1994

Keefe RS, Perkins DO, Gu H, et al: A longitudinal study of neurocognitive function in individuals at risk for psychosis. Schizophr Res 88:26–35, 2006

Lieberman J, Corcoran C: The impossible dream: can psychiatry prevent psychosis? Early Intervention in Psychiatry 1:219–221, 2007

March JS, Entusah AR, Rynn M, et al: A randomized controlled trial of venlafaxine ER versus placebo in pediatric social anxiety disorder. Biol Psychiatry 62:1149–1154, 2007

McGlashan TH, Miller TJ, Woods SW, et al: Instrument for the assessment of prodromal symptoms and states, in Early Intervention in Psychotic Disorders. Edited by Miller T, Mednick SA, McGlashan TH, et al. New York, Springer-Verlag, 2001, pp 135–149

McGlashan TH, Zipursky RB, Perkins D, et al: Randomized, double-blind trial of olan-zapine versus placebo in patients prodromally symptomatic for psychosis. Am J Psychiatry 163:790–799, 2006

McGorry PD, Yung AR, Phillips LJ, et al: Randomized controlled trial of interventions designed to reduce the risk of progression to first-episode psychosis in a clinical sample with subthreshold symptoms. Arch Gen Psychiatry 59:921–928, 2002

Miller TJ, McGlashan TH, Woods SW, et al: Symptom assessment in schizophrenic prodromal states. Psychiatr Q 70:273–287, 1999

Miller TJ, McGlashan TH, Rosen JL, et al: Prodromal assessment with the Structured Interview for Prodromal Syndromes and the Scale of Prodromal Symptoms: predictive validity, interrater reliability, and training to reliability. Schizophr Bull 29:703–715, 2003

Morrison AP, French P, Walford L, et al: Cognitive therapy for the prevention of psychosis in people at ultra-high risk: randomized controlled trial. Br J Psychiatry 185:291–297, 2004

Wechsler D: Wechsler Memory Scale—Revised. San Antonio, TX, The Psychological Corporation, 1987

Wechsler D: Wechsler Intelligence Scale for Children—Third Edition. San Antonio, TX, The Psychological Corporation, 1991

■ CHAPTER 23 ■

I Just Want to Die

Double Depression

David A. Brent, M.D.

CASE PRESENTATION

IDENTIFYING INFORMATION

Holly is a 17-year-old who lives at home with her biological parents and two younger siblings. She attends twelfth grade in a regular education classroom.

CHIEF COMPLAINT

Holly complained of increasing academic difficulties, depression, and suicidal ideation.

HISTORY OF PRESENT ILLNESS

Holly presented to the child and adolescent psychiatry clinic because of increasing difficulty with school performance and attendance. She has a history of depressed mood for "as long as I can remember," social anxiety, chronic suicidal ideation, self-cutting, some symptoms of an eating disorder, and an inflexible, perfectionistic cognitive style. Holly has been having difficulty with her sleep. She stays up late meaning to do her homework and then has difficulty falling asleep. In the mornings, she has great difficulty getting out of bed,

---

David A. Brent, M.D., is Academic Chief of Child and Adolescent Psychiatry at Western Psychiatric Institute and Clinic, and Professor of Child Psychiatry, Pediatrics, and Epidemiology and Endowed Chair of Suicide Studies at the University of Pittsburgh School of Medicine in Pittsburgh, Pennsylvania (for complete biographical information, see "About the Contributors," p. 613).

so she misses many days of school. She explained that she no longer has fun do-ing the things that she used to enjoy, such as hanging out with her friends. Her mother has been concerned and raised these concerns to her family physician several months ago. He prescribed fluoxetine, which Holly took for 20 weeks at a maximum dose of 40 mg/day. The medication did not appear to have any beneficial effect on her mood.

Holly noted that her appetite has decreased recently and she has not been very interested in eating. She is concerned about her weight; thinks she looks "fat," but is of normal weight; has regular menses; and is not nutritionally compromised. Holly has frequent suicidal ideation. On careful questioning, she can identify that the suicidal ideation appears when either she or others do not meet her very high standards; she expects peers to be loyal, doting, and respectful beyond any realistic developmental standards, and she has equally high and difficult-to-meet aca-demic and body image standards for herself. She also complained of having low motivation, guilt, low feelings of self-worth, and hopelessness.

Holly has two friends whom she sees in school, but she rarely socializes with them out of school. Her mother has encouraged her to spend time with them, but Holly says that she would rather stay home. Her mother explained that although Holly has never been particularly social, she has been even more withdrawn lately. She spends her free time on weekends watching television and doing homework. Her homework appears to take her more time than it takes her classmates. In ad-dition, Holly reported fatigue and difficulty with concentration.

Past Psychiatric History

Holly described feeling uncomfortable when speaking to peers and feeling bad about herself and sad for as long as she can remember. Initially, the symptoms were milder but became much more noticeable when she entered middle school. During puberty, she also developed body image difficulties, self-hatred, suicidal ideation, and self-cutting in response to loneliness, depression, or anxi-ety. Although she has had strong suicidal urges, she has never attempted suicide.

During the clinician's careful history taking about Holly's academic diffi-culties, Holly admitted that she has suffered from being "spacey" and inatten-tive for as long as she can remember. It was unclear if this represented the inattentive type of attention-deficit/hyperactivity disorder (ADHD) or was a be-ginning symptom of dysthymia. However, in tracing out the course of her symptomatology with the clinician, Holly indicated that her attention difficul-ties preceded her mood problems and, in fact, became exacerbated by them.

Holly has never had any prior treatment with a mental health practitioner.

Medical History

Holly is medically healthy aside from her psychiatric illnesses.

DEVELOPMENTAL HISTORY

Holly's parents denied any developmental delays.

SOCIAL HISTORY

Holly was raised by her biological parents and has two younger siblings. Her father is a busy professional, and her mother was a librarian. Her father's job has prevented him from spending much time with Holly or her mother. The patient has always had one or two close friends, but basically is a loner with few interests outside of school. She has not begun to date.

FAMILY HISTORY

Her mother suffered from untreated ongoing long-term depression and anxiety disorder.

MENTAL STATUS EXAMINATION

Holly was thin, was casually dressed, and appeared her stated age. She was cooperative with the interview. Her speech was slow, and she did not initiate any spontaneous conversation. She described her mood as down, and her affect was constricted. Her thinking was goal oriented. She denied any intent to kill herself or others but said that she often felt she would be better off dead. She was oriented and cognitively intact.

COMMENTARIES

Psychotherapeutic Perspective

Kevin D. Stark, Ph.D.

DIAGNOSTIC FORMULATION

The assessment of depression in a child such as Holly should include longitudinal information about the onset, offset, duration, and recurrence of depressive symptoms in relation to stressful life events; a thorough treatment history,

Kevin D. Stark, Ph.D., is Professor of Educational Psychology at the University of Texas in Austin, Texas (for complete biographical information, see "About the Contributors," p. 613).

including psychotropic and other medications and psychosocial therapies; and a psychosocial history, including developmental milestones, school performance and adjustment, social adjustment, and family history of psychiatric disorders. Multiple measures to assess symptoms of depression, anxiety, and ADHD would be completed by Holly, her primary caregiver, and, in the case of the ADHD, her teachers. Self-report measures would be used to assess subjective severity of the symptoms, and a semistructured interview such as the Schedule for Affective Disorders and Schizophrenia for School-Age Children—Fourth Edition, Revised (Ambrosini and Dixon 2000) would be used to complete a diagnosis. The youth version of the Beck Depression Inventory (J.S. Beck et al. 2001) would be used to monitor treatment response.

Holly reported symptoms that are common to childhood-onset double depression—episodes of major depression interspersed during a chronic course of dysthymic disorder. She reported chronic dysphoria, anhedonia, initial insomnia, appetite disturbance, guilt, low self-worth, hopelessness, fatigue, difficulty concentrating, chronic suicidal ideation, and slowed speech. She also reported symptoms consistent with a diagnosis of social phobia. She reported severe social withdrawal, including shrinking from social situations with unfamiliar people. From the historical information, Holly appears to be experiencing ADHD. Holly is experiencing academic difficulties in school that could stem from an unidentified learning disability. Thus, Holly should undergo a complete psychoeducational assessment that includes measures of IQ, achievement, and cognitive processing. She also takes an unusually long time to complete her homework, and her thinking is rigid. The longer duration to complete homework may be due to attention difficulties that stem from ADHD, or depression, or anxiety, and it could result from checking, excessive erasing, rereading, and so on, associated with obsessive-compulsive disorder. Thus, an assessment for obsessive-compulsive disorder may be useful. The Children's Yale-Brown Obsessive Compulsive Scale (Goodman et al. 1989) would be used to guide this portion of the assessment.

DSM-IV-TR DIAGNOSIS

Axis I   296.32 Major depressive disorder, recurrent, moderate, without full interepisode recovery

300.4 Dysthymic disorder, early onset

300.23 Social phobia, generalized

Rule out ADHD

Axis II   None

Axis III   None

Axis IV   Mother is experiencing major depression and an anxiety disorder

Father is absent from the family due to excessive demands at work

Axis V   Global Assessment of Functioning=45

Currently experiencing moderate impairment at school and home, and with peers

Chronic suicidal ideation and cutting behavior

TREATMENT RECOMMENDATIONS

CASE CONCEPTUALIZATION

A case conceptualization (Stark et al., in press) serves as the road map to treatment. The case conceptualization should be completed collaboratively with Holly and will continue to evolve as more is learned from each meeting. It is a hypothesis-generating and -testing process (J.S. Beck 1995). Thus, the conceptualization that follows consists of preliminary hypotheses that were generated from the description of the case and from research on depressive and anxiety disorders. Some of the hypotheses will be confirmed, others will be incorrect and altered or replaced, and additional hypotheses will be generated as new information is discovered.

Given the diagnosis of a depressive disorder, Holly's core beliefs are likely that she is unlovable, helpless, worthless, or a combination of these three (A.T. Beck 2002). Because she is chronically suicidal and cuts herself, worthlessness is likely to be one of her core beliefs. Furthermore, because her suicidal ideation, self-hatred, and cutting are triggered by loneliness, she likely possesses an unlovability core belief that is closely linked to worthlessness.

Beliefs develop as a result of repeated learning experiences. Thus, further support for the hypothesis that Holly possesses worthlessness and unlovability as core beliefs stems from the learning experiences that accrue from having a mother who is experiencing depression and anxiety. Depressed parents perceive misbehavior when it does not exist and are overly punitive and demanding of their children. They express affection contingent on achievement at a very high level of performance. Excessive punishment in combination with contingent expression of love can create a learning history that supports core beliefs of worthlessness and unlovability. Furthermore, Holly's father is too busy with work to buffer the adverse impact of her mother's behavior, and his failure to engage Holly may have further contributed to her sense of unlovability.

The core belief underlying anxiety disorders is vulnerability (A.T. Beck and Emery 1985). The anxious individual also believes that he or she lacks the skills and resources necessary to cope with a perceived threat. Holly has social anxiety disorder, so she likely fears negative evaluations by others if she reveals weaknesses. She is likely to be hypersensitive to signals regarding acceptability and to expect others to be critical and disapproving. Furthermore, she fears that when her weaknesses are revealed to other people, they will abandon or withdraw their love from her. Thus, the unlovability core belief also influences the distorted thinking that is associated with anxiety. Holly's vulnerability belief and the related expectancies may have developed as a result of her mother's anxious communications about a "dangerous world" and possibly from the negative scrutiny Holly was subject to as a result of having a depressed and anxious parent.

Intermediate beliefs reflect or grow out of core beliefs. Holly perhaps believes that if she achieves at a very high level, has the perfect figure, and treats people exceptionally well, she will then be lovable and have value. The compensatory strategies that have grown out of these intermediate beliefs include being loyal, doting on significant others, and possibly having a very close relationship with her two friends. Based on her belief that others will see through the facade and reject her, Holly withdraws from social contact and only warms up to others after an extended period of time in which she is not rejected.

MODE OF TREATMENT

A combination of cognitive-behavioral therapy (CBT) and psychopharmacologic therapy would be used to treat Holly. She would be referred to a consulting psychiatrist for consideration of additional and alternative medications for treating the depression, anxiety, and possible ADHD. Because a minimum of information is presented on the parents and family, the therapist cannot determine whether family therapy would be beneficial, so initially psychotherapy would be delivered using an individual format. Individual therapy would be the initial mode of delivery because of Holly's social anxiety. The anxiety that she would likely experience if placed initially in group therapy might be too aversive and result in either premature termination or overwhelming unpleasant affect that would prevent her from being able to benefit from group intervention. Group therapy may be used later in treatment as Holly's depression begins to lift and as her social anxiety disorder has been addressed. Interactions within the group would represent points within the hierarchy of exposure experiences. If Holly's mother is not currently in therapy and not taking an antidepressant, appropriate referrals would be made. The family would likely be referred for therapy to address her mother's depressive and anxiety disorders and any maladaptive behavior, family rules, and negative affect in the household.

TREATMENT PLAN

CBT is recommended for treating Holly because it has demonstrated efficacy with depression (Stark et al., in press) and social anxiety (Beidel 1991) and it helps to protect patients from heightened suicidal ideation that may result from taking a new selective serotonin reuptake inhibitor. CBT would follow the approach in ACTION (Stark et al. 2007a, 2007b, 2007c, 2007d). Thus, the primary treatment strategies would be goal setting, affective education, coping skills training, problem-solving training, and cognitive restructuring.

Holly presented with chief complaints of academic difficulties, depression, and suicidal ideation. One of the first steps would be to collaboratively set goals; given her chief complaints, the goals would likely be to improve academic performance and mood and to eliminate suicidal ideation. To improve Holly's academic performance and sense of self-worth and to reduce stress, the therapist would recommend that Holly set up tutoring in classes where she is experiencing the most difficulties. In addition, with Holly's permission, the therapist would consult with these teachers to establish times when Holly can get caught up on homework and take advantage of the teachers' support and the structure created by this situation. Thus, she would not stay up late ruminating about her homework and miss sleep and then school. Another strategy for helping Holly complete her homework and for getting her father more involved in her life would be to teach him how to take a positive approach to helping Holly complete her homework.

CBT for depression usually progresses from goal setting to affective education and coping skills training. This progression would enable the therapist and Holly to address the second goal of improving mood. Affective education involves discussing where emotions come from; the relationship between thoughts, feelings, and behaviors; the CBT model of depression; the client's emotional experiences; and ways to manage or improve mood. The therapist and Holly would identify the variety of emotions that Holly experiences and develop a system (e.g., a mood meter) for rating the subjective strength of her experience of each emotion. Using this information, Holly and the therapist would create a list of things that Holly does that bring her pleasure and things that she used to do that brought her pleasure. Subsequently, Holly and the therapist would complete a mood rating and then engage in one of the fun activities and then rerate her mood. Engaging in such activities produces a significant improvement in mood. The list of activities would be written down on a blank Catch the Positive Diary (see Stark et al. 2007b), and Holly would be encouraged to complete as many fun activities as possible each day and to check off which ones she completed and make a mood rating at the end of each day. Self-monitoring of engagement in pleasant events improves mood because of behavioral activation and because it helps Holly focus on the positive. Problem solving would be used to help her develop plans for overcoming potential impediments to following her plan to engage in more fun activities.

Engaging in fun and distracting activities is one of the five coping strategies that Holly would be taught. She also would learn to seek social support, use strenuous exercise, engage in relaxation, and think more positively as coping strategies for improving mood. The coping skills are used to improve mood in general, and especially when she is experiencing unpleasant affect due to being in a situation that she cannot change. Because Holly is experiencing insomnia and comorbid anxiety, the therapist would place emphasis on helping Holly to develop relaxation skills as one part of the treatment plan for helping her to overcome insomnia. Teaching her sleep hygiene and use of cognitive strategies to calm down would be other components of the treatment for insomnia. Increasing the amount of sleep should have a positive impact on Holly's mood.

Coping skills training also is central to the treatment of Holly's cutting behavior, another initial goal. Cutting is a maladaptive coping behavior that reduces stress and improves mood when she experiences loneliness, dysphoria, or anxiety. Holly would be taught to recognize the earliest signs of an experience that would lead to cutting and then to substitute an adaptive coping skill in its place. The key is to use enough coping behaviors to delay the compulsion until it passes. Because Holly has been cutting for an extended period of time, it is likely that she craves the resulting endorphin release. Thus, use of strenuous exercise would be emphasized as a healthy strategy to release endorphins. Seeking social support could be another effective strategy. Holly would be taught to talk to someone in person, over the phone, or via the Internet as a means of distracting herself from the compulsion to cut. In addition, coping statements would be recorded on cards that she can read to prevent cutting. Later in treatment, cognitive restructuring strategies would be used to help Holly to evaluate and change the negative thoughts that are elicited by the aforementioned triggers. In particular, cognitive restructuring would target her sense of worthlessness and unlovability.

Suicidal ideation is another maladaptive stress reaction. It may reflect a desire to escape from an intolerable situation or intolerable pain. Thus, Holly would be taught to use coping skills to elevate and manage her mood when she begins to feel suicidal. Coping skills would be used to help her learn that she can improve her mood using other constructive methods. Problem solving would be used to change the undesirable situations. Cognitive restructuring would be used to evaluate the thoughts that trigger suicidal ideation and to replace those thoughts with more adaptive and realistic ones. Once again, cognitive restructuring would focus on building the belief that she is loved and worthy.

Additionally, treatment of depression in general would progress. After Holly has identified specific coping behaviors within each of the five categories, added them to the Catch the Positive Diary, and experienced within the meetings the benefits of trying at least one example from each category, the focus would shift to developing problem-solving skills. Problem solving would be used both as an overarching strategy, because depressed and anxious mood and symptoms are problems to be solved, and as a strategy to change situations that produce stress when the situation is within Holly's control. Initially, Holly would be taught to distinguish between controllable and uncontrollable situations. Simultaneously, didactic teaching, modeling, and within-session activities would be used to teach a five-step problem-solving strategy. Initially, problem solving would be applied to fun problems that the therapist creates within the meetings and then to relatively easy real-life problems. Subsequently, problem solving would be applied to progressively more difficult situations.

From the first meeting forward, the therapist would be looking for opportunities to educate Holly about the relationship between thoughts, emotions, and behavior. More specifically, Holly and the therapist would begin to identify negative thoughts that lead to depressive and anxious symptoms. In addition, the therapist would be ever vigilant for opportunities to provide Holly with learning experiences that help her to believe that she is lovable, worthy, and efficacious. As Holly experiences symptom relief from coping and problem solving, the emphasis would shift to acquisition and application of cognitive restructuring strategies. Holly would be taught how to identify negative thoughts and to use a number of questions that would help her to evaluate the validity of those thoughts and then to restructure them. Evidence from her life that counters her core beliefs would be used to restructure the beliefs that she is unlovable and worthless. Holly would be given behavioral homework assignments that provide her with evidence that she is lovable and worthy. Her own definition of a worthy individual would be used to guide the restructuring.

Once Holly is experiencing relief from depression, she would begin to apply coping, problem-solving, and cognitive restructuring strategies to social anxiety. A hierarchy of exposure experiences would be constructed for each social situation that provokes anxiety, and progression through the hierarchy would begin within the sessions and continue through therapeutic homework. Holly would work through each of the hierarchies using the coping skills to manage physical upset that arises from the exposure activities. Problem solving would be used to change anxiety-provoking controllable situations, and cognitive restructuring would be used to counter negative thoughts that arise during exposure activities and to develop a core belief of self-efficacy. Holly would learn to apply cognitive restructuring to negative thoughts about herself in social situations, her perceptions of the evaluations of others, and her belief that she lacks the skills and resources necessary to cope. Her parents would be encouraged to help Holly attack situations that she normally fears and to help her ward off cutting and suicidal ideation that stem from feeling anxious.

Psychopharmacologic Perspective

Christopher J. Kratochvil, M.D.

DIAGNOSTIC FORMULATION

Holly is a 17-year-old who presents with complaints of increasing academic difficulties, depression, and suicidal ideation. On interview, she describes multiple symptoms of depression, including insomnia, decreased appetite, anhedonia, hopelessness, guilt, diminished interest, poor energy, and poor concentration. Over the past several months, these symptoms, combined with her impairment in functioning academically, socially, and within the home, would suggest that Holly likely meets criteria for major depressive disorder (MDD). Depression is common in adolescents, with approximately 5% of teens meeting criteria for MDD at any time.

Unfortunately, with this patient, as is frequently the case in youth with psychiatric disorders, once a primary diagnosis is made, the assessment is far from complete. More often than not, MDD presents with at least one comorbid psychiatric disorder, so a comprehensive psychiatric evaluation is always warranted to assess for potential additional diagnoses. Holly may suffer from ADHD, based on her chronic symptoms of inattention that preceded her mood problems, although one must always remember that many disorders can lead to poor concentration. Additionally, the case description hints at the possibility of chronic mood problems suggestive of a potential dysthymia, discomfort in social settings potentially suggestive of a social anxiety disorder, and body image difficulties with hints of an eating disorder, among other things, all of which would require careful exploration. When an adolescent presents with depressive symptoms, a substance use disorder and first presentation of bipolar disorder should also be in the differential diagnosis.

From a biopsychosocial perspective, there are several important considerations. Holly's mother has reportedly suffered from chronic anxiety and depression, so there are potential genetic underpinnings for these disorders. A physical examination and history are warranted to assess for a potential general medical condition underlying the presentation. Psychologically, her mother's

---

Christopher J. Kratochvil, M.D., is Professor in the Department of Psychiatry, and Graduate Faculty Member and Assistant Director of the Psychopharmacology Research Consortium at the University of Nebraska Medical Center in Omaha, Nebraska (for complete biographical information, see "About the Contributors," p. 613).

long-standing untreated psychiatric illnesses may contribute as well. For example, her mother's anxiety and mood disorders may have resulted in limited emotional availability and support from her mother, as well as potentially providing an unspoken message regarding the validity of psychiatric disorders and beliefs about treatment. The therapist should explore further why her mother never received treatment for her own chronic mental illnesses: Was it simply a lack of recognition, a lack of resources, a denial of MDD and anxiety as being "real" disorders, or perhaps a fear of pharmacotherapy? Additionally, Holly appears to globally lack support, not only from her mother, but also from her father, who works extended hours, and even peer support is extremely limited.

DSM-IV-TR DIAGNOSIS

Axis I   296.22 Major depressive disorder
Rule out dysthymia
Rule out ADHD
Rule out social phobia
Rule out eating disorder
Axis II   None
Axis III   None
Axis IV   Struggling academically
Chronically mentally ill mother who is not receiving treatment
Lack of social support
Axis V   Global Assessment of Functioning=50

TREATMENT RECOMMENDATIONS

After the clinician determines a primary diagnosis and identifies comorbidities, a comprehensive treatment plan can be set in place. For purposes of this discussion, I will assume that Holly is diagnosed with MDD only.

Regardless of the treatment approach, educating Holly and her parents is crucial to promote an understanding of MDD, the role of comorbidities, long-term outcomes, and the rationale for the treatment approach selected. If medication is initiated, close attention must be paid to discussions regarding what is known regarding the safety and efficacy of antidepressants, while being sensitive to the family's concerns. The clinician can provide the family with a list of reliable Web sites, such as general sites for organizations like the National Institute of Mental Health (http://nimh.nih.gov) and the American Academy of Child and Adolescent Psychiatry (http://www.aacap.org), or more specific sites such as ParentsMedGuide.org, a resource for parents with a focus on the role of pharmacotherapy in the treatment of MDD.

Close monitoring is important when treating adolescents with depression. The clinician should have an open discussion with the family regarding suicidality and the need for ongoing monitoring by family and others close to the patient, and a safety plan should be developed in case the patient presents with suicidal thoughts or behaviors. The U.S. Food and Drug Administration (FDA) issued a black box warning for antidepressants, after a meta-analysis revealed that 4% of children and adolescents taking antidepressants spontaneously reported experiencing suicidality, compared to 2% receiving placebo (Kratochvil et al. 2006b). Interestingly, when the Treatment for Adolescents with Depression Study (TADS) systematically assessed suicidality at baseline and during the study, fluoxetine, CBT, combination therapy, and placebo were all associated with decreases in suicidality (March et al. 2004).

A physical examination, review of symptoms, and drug screen are generally indicated when assessing an adolescent for a mood disorder, and a pregnancy test is generally warranted before initiating pharmacotherapy in a female adolescent.

Psychotherapy can play an important role in treating teens with depression. TADS, for example, demonstrated that CBT can provide significant improvement in acute outcomes when provided along with fluoxetine (March et al. 2006).

Because fluoxetine was prescribed to Holly at a reasonable dose yet was unsuccessful, several pharmacotherapy-related questions should be considered. Did Holly consistently take the medication? If she did and there was no effect, then the clinician should try changing the medication. Did Holly consistently take the medication but experience adverse effects that limited adherence to the dosing or perhaps experience anxiety regarding taking an antidepressant? If so, then education may resolve the issue, and restarting fluoxetine may be appropriate. Also, did Holly experience a reduction of symptoms, but was the dosing inadequate? If the medication resulted in reasonable improvements and was well tolerated, the clinician might consider an increase to fluoxetine 60 mg/day. Although fluoxetine is the only antidepressant approved by the FDA for the treatment of children and adolescents with MDD, other antidepressants (i.e., sertraline and citalopram) do have at least some evidence of efficacy in pediatric depression (Kratochvil et al. 2006a).

Throughout the treatment process, the clinician should remain vigilant for comorbid disorders that were not realized earlier or that emerge at a later date. The clinician should also consider referral for Holly's mother to address her untreated mood and anxiety disorders.

Several studies have demonstrated the benefits of fluoxetine, both alone and in combination with CBT, in the treatment of adolescents with depression. Because the data supporting the use of fluoxetine in pediatric depression are greater than for any other antidepressant, fluoxetine is a first-line pharmacotherapy for MDD (Kratochvil et al. 2006a). TADS has also highlighted the potential benefits of combining CBT with pharmacotherapy to optimize outcomes. Although combination therapy is often considered ideal, a family's limited resources or limited access to treatment may result in treatment with pharmacotherapy alone.

Integrative Perspective

David A. Brent, M.D.

DIAGNOSTIC FORMULATION

Holly suffers from double depression—that is, major depression on top of a dysthymic disorder—as demonstrated by her symptoms of low self-worth, hopelessness, difficulty sleeping, and anhedonia, antedated by her other depressive symptoms. She also has social anxiety disorder, as illustrated by her very small social circle, avoidance of class participation, and avoidance of group activities. In addition, she appears to have ADHD, predominantly inattentive type, because her difficulty with attention preceded her depression. Her attentional problems began before she had any of the symptoms of dysthymic disorder. She does not meet criteria for eating disorder not otherwise specified, but nevertheless has some symptoms and style common to the restricting type of eating disorder. Her perfectionism seems core to many of her difficulties, as she cannot feel mastery or pleasure from her activities, studies, or interpersonal relationships because they always fall short of her high standards.

DSM-IV-TR DIAGNOSIS

Axis I   296.23 Major depressive disorder

           300.4 Dysthymic disorder

           314.00 ADHD, predominantly inattentive type

           300.23 Social phobia

Axis II   None

Axis III   None

Axis IV   No current stressors

Axis V   Global Assessment of Functioning=58

TREATMENT RECOMMENDATIONS

Because of Holly's concerns about her educational problems and the possible inattentive ADHD as a contributor to her difficulties, a trial of stimulants was initiated, while carefully monitoring the patient's weight (Birmaher et al. 2007). Her academic performance improved, and her previous routine of long hours of homework with many unfinished assignments became more normalized. She began to enjoy school more, which in turn caused a lifting, to some degree, of her depression. The fluoxetine was then stopped, and citalopram begun, with some further diminution in her anxiety and depressive symptoms (Brent and Birmaher 2006). Because of fluoxetine's longer half-life, there was no need for a cross-taper, but citalopram was begun at a dosage of 10 mg/day for 1 week, during which time the fluoxetine was being cleared from her system.

CBT was initiated to focus on Holly's rigid, perfectionistic cognitive style; her low degree of distress tolerance; and her tendency to become dysregulated, resulting in self-cutting and suicidal ideation (Brent and Weersing 2008). Relief from her perfectionism also enabled her to begin to enjoy social situations. A safety plan was developed in which Holly was taught self-soothing exercises to ward off and accept negative affect, rather than resorting to self-cutting. She was taught to deal with suicidal ideation in the same way, as well as by speaking with her mother about her concerns. If those coping strategies were not efficacious, then she was to call her therapist, but for the most part, the strategies were successful. The mother was referred for her own treatment. She was reluctant to go, but was prevailed upon because of the negative impact of parental depression on children. She improved, in parallel with her daughter. Holly's high and rigid expectations about others were challenged, and she was prescribed "social experiments." Although she never became a social butterfly, she did have some successful peer relationships for the first time, participating in group activities at school.

Holly was maintained on citalopram and monthly psychotherapy for the duration of the school year. When the time came for Holly to consider colleges, the therapist advised the family to consider smaller schools, where she would be more likely to be socially successful. Also, the therapist suggested finding a school with adequate mental health services. When she graduated from high school and went to college, a transition was made to college mental health services and backup mental health expertise in the region.

REFERENCES

Ambrosini P, Dixon J: Schedule for Affective Disorders and Schizophrenia for School-Age Children (K-SADS-IVR). Philadelphia, Medical College of Pennsylvania, Eastern Pennsylvania Psychiatric Institute, 2000

Beck AT: Cognitive models of depression, in Clinical Advances in Cognitive Psychotherapy: Theory and Application. Edited by Leahy RL, Dowd TE. New York, Springer, 2002, pp 29–61

Beck AT, Emery G: Anxiety Disorders and Phobias. New York, Basic Books, 1985

Beck JS: Cognitive Therapy: Basics and Beyond. New York, Guilford, 1995

Beck JS, Beck AT, Jolly J: Beck Youth Inventories of Emotional and Social Impairment Manual. San Antonio, TX, Psychological Corporation, 2001

Beidel DC: Social phobia and overanxious disorder in school-age children. J Am Acad Child Adolesc Psychiatry 30:545–552, 1991

Brent DA, Birmaher B: Treatment resistant depression in adolescents: recognition and management. Child Adolesc Psychiatr Clin N Am 15:1015–1034, 2006

Brent DA, Weersing VR: Depressive disorders in childhood and adolescence, in Rutter's Child and Adolescent Psychiatry. Edited by Rutter M, Bishop D, Pine D, et al. Oxford, UK, Blackwell, Oxford University Press, 2008

Birmaher B, Brent D, AACAP Work Group on Quality Issues, et al: Practice parameter for the assessment and treatment of children and adolescents with depressive disorders. J Am Acad Child Adolesc Psychiatry 46:1503–1526, 2007

Goodman WK, Price LH, Rasmussen SA, et al: The Yale-Brown Obsessive Compulsive Scale, II: validity. Arch Gen Psychiatry 46:1012–1016, 1989

Kratochvil CJ, Vitiello B, Brent D, et al: Selecting an antidepressant for the treatment of pediatric depression. J Am Acad Child Adolesc Psychiatry 45:371–373, 2006a

Kratochvil CJ, Vitiello B, Walkup J, et al: Selective serotonin reuptake inhibitors in pediatric depression: is the balance between benefits and risks favorable? J Child Adolesc Psychopharmacol 16:151–164, 2006b

March J, Silva S, Petrycki S, et al; Treatment for Adolescents with Depression Study (TADS) Team: Fluoxetine, cognitive-behavioral therapy, and their combination for adolescents with depression: Treatment for Adolescents with Depression study (TADS) randomized controlled trial. JAMA 292:807–820, 2004

March JS, Silva SG, Vitiello B, et al: The Treatment for Adolescents with Depression Study (TADS): methods and message at twelve weeks. J Am Acad Child Adolesc Psychiatry 45:1393–1403, 2006

Stark KD, Schnoebelen S, Simpson J, et al: Treating Depressed Youth: Therapist Manual for "ACTION." Ardmore, PA, Workbook Publishing, 2007a

Stark KD, Simpson J, Schnoebelen S, et al: ACTION Workbook: Cognitive-Behavioral Therapy for Treating Depressed Girls. Ardmore, PA, Workbook Publishing, 2007b

Stark KD, Simpson J, Yancy M, et al: Parents' Workbook for ACTION. Ardmore, PA, Workbook Publishing, 2007c

Stark KD, Yancy M, Simpson J, et al: Treating Depressed Children: Therapist Manual for Parent Component of "ACTION." Ardmore, PA, Workbook Publishing, 2007d

Stark KD, Krumholtz L, Ridley K, et al: Treatment of depressed girls: the ACTION program, in Youth Depression. Edited by Nolen-Hoeksema S. New York, Guilford (in press)

■ CHAPTER 24 ■

Cutting Helps Me Feel Better

Nonsuicidal Self-Injury

Matthew K. Nock, Ph.D.
Tara L. Deliberto, B.S.

CASE PRESENTATION

IDENTIFYING INFORMATION

Casey is a 16-year-old girl referred for outpatient treatment after being treated at a local psychiatric emergency department for a superficial laceration to her wrist.

CHIEF COMPLAINT

Casey reported, "I didn't make a suicide attempt. Cutting helps me feel better."

HISTORY OF PRESENT ILLNESS

Casey was brought to the emergency room by her parents, who were informed via a phone call from the school nurse that Casey had cut her wrist in school. This was the first they had heard about Casey cutting herself, and on the recommendation of the nurse, they brought Casey to the local emergency depart-

Matthew K. Nock, Ph.D., is John L. Loeb Associate Professor of the Social Sciences and Director of the Laboratory for Clinical and Developmental Research in the Department of Psychology in Cambridge, Massachusetts.

Tara L. Deliberto, B.S., is Laboratory Manager of the Laboratory for Clinical and Developmental Research in the Department of Psychology at Harvard University in Cambridge, Massachusetts.

For complete biographical information, see "About the Contributors," p. 613.

ment for an evaluation. Casey reports that she did not intend to die from her self-injury, and that she engages in nonsuicidal self-injury (NSSI) approximately one time each week for the purpose of decreasing negative thoughts and feelings. Casey reports that she first started cutting herself at age 14. Although she denies any past history of suicide attempts, she endorses suicidal ideation approximately twice per month.

Casey reports a long history of intense emotional reactivity in response to stressful events, dating back to childhood. Her mother reports that Casey was often oppositional and defiant of adults and "threw tantrums when she did not get her way." Her father added that Casey is self-critical and often comments that she is "ugly" and "stupid."

Casey reports first learning about NSSI from a friend during middle school but did not think much of it at the time. Approximately 2 years later, Casey's boyfriend broke up with her, and she no longer wanted to spend time with their mutual friends. Soon after, she started spending time with a different group of teens, several of whom occasionally engage in NSSI, according to Casey. On one occasion, when she became angry at her father, Casey went to her room and scratched her wrist with a safety pin until she drew blood. She reports that the scratching made her feel less upset. She also reports that after scratching her wrist, she called her ex-boyfriend on the telephone to let him know what she had done, and she also told her new group of friends about the incident.

Since her first episode of NSSI, Casey has engaged in NSSI approximately once per week, with an increased frequency in recent weeks after a fight with a close friend. She reports engaging in NSSI when her emotions are unbearably strong, when she is lonely, and when she would like to punish herself for something. She reports that doing this always makes her feel a little better. Casey often uses a knife or razor blade to make cuts on her arms, legs, and sometimes belly. Occasionally, she will use a safety pin to prick holes in her skin to the point of drawing blood. Casey states that getting into fights with loved ones or friends, feeling that people are angry or annoyed with her, and feeling abandoned are common triggers for her NSSI.

Past Psychiatric History

Casey began seeing a psychiatrist for a major depressive episode when she was age 14 and received a prescription for fluoxetine, which she continues to take. Casey reports that although the fluoxetine helped improve her mood, it did not decrease her NSSI. Casey has never received psychosocial treatment and has never been admitted to a hospital for psychiatric treatment.

Medical History

Casey and her parents denied any significant medical history.

DEVELOPMENTAL HISTORY

Casey's parents report that as a small child, Casey was "outgoing," "smart," and "precocious." She attained all developmental milestones within normal limits. Casey's parents also report, however, that Casey was sexually abused by a relative on two occasions when she was age 10, after which she became more withdrawn than usual. Casey refused to see a clinician or counselor after these incidents, and her parents did not push her to do so; however, they report that it was around this time that Casey started to become easily upset by stressful events and increasingly emotionally reactive.

SOCIAL HISTORY

Casey lives with her biological parents, 17-year-old brother, and 8-year-old sister. Her father is an attorney, and her mother is a homemaker. Casey is currently in tenth grade at a medium-sized, suburban public school in an affluent community and has been in the same school district since kindergarten. She reports having "a lot of friends" but does not engage in any extracurricular activities. She is an A student. Casey describes her home life by saying, "I hate my parents," and she reports that she believes her parents are overly controlling in their parenting style and are extremely critical and hostile toward her and her siblings.

FAMILY HISTORY

Casey's father reports a history of alcohol abuse and problems controlling his anger on occasion, and her mother reports a history of recurrent depression. Both parents have been successfully treated and managed via outpatient psychosocial treatment. Casey's parents deny the presence of any psychopathology in her siblings and are unaware of any family history of psychopathology beyond the immediate family.

MENTAL STATUS EXAMINATION

Casey and her mother arrived on schedule at the outpatient clinic. Casey was dressed appropriately in jeans and a sweatshirt. She sat quietly in her chair for most of the interview, looking at the floor and making only occasional eye contact while giving brief one- to two-word responses to direct questions. Casey's mood was "sad and angry," and she displayed somewhat labile affect, appearing flat during much of the interview but raising her voice to the level of screaming and crying a bit when discussing problems at home and at school. Casey was oriented to time, place, and person, and her speech and thought process and content were normal. Casey denied hallucinations and delusions, denied any violent ideation or behavior, and reported twice-monthly suicidal ideation and once-daily thoughts of NSSI, with no current plan or intent to engage in self-injury of any kind.

COMMENTARIES

Psychotherapeutic Perspective

Alec L. Miller, Psy.D.
Dena A. Klein, Ph.D.

DIAGNOSTIC FORMULATION

The assessment and diagnosis of multiproblem adolescents engaging in suicidal and nonsuicidal self-injurious behaviors (NSSI) need not be as daunting as one might assume, provided one has the appropriate instruments and knowledge base. Researchers have identified evidence-based distal and proximal risk factors that, when combined, increase the likelihood of suicidal behavior among adolescents (see Miller et al. 2007). A structured diagnostic interview, such as the Schedule for Affective Disorders and Schizophrenia for School-Aged Children — Present and Lifetime Version (Kaufman et al. 1997), is useful for assessing some of these risk factors among adolescents, including the presence of diagnosable mental disorders, prior suicidal behavior, stressful life events, and relevant histories (e.g., developmental, medical, family). Self-report inventories, including the Suicidal Ideation Questionnaire (Reynolds 1987) and the Beck Suicide Intent Scale (Beck et al. 1974), as well as the interviewer-administered Columbia Suicide-Severity Rating Scale (Posner et al. 2007) and the Reasons for Living Inventory for Adolescents (Osman et al. 1998), are effective measures for evaluating the frequency, intent, and function of suicidal behavior, as well as protective factors against suicide. Other self-report measures, including the Beck Depression Inventory — Second Edition (Beck et al. 1996), Symptom Checklist–90 — Revised (Derogatis 1983), and Millon Adolescent Clinical Inventory (Millon et al. 1993), assess commonly

Alec L. Miller, Psy.D., is Professor of Clinical Psychiatry and Behavioral Sciences; Chief of Child and Adolescent Psychology; Director of the Adolescent Depression and Suicide Program; and Associate Director of the Psychology Internship Training Program at the Montefiore Medical Center/Albert Einstein College of Medicine in Bronx, New York.

Dena A. Klein, Ph.D., is Staff Psychologist and Director of the Child and Adolescent Psychological Assessment Service in the Child Outpatinet Psychiatry Department and Adolescent Depression and Suicide Program at Montefiore Medical Center in Bronx, New York.

For complete biographical information, see "About the Contributors," p. 613.

associated risk factors, including depressive symptom severity, global symptomatology, and maladaptive personality features, respectively.

Several factors suggest that Casey is at higher than average risk for crossing the threshold from suicidal ideation to action, including her twice-monthly suicidal ideation, weekly NSSI, history of sexual abuse, prior apparent major depressive episode, emotional reactivity, perceived hostile family environment, family psychiatric history of alcohol abuse and depression, modeling of self-injury by peers, and interpersonal conflicts. However, Casey's apparent NSSI, by definition, does not evidence suicidal intent; rather, it may serve other functions, such as affect regulation (e.g., emotional avoidance/escape), self-punishment, and instrumental purposes (i.e., social reinforcement) (McAuliffe et al. 2007). Assessment of intent for each behavior is critical to better understand Casey's suicide risk, as well as to better inform case formulation and subsequent interventions.

Casey's history of emotional sensitivity and reactivity predating her sexual abuse suggests that her symptom presentation is enduring and warrants consideration of DSM-IV-TR Axis II diagnoses. The Structured Clinical Interview for DSM-IV Axis II Personality Disorders (First et al. 1997) and the Structured Interview for DSM-IV Personality (Pfohl et al. 1995) are semistructured interviews useful in assessing personality disorders. Casey exhibits several features common to borderline personality disorder (BPD), including unstable interpersonal relationships, recurrent self-mutilating behavior, affective instability, and difficulty controlling anger. Furthermore, her childhood sexual abuse, perceived family conflict, critical self-thoughts, and psychiatric family history are factors commonly associated with a diagnosis of BPD (Linehan 1993). However, without administering a semistructured diagnostic clinical interview, the clinician cannot determine if Casey meets the sufficient number of DSM-IV-TR criteria (i.e., five or more) for a BPD diagnosis. Thus, further assessment of the following criteria is indicated: reaction to real or imagined abandonment; self-image; feelings of emptiness; and presence of paranoid ideation or dissociative symptoms. Although assigning personality disorder diagnoses to adolescents is considered controversial by some clinicians, a growing body of empirical evidence suggests that a BPD diagnosis is appropriate for some adolescents (Miller et al. 2007). In fact, many adolescents, especially females, diagnosed with BPD exhibit a presentation and course that are similar to those of their adult counterparts and therefore deserve a thorough diagnostic evaluation and relevant treatment (Miller et al. 2007).

Individuals with BPD have high rates of comorbidity with other disorders, particularly depression and substance abuse (Linehan 1993). Casey's "sad and angry" mood, lack of engagement in extracurricular activities, and family psychiatric history of depression are common features of a major depressive episode. However, her symptoms require further assessment to determine whether she meets criteria for major depressive disorder. Casey's history of sexual abuse and subsequent withdrawal and emotional reactivity also require further investigation to determine if she is experiencing other symptoms of posttraumatic stress disorder.

DSM-IV-TR DIAGNOSIS

Axis I   311 Depressive disorder not otherwise specified

            V61.20 Parent-child relational problem

            Rule out major depressive disorder, single episode, in partial remission

            Rule out posttraumatic stress disorder

Axis II   Rule out borderline personality disorder

Axis III   None

Axis IV   Poor relationship with parents

            Mother's history of recurrent depression

            Father's history of alcohol abuse and anger control problems

            Loss of romantic relationship

            Peer conflict

Axis V   Global Assessment of Functioning=45

TREATMENT RECOMMENDATIONS

Outpatient psychosocial interventions that directly target suicidal behavior and NSSI are considered more effective than other interventions in reducing suicide risk and associated behaviors (Lieb et al. 2004). Although few controlled studies have included adolescent samples, the efficacy of dialectical behavior therapy (DBT) for chronically suicidal adults with BPD has led to its adaptation for younger populations (Miller et al. 2007). Preliminary research has documented promising results for the usefulness of DBT in reducing NSSI and suicidal behavior among multiproblem adolescents (Goldstein et al. 2007; Rathus and Miller 2002). Informed by behavioral science, dialectical philosophy, and Zen practice, DBT relies on a collaborative, nonjudgmental approach to improve patient motivation to change, enhance patient capabilities, promote generalization of new behaviors, structure the environment, and enhance therapist capability and motivation. These functions are achieved in DBT by employing individual psychotherapy, multifamily skills training groups, family therapy, telephone consultation to teens and family members, and therapist consultation groups to comprehensively and efficiently address adolescents' suicidal behavior and their multiple life problems.

With DBT as a framework, Casey's individual therapy would employ detailed behavioral chain analyses to assess and provide insight into the emotional, behavioral, cognitive, and systemic factors contributing to and maintaining her NSSI and suicidal ideation. Subsequent solution analyses are generated to provide alternative strategies to avert the problem behaviors in the future. As she gains better control of her life-threatening behaviors, individual sessions would target any behaviors interfering in therapy, as well as behaviors interfering with Casey's quality of life, including her depression, "unbearably strong emotions," interpersonal conflicts, and self-criticism. Processing past trauma is typically addressed in DBT following the acquisition of new behavioral skills and the remission of Stage I targets, including life-threatening, therapy-interfering, and quality-of-life–interfering behaviors. The purpose of participation in a concurrent multifamily skills training group is to provide Casey and her parents with the requisite behavioral skills to manage the aforementioned life problems in a more effective manner. Parents themselves often benefit from increasing or refining their current skills repertoire to more effectively tolerate their own distress while improving family communication through more accurate validation and positive reinforcement. Telephone consultation for teens and parents is intended to enhance skills generalization in their natural environments, just as a player and coach touch base during the end of the game to strategize about a new play. For example, when suicidal crises or intense interpersonal conflicts arise, the adolescent is instructed to call the primary therapist for coaching before engaging in the default problem behavior.

Finally, DBT family therapy sessions, provided on an as-needed basis, are often used to assess and treat environmental contingencies at home (e.g., a critical and hostile family environment) that influence suicidal behavior or NSSI or interfere with quality of life. Continuous monitoring and assessment (e.g., diary cards, behavioral analyses, other self-report measures) inform the selection and emphasis of DBT strategies and should be used to update treatment goals in all modes of therapy and to evaluate outcomes. DBT is a useful treatment modality to help adolescents find the dialectical middle path and ultimately build a life worth living.

Psychopharmacologic Perspective

Niranjan S. Karnik, M.D., Ph.D.
Hans Steiner, Dr. med. univ., F.A.P.A., F.A.A.C.A.P., F.A.P.M.

DIAGNOSTIC FORMULATION

This case presents a 16-year-old female who was referred for outpatient psychiatric evaluation subsequent to treatment of superficial cutting at an emergency room. The case is quite typical of what is seen in outpatient psychiatric clinics (Jacobson and Gould 2007; Portzky and van Heeringen 2007). Casey has a history of a major depressive episode diagnosed at age 14. Her symptoms clearly extend into her childhood, and she has a significant trauma history.

Diagnostically, we would consider major depressive disorder, which has not achieved remission on her current regimen. Casey clearly exhibits stress-related exacerbations of her self-harm patterns, which would lead to consideration of whether she might be suffering from posttraumatic stress disorder or another anxiety disorder. The family history from her mother's side indicates that Casey may be at risk for anxiety spectrum disorders. Her patterns may also suggest that she is in a state of serotonergic imbalance resulting partially from her childhood trauma. Although Casey reports that the fluoxetine helped her mood, she indicates that it did not change her self-injurious patterns. Therefore, consideration needs to be given to the degree to which fluoxetine may be partially improving her mood while leading to a degree of self-harm driven by activation. Children who have a nascent bipolar affective disorder (Kim et al. 2007) can have atypical responses to selective serotonin reuptake inhibitors (SSRIs), but the likelihood of this diagnosis for Casey is low given the history that is presented and the lack of a family history of affective disorders. The ca-

Niranjan S. Karnik, M.D., Ph.D., is Assistant Adjunct Professor in the Department of Psychiatry and Department of Anthropology, History and Social Medicine at the University of California School of Medicine, San Francisco; and Staff Psychiatrist at the Palo Alto Medical Foundation in Fremont, California

Hans Steiner, Dr. med. univ., F.A.P.A., F.A.A.C.A.P., F.A.P.M., is Professor in Psychiatry and Behavioral Sciences, Child and Adolescent Psychiatry, and Human Development at Stanford University School of Medicine in Palo Alto, California.

For complete biographical information, see "About the Contributors," p. 613.

veat to this is that the father has some history of alcoholism, which may mask his own presentation of bipolar affective disorder. A detailed sleep history may provide good data to help differentiate the type of mood disorder (major depressive disorder vs. bipolar affective disorder) that Casey has.

Given her age and her peer group, some consideration must be given to substance use disorders. Her family history and to some extent her dissociative and numbing symptoms may push her toward substance use disorders, and those symptoms might also be exacerbated or caused by substance use disorders. Therefore, a careful clinician will explore this history with Casey and collateral sources, and perform laboratory screening tests where indicated.

In addition, although little in the case presentation suggests a primary dissociative disorder, the clinician might keep this possible diagnosis in the differential until it can be more definitively ruled out. Casey's history of trauma could be considered a risk factor for a primary dissociative disorder, but given the degree to which it is circumscribed and contained, the history does not fully fit the pattern generally associated with dissociative disorders.

Finally, given Casey's past trauma, mood lability, and cutting behavior, some consideration should be given to the degree to which this young person may be on a trajectory toward some type of Axis II pathology, namely BPD. Although clinicians should be wary of making judgments about characterological issues during this developmentally sensitive period before age 18, we believe that prompt intensive and integrative treatment may avoid this personality trajectory and provide Casey with a set of skills that she can better use to deal with stressors in her life.

DSM-IV-TR DIAGNOSIS

Axis I   296.3x Major depressive disorder, recurrent
          Rule out posttraumatic stress disorder
Axis II   Deferred (consider possible development of borderline qualities)
Axis III Superficial lacerations
Axis IV   Interpersonal stressors
          History of trauma
Axis V   Global Assessment of Functioning=45–50

TREATMENT RECOMMENDATIONS

The first step in treatment should be to recognize that Casey needs an integrated and multimodal strategy (Steiner 2004; Watanabe et al. 2007; Weissman 2007). Results from the Treatment for Adolescents with Depression Study support the use of medication and psychotherapy (March et al. 2006). This combined therapy is especially important because most pharmacologic interventions require several weeks to have full effect, whereas psychotherapeutic strategies are more likely to provide immediate structure and support. Given that Casey has already presented in the emergency room and that her patterns seem to be slowly escalating, we would be concerned that she may be on a path that may soon move toward true suicidal behavior. (Due to space limitations, we refer the reader to the other commentaries in this chapter, which focus on psychotherapy and integrated treatment.)

Casey presents in the midst of treatment with fluoxetine, which she has been taking for the past 2 years. Consideration should be given to whether she is taking a therapeutic dose or whether there might be potential to better optimize her dose while being attentive to side effects. Given her subjective claim of some response to this medication for her moods, she may be best classified as a partial responder to fluoxetine.

Of concern in this scenario is that the parents did not push Casey to obtain treatment and did not insist on additional interventions when her symptoms persisted. Although this inaction may represent lack of knowledge or denial, it may also be suggestive of more severe intrafamilial trauma histories that would link to her dissociative symptoms and self-injury patterns (Plattner et al. 2003).

In the context of Casey's past history of abuse, we could view her case through the lens of a stress-diathesis model whereby she has had a significant trauma that has primed her neuropsychiatric system to be more sensitive to social and interpersonal stressors. She may have some degree of serotonergic dysregulation stemming from her childhood trauma. In such cases, the use of an SSRI or a serotonin-norepinephrine reuptake inhibitor (SNRI) is potentially beneficial (Hughes et al. 2007). Caution should be exercised, however, due to the potentially activating effects of these medications and the increased potential for suicidal thoughts (Bridge et al. 2007; Perlis et al. 2007).

With a partial responder to fluoxetine, the clinician has three pharmacologic choices: 1) changing to another SSRI or SNRI, 2) adjunctive treatment with a second agent, or 3) switching to a different class of medication. When changing to another medication, the clinician should avoid agents with short half-lives. For Casey, the best option might be to use an agent with greater serotonergic effects, such as citalopram, or one that is more likely to impact multiple receptor systems, such as venlafaxine.

An adjunctive strategy would be to consider the target symptoms and select the agent based on these targets. For example, for children with depression and posttraumatic stress disorder who have significant nightmares, ruminative thoughts, or anxiety episodes, we sometimes use small doses of an atypical antipsychotic, especially at bedtime. In our experience, the combination of fluoxetine and low-dose quetiapine seems to work very well for posttraumatic stress disorder, and helps with improving quality of sleep and reduction of anxiety symptoms.

Should these sets of interventions fail to produce lower degrees of anxiety, depression, and self-harm, then consideration may be given to changing the class of medications. Mood stabilizers, such as divalproex sodium, may help Casey, and some evidence in boys indicates that this medication may be helpful in the treatment of cases with trauma (Steiner et al. 2007). Antiepileptic drugs used as mood stabilizers have good intrinsic mood-stabilizing qualities, as well as some degree of antidepressant effects. These medications also reduce impulsivity and are relatively well tolerated. Because many of these medications have black box warnings, they need to be initiated and monitored closely.

Finally, clinicians may want to avoid particular medications in a case like this one. Activating medications such as stimulants for attention-deficit/hyperactivity disorder (ADHD) or bupropion may worsen some of Casey's internal feelings of stress and produce more self-harm. Should a patient have an essential need for these medications, especially if an adolescent has ADHD and needs treatment, then careful titration should be done and secondary medications may be needed if side effects begin to exacerbate the patient's behavioral dysregulation.

Integrative Perspective

Matthew K. Nock, Ph.D.
Tara L. Deliberto, B.S.

DIAGNOSTIC FORMULATION

Engagement in self-injurious behavior is a symptom of both major depressive disorder and BPD, and prior research indicates that approximately 40% of adolescents who engage in NSSI meet criteria for major depressive disorder and 50% meet criteria for BPD (Deliberto and Nock 2008; Nock et al. 2006). However, it is important to remember that NSSI does not occur exclusively within the context of these diagnoses; individuals engaging in NSSI also meet criteria for other internalizing disorders, such as posttraumatic stress disorder (24%), externalizing disorders (63%), substance use disorders (60%), and other personality disorders (>60%). Given that NSSI occurs in the context of a wide range of diagnoses, clinicians should assess for the presence of NSSI and other forms of self-injurious thoughts and behaviors in all children and adolescents presenting for services. Community-based studies consistently report lifetime rates of NSSI at approximately 15%–20% among high school and college students (e.g., Whitlock et al. 2006).

In addition to considering the psychiatric diagnoses present in an adolescent engaging in NSSI, the clinician should consider the function or purpose of the behavior. Prior work reveals that adolescents engage in NSSI in the service of four primary functions. NSSI for *automatic negative reinforcement* is that performed to relieve or distract from negative thoughts or feelings. This is the function endorsed most frequently in virtually all studies on this topic. NSSI for *automatic positive reinforcement* is that performed for feeling generation, such as in response to dissociation or numbness. NSSI for *social positive reinforcement* is that performed to get attention or access to resources (e.g., hospital admission). Finally, *social negative reinforcement* is that performed to escape from social demands or situations (e.g., to get out of having to attend school, to get parents to stop fighting). Research has elucidated the ways in which these behavioral functions of NSSI relate to different diagnoses and related problems (see Nock and Prinstein 2005). NSSI for automatic negative reinforcement is most strongly related to suicidal ideation and attempts, which also are believed to serve a negative reinforcement function. NSSI for automatic positive reinforcement is uniquely related to symptoms of posttraumatic stress disorder, which is characterized by numbness and dissociation. Finally, NSSI for either positive or negative social reinforcement is strongly and uniquely related to the experience of social problems.

Casey reported engaging in NSSI to get rid of bad feelings, which suggests an automatic negative reinforcement function for this behavior. Her suicidal ideation may also be understood in this light, and the occurrence of both of these phenomena may be similar in that they could function to help Casey escape from aversive cognitive and emotional states. The fact that Casey called her ex-boyfriend and friends to inform them of her NSSI after doing it *suggests* that social factors may also be motivating her desire to engage in NSSI; however, the clinician should be careful not to infer that social factors motivate Casey and would be wise to monitor potential social influences on Casey's NSSI over time.

Several other correlates of NSSI that have been identified in the literature are notable in Casey's history. A history of childhood abuse (especially sexual and emotional abuse) has been associated with subsequent engagement in NSSI (Glassman et al. 2007). Moreover, heightened emotional reactivity, as measured both subjectively and via physiological measures, has been linked to engagement in NSSI, especially to that performed for automatic negative reinforcement (Nock and Mendes 2008). Finally, elevated levels of parental hostility and criticism have been associated with engagement in NSSI, as has the adoption of a self-critical cognitive style (Glassman et al. 2007; Wedig and Nock 2007). Casey's early experience of sexual abuse may have contributed to her heightened emotional reactivity, and Casey's self-critical style may further increase the likelihood that she will respond to stressful events by hurting herself as an extreme means of self-punishment. Casey's NSSI may have been maintained over time both by the decrease in negative feelings it produces and via the way in which it might influence the behavior of her peers, although each of these factors remains a question for assessment and treatment.

Administration of a semistructured diagnostic interview reveals the following five-axis diagnosis.

DSM-IV-TR DIAGNOSIS

Axis I   296.32 Major depressive disorder, recurrent, moderate

Axis II   Borderline personality disorder

Axis III No diagnosis

Axis IV Problems with primary support group (history of sexual abuse, family conflict)

        Problems with social environment (peer conflicts)

Axis V   Global Assessment of Functioning=55

TREATMENT RECOMMENDATIONS

The evidence-based assessment of self-injurious thoughts and behaviors should include 1) assessing for the presence, frequency, and severity of suicidal and nonsuicidal self-injurious thoughts and behaviors; 2) drawing on multiple informants and measurement methods (e.g., parent, adolescent, self-report, interview); 3) assessing known risk and protective factors for each self-injurious thought and behavior; and 4) assessing the function of self-injury (Nock et al. 2008). Given that self-injurious thoughts and behaviors are often transient in nature, assessment should be conducted on a regular basis and not solely during the initial evaluation. One excellent tool for ongoing assessment is a one-page diary card; the adolescent records self-injurious thoughts and behaviors (as well as other target behaviors) on the card daily and brings this information to treatment sessions.

The results of the assessment and case conceptualization should guide treatment procedures in an ongoing way. We encourage the use of an analysis of the functions of NSSI to guide the choice of treatment procedures. This involves assessing the antecedent(s) and consequence(s) of each episode of NSSI to determine what factors influence a patient's engagement in this behavior. Interventions can then be developed that address these controlling factors. For instance, if the assessment indicates that NSSI is being performed for the purposes of automatic negative reinforcement, then the use of antidepressant medication or psychosocial treatment procedures aimed at teaching emotion regulation and distress tolerance skills may prove most effective. If the assessment finds that NSSI is serving a social communication function, then medication is less likely to be as useful as a psychosocial intervention that teaches interpersonal communication skills. The clinician should work with parents, teachers, and other clinicians involved in the case to learn what factors may be driving the NSSI and to develop interventions to decrease this behavior. If agreeable, parents, teachers, and clinicians may benefit from brief education about and instruction in the skills that the adolescent is learning so they can provide encouragement or even coaching in the use of these skills in the adolescent's natural environment.

Unfortunately, no research evidence exists demonstrating the superiority of any one approach for the treatment of NSSI among adolescents (see Nock et al. 2007). Some evidence supports the use of cognitive-behavioral therapy and DBT for the treatment of adolescent suicide attempts, so these treatments should be considered among the best treatments currently available for adolescent self-injury. One of the useful features of using modular approaches such as cognitive-behavioral therapy and DBT in the treatment of NSSI is that they can be flexibly modified to treat unique cases (see Nock et al. 2004). Simpler interventions, such as the use of aerobic exercise, also have shown impressive effects in the treatment of NSSI and can be easily incorporated into any existing treatment regimen (see Wallenstein and Nock 2007).

REFERENCES

Beck A, Schuyler D, Herman I: Development of suicidal intent scales, in The Prediction of Suicide. Edited by Beck A, Resnik A, Lettieri D. Bowie, MD, Charles Press, 1974

Beck AT, Steer RA, Brown GK: Manual for the Beck Depression Inventory, 2nd Edition. San Antonio, TX, Psychological Corporation, 1996

Bridge JA, Iyengar S, Salary CB, et al: Clinical response and risk for reported suicidal ideation and suicide attempts in pediatric antidepressant treatment: a meta-analysis of randomized controlled trials. JAMA 297:1683–1696, 2007

Deliberto T, Nock M: Exploratory study of the correlates, onset, and offset of nonsuicidal self-injury. Arch Suicide Res 12:219–231, 2008

Derogatis LR: SCL-90-R: Administration, Scoring and Procedures Manual, 2nd Edition. Towson, MD, Clinical Psychometric Research, 1983

First MB, Gibbon M, Spitzer RL, et al: The Structured Clinical Interview for DSM-IV Axis II Personality Disorders (SCID-II), Version 2.0. Washington, DC, American Psychiatric Press, 1997

Glassman LH, Weierich MR, Hooley JM, et al: Child maltreatment, non-suicidal self-injury, and the mediating role of self-criticism. Behav Res Ther 45:2483–2490, 2007

Goldstein TR, Axelson DA, Birmaher B, et al: Dialectical behavior therapy for adolescents with bipolar disorder: a 1-year open trial. J Am Acad Child Adolesc Psychiatry 46:820–830, 2007

Hughes CW, Emslie GJ, Crismon ML, et al; Texas Children's Medication Algorithm Project: update from Texas Consensus Conference Panel on Medication Treatment of Childhood Major Depressive Disorder. J Am Acad Child Adolesc Psychiatry 46:667–686, 2007

Jacobson CM, Gould M: The epidemiology and phenomenology of non-suicidal self-injurious behavior among adolescents: a critical review of the literature. Arch Suicide Res 11:129–147, 2007

Kaufman J, Birmaher B, Brent D, et al: Schedule for Affective Disorders and Schizophrenia for School-Aged Children (6–18 years)—Present and Lifetime Version (K-SADS-PL). Pittsburgh, PA, University of Pittsburgh School of Medicine, Department of Psychiatry, 1997

Kim EY, Miklowitz DJ, Biuckians A, et al: Life stress and the course of early onset bipolar disorder. J Affect Disord 99:37–44, 2007

Lieb K, Zanarini M, Linehan MM, et al: Seminar section: borderline personality disorder. Lancet 364:453–461, 2004

Linehan MM: Cognitive-Behavioral Treatment of Borderline Personality Disorder. New York, Guilford, 1993

March J, Silva S, Vitiello B: The Treatment for Adolescents with Depression Study (TADS): methods and message at 12 weeks. J Am Acad Child Adolesc Psychiatry 45:1393–1403, 2006

McAuliffe C, Arensman E, Keeley HS, et al: Motives and suicide intent underlying hospital treated deliberate self-harm and their association with repetition. Suicide Life Threat Behav 37:397–408, 2007

Miller AL, Rathus JH, Linehan MM: Dialectical Behavior Therapy With Suicidal Adolescents. New York, Guilford, 2007

Millon T, Millon C, Davis R, et al: The Millon Adolescent Clinical Inventory. Minneapolis, MN, National Computer Systems, 1993

Nock MK, Mendes WB: Physiological arousal, distress tolerance, and social problem solving deficits among adolescent self-injurers. J Consult Clin Psychol 76:28–38, 2008

Nock MK, Prinstein MJ: Contextual features and behavioral functions of self-mutilation among adolescents. J Abnorm Psychol 114:140–146, 2005

Nock MK, Goldman, JL, Wang Y, et al: From science to practice: the flexible use of evidence-based treatments in clinical settings. J Am Acad Child Adolesc Psychiatry 43:777–780, 2004

Nock M, Joiner T, Gordon K, et al: Non-suicidal self injury among adolescents: diagnostic correlates and relation to suicide attempts. Psychiatry Res 144:65–72, 2006

Nock MK, Teper R, Hollander M: Psychosocial treatment of self-injury among children and adolescents. J Clin Psychol 63:1081–1089, 2007

Nock MK, Wedig MM, Janis IB, et al: Self-injurious thoughts and behaviors, in A Guide to Assessments That Work. Edited by Hunsley J, Mash E. New York, Oxford University Press, 2008

Osman A, Downs WR, Kopper BA, et al: The Reasons for Living Inventory for Adolescents (RFL-A): development and psychometric properties. J Clin Psychol 54:1063–1078, 1998

Perlis RH, Beasley CM Jr, Wines JD Jr, et al: Treatment-associated suicidal ideation and adverse effects in an open, multicenter trial of fluoxetine for major depressive episodes. Psychother Psychosom 76:40–46, 2007

Pfohl B, Blum N, Zimmerman M: The Structured Interview for DSM-IV Personality. Iowa City, IA, University of Iowa, 1995

Plattner B, Silvermann MA, Redlich AD, et al: Pathways to dissociation: intrafamilial versus extrafamilial trauma in juvenile delinquents. J Nerv Ment Dis 191:781–788, 2003

Portzky G, van Heeringen K: Deliberate self-harm in adolescents. Curr Opin Psychiatry 20:337–342, 2007

Posner K, Oquendo M, Davies M, et al: Columbia Classification Algorithm of Suicide Assessment (C-CASA): classification of suicidal behavior and related events in the FDA's pediatric suicidal risk analysis of antidepressants. Am J Psychiatry 164:1035–1043, 2007

Rathus JH, Miller AL: Dialectical behavior therapy adapted for suicidal adolescents. Suicide Life Threat Behav 32:146–157, 2002

Reynolds WM: Suicidal Ideation Questionnaire: Professional Manual. Odessa, FL, Psychological Assessment Resources, 1987

Steiner H: Handbook of Mental Health Interventions in Children and Adolescents: An Integrated Developmental Approach. San Francisco, CA, Jossey-Bass, 2004

Steiner H, Saxena KS, Carrion V, et al: Divalproex sodium for the treatment of PTSD and conduct disordered youth: a pilot randomized controlled clinical trial. Child Psychiatry Hum Dev 38:183–193, 2007

Wallenstein MB, Nock MK: Physical exercise for the treatment of non-suicidal self-injury: evidence from a single-case study. Am J Psychiatry 164:350–351, 2007

Watanabe N, Hunot V, Omori IM, et al: Psychotherapy for depression among children and adolescents: a systematic review. Acta Psychiatr Scand 116:84–95, 2007

Wedig MM, Nock MK: Parental expressed emotion and adolescent self-injury. J Am Acad Child Adolesc Psychiatry 46:1171–1178, 2007

Weissman MM: Recent non-medication trials of interpersonal psychotherapy for depression. Int J Neuropsychopharmacol 10:117–122, 2007

Whitlock J, Eckenrode J, Silverman D: Self-injurious behaviors in a college population. Pediatrics 117:1939–1948, 2006

■ CHAPTER 25 ■

From Foster Care to the State Hospital

Psychotic Symptoms in a Child Who Is the Victim of Neglect

Patricia K. Leebens, M.D.

CASE PRESENTATION

IDENTIFYING INFORMATION

Lena is a 14-year-old Hispanic eighth grader in special education who has been a ward of the state and in various foster care placements for the last 2 years since removal for neglect from her single mother. She was recently hospitalized for running away from foster placement, suicidal ideation, and agitation, and has been transferred to the state psychiatric hospital for a comprehensive assessment and to await placement in a residential facility.

CHIEF COMPLAINT

Lena reports, "I always get into trouble because I want to live with my mom."

Patricia K. Leebens, M.D., is Consulting Child and Adolescent Psychiatrist at Family and Children's Aid in Danbury, Connecticut, and Assistant Clinical Professor of Child Psychiatry at the Yale Child Study Center in New Haven and the University of Connecticut School of Medicine in Farmington, Connecticut (for complete biographical information, see "About the Contributors," p. 613).

History of Present Illness

Prior to her most recent hospitalization, Lena ran away from her foster placement and was brought to a local emergency room by the police, when she was
found pacing, disheveled, and agitated at a bus station. She threatened to kill
herself if the police did not take her to her mother. At the emergency room,
her toxicology screen was negative, but she was thought to be psychotic and/or
traumatized. In the emergency room, she was treated with haloperidol (Hal-
dol) and lorazepam (Ativan) for agitation. Because of her persistent suicidal
threats and her agitation, she was hospitalized for 3 weeks and treated with
risperidone (Risperdal) up to 4 mg/day and chlorpromazine (Thorazine) as
needed; the treatment resulted in limited periods of stabilization. Lena also
continued taking the medications she had been taking at admission: fluoxetine
(Prozac) 40 mg/day, methylphenidate (Ritalin) 60 mg/day, and divalproex sodium (Depakote) 450 mg twice a day. Risperidone was discontinued prior to
transfer because of weight gain and constipation.

Past Psychiatric History

Lena was first noted to be hypermotoric, inattentive, and aggressive with peers
in her Head Start program at age 4. Her pediatrician diagnosed attention-
deficit/hyperactivity disorder (ADHD), combined type, and prescribed Ritalin,
with modest benefit. Lena was also noted to be very anxious, prior to the use of
Ritalin, often having great difficulty separating from her mother. Because of
her limited academic progress, language delays, and excessive absences in first
grade, Lena was held back and repeated the grade.

Lena was referred for a comprehensive psychiatric and psychological evaluation at age 8 because of persistent difficulties at home and in school. Her Full
Scale IQ was 82, with significantly greater Performance IQ than Verbal IQ
(Wechsler Intelligence Scale for Children—Third Edition [WISC-III]; Wechsler 1991). A speech and language evaluation suggested that she had some expressive language delays. Academic achievement testing indicated that Lena
was 12–14 months behind in writing and spelling, but nearly at grade level for
math computation. The neurological examination was nonfocal, with some soft
neurological signs, including left-right confusion and clumsiness. Projective
testing revealed an anxious, easily overwhelmed girl, excessively preoccupied
with body integrity and aggression, with many images referring to "blood dripping down walls." Some of Lena's responses on the Rorschach were unusual but
were not thought to be frankly psychotic. Her psychiatric examination was notable for extreme hyperactivity, aggressive play, excessive anxiety, and limited
eye contact, although she was evaluated while on Ritalin. She was diagnosed
with ADHD, combined type, and possible posttraumatic stress disorder (PTSD).

Lena received no ongoing treatment until she was hospitalized psychiatri-
cally at age 12 for extreme aggression and suicidal ideation (plan to stab her-

self), following the removal from her mother's care. Between ages 12 and 14, she had three more psychiatric hospitalizations for threatening to kill herself if she were not sent back to her mother. She was treated with a variety of stimulants, without much benefit, as well as Risperdal, Depakote, Prozac, paroxetine (Paxil), sertraline (Zoloft), guanfacine (Tenex), and clonidine (Catapres), with mixed results.

SUBSTANCE ABUSE HISTORY

All informants deny that Lena uses substances, and previous toxicology screens have been negative.

MEDICAL HISTORY

Lena had recurrent otitis media from age 18 months to age 4 years and had tubes placed in her ears at age 3. She had four "febrile seizures" before age 3. She was diagnosed with mild asthma at age 5 and treated with albuterol (Proventil) as needed. She has had no serious illnesses, surgeries, broken bones, head trauma, or loss of consciousness. She was in a minor motor vehicle accident with her mother at age 8, with no injury. Menses began at age 11 and have been regular. She is not sexually active, although she may have been touched inappropriately by a boyfriend of her mother's (allegation unsubstantiated) between ages 8 and 10.

DEVELOPMENTAL HISTORY

Lena's mother's pregnancy was significant for a maternal diagnosis of schizophrenia. Her mother was taking fluphenazine (Prolixin) and Prozac when she became pregnant but did not take her antipsychotic medications the last 5 months of the pregnancy. Lena was exposed to cocaine and alcohol in utero, but her mother claimed that she stopped using substances when she learned she was pregnant. Lena was born 3 weeks early. The labor and delivery were uncomplicated, and Lena's birth weight was 6 lbs 9 oz. Lena's mother became psychotically depressed and was hospitalized 3 weeks after Lena's birth. Lena lived with her maternal grandmother for the first 4 months of life. Lena's developmental milestones were described as "normal." She was an "active" baby who did not sleep much. She had delayed expressive language, which was attributed to speech confusion, as her grandmother spoke Spanish and her mother spoke English. A Birth to Three developmental evaluation at 30 months did not indicate the need for intervention.

SOCIAL HISTORY

Lena, the youngest of three children, was born to a 39-year-old woman of Dominican heritage. Lena's mother currently lives with her boyfriend. Lena's 19-

year-old half brother is incarcerated on drug charges; and her 22-year-old half sister is employed and lives independently with her three small children.

When she was younger, Lena lived with her mother, her maternal grandmother, and her siblings. Her mother was hospitalized multiple times due to psychiatric illness and substance use. The mother lost custody during her hospitalizations and periods of illness, and Lena's grandmother often cared for the children. Lena went into long-term foster care 2 years ago during one of her mother's hospitalizations, following the death of the maternal grandmother (due to complications from diabetes and heart disease). Neither Lena nor her siblings have any contact with their respective fathers.

FAMILY HISTORY

The maternal family psychiatric history is remarkable for ADHD (half brother, cousins, uncles), dyslexia (mother, maternal uncle), substance abuse (mother, uncles, half brother), depression (mother, grandmother, half sister), anxiety (mother), psychosis (mother, great uncle), incarceration (half brother, uncles), and psychiatric hospitalizations (mother, great uncle). Medical history is notable for diabetes (grandmother, great-uncle), heart disease (grandmother, great-uncles), asthma (half sister), and epilepsy (great-aunt). Nothing is known about the paternal family.

MENTAL STATUS EXAMINATION

Lena presented as an attractive but unkempt 14-year-old Hispanic girl in age-appropriate clothing. She spoke English with a slight accent. She often answered in one word or short sentences to end further discussion. She sat between her biological mother and her state caseworker, who both provided warm support. She cooperated with an hour-long intake interview, although she seemed guarded and was restless at times. She often shifted back and forth in her chair. On two occasions, she stood up and looked as though she were going to leave the room, until her mother took her hand and asked her to sit. She had fleeting eye contact and appeared quite anxious, often looking about the room and pushing her chair against the wall. She described her mood as "fine," although she looked dysphoric and distressed. She denied current suicidal or homicidal ideations or plans but admitted that she had felt that way in the past. She also acknowledged that she did not want to be at this hospital and that she thought she was going to get to go home to her mother from the other hospital. She had a flattened affect, which was generally appropriate to the content of her speech, although she sometimes laughed nervously and at times inappropriately when discussing her current symptoms. She initially denied auditory or visual hallucinations, but later said, "Well, maybe sometimes." She refused to participate in a formal mental status examination, saying, "I'm not very good at that." She refused to look at her hospital room, until her mother agreed to go with her. She paced and was agitated at the departure of her mother following the intake process.

COMMENTARIES

Psychotherapeutic Perspective

Nancy C. Winters, M.D.

DIAGNOSTIC FORMULATION

The assessment of a child or adolescent presenting with disorganization, agitation, suicidality, and symptoms suggestive of psychosis is always complex, and diagnostic certainty is often not achieved for some time, particularly when a youngster has a complicated developmental, psychiatric, and social history, as Lena does. Assessing the validity of psychotic-like symptoms can be a challenge in a youth with a mixture of developmental delay and mood lability (Frazier et al. 2007). Moreover, differentiating psychotic mood disorders from schizophrenia can be problematic in an adolescent and may only become possible as the course unfolds (Calderoni et al. 2001).

Therefore, a comprehensive evaluation that assesses the contribution of medical, neurodevelopmental, psychological, interpersonal, and sociocultural factors is essential (Birmaher et al. 2007). The evaluation should include a detailed, longitudinal history of depressive and manic symptoms based on interviews with Lena and her caregivers. The presence of psychotic symptoms, both positive and negative, and their concurrence with mood symptoms should be carefully examined. Additional developmental information should include age at onset of mood symptoms and their relation to negative life events, as well as an understanding of Lena's exposure to neglect, abuse, and violence, and the impact of these experiences on her psychological development. A culturally sensitive family assessment should be performed to understand the key relationships in Lena's social network and the strengths of family members that may be

Nancy C. Winters, M.D., is Associate Professor in the Department of Psychiatry, Division of Public Psychiatry, at Oregon Health and Science Universit in Portland, Oregon, and Chief Psychiatrist, Children's Mental Health and Addictions, of the State of Oregon (for complete biographical information, see "About the Contributors," p. 613).

helpful to her treatment. It is also of great importance to understand Lena's motivation for making suicidal threats and her mother's responses to the threats: Does Lena believe that making threats may result in a return to her mother? Is her mother most involved with Lena when Lena is hospitalized and thereby unwittingly reinforcing this behavior? The evaluation should explore any specific traumatic events that may have precipitated Lena's running away or that may have occurred while she was at large. Neuropsychological and projective testing will be helpful to gain more information about how Lena understands her internal and external experience and whether a psychotic disorder is likely to be present. No less important is an examination of why previous attempts at treatment have failed such that Lena is now in her fifth hospitalization.

Lena has many risk factors for severe mood disorder, including comorbid conditions of anxiety (including possible PTSD), ADHD, and learning disorder. Other significant risk factors for severe depression include Lena's exposure to major negative life events, including neglect, attachment disturbance, and separation from her mother (DiFilippo and Overholser 2000). Lena currently presents with symptoms of suicidality, running away, psychomotor agitation, dysphoric and anxious affect, disheveled appearance, and guarded communication, and she reports that "maybe sometimes" she has hallucinations. The case presentation contains no specific information indicating a history of manic symptoms or of psychosis in the absence of mood symptoms. Thus, this presentation is best described as a recurrent major depression with psychotic features. However, given the increased risk of bipolar disorder in adolescents with psychotic depression, as well as the history of psychosis (possibly schizoaffective disorder) in Lena's mother, Lena is at high risk of developing either bipolar disorder or a schizophrenic spectrum disorder such as schizophrenia or schizoaffective disorder (Birmaher et al. 2007). Finally, although personality factors cannot be definitively evaluated in the context of Lena's young age and in the context of her major depression, especially in the presence of psychotic symptoms, the clinician needs to be aware of personality development as it relates to behavior. Lena's emerging pattern of dysfunctional affect regulation, self-endangering impulsivity, suicidality, difficulty controlling anger, and efforts to avoid abandonment could signal that she is at risk for borderline personality disorder.

DSM-IV-TR DIAGNOSIS

Axis I   296.34 Major depressive disorder, recurrent, severe with psychotic features

314.01 ADHD, combined type

315.00 Reading disorder

315.2 Disorder of written expression

Axis II   Features of borderline personality disorder

Axis III   None

Axis IV   Separation from her mother and placement in foster care at age 12

           History of neglect and disrupted attachment

           Mother has history of schizoaffective disorder, substance abuse, and multiple psychiatric hospitalizations

Axis V   Global Assessment of Functioning=30

           Currently has impaired communication and judgment and inability to function in almost all areas

TREATMENT RECOMMENDATIONS

Lena's psychotic depression and impulsive self-endangering behavior would be most safely addressed in a secure psychiatric setting until she is stable. Her suicidality needs to be monitored closely, along with her depression and psychotic symptoms. Lena has many of the predictors of poor outcome in depression, including greater severity, chronicity, multiple recurrent episodes, comorbidity, family problems, low socioeconomic status, and exposure to ongoing negative events such as abuse and family conflict (Birmaher et al. 2002; Lewinsohn et al. 1998). Therefore, she needs an intensive multimodal treatment plan that addresses these issues. Given the severity of her depressive symptoms, medication will be an important part of her treatment and may be the most effective initial intervention (as discussed below in "Psychopharmacologic Perspective").

With regard to psychosocial treatments, Lena may initially be able to benefit only from supportive interventions. As her thinking improves, other psychosocial interventions should be considered. Although no specific guidelines exist for psychosocial treatment of psychotic depression in adolescents, the consensus is that psychoeducation, supportive management, and family involvement are important in the treatment of depression disorders (Birmaher et al. 2007). Because Lena's concerns about her relationship with her mother are quite prominent, family intervention should be started immediately, and Lena should participate to the extent that she is able unless doing so worsens her symptoms. The initial phase should involve psychoeducation about Lena's symptoms and how to best support her recovery. If further investigation indicates that Lena's mother will be unable to take care of Lena, family intervention should have the goal of exploring how Lena and her mother can have a closer relationship without living together. If Lena will be returning to live with a particular foster parent, the foster parent should also be involved in the family intervention at a point decided upon by the family and therapist. The wraparound planning process, a community-based model of intervention used for youth with serious emotional disturbance, may be helpful for Lena and her family (Winters et al. 2007). A specialist facilitator would help Lena and her family to form a team that will have an ongoing role in planning an individualized array of services and supports that build on Lena's and her family's strengths and meet their needs as the family perceives them. When Lena's thought process is amenable to engaging in her own psychotherapy, her somewhat limited verbal abilities would have to be considered in selecting treatment. She may benefit from adaptations of cognitive-behavioral therapy, interpersonal psychotherapy, and psychodynamic techniques that are used with younger children (Birmaher et al. 2007). If her mental status improves enough, she might find the relationship orientation of interpersonal psychotherapy beneficial (Klomek and Mufson 2006). Cultural factors should also be taken into account in adapting psychotherapeutic interventions for Lena, because minority status may increase the risk for depression and suicidality (Roberts and Chen 1995). Because Lena's suicidal thinking and threats have led to her hospitalizations, she needs some very specific help in managing these thoughts and impulses. Dialectical behavior therapy, which some evidence indicates can be useful for suicidal adolescents, would be important to consider for Lena if a trained therapist is available (Katz et al. 2004).

Given Lena's language-based learning disorder, ADHD, and emotional problems, she is likely to have significant challenges in school and will require an individualized education program. During her residential psychiatric treatment, her academic functioning and ability to relate to peers need to be carefully assessed. Because some evidence indicates that peer attachments are particularly relevant to depressive symptoms and suicide in girls (DiFilippo and Overholser 2000), enhancing these relationships may be protective. When Lena's depression and psychotic symptoms resolve, her need for medication for ADHD should also be reassessed. Before she returns to school, conjoint planning should be done to determine whether she needs a day treatment program or other school-based mental health service. Her teachers need to be involved in recognizing symptoms in Lena that may be warning signs and developing a crisis plan allowing for preventive action.

Psychopharmacologic Perspective

Harvey N. Kranzler, M.D.

DIAGNOSTIC FORMULATION

Lena's case is representative of many of the cases of children and adolescents referred for inpatient treatment who present on admission with diagnostic questions and incomplete information about their past psychiatric treatment. Lena was transferred to the state psychiatric hospital from the local hospital after having been found pacing, disheveled, agitated, and threatening to kill herself if not taken to her mother. She had a negative toxicology screen; had been evaluated to be psychotic, possibly traumatized; and was stabilized, before being transferred, with Risperdal up to 4 mg/day and Thorazine as needed, in addition to her previous maintenance medications of Prozac 40 mg/day, Ritalin 60 mg/day, and Depakote 450 mg twice a day. (The case presentation does not indicate whether the Ritalin was short- or long-acting.) This was Lena's fifth psychiatric hospitalization in the last 3 years, and her past medication history includes a number of unspecified stimulants, as well as Paxil, Zoloft, Tenex, and Catapres, with mixed or no benefit. The lack of specific data concerning past medication treatment is a frequent occurrence on admission, and obtaining this information is an important part of the assessment and treatment planning.

Lena has a long-past psychiatric history with a diagnosis of ADHD as early as age 4. At age 8, she had a comprehensive psychiatric evaluation due to unspecified difficulty at home and school. On psychological testing, she had a Full Scale IQ of 82, with Performance IQ greater than Verbal IQ; she was noted to have an expressive language delay on speech and language evaluation; she had soft neurological signs on neurological evaluation; and projective testing showed evidence of anxiety and possible psychotic ideation in her preoccupation with body integrity, aggression, and images of "blood dripping down walls." She was noted to be hyperactive and aggressive, with excessive anxiety, and maintained limited eye contact. The history did not mention further psychiatric assessment or treatment until her first hospitalization at age 12 for suicidal ide-

Harvey N. Kranzler, M.D., is Professor of Clinical Psychiatry and Director of the Division of Child and Adolescent Psychiatry at Albert Einstein College of Medicine, and Clinical Director of the Bronx Children's Psychiatric Center in Bronx, New York (for complete biographical information, see "About the Contributors," p. 613).

ation and severe aggression, with three subsequent hospitalizations for similar symptoms. Family psychiatric history is significant, with her mother having a diagnosis of schizophrenia and substance abuse disorder and other family members having ADHD, learning disabilities, depression, anxiety, psychosis, psychiatric hospitalizations, and incarcerations. Lena was exposed to drugs in utero and her mother developed postpartum psychotic depression after her birth, for which mother was hospitalized. For much of her early life, Lena was cared for by her maternal grandmother. After her grandmother died, Lena was placed in long-term foster care. Lena's loss of primary caretakers and her constant wish to be returned to her mother are important factors in her psychological and behavioral difficulties. Lena has a possible history of sexual abuse, but this allegation was unsubstantiated. Lena's medical history includes frequent otitis media as an infant and toddler, four febrile seizures before age 3, and a present diagnosis of mild asthma treated symptomatically.

On admission, Lena was guarded and restless, and made only fleeting eye contact with the admitting clinician, yet related well both to her mother and the state caseworker who accompanied her. She was noted to have flat affect, anxiety, dysphoria, and occasional inappropriate laughter. Lena was uncooperative during the formal mental status examination, but she demonstrated no evidence of overt thought disorder or paranoid delusions. She initially denied auditory and visual hallucinations, but eventually hinted that she may have experienced hallucinations in the past. The clinician saw no evidence of pressured speech, flight of ideas, manic symptoms, or vegetative symptoms of depression.

Lena presents with enough evidence to make a diagnosis of psychosis, because of her flat affect, guardedness, inappropriate laughter, and possible auditory and visual hallucinations. Her past history of being found unkempt, disheveled, and agitated, as well as the images of blood dripping down walls on projective testing, points toward past psychotic symptoms. At this time, a definitive diagnosis of childhood-onset schizophrenia cannot be made because Lena does not meet the full DSM-IV-TR criteria based on the admitting data (Kumra 2000). However, her learning disabilities, her disruptive behavior, and her premorbid functioning in social, motor, and language domains point in the direction of a schizophrenic process that has been ongoing (Gogtay and Rapoport 2007). Her mother's diagnosis of schizophrenia adds further weight to this diagnosis. One cannot rule out an affective component to her diagnosis, even though the case presentation includes no evidence of overt manic symptoms or of overt depression except for dysphoric appearance and a history of suicidal threats. Lena's family history of significant mood disorder, her irritability, her past history of suicidal ideation, and her dysphoria may indicate a diagnosis of schizoaffective disorder or a mood disorder with psychosis. There is no evidence of a medical condition or substance abuse contributing to her psychosis, and her relatedness to her mother and the caseworker point away from a diagnosis of pervasive developmental disorder or autistic spectrum disorder. One needs to rule out a diagnosis of atypical psychosis, known as multidimensionally impaired disorder (Kumra et al. 1998), because of evidence of previous brief transient psychotic symptoms in response to stress, emotional lability, cognitive deficits, and comorbid ADHD, although Lena has no known history of impaired interpersonal skills. Lena has a vague past history of anxiety but no evidence of an anxiety disorder at present. Although Lena has had significant losses and may have been exposed to traumatic experiences while growing up, she does not meet the DSM-IV-TR criteria of PTSD because she has no history of persistent avoidance, numbing, or increased arousal secondary to traumatic stimuli, despite her being irritable and hypervigilant. Lena does have a past history of ADHD and she does manifest impulsivity, distractibility, fidgetiness, and oppositionality, but these behaviors may also be explained by her primary psychiatric diagnosis. Once the psychotic and affective symptoms are ameliorated, one needs to assess if any symptoms of ADHD are still evident.

DSM-IV-TR DIAGNOSIS

Axis I   298.9 Psychotic disorder not otherwise specified

314.01 History of ADHD

Rule out childhood-onset schizophrenia

Rule out schizoaffective disorder

Rule out mood disorder with psychosis

Axis II   None

Axis III   History of febrile seizures before age 3

Mild asthma

Axis IV   Exposure to drugs in utero

Separation from mother

Death of maternal grandmother

Family history of significant psychiatric illness, substance abuse, and incarceration

Axis V   Global Assessment of Functioning=40

Current runaway behavior, suicidal ideation, possible auditory and visual hallucinations, and impairment in judgment

TREATMENT RECOMMENDATIONS

The treatment of Lena requires a team approach to gather important past psychiatric and medical information not available at the time of admission, including a better medication history and more specific information about response to, adverse effects of, duration of treatment with, and maximum dosages of previous medications tried. Continued mental status evaluation may clarify whether Lena has either delusions or actual auditory or visual hallucinations. A full medical and psychiatric evaluation is necessary, including blood workup with complete blood count and differential, fasting glucose, chemistries, liver function studies, a full lipid panel, and a thyroid profile with thyroid-stimulating hormone. One should also obtain baseline height, weight, and body mass index; vital signs; Abnormal Involuntary Movement Scale (AIMS); electrocardiogram; psychological testing, including neurocognitive and projective tests; a neurological evaluation, including magnetic resonance imaging and electroencephalography, to assess for potential lower seizure threshold; a hearing evaluation to rule out any loss of hearing secondary to history of otitis media; and a speech and language screening. Structured assessment instruments, such as the Brief Psychiatric Rating Scale for Children (Overall and Pfefferbaum 1982) and the Kiddie Schedule for Affective Disorders and Schizophrenia in School-Aged Children (Ambrosini 2000), may be helpful (Pappadopulos et al. 2003).

At least two of the medications that Lena has been receiving—Prozac 40 mg/day and Ritalin 60 mg/day—should be tapered and discontinued because they have the potential for exacerbating an underlying psychotic process or may be contributing to activation, irritability, akathisia, and possible suicidal ideation. The Risperdal is an appropriate antipsychotic for her diagnosis, but 4 mg/day is a relatively high dose, which may be a factor in her flat affect, restlessness, and irritability secondary to extrapyramidal symptoms. The Depakote, 450 mg twice a day, is an appropriate mood stabilizer to treat Lena's agitation and aggression, but a Depakote blood level should be obtained. The clinician may want to consider careful tapering and discontinuing of the Depakote and then the Risperdal in a washout effort to assess more accurately the diagnosis and side-effect profile. This may not be possible if Lena has a recurrence of severe psychosis or agitation, but at least a careful tapering and monitoring of emerging symptoms or resolution of side effects may provide useful information. One cannot review in this chapter all of the alternative antipsychotic and mood-stabilizing medications that may be considered for the treatment of Lena's symptoms. The reader is referred to Correll (2008) for a review of the efficacy of antipsychotic medications, as well as a description of the ongoing monitoring for adverse reactions that is essential in a treatment plan that will allow Lena to be discharged from the state hospital. The psychopharmacologic management of her psychiatric symptoms will enable her to become a partner with the ongoing psychotherapeutic modalities in her treatment and allow her development to continue in a more normal trajectory.

In dealing with the pharmacologic treatment of children and adolescents such as Lena, the recommendation is to select a particular medication and dosing regimen based on clearly identified target symptoms and evidence-based data of efficacy and tolerability for the individual's age and stage of development. The clinician needs to monitor vital signs at least weekly, weight and body mass index at least monthly, and full blood work at least every 3–4 months (Correll 2008; Correll and Carlson 2006). Furthermore, the clinician should make one change at a time, with a "start low and go slow" medication algorithm to achieve the lowest effective dose with the maximum benefit. At all times, the clinician should provide clear explanations of the rationale for each test or change in medication and obtain informed consent from the legal guardian, as well as educated assent from the adolescent (Correll 2008; Pappadopulos et al. 2003). A standardized pediatric side-effect scale (Correll 2008; Pappadopulos et al. 2003) should be used at baseline and at regular intervals to assess ongoing potential side effects. The use of scales such as the Clinical Global Improvement Scale (Guy et al. 1970) or the Brief Psychiatric Rating Scale for Children (Overall and Pfefferbaum 1982) to assess the patient's progress, either monthly or at least quarterly, may be helpful in monitoring improvement or lack thereof (Pappadopulos et al. 2003).

If at least two trials of antipsychotic medications do not treat the underlying psychotic process, Lena's condition may be refractory to treatment with the usual antipsychotic and mood-stabilizing medications. In this case, the clinician should consider a trial of clozapine (Clozaril) (Kranzler et al. 2006; Sporn et al. 2007), which has the potential to ameliorate her symptoms and treat her psychosis and mood symptoms with a decreased need for polypharmacy. Although this medication requires increased blood work, medical monitoring, and management of side effects, when other antipsychotic medications and mood stabilizers are insufficient to improve or resolve her symptoms, Clozaril may allow Lena to be discharged to a less restrictive residential treatment facility or home, despite her serious psychiatric condition.

Integrative Perspective

Patricia K. Leebens, M.D.

DIAGNOSTIC FORMULATION

At admission, Lena was diagnosed with ADHD, combined type, by history; PTSD; expressive language disorder; and psychotic disorder not otherwise specified. Her medications at admission were Ritalin 60 mg/day, Prozac 40 mg/day, and Depakote 450 mg twice a day. Her Risperdal had been stopped prior to transfer because of severe constipation and weight gain. Although schizophrenia was a consideration because of her family history, her complex history of cognitive and social delays as well as aggression, and her mental status on presentation, Lena did not meet the full DSM-IV-TR criteria for schizophrenia at the time of admission.

Consideration was also given to the diagnosis of major depressive disorder, recurrent, severe with psychotic features, because mood disorders are the most frequent condition associated with psychosis (Cepeda 2007). However, depressive or irritable symptoms had not been described as major concerns by Lena or her caretakers, despite her suicidal statements. According to past records, Lena had received prescriptions for Depakote and Prozac for aggression and mood lability, which worsened with stimulant treatment.

Although Lena had disturbances of language, cognition, and interpersonal relationships—symptoms also seen in pervasive developmental disorders—her symptoms appeared to begin in latency, not during infancy or early childhood, as one would see with pervasive developmental disorders. She also appeared to have hallucinations and paranoid delusions, which are symptoms more related to a primary psychotic disorder than a pervasive developmental disorder.

For a schizophrenia diagnosis, DSM-IV-TR requires the patient to have had at least two of the following symptoms for most of a 1-month period: delusions; hallucinations; disorganized speech; catatonia or disorganized behavior; and negative symptoms such as affective flattening, alogia, or avolition. The patient also needs to have a level of social or occupational dysfunction, which in children is described as a failure to achieve the expected level of interpersonal, academic, or occupational achievement. Impairment should persist for at least 6 months, during which at least 1 month of active phase symptoms are present. The diagnosis of schizophrenia also requires the exclusion of mood disorders with psychotic features, substance-induced psychosis, and psychosis due to medical or organic conditions.

Schizophrenia is a complex neurodevelopmental disorder, with deficits in cognition (including language and executive function deficits, as well as psychotic processing), social functioning, and affect (American Academy of Child and Adolescent Psychiatry 2001). Given the rarity of the disorder in youth, clinical presentations of schizophrenia are less known and misdiagnosis of childhood schizophrenia is common. Also, given the complicated nature of the dysfunction in schizophrenia, as well as the multiplicity of symptoms that may overlap with other diagnoses, children with the disorder may be misdiagnosed with many other disorders, including pervasive developmental disorders, affective disorders, anxiety disorders, personality disorders, and externalizing disorders such as ADHD and conduct disorder (DelBello 2004; Gogtay 2007). Another confusion comes from the symptom of hallucinations, which about 8%–10% of all children will report, even though they may not have schizophrenia or even a psychotic disorder (American Academy of Child and Adolescent Psychiatry 2001; Cepeda 2007; Masi et al. 2006).

Although a genetic predisposition appears to exist for schizophrenia, neurohormonal systems that govern the response to stress—particularly the hypothalamic-pituitary-adrenal axis—may influence the expression of the core vulnerability to psychosis (Walker et al. 2007). Thus, stressful life events that increase levels of cortisol—that is, trauma, neglect, abuse, and effects of chronic illness—increase the risk of psychosis in genetically vulnerable children.

Although Lena acknowledged auditory hallucinations, appeared to be paranoid, and had blunting of affect, she had experienced an extensive history of neglect (and possible abuse during the times of her mother's substance use and psychotic illness), as well as exposure to domestic violence, resulting in a history of anxiety, hypervigilance, and nightmares, which had been diagnosed as PTSD. Her current dysfunction also may have resulted from the stress that resulted following the death of her grandmother and the removal from her mother's care because of her mother's psychiatric hospitalization.

Lena also had not met expected social, interpersonal, and academic levels; her borderline intelligence and possible attentional and language disorders, as well as frequent school absences, were possible contributors to her many delays. Her current medication regimen, including the stimulant Ritalin, which would increase her cortisol levels and could increase psychotic symptoms (Walker et al. 2007), may have contributed to her mental status at admission. The history was not complete enough to confirm the presence of acute psychotic symptoms for at least 1 month as well as impairment for 6 months due, primarily, to schizophrenia.

Clarifying Lena's diagnoses required systematic assessment and reevaluation during the ongoing attempts to treat her complex symptoms. Her assessment included a complete physical examination, including a thorough neurological assessment by a pediatric neurologist; toxicology screens for substance use (even though she was in a hospital setting, she had family visitors who were substance abusers, and other patients who were substance abusers resided on her inpatient unit); and laboratory tests to assess routine functioning and medication levels (complete blood count, liver function tests, thyroid function tests, fasting glucose, electrolytes, blood urea nitrogen to creatinine ratio, lipid panel, Depakote level) and to rule out metabolic disturbances, Lyme's disease, mononucleosis, pregnancy, and the presence of heavy metals (for additional rule-outs, see Cepeda 2007).

Lena's physical examination and lab tests were within normal limits. An electrocardiogram and computed tomography scan of the head had been done and were normal at age 13 and were not repeated at this admission. Consideration was given to performing an electroencephalogram because Lena had a history of febrile seizures in childhood and had a maternal aunt with epilepsy; however, she was too unstable to take out of the state hospital for completing the procedure in a local general hospital.

Cognitive testing and projective testing were attempted, but were abandoned due to Lena's recurrent agitation and difficulties cooperating with the clinical psychologist. Instruments such as the Kiddie Schedule for Affective Disorders and Schizophrenia in School Age Children—Present and Lifetime Version (Kaufman et al. 1997), Brief Psychiatric Rating Scale for Children (Overall and Pfefferbaum 1982), and Positive and Negative Syndrome Scale (Kay et al. 1992) are recommended for use in the initial assessment of schizophrenia and for monitoring symptoms during follow-up (Cepeda 2007; Kalapatapu and Dunn 2008); however, Lena was not tested with these instruments.

Close observation of Lena helped sort out whether her symptoms were due to a primary PTSD, a primary mood disturbance, or externalizing disorders such as ADHD or conduct disorder. Lena slept well most nights, did not have nightmares of past traumas, and did not appear to dissociate disclosing fragments of past traumas; also, her agitation and assaultiveness did not appear to arise out of reenactments of past traumas. She had flattened affect, demonstrated clear paranoia about eating certain foods (initially she only ate foods that came to her wrapped or in packages), and clearly had bizarre thoughts and fears (she expressed worry about what might come out of the toilet or shower-heads in the bathroom and frequently complained that there was blood running down the walls of her bedroom).

Although she was clearly hypermotoric and distractible, these behaviors worsened when her paranoia and anxiety worsened, and were often observed when she was talking to herself or staring at walls (i.e., when she was seemingly responding to internal stimuli). Her assaults were not planned or calculated, but rather were spontaneous and defensive, often occurring when she was backed into a corner or encouraged to do something that increased her anxiety and paranoia. This evidence of positive and negative psychotic symptoms and bizarre thoughts and behavior was much more suggestive of schizophrenia than of PTSD, personality disorders, or externalizing disorders (American Academy of Child and Adolescent Psychiatry 2001).

Simplifying her medication regimen was necessary to determine if the medications themselves were contributing to her current symptoms. Because Ritalin (Cepeda 2007) and Prozac at their current doses may have contributed to Lena's psychotic and anxious symptoms (Walker et al. 2007), the clinician discontinued the Ritalin and decreased the Prozac to 20 mg/day. Lena showed some modest improvement in her anxiety and psychosis, but her hyperactivity and impulsivity increased excessively. The Prozac was discontinued, and Lena did become somewhat more dysphoric, but the psychotic symptoms improved.

DSM-IV-TR DIAGNOSIS AT DISCHARGE

Axis I   295.30 Schizophrenia, paranoid type, episodic with interepisode residual symptoms
Axis II   V62.89 Borderline intellectual functioning
Axis III   History of recurrent otitis media
           Febrile seizures
           Mild asthma in early childhood
Axis IV   Problems with primary support: mother with mental illness, death of maternal grandmother/caretaker, neglect and possible abuse, placement in foster care
Axis V   Global Assessment of Functioning=25 (at admission)
           Global Assessment of Functioning=53 (at discharge)

TREATMENT RECOMMENDATIONS

Treatment of schizophrenia requires multiple therapeutic interventions, including pharmacotherapy, with atypical antipsychotic agents generally as the initial drugs of choice, with supplemental mood stabilizers, antidepressants, or anxiolytics to help alleviate mood or anxiety symptoms that may accompany the psychosis; psychosocial care, including a supportive environment, social skills training, and an individualized special education program, as well as speech and language therapy and occupational, vocational, and physical therapy as needed; and psychoeducation for the patient and family members to become educated about the nature of schizophrenia, the signs of impending relapse, the importance of medication and treatment compliance, and the importance of low levels of expressed emotion in the home setting to decrease the risk of relapse (American Academy of Child and Adolescent Psychiatry 2001; Cepeda 2007; Kalapatapu and Dunn 2008). An interdisciplinary treatment team is often needed to address these complex treatments adequately.

Individual patient responses to these interventions, as well as the ability of the family, school district, and local community to provide appropriate support and structure to the child with schizophrenia, will determine whether or not the child can live successfully at home. Children with treatment-resistant schizophrenia may require longer hospitalizations or out-of-home care (American Academy of Child and Adolescent Psychiatry 2001; Cepeda 2007). However, practitioners should be aware that even with extensive interventions, children and adolescents with early-onset schizophrenia often have extensive residual impairment at follow-up years later (American Academy of Child and Adolescent Psychiatry 2001).

Antipsychotic agents—usually second-generation, or atypical, antipsychotics—are recommended as first-line agents for the treatment of psychotic symptoms associated with schizophrenia (American Academy of Child and Adolescent Psychiatry 2001; Cepeda 2007). However, weight gain, metabolic disturbances, and cardiac side effects may limit the use of these medications in certain patients. The second-generation antipsychotics also appear to impact mood and have been approved for antimanic and antidepressant indications (Cepeda 2007).

The use of antipsychotic agents requires adequate informed consent from the parent or guardian, as well as assent from the child when appropriate; delineation of clear target symptoms; documentation of baseline and follow-up medical monitoring; and documentation of treatment response and suspected side effects. Therapeutic trials of at least 4–6 weeks at adequate doses are recommended (American Academy of Child and Adolescent Psychiatry 2001). Schizophrenia is considered to be treatment resistant following two failed trials of different antipsychotic medications at adequate doses for adequate periods of time. Medical monitoring with antipsychotic agents is imperative, with guidelines being updated often (see Cepeda 2007).

Clozaril has documented efficacy for treatment-resistant schizophrenia in adults and children with early-onset schizophrenia (American Academy of Child and Adolescent Psychiatry 2001; Sporn et al. 2007). However, because serious adverse events are possible (agranulocytosis and severe weight gain and diabetes), frequent medical monitoring is required (Cepeda 2007).

The clinician prescribed Risperdal, an atypical antipsychotic, because Lena had gotten benefit from the medication in the past. (Aripiprazole [Abilify] was not yet on the market; ziprasidone [Geodon] was not approved for use with children in state care at that time; and olanzapine [Zyprexa] was not prescribed because of Lena's tendency for weight gain and the family history of diabetes.) The Risperdal helped with some of Lena's paranoia but did not reduce her auditory or visual hallucinations. She often looked tortured and afraid, even during visits with her much beloved mother or with favorite staff members. In addition to increasing doses of Risperdal, she often required multiple as-needed administrations of the first-generation antipsychotic agent Thorazine (the only antipsychotic medication that Lena's guardians allowed the clinician to administer intramuscularly during acute psychotic episodes).

The Depakote was increased to high therapeutic dosage. With the Depakote, Risperdal, and as-needed administration of Thorazine, Lena was more stable, but she still required one-to-one observation and unit restrictions. She continued to complain of auditory hallucinations, appeared hypervigilant, and often laughed inappropriately, despite her two antipsychotic medications.

Milieu management of Lena in the inpatient setting was challenging: Lena's paranoia, high anxiety, and frequent agitation, self-abuse, and assaultiveness resulted in her being moved to the single bedroom closest to the nurses' station. She was placed on one-to-one observation (out of arm's reach) and had a small number of items in her bedroom, to limit her access to items for assault and self-abuse. A limited number of female staff members attended to Lena, talking to her in calm, reassuring voices. Although Lena was restricted to the unit, she had a structured daily routine, which included schooling, exercise, access to the outdoors, regular meals in a side conference room, and semi-weekly visits from her mother and caseworker. Lena would earn points for trying and succeeding at these daily activities, which resulted in increased opportunities on the unit.

Lena was often quite paranoid in the bathroom and often refused to shower or complete her daily hygiene tasks. Over time, Lena agreed to sponge baths in her room and to semiweekly shampoos and hair combing by her mother.

A trial of Clozaril was recommended by her treatment team when Lena remained psychotic after more than 6 months of pharmacologic and psychosocial interventions.

Following baseline assessment of electrocardiogram, complete blood count, fasting glucose, cholesterol, triglycerides, electroencephalogram (normal on Depakote), liver function tests, weight, blood pressure and heart rate, and thyroid function tests, all of which were normal, Lena started taking Clozaril, titrated in 25-mg aliquots every 4 days up to 225 mg/day, while maintaining therapeutic Depakote levels. As Clozaril was increased, Risperdal was tapered off. Staff weighed Lena weekly, checked her vitals (including temperature) daily during the Clozaril increases, and asked her twice a day whether she had had a bowel movement or started her menses. She was maintained on stool softeners and prune juice. Weekly blood draws became difficult, because Lena became more oppositional as she became less psychotic.

The Clozaril was a miracle drug. Lena's grooming and hygiene improved remarkably, and her anxiety and assaultiveness were reduced to almost nothing. Her auditory hallucinations broke through on occasion, but she could use her therapeutic relationships to obtain support when the hallucinations were troublesome. Her hallucinations abated with the addition of Risperdal 1 mg twice a day to her Clozaril 225 mg/day and therapeutic Depakote levels. Staff monitored her vital signs and labs religiously; an absolute neutrophil count (ANC) down to 800–1,000 was tolerated. Over time, her ANC increased into the normal range on the three-drug regimen, with Clozaril maintained at a dosage of 225 mg/day because dosages above that amount led to precipitous drops in her ANC.

Psychotic disorders such as schizophrenia may present complex ethical and legal dilemmas to the practitioner. Because a patient with schizophrenia may have paranoid delusions and disordered thinking, the clinician may have difficulty obtaining full cooperation from the patient in initiating and maintaining treatment interventions. Issues of informed consent and involuntary treatment interventions may be difficult to resolve without court involvement. In children and adolescents, particularly for those in foster care or those who are wards of the state, these issues may be complicated by guardianship issues. Before initiating such treatment measures, the clinician may have to present treatment plans—particularly those that may include use of involuntary medication or intrusive methods of dispensing medications (i.e., intramuscular injections or medications via nasogastric [NG] tube)—to state medical review boards and/or to probate courts. To anticipate these complicated medical-legal treatment issues, psychiatrists treating children with schizophrenia or other psychotic disorders must be aware of their state's statutes regarding involuntary treatment and treatment of children in state custody or foster care.

As Lena improved, her world expanded: she went to school on the hospital grounds, she had grounds passes for recreation and visits with her mother, and then she went home on day passes. However, she became frustrated and discouraged over her difficulties being accepted into a residential treatment center. One day she refused her Clozaril—a "strike" that continued for 3 more days, despite maximal therapeutic support. The reemergence of her symptoms was dramatic, with paranoia, hallucinations, and visions of blood running down the walls appearing within days. She refused all medications and became withdrawn, paranoid, and increasingly assaultive. Through the use of as needed Thorazine (often given intramuscularly), Lena became more stable and less psychotic, and staff were able to convince her to start her medications again, at least for a short time.

Lena had been at the hospital for 18 months when she first refused her medications, and it became clear that her chances of ever getting out of the hospital without the Clozaril to stabilize her were very slim. The significant adults in her life tried to convince her of the importance of taking her medications, but to no avail. Numerous behavioral plans were devised to encourage Lena to work toward various rewards or privileges if she took her medications. All such interventions worked for a short time, until she again would go on "strike." Each time, she would have to start the Clozaril trial all over again at 25 or 50 mg/day and slowly taper up. This yo-yo process went on for over 3 months before it was clear that involuntary medication administration needed to be considered to treat her psychosis.

Lena's treatment team reviewed the issues with her biological mother, who agreed with the decision to try to administer the Clozaril involuntarily to Lena. Because Lena was under age 16, her guardian, in this case the state, could agree to give her the medication involuntarily. Lena's case was presented to the state's medical review board, and permission was gained to give her (as a ward of the state) the Clozaril involuntarily (crushed in liquid via an NG tube). Her case was also presented to probate court, and permission was granted to give the medication involuntarily.

On the day of the NG tube placement, Lena's mother held one hand and her favorite staff member held the other hand. The hospital's pediatrician—another favorite person of Lena's—placed the NG tube and explained to Lena that she would replace the tube each time, if Lena pulled out the tube. The Clozaril was given by NG tube for over 2 weeks, at which time Lena announced that the tube could be removed because she had decided to take all of her medications. She never needed the NG tube again during the last 5 months of her hospitalization, and she never refused her medications again.

Five months later, Lena left the hospital to residential treatment, taking Clozaril, Depakote, Risperdal, and as-needed administrations of Thorazine (about once every 2 weeks). Seven years since this treatment, Lena remains out of the hospital, living at home with her mother, following a year in residential treatment, and is involved in an intimate relationship with a longtime friend. She has recently gotten pregnant, which resulted in the cessation of her medication regimen.

REFERENCES

Ambrosini PJ: Historical development and present status of the Schedule for Affective Disorders and Schizophrenia for School Age Children (K-SADS). J Am Acad Child Adolesc Psychiatry 39:49–58, 2000

American Academy of Child and Adolescent Psychiatry: Practice parameter for the assessment and treatment of children and adolescents with schizophrenia. J Am Acad Child Adolesc Psychiatry 40 (suppl 7):4–23, 2001

Birmaher B, Arbelaez C, Brent D: Course and outcome of child and adolescent major depressive disorder. Child Adolesc Psychiatr Clin N Am 11:619–637, 2002

Birmaher B, Brent D; AACAP Work Group on Quality Issues, et al: Practice parameter for the assessment and treatment of children and adolescents with depressive disorders. J Am Acad Child Adolesc Psychiatry 46:1503–1526, 2007

Calderoni D, Wudarsky M, Bhangoo R: Differentiating child-onset schizophrenia from psychotic mood disorders. J Am Acad Child Adolesc Psychiatry 40:1190–1196, 2001

Cepeda C: Psychotic Symptoms in Children and Adolescents: Assessment, Differential Diagnosis, and Treatment. New York, Routledge Mental Health, 2007

Correll CU: Antipsychotic use in children and adolescents: minimizing adverse effects to maximize outcomes. J Am Acad Child Adolesc Psychiatry 47:9–20, 2008

Correll CU, Carlson HE: Endocrine and metabolic adverse effects of psychotropic medications in children and adolescents. J Am Acad Child Adolesc Psychiatry 45:771–791, 2006

DelBello MP: Role of atypicals in the treatment of pediatric psychotic disorders and common comorbidities. June 15, 2004. Available at: http://www.medscape.com/viewarticle/479929_19. Accessed December 3, 2007.

DiFilippo JM, Overholser JC: Suicidal ideation in adolescent psychiatric inpatients as associated with depression and attachment relationships. J Clin Child Psychiatry 29:155–166, 2000

Frazier J, McClellan J, Findling R: Treatment of early-onset schizophrenia spectrum disorders (TEOSS): demographic and clinical characteristics. J Am Acad Child Adolesc Psychiatry 46:979–988, 2007

Gogtay N, Rapoport J: Childhood onset schizophrenia and other early onset psychotic disorders, in Lewis's Child and Adolescent Psychiatry: A Comprehensive Textbook. Edited by Martin A, Volkmar FR. New York, Lippincott Williams & Wilkins, 2007, pp 493–503

Guy W, Bonato RR (eds): Manual for the ECDEU Assessment Battery, Revised Edition. Chevy Chase, MD, National Institute of Mental Health, 1970, 12–1 to 12–6

Kalapatapu RK, Dunn DW: Schizophrenia and other psychoses. March 10, 2008. Available at: http://www.emedicine.com/ped/topic2057.htm. Accessed July 29, 2008.

Katz LY, Cox BJ, Gunasekara S, et al: Feasibility of dialectical behavior therapy for suicidal adolescent inpatients. J Am Acad Child Adolesc Psychiatry 43:276–282, 2004

Kaufman J, Birmaher B, Brent D, et al: Schedule for Affective Disorders and Schizophrenia for School Age Children—Present and Lifetime Version (K-SADS-PL): initial reliability and validity data. J Am Acad Child Adolesc Psychiatry 36:980–988, 1997

Kay SR, Opler LA, Fiszbein A: Positive and Negative Syndrome Scale. North Tonawanda, NY, Multi-Health Systems, 1992

Klomek AB, Mufson L: Interpersonal therapy for depressed adolescents. Child Adolesc Psychiatr Clin N Am 15:959–975, 2006

Kranzler HN, Kester BA, Gerbino-Rosen G, et al: Treatment-refractory schizophrenia in children and adolescents: an update on clozapine and other pharmacologic interventions. Child Adolesc Psychiatric Clin N Am 15:135–159, 2006

Kumra S: The diagnosis and treatment of children and adolescents with schizophrenia: "my mind is playing tricks on me." Child Adolesc Psychiatr Clin N Am 9:183–199, 2000

Kumra S, Jacobsen LK, Lenane M, et al: "Multidimensionally impaired disorder": is it a variant of very early-onset schizophrenia? J Am Acad Child Adolesc Psychiatry 37:91–99, 1998

Lewinsohn PM, Rohde P, Seeley JR: Major depressive disorder in older adolescents: prevalence, risk factors, and clinical implications. Clin Psychol Rev 18:765–794, 1998

Masi G, Mucci M, Pari C: Children with schizophrenia: clinical picture and pharmacological treatment. CNS Drugs 20:841–866, 2006

Overall JE, Pfefferbaum B: The Brief Psychiatric Rating Scale for Children. Psychopharmacol Bull 18:10–16, 1982

Pappadopulos E, Macintyre JC, Crismon LM, et al: Treatment recommendations for the use of antipsychotics for aggressive youth (TRAAY), part II. J Am Acad Child Adolesc Psychiatry 42:145–161, 2003

Roberts RE, Chen Y-W: Depressive symptoms and suicidal ideation among Mexican-origin and Anglo adolescents. J Am Acad Child Adolesc Psychiatry 34:81–90, 1995

Sporn AL, Vermani A, Greenstein DK, et al: Clozapine treatment of childhood-onset schizophrenia: evaluation of effectiveness, adverse effects and long-term outcome. J Am Acad Child Adolesc Psychiatry 46:1349–1356, 2007

Walker EF, McMillan A, Mittal V: Neurohormones, neurodevelopment, and the prodrome of psychosis in adolescence, in Adolescent Psychopathology and the Developing Brain: Integrating Brain and Prevention Science. Edited by Romer D, Walker EF. New York, Oxford University Press, 2007, pp 264–285

Wechsler D: Manual for the Wechsler Intelligence Scale for Children—Third Edition. San Antonio, TX, The Psychological Corporation, 1991

Winters NC, Pumariga A; Work Group on Community Child and Adolescent Psychiatry; Work Group on Quality Issues: Practice parameter on child and adolescent mental health care in community systems of care. J Am Acad Child Adolesc Psychiatry 46:284–299, 2007

▪ P a r t I V ▪

KIDS IN CRISIS
Psychopathology in the
Context of Social Stressors

Introduction to Kids in Crisis

Peter S. Jensen, M.D.
Cathryn A. Galanter, M.D.

In this section, we deliberately present cases in which moderate to severe environmental stressors are part of the clinical presentation. Important in such cases is the understanding of the potential role played by environmental factors, any biological or constitutional factors related to the preexisting vulnerabilities, the presence of full-blown DSM-IV-TR conditions, and the degree of impairment. Another critical factor is how the clinician chooses to cobble together the necessary psychotherapeutic, environmental, supportive, and psychopharmacologic approaches to provide an optimal intervention.

In "Suicidal Ideation After Supervised Visits With Biological Mom: Depressed Mood in a Child in Foster Care" (Chapter 26), all commentators identify the precipitating role of the visit to the child's biological mother on the child's suicidal ideation. Of greater interest are the differences among commentators in how they recommend addressing attention-deficit/hyperactivity disorder (ADHD) and treating it and the other disorders. The experts take somewhat different approaches in the extent to which they prioritize the use of trauma-focused cognitive-behavioral therapy (CBT), medication adjustments, and/or family support. Even among medication recommendations, differences emerge in prioritization of adjustments to the stimulants versus the use of a selective serotonin reuptake inhibitor. Differences are also noted in the extent to which the importance of the environment (including a loving foster mother) was supported, reinforced, and acknowledged as the key aspect of the overall approach to helping the child in the context of treatment.

As with earlier cases, any differences between commentators do not reflect differences in expertise, because all are internationally prominent experts, but rather differences in how the professionals tend to approach their cases, given their different backgrounds, therapeutic persuasions, and previous experiences. What would be interesting would be to conduct a multisite trial of cases

461

similar to that discussed in Chapter 26, and to compare and contrast the benefits of the commentators' three treatment approaches. In the meantime, the best we can do is widen our perspective by becoming aware of other treatment approaches and considering them fully as a part of our therapeutic armamentarium, and discuss all of these options in the context of a supportive, problem-solving approach with the parent and family.

In "The Legacy of War: Irritability and Anger in an Adolescent Refugee" (Chapter 27), all commentators emphasize the role of trauma-focused CBT in what appears to be the child's clear response to a traumatic history. Important differences do emerge, however, in the extent to which the conduct and oppositional problems are seen as key targets of the intervention. Differences also emerge in the extent to which commentators identify other key stressors in the environment as potential targets of intervention, or at least in understanding the roles of the stressors as possible etiological factors.

In the case of "Moody Child: Depressed in Context of Parental Divorce" (Chapter 28), it is unclear whether the patient meets the full criteria for major depressive disorder. Of course, life stressors in and of themselves cannot be used to rule out whether the diagnosis of depression should be made. One clinician might make the diagnosis of major depressive disorder; another might refer to depression not otherwise specified; and a third might favor a diagnosis such as adjustment disorder with depressed mood. Such differences in depressive diagnoses are seen in this chapter. Note, however, that CBT methods are used for both prevention and treatment approaches, regardless of whether the commentator diagnosed major depressive disorder, adjustment disorder, or a V-code diagnosis for a parent-child relational problem.

In "It Should Have Been Me: Childhood Bereavement" (Chapter 29), the experts draw distinctions between major depressive disorder and pathological grief. The role of environmental factors, such as the loss of the grandmother in this case, illustrates how conditions within the child (depressive disorder) may at least in part arise from circumstances outside of the child (loss of the grandmother).

Nowhere in child psychopathology does assessment of the environment take on more form and force than in cases of very young children. In "Won't Settle Down: Disinhibited Attachment in a Toddler" (Chapter 30), all commentators express reluctance to use medications, and all discuss the implicit importance of addressing the child's attachment difficulties. Although these similarities may be due in part to our choice of commentators, the commonalities of their opinions indicate that the use of medications in very young children remains problematic and controversial, except in selected cases of autism or extreme aggression, or in children ages 3–5 with severe ADHD, as demonstrated by the recent multisite preschool ADHD treatment study (Abikoff et al.

2007). Even with ADHD, however, there is no unambiguous green light, because young children's responses to medication are more variable than those seen in older children with ADHD. In young children, ADHD is also moderated by comorbidity, side effects are more common, and response to treatment is often less than optimal (Abikoff et al. 2007; Ghuman et al. 2007; Posner et al. 2007; Swanson et al. 2006; Vitiello et al. 2007).

REFERENCES

Abikoff HB, Vitiello B, Riddle MA, et al: Methylphenidate effects on functional outcomes in the Preschoolers With Attention-Deficit/Hyperactivity Disorder Treatment Study (PATS). J Child Adolesc Psychopharmacol 17:581–592, 2007

Ghuman JK, Riddle MA, Vitiello B, et al: Comorbidity moderates response to methylphenidate in the Preschoolers With Attention-Deficit/Hyperactivity Disorder Treatment Study (PATS). J Child Adolesc Psychopharmacol 17:563–580, 2007

Posner K, Melvin GA, Murray DW, et al: Clinical presentation of attention-deficit/hyperactivity disorder in preschool children: the Preschoolers With Attention-Deficit/Hyperactivity Disorder Treatment Study (PATS). J Child Adolesc Psychopharmacol 17:547–562, 2007

Swanson J, Greenhill L, Wigal T, et al: Stimulant-related reductions of growth rates in the PATS. J Am Acad Child Adolesc Psychiatry 45:1304–1313, 2006

Vitiello B, Abikoff HB, Chuang SZ, et al: Effectiveness of methylphenidate in the 10-month continuation phase of the Preschoolers With Attention-Deficit/Hyperactivity Disorder Treatment Study (PATS). J Child Adolesc Psychopharmacol 17:593–604, 2007

■ CHAPTER 26 ■

Suicidal Ideation After Supervised Visits With Biological Mom

Depressed Mood in a Child in Foster Care

Paramjit T. Joshi, M.D.
Lisa M. Cullins, M.D.

CASE PRESENTATION

IDENTIFYING INFORMATION

Timothy is an 11-year-old black male who has been in foster care for 2 years.

CHIEF COMPLAINT

Timothy has repeatedly said, "I want to kill myself."

Paramjit T. Joshi, M.D., is Endowed Professor and Chair, Department of Psychiatry and Behavioral Sciences, Children's National Medical Center; Professor of Psychiatry, Department of Behavioral Sciences and Pediatrics, George Washington University School of Medicine, Washington, D.C.

Lisa M. Cullins, M.D., is Corporate Medical Director of EMQ Children and Family Services in Campbell, California, and Adjunct Assistant Clinical Professor of Psychiatry at the University of California, San Francisco.

For complete biographical information, see "About the Contributors," p. 613.

History of Present Illness

Timothy was removed from his biological mother's care secondary to neglect and alleged sexual abuse by an older brother. Timothy was placed in foster care at that time and has remained in the same foster home for the past 2 years. After two consecutive missed visits with his biological mother, Timothy began to express suicidal ideation, stating, "I want to kill myself," with a plan to either jump off a building or set himself on fire. He was subsequently hospitalized in an acute inpatient unit for stabilization.

Approximately 2 years prior to his inpatient admission and shortly after he was removed from his biological mother's care, Timothy was taken for an initial outpatient psychiatric evaluation for his disruptive behaviors. At that time, Timothy was experiencing difficulty in following directions and waiting his turn, poor attention and concentration, forgetfulness, hyperactivity and impulsivity, and decreased focus and distractibility both at home and at school. Timothy also reported receiving more than 10 school suspensions for "fighting."

According to the social worker, prior to his initial outpatient evaluation, Timothy had been evaluated in our child and adolescent protection center secondary to allegations of sexual abuse. The social worker states that when the children were left unsupervised by their mother, Timothy's older brother would reportedly fondle Timothy and coerce him to fondle his younger sister. Although Timothy had reported this information during his initial comprehensive evaluation in the child and adolescent protection center, he denied any sexual or physical abuse during his initial evaluation in the outpatient clinic. Timothy did endorse symptoms of hypervigilance, increased startle response, fear of the dark, difficulty falling asleep, and nightmares of suffocation.

Timothy endorses intermittent irritability and anger during the initial outpatient psychiatric evaluation but denies any neurovegetative symptoms or mania. Timothy also denies a history of suicidal and homicidal ideation, perceptual disturbances, phobias, and obsessive-compulsive disorder. Timothy's foster mother states, "Timothy is fine when he gets his way; when he doesn't, then he acts up." She reports some lying and "taking things without asking for them" but denies any arrests or legal problems. Timothy denies a history of setting fires and animal cruelty. His foster mother states that whether he does or does not see his family at a scheduled visit, his behavior "is much worse for at least a day or two after." She says that Timothy becomes slightly more irritable and oppositional and defiant at home and school. She states, "If his mother can't do what she is supposed to do to get him back, they should just stop the visits."

Two days prior to his recent inpatient admission, Timothy was eagerly awaiting his scheduled supervised visit with his mother at the agency. According to Timothy, he was really excited about this visit because it was 4 days before his birthday, and the previous year his mother had missed his birthday and scheduled visit because his sister had been hospitalized. Timothy reports that his mother also had missed the visit the week before, and he was certain she would come to this scheduled visit. Timothy states that his mother did not show for this prebirthday visit and did not call. His foster mother says that his behavior then became more disruptive at school and home, with increased irritability, aggression, and agitation. She also states that Timothy began to wet the bed and impulsively jut into major streets with cars oncoming. She describes him as "out of control." She reports that he began to make comments like "I shouldn't be alive anyway." As instructed, she brought him to the emergency room, where he was evaluated and subsequently hospitalized.

Past Psychiatric History

Timothy received no psychiatric treatment prior to placement in foster care. He has made no prior suicide attempts. Two years ago, after his initial outpatient psychiatric examination, he started weekly individual therapy, which he has continued for 2 years. He also has been taking methylphenidate (Concerta) with good response and no side effects for the past 2 years. This hospitalization is Timothy's first inpatient treatment.

Current Medications

Timothy is currently taking Concerta 36 mg every morning.

Substance Abuse History

Timothy denies substance abuse.

Medical History

Timothy's medical history is unremarkable, and he has no known drug allergies.

Developmental History

Neither the social worker nor the foster parents are able to provide Timothy's developmental history.

Social History

Timothy has lived with his foster parents and their foster daughter, age 17, since removal from his biological mother 2 years ago. Timothy has a 17-year-old biological brother and a 10-year-old biological sister who live in separate foster homes. Timothy denies a history of physical or sexual abuse but reportedly was sexually abused by his older brother and coerced to fondle his younger sister. Timothy's biological mother was sexually abused by her uncle, and her eldest son is the product of this sexual assault. Timothy attends a public special education school program and is reportedly functioning at a third-grade level academically. No current psychoeducational test results are available. Approximately 2 years ago, his Full Scale IQ on the Wechsler Intelligence Scale for Children—Third Edition (Wechsler 1991) was 71, and his performance on the Vineland Adaptive Behavior Scales (Sparrow et al. 1984) was average.

FAMILY HISTORY

Timothy's biological sister has been diagnosed with disruptive behavior disorder and posttraumatic stress disorder (PTSD). She is being treated with bupropion (Wellbutrin). His biological brother has a history of individual therapy. His biological mother has a history of depression, also treated with Wellbutrin.

MENTAL STATUS EXAMINATION

Timothy appeared his stated age. He was cooperative with the clinician. No psychomotor agitation or retardation was noted, but his mood was dysphoric. His affect was constricted. His thought processes were grossly linear. His thought content was positive for suicidal ideation with a plan to jump off a building or set himself on fire. He denied homicidal ideation or perceptual disturbances. Timothy was alert and oriented to person, place, and time. The clinician estimated Timothy's intelligence to be below average. The boy's insight and judgment were poor.

COMMENTARIES

Psychotherapeutic Perspective

Anthony P. Mannarino, Ph.D.

DIAGNOSTIC FORMULATION

Timothy, an 11-year-old with below-average intelligence, has been in foster care for 2 years because of neglect in the family of origin and alleged sexual

---

Anthony P. Mannarino, Ph.D., is Director of the Center for Traumatic Stress in Children and Adolescents; Vice President of the Department of Psychiatry at Allegheny General Hospital, Pittsburgh, Pennsylvania; and Professor of Psychiatry at Drexel University College of Medicine in Philadelphia, Pennsylvania (for complete biographical information, see "About the Contributors," p. 613).

abuse by an older brother. His two siblings live in different foster homes. Timothy has supervised visits with his biological mother, but she missed the two most recent visits, including the one just prior to his birthday. Over an extended period, he has exhibited symptoms consistent with attention-deficit/ hyperactivity disorder (ADHD). Also, he displays oppositional behaviors, which increase markedly after visits with his biological family. After the most recent missed visit with his mother, Timothy has become depressed and expressed suicidal ideation with a plan.

DSM-IV-TR DIAGNOSIS

Axis I   314.01 ADHD (by history)

           309.4 Adjustment disorder with mixed disturbance of emotions and conduct

           Rule out major depressive disorder, single episode

           Rule out posttraumatic stress disorder

           Rule out oppositional defiant disorder

Axis II   Rule out mild mental retardation

Axis III None

Axis IV Alleged sexual abuse

           Neglect

           Removal from biological family

           Foster care placement

           Academic problems

           Behavior problems at school

Axis V   Global Assessment of Functioning=50 (current)

RATIONALE FOR DIAGNOSIS

Timothy's diagnosis of ADHD seems reasonably clear from the history, although a complete developmental and social history was not available. He presents with both serious internalizing problems (depressive symptoms) and ongoing externalizing difficulties (oppositional and defiant behaviors) but does not yet meet full criteria for either a major depressive disorder or oppositional defiant disorder. Hence, the current diagnosis is adjustment disorder with mixed disturbance of emotions and conduct. Additionally, PTSD is a possible diagnosis for Timothy given his history of neglect and alleged sexual abuse and presence of traumatic stress symptoms (hypervigilance, increased startle response, difficulty falling asleep, nightmares, possible avoidance because of current denial of sexual abuse).

ADDITIONAL RULE-OUT DIAGNOSES

To make a more definitive diagnosis related to depression, I would recommend that Timothy be administered the Children's Depression Inventory (Kovacs 1992) and that his foster mother complete the parent version of the inventory. Also, I believe that additional information should be sought about the traumatic events to which Timothy may have been exposed. The clinician should try to learn whether other kinds of violence occurred in the family of origin, in addition to the documented neglect and possible sexual abuse, as well as assess Timothy for symptoms in relation to these possible events. In this regard, I would recommend that Timothy be administered either the Traumatic Events Screening Inventory for Children (Ford et al. 1999) or the UCLA PTSD Index for DSM-IV (Pynoos et al. 1998) and that the foster mother be asked to complete the parent version of the UCLA PTSD Index.

TREATMENT RECOMMENDATIONS

Although Timothy likely should continue to take stimulant medication for his ADHD symptoms, his symptoms of distractibility, irritability, and angry outbursts may be related to his trauma history, in which case trauma-focused treatment will result in a reduction of these symptoms. Therefore, as the primary intervention, I would recommend trauma-focused cognitive-behavioral therapy (TF-CBT) for Timothy and his foster mother (Cohen et al. 2006). TF-CBT has the most empirical support of any treatment for children and adolescents who have been sexually abused and is effective in reducing depressive symptoms, PTSD symptoms, and moderate behavioral problems (Cohen et al. 2004). Also, research demonstrates that these treatment gains are sustained for at least 1 year following the end of the intervention (Deblinger et al. 2006). Importantly, TF-CBT is appropriate for children who have experienced multiple traumatic events, as appears to be true with Timothy.

TF-CBT is a components-based model that is derived from cognitive-behavioral principles but also draws from attachment theory, developmental neurobiology, family therapy, and humanistic therapy (Cohen et al. 2006). It is a short-term treatment approach (12–20 sessions), with a significant parenting component. In Timothy's case, it would be appropriate for the foster mother to participate in TF-CBT with him. The components of TF-CBT can be summarized by the PRACTICE acronym: psychoeducation and parenting skills, relaxation, affective regulation, cognitive processing, trauma narrative, in vivo desensitization, conjoint sessions, and enhancing safety.

The early treatment sessions with Timothy would be devoted to the skills components of TF-CBT. Psychoeducation could be beneficial to Timothy to help him to understand the impact of sexual abuse and other traumatic events, to shed light on his pattern of disclosure (i.e., acknowledging sexual abuse and then retracting his allegation), and to normalize his traumatic stress symptoms. The relaxation component could assist in reducing hyperarousal symptoms. The affective regulation component would focus on Timothy's angry feelings and would be geared toward helping him to use words to express his disappointment and anger, instead of using externalizing behaviors. The foster mother would also receive the psychoeducation component and work with the therapist to develop appropriate behavioral interventions for Timothy's externalizing problems in the foster home (parenting skills).

The cognitive processing component would focus on the connection between thoughts, feelings, and behaviors. Timothy's depressive symptoms may be related to self-blame for his biological mother's missing visits, and this component would be geared toward helping him to identify inaccurate cognitions and to replace them with more accurate and helpful thoughts. Assuming that Timothy was indeed sexually abused by his older brother, the trauma narrative would be the opportunity for him to tell his story about what occurred, including associated secondary adversities. The major goal of the trauma narrative is to help children to overcome their avoidance, which is the hallmark of PTSD.

In addition to medication treatment and psychotherapy, I would strongly recommend that Timothy's therapist consult with the local child protective service system regarding his ongoing visitation with his biological mother. Because he has been in foster care for 2 years, a permanent placement plan needs to be devised. Also, the child protective service system caseworker needs to be apprised of the detrimental impact of missed visits with his biological mother.

If this initial treatment were not successful, and the placement plan was for Timothy to return to his biological mother's care, I would recommend family sessions for him and his mother, possibly including his siblings for some sessions. These sessions should address abuse and neglect issues, attachment concerns, and permanency planning.

Psychopharmacologic Perspective

Sandra J. Kaplan, M.D.

DIAGNOSTIC FORMULATION

Axis I

ADHD

The diagnosis of ADHD is likely because Timothy has core symptoms of this disorder, including a history of poor school functioning with academic delay, problems following directions and waiting his turn, poor attention span and concentration, forgetfulness, hyperactivity, impulsivity, and distractibility both at home and in school.

Conduct Disorder

A diagnosis of conduct disorder is suggested by the history of Timothy's more than 10 suspensions from school for fighting, as well as his foster mother's comments that he "acts up" if he does not get his way, lies, and takes things without asking for them.

Probable Adjustment Disorder With Depressed Mood and Suicidal Behavior

Timothy's dysphoric mood and suicidal behavior began after he experienced the stress of his biological mother's missing her second consecutive visit with him. Timothy also has the risk factors for having an affective disorder, including maternal depression, prolonged separation from his mother and siblings, and sexual abuse. The diagnostic classification adjustment disorder with depressed mood should be used if he does not meet the duration of dysphoria and other criteria required for major depressive disorder or dysthymic disorder.

Sandra J. Kaplan, M.D., is Director of the Division of Trauma Psychiatry at North Shore University Hospital–The Zucker Hillside Hospital, Long Island Jewish Medical Center, Manhasset, New York; Professor of Psychiatry at New York University School of Medicine; and Director of the Adolescent Trauma Treatment Development Center in the National Child Traumatic Stress Network and of the Florence and Robert A. Rosen Center for Law Enforcement and Military Personnel and Their Families (for complete biographical information, see "About the Contributors," p. 613).

Rule Out Major Depressive Episode and Dysthymic Disorder With Suicidal Behavior

Additional history from Timothy, his foster mother, and his teacher is needed to determine if he 1) had a 2-week or continuous duration of dysphoric mood as required, respectively, for a diagnosis of major depressive episode or dysthymic disorder, and 2) has functional impairment. Timothy's risk factors for these disorders include separation from his family of origin and a history of maternal depression (American Academy of Child and Adolescent Psychiatry 1998).

Rule Out Posttraumatic Stress Disorder

Sexual abuse, which was a stressor for Timothy, has been associated with PTSD (Cohen et al. 2007). His history of hypervigilance, increased startle, fear of the dark, nightmares of suffocation, and difficulty falling asleep is suggestive of this disorder. A score of 40 or greater on the UCLA PTSD Reaction Index for DSM-IV (Steinberg et al. 2004) would provide additional confirmation of the presence of this disorder. Most important, Timothy needs to be asked about avoidance behaviors, intrusive thoughts of traumatic events, traumatic reminders that trigger anxiety, and symptoms of dissociation.

Rule Out Learning Disorders

Because Timothy's Vineland performance was average, despite his IQ in the mild mental retardation range, his poor school functioning may be related to his having undiagnosed learning disorders, and also cognitive impairment secondary to depressive and anxious symptoms. Learning disorders are often comorbid with ADHD. Timothy needs a repeat psychoeducational assessment to understand his current cognitive capacity and academic functioning.

Axis II

Mild mental retardation is a possibility in Timothy's case. Psychological testing 2 years ago indicated that Timothy had a Full Scale IQ of 71. This assessment needs to be repeated after Timothy's suicidal ideation and behavior and depressive symptoms have subsided to understand his current functioning, particularly in light of his comorbid disorders. His disruptive behavior and his depressive and anxious symptoms and disorders can all be associated with difficulties concentrating and impairment of cognitive functioning. Treatments for these disorders and symptoms may lead to improvement in cognitive functioning.

Axis III

Timothy has no general medical conditions.

Axis IV

Timothy's foster care placement has continued for 2 years and resulted in his residing separately from his mother, sister, and brother. His mother has missed two consecutive visitations with him. Also, child sexual abuse and neglect are significant stressors.

Axis V
Global Assessment of Functioning = 50

EPIDEMIOLOGY AND COMORBIDITY

Comorbidity is present. ADHD is likely present, as mentioned above and as indicated by history from Timothy and his foster mother and from outpatient psychiatric records. Timothy has also been treated with Concerta and was reported in the psychiatric outpatient records to have responded to that stimulant medication with no side effects. Timothy's dysphoric mood, suicidal ideation and plan, and impulsive risk-taking behavior of jutting into the street with oncoming cars were precipitated by his mother's lack of visitation. These symptoms suggest that Timothy was also having a depressive mental health disorder. Up to 33% of persons with ADHD have a comorbid depressive disorder (Pliszka et al. 1999). Also, conduct disorder frequently co-occurs with ADHD (Dulcan 1997). This disorder is suggested, as stated above, by history from Timothy's foster mother and his psychiatric outpatient records. Possible PTSD is also suggested, as stated above, by Timothy's history of sexual abuse exposure and his symptoms at the time of his initial outpatient psychiatric visit.

DIAGNOSTIC INSTRUMENTS AND ADDITIONAL SOURCES OF INFORMATION FOR DIAGNOSTIC AND TREATMENT NEEDS CLARIFICATION

ADHD

The following assessments would help to clarify the presence of ADHD symptoms, as well as Timothy's response to his regimen of Concerta 36 mg daily. This testing would also clarify whether he needs a medication adjustment for ADHD to optimize his school and home functioning upon discharge from the hospital.

- Conners' Parent Rating Scale—Revised (Conners 1997), to be completed by his foster mother.
- Conners' Teacher Rating Scale—Revised (Conners et al. 1998), to be completed by his teacher.
- Academic Performance Rating Scale (DuPaul et al. 1991), to screen for academic achievement.

The Conners' Parent and Teacher Rating Scales should be administered every 3 months while Timothy continues ADHD treatment with Concerta, to monitor the effectiveness of this medication. In addition, Timothy's school records prior to and since entering foster care should be obtained to review schools attended, school attendance, grades, and standardized test results. This review will clarify his academic progress, demonstrate his responses to medication for ADHD during the past 2 years, and establish whether all special education recommendations, such as after-school tutoring, have been implemented. His schools should also be asked about the circumstances and timing of his school suspensions. Because learning disorders often co-occur with ADHD, repeated psychoeducational testing should be done to clarify if these disorders are present and if additional specific educational remediation is needed.

DEPRESSIVE DISORDER

Any one of the following measures would help to clarify the severity of Timothy's depressive symptoms and whether he has a clinical depressive disorder.

- Children's Depression Rating Scale — Revised: A score >28 suggests a clinical depressive disorder (Poznanski and Mokros 1996).
- Children's Depression Inventory: A score ≥65 is associated with a clinical depressive disorder (Kovacs 1992).
- Beck Depression Inventory: A score >9 suggests a clinical depressive disorder (Beck et al. 1996).
- K-SADS (Orvaschel et al. 1982): Results can be used to confirm whether major depressive disorder or dysthymic disorder is present.

POSTTRAUMATIC STRESS DISORDER

Administration of the following self-report measure would contribute systematic information needed for a diagnosis of PTSD.

- UCLA PTSD Reaction Index for DSM-IV: A score ≥40 would be consistent with a diagnosis of PTSD (Steinberg et al. 2004).

FUNCTIONAL IMPAIRMENT

The following scale would assist in the assessment of need for treatment.

- Children's Global Assessment Scale: A score of 60 or less indicates impairment of functioning warranting treatment services (Shaffer et al. 1983).

DSM-IV-TR DIAGNOSIS

Axis I   314.01 ADHD, combined type

312.81 Conduct disorder, childhood-onset type

Probable adjustment disorder with depressed mood and suicidal behavior

Rule out major depressive episode and dysthymic disorder with suicidal behavior

Rule out PTSD

Rule out learning disorders

Axis II   Rule out mild mental retardation

Axis III   None

Axis IV   Severe stressors: child sexual abuse

Child neglect

Foster care placement

Axis V   Global Assessment of Functioning=50

TREATMENT RECOMMENDATIONS

I would recommend the following treatments for Timothy: individual psychotherapy, psychoeducational and parenting sessions for Timothy's foster mother, educational remediation, continuation of Concerta for ADHD, and consideration of antidepressant medication if indicated. Individual psychotherapy for Timothy should use TF-CBT and focus on sexual abuse and his depressive and PTSD symptoms. Following discharge from the hospital, Timothy needs to be seen weekly for at least 6 months to monitor his depressive symptoms, disruptive behavior, and anxiety.

Timothy's foster mother should attend psychoeducational and parenting sessions both during Timothy's hospitalization and after his discharge to outpatient status. This intervention is necessary for effective treatment of the co-morbidities of disruptive behavioral problems, such as are found in Timothy's childhood-onset conduct disorder (Patterson and Narrett 1990), as well as for treatment of his ADHD (Dulcan 1997), depressive symptoms (Brent et al. 1993), and PTSD symptoms (Cohen et al. 2007).

Educational remediation should be planned on the basis of input from Timothy's school and repeated psychoeducational testing. Enhancement of Timothy's school functioning will likely lead to increased self-esteem and increased protection against suicidal behavior.

Because Timothy has a history of responding to Concerta for ADHD, Timothy should continue taking it. Every 3 months during Timothy's outpatient visits, this medication should be monitored. Additionally, school records and the Conners' Parent and Teacher Rating Scales should be obtained and reviewed; Timothy's height and weight should be monitored because anorexia and a slight decrease in body growth have been reported as side effects associated with use of stimulant medication in children (Schatzberg et al. 2007); and Timothy should be observed for possible onset of tics, another possible side effect associated with stimulant medication.

Timothy should begin taking antidepressant medication if his depressive and PTSD symptoms do not subside after a course of at least 3 months of TF-CBT, or if his symptoms exacerbate and his functioning declines during this time and diagnostic interviewing and assessments confirm the presence of major depressive disorder, dysthymic disorder, or PTSD. Sertraline (Zoloft) has been used for both pediatric depression (Wagner et al. 2003) and PTSD (Cohen et al. 2007). The UCLA PTSD Reaction Index for DSM-IV should be readministered monthly to monitor for reduction in PTSD symptoms. The Children's Depression Rating Scale or the Beck Depression Inventory should also be administered monthly to monitor reduction of depressive symptoms.

If Timothy does not respond to Zoloft, the clinician should consider Wellbutrin because both Timothy's mother and his sister have histories of taking this medication. Wellbutrin has been used in adolescents with depression and ADHD (Daviss et al. 2006). If Wellbutrin is used, prior seizure disorder needs to be ruled out before beginning this medication, and monitoring for anorexia and seizure needs to take place during his visits. Both of these symptoms have been reported as associated with use of this medication.

In addition to the previous treatment recommendations, a consultation is needed with Timothy's child welfare caseworker and attorneys assigned to represent him in a state-mandated judicial hearing relating to termination of parental rights for children in foster care. Advocacy for a cessation of maternal visitation rights and for permanency of placement and hopefully adoption of Timothy is essential. Child suicidal behavior is associated with parent-child communication problems as well as with abuse (American Academy of Child and Adolescent Psychiatry 1998). The missing of visitation by Timothy's biological mother has been a repeated stressor, which has already precipitated his suicidal behavior and must be stopped to decrease his risk for suicide.

Integrative Perspective

Paramjit T. Joshi, M.D.
Lisa M. Cullins, M.D.

DIAGNOSTIC FORMULATION

Timothy is an 11-year-old black male who was admitted for acute inpatient hospitalization secondary to suicidal ideation with a plan to harm himself. The major biological factor contributing to Timothy's clinical picture is the family history of mood and anxiety disorders and sexual abuse. The developmental history is unknown but, if Timothy was exposed to substances in utero, could be a contributing factor to any cognitive delays, ADHD symptoms, and emotional dysregulation. The major psychosocial factors contributing to Timothy's psychopathology are his history of neglect and sexual abuse, placement in foster care, and ongoing educational difficulties. Given all of these significant contributing factors, the following are the diagnoses to be considered.

POSTTRAUMATIC STRESS DISORDER

Timothy suffered significant trauma at a young age. The sexual abuse has been recounted once in a clinical interview, and he has either avoided or had difficulty recalling this traumatic event since then. Neglect is the most common reason for placement in foster care and is a traumatic event whose magnitude and pervasiveness are often overlooked (The David and Lucile Packard Foundation 2004). Timothy experienced symptoms including hypervigilance, recurrent nightmares of suffocation, increased startle response, difficulty concentrating, irritability and anger, and fear of the dark with difficulty falling asleep, all of which are consistent with PTSD (Cohen et al. 2004).

MAJOR DEPRESSIVE DISORDER

Timothy mostly experienced intermittent, reactive mood, with occasional sustained periods of unprovoked irritability and anger lasting from several days to a week. He denied neurovegetative symptoms except some difficulty with sleep and concentration, which could be symptoms of PTSD. Only during that 2-day period prior to inpatient hospitalization did he ever endorse suicidal ideation. Although Timothy does exhibit some symptoms of major depressive disorder, he does not appear to meet full criteria.

ADJUSTMENT DISORDER WITH DEPRESSED MOOD

Missed visits with his mother seemed to be a chronic stressor for Timothy. However, the two consecutive missed appointments coupled with the prospect of yet another missed birthday magnified this chronic stressor. Never before had Timothy expressed suicidal ideation, recklessly run into traffic, and been "out of control." He appeared to have an adjustment disorder secondary to this intensified chronic stressor. However, in the presence of a preexisting Axis I disorder such as PTSD, these symptoms may have been an exacerbation of his PTSD when this stressor triggered traumatic memories.

ADHD

Although Timothy appeared to have classic symptoms of ADHD, the history was not clear as to whether these symptoms were present prior to age 7. After speaking with the teacher and foster parent, having them complete SNAP forms (Swanson 1992), and making clinical observations, the clinician confirmed a diagnosis of ADHD.

LEARNING DISORDER

Timothy's Full Scale IQ was 71 and his adaptive functioning was average. Commonly, children who have suffered trauma and deprivation have unmet educational needs and significant cognitive delays (The David and Lucile Packard Foundation 2004). However, once placed in a nurturing, structured environment, children may begin to thrive academically (Centers for Disease Control and Prevention 2004). A child who has difficulty learning often externalizes his or her feelings of worthlessness, failure, and frustration. To discern the presence of learning disorders alone or comorbidly with ADHD, the clinician can use clinical observations, teacher and parent reports, psychoeducational testing, and screening instruments such as the SNAP, Conners' Rating Scale (Conners 1997), and Child Behavior Checklist (Achenbach 1991). Timothy's symptoms are consistent with a significant learning disorder and ADHD.

DSM-IV-TR DIAGNOSIS

Axis I   309.81 Posttraumatic stress disorder

             314.01 ADHD, combined type

             315.9 Learning disorder NOS

Axis II   Deferred

Axis III   None

Axis IV   Moderate to severe

             Educational difficulties

             Foster care

             Separation/grief and loss from biological family

Axis V   Global Assessment of Functioning=35–40

TREATMENT RECOMMENDATIONS

Timothy was stabilized in an acute inpatient unit to monitor his safety and symptoms. He responded well to the therapeutic milieu and did not report any further suicidal ideation. He started taking a trial of antidepressants to better target his mood and anxiety symptoms. After considerable deliberation, the clinician had Timothy start taking Wellbutrin, a second-line treatment, because both his mother and sister had responded well to this medication. Selective serotonin reuptake inhibitors (SSRIs) are considered first-line antidepressant treatment in children (Donnelly 2003). However, given the dearth of literature on pharmacologic treatment of PTSD in children, the similar clinical history of his mother and sister, and their positive response to Wellbutrin, it was tried first, with the plan to switch to an SSRI if Timothy did not respond. Follow-up with an outpatient psychiatrist was essential to monitor his symptomatology and medication response. Timothy did respond well to Wellbutrin, with improved mood and decreased irritability.

A critical element in Timothy's treatment plan is individual therapy, both inpatient and outpatient, utilizing techniques from both cognitive-behavioral therapy and psychodynamic psychotherapy to address ongoing issues of separation and loss, mood and anxiety symptoms, self-esteem, and coping skills. In conjunction with his individual therapy, collateral sessions were recommended with his foster mother (and his biological mother, given reunification status) to provide psychoeducation regarding Timothy's diagnosis and treatment, as well as effective parenting strategies fostering improved communication and positive behavior.

Timothy underwent a full battery of psychoeducational testing during hospitalization and received a Full Scale IQ of 81 on the Wechsler Intelligence Scale for Children—Third Edition (Wechsler 1991), demonstrating improvement. The clinician recommended that the social worker collaborate with an educational advocate and have Timothy transferred to a small, structured private educational setting that could better meet his educational needs and build on the gains already made. Foster children often languish in meager educational environments because they have no one to advocate on their behalf or because they live in disadvantaged neighborhoods where resources are dismal (The David and Lucile Packard Foundation 2004).

Despite numerous challenges, Timothy has many things going for him. He has remained in the same loving foster home for 2 years, a period of time during which foster children experience an average of four to five placement disruptions (Carpenter et al. 2001). He has had the same outpatient treatment team for 2 years, whereas foster children typically have poor access to health care, which is at best fragmented (Staudt 2003). What he shares with most foster children is the yearning to be loved, nurtured, protected, and taken care of unconditionally. As the uncertainty of reunification, adoption, or long-term foster care ensues, so does the child's symptomatology. The uncertainty, broken promises, and inconsistencies fuel feelings of anger, resentment, sadness, frustration, ambivalence, and confusion, which are internalized and externalized. Timothy's symptoms of anxiety, moodiness, and disruptive behaviors were intricately connected to these feelings. The clinician recommended to the social worker that the court come to a decision about Timothy's reunification status within a clear time frame and identify whether Timothy's current foster placement of 2 years is temporary or permanent so he might begin to believe that he is good enough to be wanted in somebody's family.

REFERENCES

Achenbach TM: Integrative Guide for the 1991 Child Behavior Checklist/4–18 YSR and TRF profiles. Burlington, VT, University of Vermont, Department of Psychiatry, 1991

American Academy of Child and Adolescent Psychiatry. Practice parameters for the assessment and treatment of children and adolescents with depressive disorders. J Am Acad Child Adolesc Psychiatry 37 (suppl 10):63S–83S, 1998

Beck AT, Steer RA, Brown GK: Beck Depression Inventory–II. San Antonio, TX, Psychological Corporation, 1996

Brent DA, Poling K, McKain B, et al: A psychoeducational program for families of affectively ill children and adolescents. J Am Acad Child Adolesc Psychiatry 32:770–774, 1993

Carpenter SC, Clyman RB, Davidson AJ, et al: The association of foster care or kinship care with adolescent sexual behavior and first pregnancy. Pediatrics 108:1–6, 2001

Centers for Disease Control and Prevention: Therapeutic Foster Care for the Prevention of Violence: A Report on Recommendations of the Task Force on Community Preventive Services. July 2, 2004. Available at: http://www.cdc.gov/mmwr/PDF/rr/rr5310.pdf. Accessed August 1, 2008.

Cohen JA, Deblinger E, Mannarino AP, et al: A multisite, randomized controlled trial for children with sexual abuse-related PTSD symptoms. J Am Acad Child Adolesc Psychiatry 43:393–402, 2004

Cohen JA, Mannarino AP, Deblinger E: Treating Trauma and Traumatic Grief in Children and Adolescents. New York, Guilford, 2006

Cohen JA, Mannarino AP, Perel JM, et al: A pilot randomized controlled trial of combined trauma-focused CBT and sertraline for childhood PTSD symptoms. J Am Acad Child Adolesc Psychiatry 46:811–819, 2007

Conners CK: A teacher rating scale for use in drug studies with children. Am J Psychiatry 126:884–888, 1969

Conners CK: Conners' Rating Scales—Revised: Technical Manual. New York, Multi-Health Systems, 1997

Conners CK, Sitarenios G, Parker JD, et al: Revision and restandardization of the Conners' Teacher Rating Scale (CTRS-R): factor structure, reliability, and criterion validity. J Abnorm Child Psychol 26:279–291, 1998

The David and Lucile Packard Foundation: Children, families, and foster care. The Future of Children 14(1):1–193, 2004

Daviss WB, Perel JM, Birmaher B, et al: Steady-state clinical pharmacokinetics of bupropion extended-release in youths. J Am Acad Child Adolesc Psychiatry 45:1503–1509, 2006

Deblinger E, Mannarino AP, Cohen JA, et al: A follow-up study of a multisite, randomized, controlled trial for children with sexual abuse-related PTSD symptoms. J Am Acad Child Adolesc Psychiatry 45:1474–1484, 2006

Donnelly CL: Pharmacologic treatment approaches for children and adolescents with posttraumatic stress disorder. Child Adolesc Psychiatr Clin N Am 12:251–269, 2003

Dulcan M: Practice parameters for the assessment and treatment of children, adolescents, and adults with attention-deficit/hyperactivity disorder. American Academy of Child and Adolescent Psychiatry. J Am Acad Child Adolesc Psychiatry 36 (suppl 10):85S–121S, 1997

DuPaul G, Rapport MD, Perriello LM: Teacher ratings of academic skills: the development of the Academic Performance Scale. School Psychology Review 20:284–300, 1991

Ford JD, Racusin R, Daviss WB, et al: Trauma exposure among children with oppositional defiant disorder and attention-deficit/hyperactivity disorder. J Consult Clin Psychol 67:786–789, 1999

Kovacs M: The Children's Depression Inventory. North Tonawanda, NY, Multi-Health Systems, 1992

Orvaschel H, Puig-Antich P, Chambers W, et al: Retrospective assessment of prepubertal major depression with the Kiddie SADS. J Am Acad Child Adolesc Psychiatry 21:392–397, 1982

Patterson G, Narrett C: The development of a reliable and valid treatment program for aggressive young children. Int J Ment Health 19:19–26, 1990

Pliszka SR, Carlson CL, Swanson JM: ADHD With Comorbid Disorders: Clinical Assessment and Management. New York, Guilford, 1999

Poznanski EO, Mokros HB: Children's Depression Rating Scale, Revised. Los Angeles, CA, Western Psychological Services, 1996

Pynoos RS, Rodriguez N, Steinberg A, et al: The UCLA PTSD Reaction Index for DSM-IV. 1998. Available from the National Child Traumatic Stress Network Web site: http://www.nctsnet.org. Accessed on December 1, 2007.

Schatzberg AF, Cole JO, DeBattista C: Manual of Clinical Psychopharmacology, 6th Edition. Washington, DC, American Psychiatric Publishing, 2007

Shaffer D, Gould MS, Brasic J, et al: A children's global assessment scale (CGAS). Arch Gen Psychiatry 40:1228–1231, 1983

Sparrow SS, Balla DA, Cicchetti DV: Vineland Adaptive Behavior Scales. Circle Pines, MN, American Guidance Service, 1984

Staudt M: Mental health services utilization by maltreated children: research findings and recommendations. Child Maltreat 8:195–203, 2003

Steinberg AM, Brymer MJ, Decker KB, et al: The University of California at Los Angeles Post-traumatic Stress Disorder Reaction Index. Curr Psychiatry Rep 6:96–100, 2004

Swanson JM: School-Based Assessments and Interventions for ADD Students. Irvine, CA, KC Publications, 1992

Wagner KD, Ambrosini P, Rynn M, et al: Efficacy of sertraline in the treatment of children and adolescents with major depressive disorder: two randomized controlled trials. JAMA 290:1033–1041, 2003

Wechsler D: Wechsler Intelligence Scale for Children—Third Edition (WISC-III). San Antonio, TX, The Psychological Corporation, 1991

■ CHAPTER 27 ■

The Legacy of War

Irritability and Anger in an Adolescent Refugee

Brian L. Isakson, Ph.D.
Christopher M. Layne, Ph.D.

CASE PRESENTATION

IDENTIFYING INFORMATION

Ibrahim is a 15-year-old boy from Somalia. He lives with his grandmother and 23-year-old uncle.

CHIEF COMPLAINT

Ibrahim was referred by his grandmother to the staff psychologist at a refugee center because of anger problems and episodes of dissociation. He complains, "School is too hard; I can't learn like I used to. I get so mad when the kids make fun of me because of my accent."

HISTORY OF PRESENT ILLNESS

Ibrahim's grandmother took him to a psychologist at the refugee community center where she attends English classes and where Ibrahim receives after-

Brian L. Isakson, Ph.D., is a clinical psychology postdoctoral fellow at the Center for Rural and Community Behavioral Health in the Department of Psychiatry at the University of New Mexico Health Science Center in Albuquerque, New Mexico.

Christopher M. Layne, Ph.D., is Director of Treatment and Intervention Development at the University of California, Los Angeles/Duke National Center for Child Traumatic Stress in Los Angeles, California.

For complete biographical information, see "About the Contributors," p. 613.

school tutoring. She asked that Ibrahim be assessed after he was suspended from school for 2 days because of fighting. According to his grandmother's report, Ibrahim has not been the same since they fled from Somalia. He is much more irritable and angry and is not interested in soccer or reading, which he enjoyed before his parents were killed. He is becoming more difficult for her to handle. She attributes his behavior to the influence of his friends, who lack supervision at home because their parents are always working. Ibrahim stays out with his friends until midnight on some school nights and sometimes does not come home at night on weekends. He has had difficulty transitioning into mainstream classes from his English-intensive classes. Ibrahim is often teased by youths in the mainstream classes he attends. They make fun of his accent and, because he is 2 years behind his age group, they call him "stupid." Ibrahim and his group of friends have also been in several fights with some Bosnian refugee boys who live in his apartment complex. Ibrahim reported that the boys were "disrespecting" them by mocking their language and clothes.

Ibrahim has a difficult time paying attention in class. His mind often wanders and sometimes goes blank. Time passes without his being aware of it. He often thinks about his family, particularly about the night when his parents were killed, although he tries not to think about what happened. When he thinks about the experience, he becomes frightened. Ibrahim feels very guilty that he survived when other members of his family did not. His teachers must call his name in class several times to get his attention, and when he mentally refocuses on the present, he still feels confused. Even though he tries hard to concentrate, he has difficulty remembering what he just learned. He does not consider obtaining an education important, because he does not plan to have a job in the future that will require much education and he has no plans to have a family of his own that he will need to support.

PAST PSYCHIATRIC HISTORY

While he was age 10 and living in Somalia, Ibrahim witnessed the brutal murder of his parents by an antigovernment rebel group. His father was a police officer for the government and was thus targeted by the rebel group. The rebels entered the family home in the middle of the night and shot the father point-blank in front of the family. When the mother threw herself onto her husband to protect him, they also shot her. Ibrahim witnessed these events and feared that he would be killed as well. The rebels took his older sister, most likely as a "war bride." The rebels broke Ibrahim's arm with the dull edge of a machete as a warning to the young man to flee and not seek retribution. The rebels forced Ibrahim and his grandmother to flee, and the two fled across the border to Kenya in a refugee caravan. During this refugee flight, the pair became involuntarily separated after the rebels began to pursue their caravan. Alone and afraid, Ibrahim was taken in by other members of his tribe, who allowed him to travel with them. The group hid from the rebels by traveling mostly at night. After arriving at a refugee camp in Kenya, Ibrahim was reunited with his grandmother and lived there with her for the next 3 years. While living in the refugee camp, Ibrahim and his grandmother lived in fear that rebels would come across the border to attack them or that local inhabitants would rob them. Although Ibrahim has participated in a mentoring program supervised by a clinical psychologist, he has never participated in therapy or been prescribed any psychotropic medication.

SUBSTANCE ABUSE HISTORY

Ibrahim has experimented with alcohol with his friends. He has stolen beer on occasion from his uncle and drunk it.

MEDICAL HISTORY

Ibrahim's arm was broken when his family was attacked by the rebels. He did not receive proper medical treatment for several weeks, until he received treatment by the Red Cross in the refugee camp. He cannot fully extend his arm as a result. This physical disability evokes intrusive thoughts of the night his parents were killed, his sister was abducted, and he and his grandmother were forced to flee. He tries to distract himself from these memories by listening to loud music.

DEVELOPMENTAL HISTORY

According to his grandmother, Ibrahim met all developmental milestones at the appropriate ages.

SOCIAL HISTORY

Ibrahim lives with his grandmother and 23-year-old uncle, who was in the Somali army at the time Ibrahim's family was attacked. Ibrahim has an older sister who has been missing since his parents were killed. When he was age 13, Ibrahim and his grandmother moved from Kenya to Denver, Colorado, where they have lived for the past 2 years. Ibrahim immigrated to the United States with his grandmother; his uncle joined the family in Denver a year later after being released from prison for opposing a local warlord in Somalia. Ibrahim's grandmother reports that her son, Ibrahim's uncle, drinks too much and yells at Ibrahim.

The grandmother works part-time at a local hotel, where she cleans rooms, and the uncle works at a local food-processing factory. Ibrahim is consequently unmonitored after school. He is enrolled in an after-school tutoring program at the refugee center but attends only several times a week. Ibrahim has several close Somali friends who live in his apartment complex. Ibrahim states that he "gets along fine" with his grandmother but considers her "old-fashioned" and says that she "does not understand what life is like for teenagers here in the United States." His grandmother, on the other hand, worries that Ibrahim is becoming "too American and forgetting his native culture." Ibrahim must often translate for his grandmother because he has learned English much more quickly than she has. He finds it stressful to translate for her at the bank, at stores, and with his teachers during parent-teacher conferences.

FAMILY HISTORY

Ibrahim's grandmother reports that she has had intermittent episodes of depression since immigrating to the United States. She attributes these depressed thoughts and feelings to the family's poor financial situation, the need to adapt to a new setting and culture, and her inability to help her grandson in school. Ibrahim's uncle has abused alcohol since immigrating. His alcohol use has led to inconsistent work attendance and the loss of a job because of frequent absences and poor work performance.

MENTAL STATUS EXAMINATION

Ibrahim met with the psychologist during a tutoring session. He was dressed in baggy clothes that made it difficult to gauge his body weight. He was quiet, giving brief answers when asked direct questions. He appeared sullen and mildly agitated, making little eye contact throughout the discussion. He did not display evidence of psychosis, and his thinking appeared logical and coherent. He reported that he would never hurt himself or try to kill himself because it would be "against my religious beliefs."

COMMENTARIES

Psychotherapeutic Perspective

Judith A. Cohen, M.D.

This commentary addresses Ibrahim's trauma and traumatic/complicated grief psychosocial treatment issues. If I were his therapist, I would also consider systemic issues, but these considerations are beyond the scope of this commentary.

Judith A. Cohen, M.D., is Medical Director of the Center for Traumatic Stress in Children and Adolescents at Allegheny General Hospital in Pittsburgh, Pennsylvania (for complete biographical information, see "About the Contributors," p. 613).

DIAGNOSTIC FORMULATION

Ibrahim displays symptoms of posttraumatic stress disorder (PTSD) as they are commonly manifested in children and teens who have experienced severe and/or repeated traumatic events, complicated by multiple deaths; loss of cultural, familial, and peer supports; and economic and other psychosocial stressors. Ibrahim's DSM-IV-TR symptoms of PTSD include the following:

- *Criterion A*—exposure to multiple life-threatening traumas, including witnessing the brutal murders of his parents
- *Criterion B*—intrusive thoughts about his family and the night when his family were killed, accompanied by psychological distress; dissociative episodes
- *Criterion C*—avoidance of thinking about his parents' murder; not participating in activities that remind him of his life with his parents (soccer, reading) and other trauma reminders (e.g., listens to music to avoid intrusive thoughts); decreased interest in school and learning; restricted affective range; sense of foreshortened future (does not think education is important because does not plan to have a family or a job that requires education)
- *Criterion D*—possible decreased sleep; irritability and angry outbursts (fighting); difficulty concentrating; possible hypervigilance or increased startle (mental status examination indicates mild agitation)

Impairment is present in school and possibly with peers and at home.

EPIDEMIOLOGY AND COMORBIDITY

A majority of children and teens with PTSD also have another DSM-IV-TR diagnosis. The most common comorbid conditions include another anxiety disorder, depressive disorders, and externalizing disorders such as substance use disorders, oppositional defiant disorder, or attention-deficit/hyperactivity disorder (ADHD).

Although Ibrahim has used alcohol and has some problems with fighting, I have more concerns about the possibility that he is depressed. When asked about suicidality, he does not give a more typical adolescent response (e.g., "Are you crazy?") but instead says that this would be "against my religious beliefs," suggesting that perhaps he has thought about this and would even consider suicide if it were not proscribed by his religion. In addition to his difficulty concentrating, survivor guilt, irritability, and substance use (which might represent an attempt to self-medicate affective symptoms), I would more thoroughly assess this young man for depressive and suicidal symptoms.

INSTRUMENTS

Self-report instruments such as the UCLA PTSD Reaction Index for DSM-IV (Steinberg et al. 2004) or the Child PTSD Symptom Scale (Foa et al. 2001) are helpful for assessing PTSD symptoms in teens. However, the clinician should also ask caretakers and other adults, such as Ibrahim's grandmother or teachers who know him, to complete the caregiver version of the UCLA PTSD Reaction Index. A depression screen such as the Beck Depression Inventory–II (Beck et al. 1996) would also be helpful. Although inadequate information is provided in the case presentation, Ibrahim might also be experiencing traumatic or complicated grief, resulting from unresolved issues related to witnessing the traumatic death of his parents, the abduction of his sister, and perhaps other experiences. The Extended Grief Inventory (Layne et al. 2001) may be useful in assessing this condition.

DSM-IV-TR DIAGNOSIS

Axis I   309.81 Posttraumatic stress disorder
          Rule out alcohol use D/O
          Rule out major depressive disorder
          Rule out oppositional defiant disorder
Axis II   None
Axis III Status post-fractured arm with residual disability
Axis IV   Severe to extreme: witness to murder of parents, war, refugee status, economic hardship
Axis V   Global Assessment of Functioning=40

TREATMENT RECOMMENDATIONS

Several evidence-based or evidence-informed treatments for childhood trauma are available. Depending on whether Ibrahim would be more amenable to receiving individual or group treatment and whether an appropriate cohort of traumatized youth would be available with whom he could participate in treatment, trauma-focused cognitive-behavioral therapy (TF-CBT; Cohen et al. 2006), cognitive-behavioral intervention for trauma in schools (Jaycox 2004), or trauma/grief-focused group psychotherapy (Layne et al. 2001a, 2001b) would be appropriate to address his trauma, traumatic grief, and, if present, depressive symptoms. If Ibrahim were agreeable and his grandmother's English were up to it, I would recommend TF-CBT, because this would give his grandmother a chance to understand more about what her grandson is dealing with, particularly in terms of his current PTSD and/or traumatic grief symptoms. Because Ibrahim complains that his grandmother does not understand what life is like for teens in the United States, perhaps this therapy could give them a chance to become closer.

Ibrahim's grandmother thinks that he is "forgetting his native culture" when in fact he is trying not to think about his traumatic memories. Providing his grandmother with psychoeducation about PTSD and how this disorder is affecting her grandson might help her understand why he does not want to think about his native land or his family right now—these are all trauma reminders for him.

When Ibrahim's mother showed an emotional reaction to the shooting of his father, the rebels murdered her, so Ibrahim learned to be silent and not express his feelings. Ibrahim has not learned that it is now safe to express emotions and that they do not have to be suppressed or acted out. TF-CBT (or the group models mentioned above) addresses affective expression skills that could assist Ibrahim in this regard. TF-CBT can also target his survivor guilt through cognitive processing (examining and reframing dysfunctional thoughts, such as survivor guilt).

After Ibrahim and his grandmother individually master these skills in TF-CBT, I would assist Ibrahim in gradually developing a trauma narrative (i.e., telling the story of what he experienced during the war), without allowing him to be overwhelmed with trauma reminders. If he and I agreed that this would be helpful, he might then share his narrative with his grandmother. Although this might be painful, I believe it would ultimately be healing for both of them. Certainly, the narrative would reassure his grandmother that Ibrahim has not forgotten his native culture and hopefully would improve their ability to communicate about other issues. Perhaps being able to talk about this would decrease the grandmother's depression and make her more available to Ibrahim as well, thereby possibly making her better able to address family issues, including the uncle's behaviors.

If Ibrahim has symptoms of traumatic grief, both TF-CBT and trauma/grief-focused group psychotherapy (Layne et al. 2001a, 2001b) include grief-focused components that can be used to address unresolved grief issues. The TF-CBT model provides these treatments conjointly to children/teens and their caregivers, which might be ideal for this family, providing Ibrahim were willing to allow his grandmother to participate.

TF-CBT also addresses issues related to safety, including making optimal choices about when and whether to fight, using drugs and alcohol for affective regulation, and so on. Hopefully, if Ibrahim has less dissociation and better concentration, he will have more success and interest in school. If not, educational alternatives may need to be addressed.

Psychopharmacologic Perspective

Frank W. Putnam, M.D.

DIAGNOSTIC FORMULATION

Ibrahim fulfills the DSM-IV-TR criteria for PTSD. The witnessed death of his parents satisfies Criterion A (traumatic stressor). The intrusive thoughts of his parents' death, which he attempts to block out with loud music, satisfy Criterion B (persistent reexperiencing). His loss of interest in favorite activities, such as playing soccer and reading, and his foreshortened sense of the future meet Criterion C (persistent avoidance). His difficulties with anger and his problems concentrating in school fulfill Criterion D (persistent increased arousal). Rates of PTSD are reported to range from 50% to 90% in refugee children exposed to war or civil conflict (Lustig et al. 2004).

Psychiatric comorbidity is high in multiply traumatized individuals of all ages. The prospective Great Smoky Mountain study of a representative U.S. population sample of 1,420 children up to age 16 found high rates of comorbidity for those children with posttraumatic stress symptoms (Copeland et al. 2007). Affective and anxiety disorders were the most common, but rates of ADHD and conduct disorder were at least three times greater than for children with no posttraumatic symptoms.

A number of additional clinical issues are raised by this case. Ibrahim and his family have been permanently displaced from their homeland and culture and are experiencing resettlement and acculturation issues common in such cases. In addition to their daily struggles to meet basic needs and create a new life, they must learn a new language and adapt to a radically different culture, often with little or no social support. Children and adolescents usually acculturate more quickly than adults because they are cognitively and socially more flexible and because they are more thoroughly immersed in the new culture through school, sports, and peer activities. As often occurs in such families, Ibrahim must translate for his grandmother in all manner of transactions, including parent-teacher discussions about his own behavior. This dependence

Frank W. Putnam, M.D., is Professor of Pediatrics and Psychiatry and Director of the Mayerson Center for Safe and Healthy Children at Cincinnati Children's Hospital Medical Center in Cincinnati, Ohio (for complete biographical information, see "About the Contributors," p. 613).

undercuts his grandmother's authority and exacerbates their generational conflict about what constitutes appropriate behavior on his part.

DSM-IV-TR DIAGNOSIS

Axis I   309.81 Posttraumatic stress disorder

        Rule out adjustment disorder

        Rule out acute stress disorder

        Rule out conduct disorder

Axis II   No diagnosis

Axis III   None

Axis IV   Educational problems

Axis V   Global Assessment of Functioning=57

        Moderate difficulties in school functioning

TREATMENT RECOMMENDATIONS

Although I was asked to address the psychopharmacologic treatment of Ibrahim, my treatment of choice for Ibrahim would be TF-CBT (Cohen et al. 2006). Selective serotonin reuptake inhibitors (SSRIs) are approved for use by adults with PTSD and are the only medications proven to reduce all three adult PTSD symptom clusters. No randomized trials have been published documenting the efficacy of any class of medications for children or adolescents with PTSD. TF-CBT has been shown to be effective in more than 10 randomized clinical trials, including studies with multiply traumatized children. A meta-analysis found effect sizes of $d=0.50$ for posttraumatic stress symptoms, $d=0.29$ for depression, and $d=0.24$ for externalizing behavior problems (Silverman et al. 2008). Follow-up has found that outcomes are maintained for at least 2 years posttreatment (Deblinger et al. 1999).

TF-CBT is a manualized treatment that is typically delivered in 12–15 sessions but occasionally requires as many as 30–40 sessions. The manual is considered a guide and allows clinical flexibility in choosing the focus, range, and intensity of the treatment (Cohen et al. 2006). The essential components of a child's treatment include psychoeducation about trauma and PTSD, emotional regulation skills, individualized stress management skills, connecting thoughts and behaviors with traumatic experiences, constructing and sharing a narrative about a self-selected traumatic experience, cognitive and affective processing of the trauma experience(s), and education about healthy relationships. A variation of TF-CBT can be delivered in group settings for adolescents (Stein et al. 2003; see also Layne et al. 2008a). Information on training in TF-CBT is available through the National Child Traumatic Stress Network, and a

Web-based course is hosted by the Medical University of South Carolina (http://tfcbt.musc.edu).

An important component of TF-CBT is its inclusion of individual sessions for both the child and a parent or caretaker, as well as conjoint parent-child sessions. Work with the parent or caregiver focuses on parenting skills and enhanced trauma discussions and future coping with traumatic reminders. In one or more conjoint sessions, the child shares his or her trauma narrative with the parent or caregiver, who has been previously prepared for the content by the therapist. Research has shown that including the parent or caretaker is more effective than treating the child alone (Deblinger et al. 1996). Ibrahim should be consulted regarding whether he wants his grandmother or uncle to participate in this role. I would recommend his uncle, who is closer in age, and who may also receive some benefit and subsequently be more open to pursuing his own treatment. If willing, his grandmother should be referred for treatment of her depression.

Ibrahim's treatment will have to accommodate his family's cultural differences as well as address the many forms of trauma and loss that he has endured. Ibrahim witnessed the murder of his parents at close range, which is perhaps the single most traumatizing experience a child can have. Subsequently, he repeatedly experienced threats to his own life and separations from his family during their escape and later in the Kenyan refugee camp. His sister is still missing. At the time of his parents' murder, he had his arm broken, resulting in a partial disability that serves both to remind him of the incident and as a source of embarrassment with peers. The therapy does not have to focus on every trauma, but it should include work on grief and loss as well as his experiences of terror and violence.

Ibrahim has a number of important strengths to build on. Prior to the trauma, he was interested in reading and sports. He has participated to some extent in a mentoring program at the refugee center. He has several friends. He has only experimented with alcohol. He has learned English sufficiently well to translate for his grandmother and to be mainstreamed in school. He was at least cooperative with psychological assessment and is not suicidal. He currently uses a coping strategy (loud music) to deal with his intrusive thoughts and thus may be open to trying more adaptive strategies as part of TF-CBT.

If Ibrahim remains significantly symptomatic after TF-CBT is completed, I would consider a medication trial. My first choice would be sertraline because limited evidence shows its efficacy (Cohen et al. 2007). If children or adolescents have a comorbid major depressive disorder, generalized anxiety disorder, or obsessive-compulsive disorder, the addition of an SSRI early in treatment may be beneficial.

Integrative Perspective

Brian L. Isakson, Ph.D.
Christopher M. Layne, Ph.D.

DIAGNOSTIC FORMULATION

Ibrahim meets DSM-IV-TR criteria for PTSD due to witnessing a traumatic event—the murder of his parents—and directly experiencing one or more traumatic events—fleeing from the rebels and receiving a broken arm (Criterion A1). He experienced terror and horror in fearing that he would be killed as well (Criterion A2). Ibrahim reports persistently reexperiencing traumatic events from his past in the form of thoughts and images relating to his parents' violent death (Criterion B1). He displays signs of avoidance and numbing of responsiveness. Although unbidden, intrusive memories of these traumatic experiences often pop into his mind, he tries not to think about what happened (Criterion C1). He reports diminished interest in activities he once enjoyed (Criterion C4) and describes having a sense of a foreshortened future in that he does not think he will have a career or a family (Criterion C7). He displays increased arousal in the form of irritability and outbursts of anger, which sometimes leads to fights with other boys (Criterion D2). He also reports difficulties with concentrating at school and remembering what he recently learned (Criterion D3). Ibrahim has been experiencing these symptoms for several years (Criterion E), and his symptoms are linked to significant impairment in his social and school functioning (Criterion F).

DIFFERENTIAL DIAGNOSIS

Not all children exposed to traumatic events develop PTSD. However, PTSD, other anxiety disorders, depression, and behavior disorders are common in trauma survivors and often co-occur, leading to significant comorbidity (Joshi and O'Donnell 2003). Because of the onset of Ibrahim's behavior and attention problems *after* the traumatic event, oppositional defiant disorder, conduct disorder, and ADHD can be ruled out as possible diagnoses. Ibrahim does not appear to display either the broad anxiety characteristic of generalized anxiety disorder or the fear in relation to a specific object or situation that is characteristic of specific phobia. Although he reports recurrent intrusive thoughts relating to the death of his parents, these thoughts are related to an objective traumatic event and are not inappropriate, which distinguishes his symptoms from obsessive-compulsive disorder. Furthermore, although Ibrahim is having difficulty adjusting to life in the United States, he has been exposed to extreme stressors in which his life and the lives of people he cared about were in objective danger; this rules out a simple adjustment disorder. Ibrahim reports forms of distress that also characterize diagnostic criteria for major depressive disorder, including irritable mood, loss of interest in activities he formerly enjoyed, diminished ability to concentrate, and excessive or inappropriate guilt. Thus, major depressive disorder is important to rule out.

DSM-IV-TR DIAGNOSIS

Axis I   309.81 Posttraumatic stress disorder, chronic

           Rule out major depressive disorder

Axis II   None

Axis III   None reported

Axis IV   Primary support problems: death of family members, inadequate parental monitoring, disruption of the family system produced by involuntary separation from family members

           Social environment problems: difficulties with acculturation, discrimination, taunting by schoolmates and peers

           Economic problems: inadequate income, financial strain

           Other environmental problems: exposure to war, refugee flight

Axis V   Global Assessment of Functioning=43

TREATMENT RECOMMENDATIONS

INITIAL ASSESSMENT

In considering how best to proceed, the school psychologist may find it useful to administer a number of assessment instruments. These include, given Ibrahim's history of trauma exposure and traumatic bereavement, the self-report UCLA PTSD Reaction Index (Steinberg et al. 2004) and a grief measure, such as the Extended Grief Inventory (Layne et al. 2001, 2007). A measure of war trauma exposure, such as the War Trauma Exposure Index (described in Layne et al. 2001, 2008a), may also be useful. A depression measure, such as the Beck Depression Inventory–II (Beck et al. 1996), may also be profitably added. Assessment by the school psychologist focusing on academic strengths and weaknesses may also be needed to identify focal areas of difficulty, rule out other potential causes or areas of difficulty, and develop an intervention plan.

FORMING A TREATMENT PLAN

Treatment for PTSD in refugee youth should utilize an interdisciplinary, multimodal approach that addresses as needed the adolescent's biological, psychological, social, and physical needs (Brymer et al. 2008; Lustig et al. 2004). Cultural issues are an integral part of all such interventions (Marsella et al. 1996). More generally, resilience-promoting factors in an adolescent and his or her surrounding social and physical environment, though too often overlooked, should be incorporated as valuable components of treatment (Layne et al. 2007, 2008b, 2009; Papadopoulos 2001). Among these beneficial factors are Ibrahim's pretrauma interests in soccer and reading. Although they may serve as a powerful protective agent, Ibrahim's social ties with members of his family may also generate significant persisting stress, arising from his conflicted relationship with his uncle and ongoing concerns over his missing sister (Layne et al. 2008b). To date, few interventions currently used to treat refugee adolescents (e.g., cognitive-behavioral therapy, art therapy, group therapy) have been manualized, and even fewer have been empirically validated (Birman et al. 2005; Ehntholt and Yule 2006; Layne et al. 2004). Given this limited evidence base, candidate interventions for Ibrahim and his family are probably best approached as evidence informed rather than evidence based.

One promising intervention is trauma and grief component therapy (TGCT; Layne et al. 2000; Saltzman et al. 2006), as delivered in either an individual-based or preferably a group-based modality (Davies et al. 2006). In a randomized controlled field trial of TGCT with severely war-traumatized and traumatically bereaved Bosnian adolescents, Layne et al. (2008a; see also Cox et al. 2007) found that the percentages of youths who completed group-based TGCT and showed significant reductions in PTSD symptoms compared favorably to those percentages reported in carefully controlled treatment efficacy trials, whereas the percentages who reported significant reductions in traumatic grief reactions and depression symptoms compared favorably to percentages achieved in community treatment settings. The primary aims of TGCT are to reduce distress and dysfunction, enhance current positive adaptation, and promote healthy developmental progression and preparation for the roles and responsibilities of adulthood.

Features of TGCT that may be helpful in Ibrahim's case include (see Layne et al. 2008a) the following:

1. Providing psychoeducation concerning trauma and loss reminders and the traumatic stress and grief reactions they continue to evoke over time (see Layne et al. 2006)
2. Enhancing coping with intense negative emotions to address adolescent social withdrawal and attempts to reduce distress through substance use
3. Trauma processing, giving special attention to existential dilemmas (i.e., painful quandaries during traumatic events in which one is forced to choose between self-protection and assisting others in distress; see Layne et

al. 2001a) and intervention thoughts (i.e., distressing ongoing preoccupations with how the traumatic injury or loss could have been prevented, protected against, or repaired—including thoughts linked to severe guilt, shame,
rage, and desires for revenge)

4. Grief processing designed to help traumatic grief reactions to recede, while
addressing the impact of the loss on adolescent identity, life plans, and future outlook

5. Building social support skills to bridge social estrangement and facilitate
coping with adversities

6. Enhancing problem-solving skills, including those needed to address lost
developmental opportunities and age-appropriate developmental tasks

7. Engaging adolescent capacities for insight to understand the links between
past traumatic experiences and losses, trauma and loss reminders, and current behavior problems

8. Reappraising traumatic expectations (i.e., trauma-induced pessimistic
alterations in basic belief systems and core values that are dysfunctional
given one's current life context) that interfere with life plans and activities
that promote a healthy transition to adulthood (see Layne et al. 2001a;
2001b)

Other potentially relevant war-focused interventions include a psychoeducational program for mothers who have been internally displaced within war-
ravaged Bosnia (Dybdahl 2001). Biweekly group treatment sessions address
maternal mental health– and trauma-related issues, as well as facilitating positive caregiver-child interaction. The author reported that the intervention led
to better maternal mental health outcomes than in a control group that addressed only medical concerns. Although children were not the direct focus of
treatment in either treatment condition, children in the treatment group
showed greater improvements in their psychosocial well-being, cognitive abilities, and physical health compared to children in the control group. Weine et
al.'s (2003) family support and education group intervention for Kosovar refugees may also be relevant for Ibrahim and his family. Although a control group
was not included in the design, pre-post analyses found that participation in
the intervention was associated with increased social support, use of psychiatric
services, understanding of trauma reactions, and family hardiness.

In addition to the interventions for war-exposed youths and families described above, a number of interventions described in the general child and
adolescent trauma treatment literature, including such cognitive-behavioral
approaches as TF-CBT (described previously in this chapter; see Brown et al.
2004; Cohen et al. 2006; Goodman et al. 2004), may also be useful. A multisystemic intervention may be helpful, consisting of individual or group therapy

at school or at a local youth club to strengthen adaptive coping skills, enhance emotional and behavioral regulation skills, increase social support, address social challenges with peers, and remove barriers to learning (see Brymer et al. 2008; Saltzman et al. 2001; Stein et al. 2003). In addressing Ibrahim's problems from a multisystemic perspective, the psychologist could organize an interdisciplinary team to address Ibrahim's biological, psychological, social, and physical needs (Brymer et al. 2008; Saxe et al. 2006). One component might be a routine medical examination to address Ibrahim's medical concerns, including problems that may be attributable to general medical conditions. Given that Ibrahim's grandmother expressed concern primarily about her grandson's school performance and interpersonal conflicts, the psychologist could work with Ibrahim's school counselor to implement interventions that address Ibrahim's difficulties with concentration and learning, as well as his difficulties with assimilation. Adult mentoring intervention may also serve as an appropriate adjunct intervention (Silove and Zwi 2005). Pharmacotherapy may also be considered to address specific symptoms of anxiety, depression, and arousal (see Brown et al. 2004; Saxe et al. 2006), and thus pharmacologic consultation may be warranted to address Ibrahim's irritability, PTSD symptoms, and depressed mood (Brown et al. 2004). Multisystemic intervention may also extend to Ibrahim's family and broader community. Possible interventions, particularly given the grandmother's descriptions of recurrent episodes of depression and her son's drinking problems, include referring Ibrahim's grandmother and uncle for assessment relating to their own trauma exposure histories and subsequent adversities, as well as interventions focused on strengthening connections between Ibrahim's family and the larger Somali community (Lustig et al. 2004; Saxe et al. 2006). TGCT offers several caregiver-focused sessions on increasing awareness of trauma and loss reminders and the distress reactions they evoke, improving communication, and enhancing social support (Layne et al. 2008a).

REFERENCES

Beck AT, Steer RA, Brown GK: Beck Depression Inventory–II. San Antonio, TX, Harcourt Assessment, 1996

Birman D, Ho J, Pulley E, et al: Mental Health Intervention for Refugee Children in Resettlement: White Paper II from the National Child Traumatic Stress Network Refugee Task Force. Boston, MA, National Child Traumatic Stress Network, 2005

Brown EJ, Albrecht A, McQuaid J, et al: Treatment of children exposed to trauma, in Posttraumatic Stress Disorders in Children and Adolescents: Handbook. Edited by Silva RR. New York, WW Norton, 2004, pp 257–286

Brymer MJ, Steinberg AM, Sornborger J, et al: Acute interventions for refugee children and families. Child Adolesc Psychiatr Clin N Am 17:625–640, 2008

Cohen JA, Mannarino AP, Deblinger E: Treating Trauma and Traumatic Grief in Children and Adolescents. New York, Guilford, 2006

Cohen JA, Mannarino AP, Perel JM, et al: A pilot randomized controlled trial of combined trauma-focused CBT and sertraline for childhood PTSD symptoms. J Am Acad Child Adolesc Psychiatry 46:811–819, 2007

Copeland W, Keeler G, Angold A, et al: Traumatic events and posttraumatic stress in childhood. Arch Gen Psychiatry 64:577–584, 2007

Cox J, Davies DR, Burlingame GM, et al: Effectiveness of a trauma/grief-focused group intervention: a qualitative study with war-exposed Bosnian adolescents. Int J Group Psychother 57:319–345, 2007

Davies DR, Burlingame GM, Layne CM: Integrating small-group process principles into trauma-focused group psychotherapy: what should a group trauma therapist know? in Psychological Effects of Terrorist Disasters: Group Approaches to Treatment. Edited by Schein LA, Spitz HI, Burlingame GM, et al. New York, Haworth, 2006, pp 385–424

Deblinger E, Lippmann J, Steer R: Sexually abused children suffering posttraumatic stress symptoms: initial treatment outcome findings. Child Maltreat 1:310–321, 1996

Deblinger E, Steer R, Lippmann J: Two-year follow-up study of cognitive behavioral therapy for sexually abused children suffering post-traumatic stress symptoms. Child Abuse Negl 23:1371–1378, 1999

Dybdahl R: Children and mothers in war: an outcome study of a psychosocial intervention program. Child Dev 72:1214–1230, 2001

Ehntholt KA, Yule W: Practitioner review: assessment and treatment of refugee children and adolescents who have experienced war-related trauma. J Child Psychol Psychiatry 47:1197–1210, 2006

Foa EB, Treadwell K, Johnson K, et al: The Child PTSD Symptom Scale: a preliminary examination of its psychometric properties. J Clin Child Psychol 30:376–384, 2001

Goodman RF, Morgan AV, Juriga S: Letting the story unfold: a case study of client-centered therapy for childhood traumatic grief. Harv Rev Psychiatry 12:199–212, 2004

Jaycox L: Cognitive-Behavioral Intervention for Trauma in Schools. Longmont, CO, Sopris West Educational Services, 2004

Joshi PT, O'Donnell DA: Consequences of child exposure to war and terrorism. Clin Child Fam Psychol Rev 6:275–292, 2003

Layne CM, Saltzman WR, Steinberg AM, et al: Trauma and Grief Component Therapy for Adolescents: Group Treatment Manual. Sarajevo, Bosnia, UNICEF Bosnia and Herzegovina, 2000

Layne CM, Pynoos RS, Cardenas J: Wounded adolescence: school-based group psychotherapy for adolescents who have sustained or witnessed violent interpersonal injury, in School Violence: Contributing Factors, Management, and Prevention. Edited by Shafii M, Shafii S. Washington, DC, American Psychiatric Press, 2001a, pp 163–186

Layne CM, Pynoos RS, Saltzman WR, et al: Trauma/grief-focused group psychotherapy: school-based post-war intervention with traumatized Bosnian adolescents. Group Dyn 5:277–290, 2001b

Layne CM, Murray L, Saltzman WR: An overview of evidence-based group approaches to trauma with children and adolescents, in Group Interventions for Treatment of Psychological Trauma. Edited by Buchele BJ, Spitz HI. New York, American Group Psychotherapy Association, 2004, pp 169–179

Layne CM, Warren JS, Saltzman WR, et al: Contextual influences on post-traumatic adjustment: retraumatization and the roles of distressing reminders, secondary adversities, and revictimization, in Group Approaches for the Psychological Effects of Terrorist Disasters. Edited by Schein LA, Spitz HI, Burlingame GM, et al. New York, Haworth, 2006, pp 235–286

Layne CM, Warren J, Watson P, et al: Risk, vulnerability, resistance, and resilience: towards an integrative model of posttraumatic adaptation, in PTSD: Science and Practice—A Comprehensive Handbook. Edited by Friedman MJ, Kean TM, Resick PA. New York, Guilford, 2007, pp 497–520

Layne CM, Saltzman WR, Poppleton L, et al: Effectiveness of a school-based group psychotherapy program for war-exposed adolescents: a randomized controlled trial. J Am Acad Child Adolesc Psychiatry 47:1048–1062, 2008a

Layne CM, Warren JS, Hilton S, et al: Measuring adolescent perceived support amidst war and disaster: the Multi-Sector Social Support Inventory, in Adolescents and Violence. Edited by Barber BK. New York, Oxford University Press, 2008b, pp 145–176

Layne CM, Beck CJ, Rimmasch H, et al: Promoting "resilient" posttraumatic adjustment in childhood and beyond: "unpacking" life events, adjustment trajectories, resources, and interventions, in Treating Traumatized Children: Risk, Resilience, and Recovery. Edited by Brom D, Pat-Horenczyk R, Ford J. New York, Routledge, 2009, pp 13–47

Lustig SL, Kia-Keating M, Grant-Knight W, et al: Review of child and adolescent refugee mental health. J Am Acad Child Adolesc Psychiatry 43:24–36, 2004

Marsella AJ, Friedman MJ, Gerrity ET, et al: Ethnocultural Aspects of Posttraumatic Stress Disorder: Issues, Research, and Clinical Applications. Washington, DC, American Psychological Association, 1996

Papadopoulos RK: Refugee families: issues of systematic supervision. Journal of Family Therapy 23:405–422, 2001

Saltzman WR, Pynoos RS, Layne CM, et al: Trauma/grief-focused intervention for adolescents exposed to community violence: results of a school-based screening and group treatment protocol. Group Dyn 5:291–303, 2001

Saltzman WR, Layne CM, Steinberg AM, et al: Trauma/grief-focused group psychotherapy with adolescents, in Psychological Effects of Terrorist Disasters: Group Approaches to Treatment. Edited by Schein LA, Spitz HI, Burlingame GM, et al. New York, Haworth, 2006, pp 669–730

Saxe GN, Ellis HB, Kaplow JB: Collaborative Treatment of Traumatized Children and Teens: The Trauma Systems Therapy Approach. New York, Guilford, 2006

Silove D, Zwi AB: Translating compassion into psychosocial aid after the tsunami. Lancet 365:269–271, 2005

Silverman WK, Ortiz CD, Viswesvaran C, et al: Evidence-based psychosocial treatments for children and adolescents exposed to traumatic events. J Clin Child Adolesc Psychol 37:156–183, 2008

Stein BD, Jaycox LH, Kataoka SH, et al: A mental health intervention for schoolchildren exposed to violence: a randomized controlled trial. JAMA 290:603–611, 2003

Steinberg AM, Brymer MJ, Decker KB, et al: The University of California at Los Angeles Posttraumatic Stress Disorder Reaction Index. Curr Psychiatry Rep 6:96–100, 2004

Weine SM, Raina D, Zhubi M, et al: The TAFES multi-family group intervention for Kosovar refugees: a feasibility study. J Nerv Ment Dis 191:100–107 2003

■ CHAPTER 28 ■

Moody Child

Depressed in Context of Parental Divorce

Sharlene A. Wolchik, Ph.D.
Irwin N. Sandler, Ph.D.

CASE PRESENTATION

IDENTIFYING INFORMATION

Jamie is an 11-year-old girl who was brought for an evaluation by her mother because of concerns about moodiness and clinginess. She lives with her mother and her 7-year-old brother and attends fifth grade in a regular education class.

CHIEF COMPLAINT

Jamie has become increasingly emotional and moody over the last couple of months. Also, she becomes distressed when her mother spends time with adults rather than with Jamie.

HISTORY OF PRESENT ILLNESS

During the past few months, Jamie has frequently experienced sudden changes in moods and has been increasingly sullen and irritable. She often fights with her

---

Sharlene A. Wolchik, Ph.D., is Professor in the Department of Psychology at Arizona State University in Tempe, Arizona.

Irwin N. Sandler, Ph.D., is Regents' Professor in the Department of Psychology, and Director of the Prevention Research Center for Families in Stress at Arizona State University in Tempe, Arizona.

For complete biographical information, see "About the Contributors," p. 613.

brother and argues with her mother. Also, Jamie gets upset whenever her mother wants to spend time with adult friends outside the house. When her mother talks about such plans, Jamie pleads with her mother to change her plans. Jamie frequently cries as her mother gets ready to leave the house to meet friends. In addition, she has seemed sad and unhappy or tense and anxious a lot of the time over the past couple of months. On several occasions during the last month when she has been angry with her mother, Jamie has made statements like "I wish I were dead" or "I am going to run away." However, Jamie has neither talked about specific plans to commit suicide nor run away from home.

Jamie's moodiness began about 1½ years ago, shortly after her parents decided to divorce and her father moved out of the family's home. Jamie's symptoms have become more frequent and intense over the last few months. Although her mother cannot identify an environmental precipitant for the increase in symptoms, she noted that after her ex-husband moved out of the house, she herself went through about a year when she was depressed and struggling with adjusting to life as a single mother. She also noted that although she was very worried about the effects of the divorce on her children, she probably did not spend as much time with Jamie as she should have during this period and that she did not have the patience or mental energy to really "be there" for either of her children. Jamie's mother also reported that since the divorce was finalized, she has been trying to reestablish her own social network, so she has been spending more time outside the home than she did before the divorce. She also mentioned that about 4 months ago, the family moved and the children enrolled in a new school.

PAST PSYCHIATRIC HISTORY

Jamie has never participated in therapy and has never been given a prescription for psychotropic medication.

MEDICAL HISTORY

Jamie's medical history is unremarkable.

DEVELOPMENTAL HISTORY

As an infant and toddler, Jamie was somewhat reserved and shy in new situations, although this was never seen as an indicator of pathology and did not impair her functioning.

SOCIAL HISTORY

Jamie lives with her biological mother and her 7-year-old brother. Her parents physically separated about 1½ years ago and were legally divorced 6 months ago. Her mother, an accountant at a small company, has sole legal custody of both children. The family moved about 4 months ago, and the children enrolled in a new school. Jamie spends time with her father at least once a week. These visits are not scheduled; the father drops by the house and, if the children are there, spends time with them. The frequency and nature of the contact between Jamie and her father have been stable since he moved out of the house. Jamie's mother noted that over the last year or so, she and her ex-spouse have rarely argued or fought. The family has no history of neglect or abuse. Jamie is currently in fifth grade. Last year, she received mostly A's and B's in school; this year she received mostly C's. After her typical summer break from piano lessons, Jamie refused to start taking lessons this fall, despite seeming to enjoy her lessons over the last 3 years. She also dropped out of her Girl Scout troop recently.

FAMILY HISTORY

Jamie's parents and brother have never been treated for psychological problems. Jamie's maternal grandfather has a history of alcohol abuse.

MENTAL STATUS EXAMINATION

Jamie was well dressed for the interview. She appeared her stated age. She provided brief responses to the questions. Jamie's affect was sad and somewhat anxious. She denied current suicidal ideation but stated that she sometimes wishes she were dead. Her thinking was logical and coherent. There was no evidence of psychosis.

COMMENTARIES

Psychotherapeutic Perspective

Clarice J. Kestenbaum, M.D.

DIAGNOSTIC FORMULATION

At first glance, Jamie's problems seem straightforward: the case of a sad and anxious preteen girl in the wake of her parents' divorce. However, 18 months after her father left home, Jamie continues to have symptoms that indicate psychopathology: anxiety and anger when her mother goes out; tearfulness and

Clarice J. Kestenbaum, M.D., is Professor of Clinical Psychiatry and Director of Training Emerita in the Division of Child and Adolescent Psychiatry at the Columbia University College of Physicians and Surgeons in New York, New York (for complete biographical information, see "About the Contributors," p. 613).

loss of interest in formerly enjoyable activities, such as Girl Scouts and piano lessons; social withdrawal; a drop in academic performance; and statements such as "I wish I were dead."

To evaluate Jamie's current state, I would need to know more about her early development. Did Jamie, a quiet and shy little girl, have difficulty separating from her mother in the preschool years? Was her attachment secure or insecure (Kestenbaum 2003)? Was her mother depressed prior to the divorce (Olfson et al. 2003; Weissman 2002)? Did Jamie's symptoms predate the divorce?

Although the negative effects of divorce on children are well established, as noted by Huurre et al. (2006), Kelly (2000) noted in a 10-year review that children of divorced parents, compared with children from intact homes, have many psychological symptoms that can be accounted for in the years prior to the divorce.

I would also want to know whether Jamie has a nonverbal learning disability that impairs her organizational skills necessary for academic success in middle and high school. I would obtain a neuropsychological test battery before beginning treatment to determine whether Jamie's academic problems result from psychological conflict or neuropsychiatric deficits.

DSM-IV-TR DIAGNOSIS

Axis I   300.4 Dysthymic disorder

Rule out generalized anxiety disorder

Rule out learning disorder not otherwise specified (NOS)

Axis II   Deferred

Axis III   Deferred

Axis IV   Parental divorce

Academic problems

Axis V   Global Assessment of Functioning=60

TREATMENT RECOMMENDATIONS

Of the several treatment options I could recommend, my first choice for Jamie would be individual psychodynamic psychotherapy. Although recent literature has provided few evidence-based studies describing the benefits of psychodynamic therapy for adolescent disorders, clinical illustrative vignettes have been described for 60 years (Freud 1958). Interpersonal therapy and cognitive-behavioral therapy (CBT) have been researched more assiduously during the past decade. Nevertheless, I believe Jamie would benefit from an in-depth examination of her life in twice-weekly psychodynamic psychotherapy. I would explore unconscious conflicts, utilize the transference plus real relationship, analyze resistance, and help her gain insight into her behavior and feelings of loss of "the way things were" that contribute to her depression, while establishing a strong therapeutic alliance. The therapy would involve her dreams and fantasies using a variety of techniques such as storytelling and narrative therapy that I have found useful in working with adolescents (Kestenbaum 1985). The ability to put one's life into perspective is a process that young children do not possess, most likely not until adolescence. Most children can recall life events in sequential fashion unless the process of recall is interrupted by a traumatic event such as death or divorce.

The use of narrative and storytelling is suitable for exploring the inner lives of children, particularly those who do not wish to talk about their feelings and behaviors. In this technique, the young child dictates a story to the therapist so that spontaneity and flow will not be hampered by the rules of spelling or grammar. I keep a special loose-leaf notebook for each child who wants to write a "book," with plenty of space for illustrations. I ask questions about the characters, their backgrounds, and their motives, and record the information in a separate notebook for future reference. Thus, a dual purpose is served: the child has a store of information to include in his or her book, and I have psychodynamic material to help me plan the direction of the treatment. Occasionally, young adolescents are willing to engage in "talk therapy" as well.

In Jamie's case, I would add a family component, either seeing the parents on a regular basis or referring them to a family therapist to ascertain whether the mother is still depressed and needs her own treatment. The parents could be seen together or, as in many divorce cases, on an individual basis. The father needs to have regular planned visits with Jamie rather than hit-or-miss appearances. Without treatment, I believe Jamie is at risk of developing major depression in adult life (Weissman 2002).

If the neuropsychological tests indicate that Jamie has learning difficulties, I would recommend remediation by a learning specialist.

If these measures fail to demonstrate improvement in Jamie's mood and behavior within 2 months, I would then add an antidepressant medication to the therapy, most likely a U.S. Food and Drug Administration (FDA)–approved selective serotonin reuptake inhibitor (SSRI).

Psychopharmacologic Perspective

Bruce Waslick, M.D.

DIAGNOSTIC FORMULATION

The case as presented represents a child with escalating mood and anxiety symptoms over the past few months. Jamie has become increasingly emotional, sullen, and irritable over the past few months. Irritability is a nonspecific symptom that occurs in a variety of pediatric (and adult) psychopathological conditions, but it can be the primary identifiable symptom of a developing mood disorder in a child. Jamie's statements of wanting to be dead may be indicative of increasing suicidality, another hallmark of a developing mood disorder. Some of her symptoms point toward features of escalating anxiety as well. Jamie's increasing clinginess, her difficulty tolerating her mother's going out on her own, the possibility of a baseline anxious or shy temperament, and her anxious affect during the initial mental status examination all suggest the possibility of a developing anxiety disorder, specifically separation anxiety disorder. This child also has been through a variety of major life changes recently (finalization of the parents' divorce, the family moving, changing of schools, mother spending more time out of the home), so the clinician would certainly have to consider the possibility that Jamie has developed an adjustment disorder with mood and anxiety symptom manifestations.

The evidence of significant change in the child's level of functioning suggests that she may be developing a serious psychiatric disorder. Her symptoms are having a worsening impact on her ability to function as a family member. She also is deteriorating in terms of her academic function, and she appears to be losing interest in activities she formerly enjoyed, specifically the piano lessons, but perhaps her Girl Scout troop as well.

The challenge diagnostically is to sort out the severity and stability of Jamie's affective and anxiety symptoms. "Moodiness" can range from normative development to the affective presentation of transient psychopathological states (i.e., adjustment disorders) to major pediatric mood disorders, such as major depres-

Bruce Waslick, M.D., is Staff Child Psychiatrist in the Division of Child Behavioral Health at Baystate Medical Center in Springfield, Massachusetts, and Associate Professor of Psychiatry at Tufts University School of Medicine in Boston, Massachusetts (for complete biographical information, see "About the Contributors," p. 613).

sion or bipolar disorder. The vignette includes no descriptions of major neuroveg-etative symptoms, such as sleep changes or appetite changes, and does not clearly indicate whether the mood symptoms mainly present in response to environmen-tal triggers (her mother's going out) or are pervasively present throughout the day. According to DSM-IV-TR, for the establishment of a diagnosis of major depres-sion in adults and youth, the affective presentation should be consistent nearly ev-ery day for most of the day, rather than primarily being reactive to environmental triggers. Not enough information is provided to conclusively make a diagnosis, but the available information is worrisome. Similarly, Jamie's anxiety symptoms need to be better characterized in terms of persistence and severity.

A variety of collateral information would be helpful in sorting out the di-agnosis. Having the opportunity to interview or gather information from other adults who know the child well could be helpful. An interview with the child's father could shed light on her symptoms and functional changes. Collecting information from the girl's teachers at school would be helpful to assess her ac-ademic and social functioning. Communication with the child's primary care provider and an updated health status report could be important in learning about any recent health changes.

An important source of information would be rating scales that have been adequately studied in terms of differentiating normal development from psychopathology in children (see King 1997). These scales include broad-spectrum instruments that assess for psychopathology across the range of diag-noses common in youth, as well as more narrow–spectrum instruments to as-sess specifically mood and anxiety symptoms in Jamie's case. Determining the extent to which the child's symptoms are outside the range of normal can be aided by the use of age- and gender-normed instruments. A combination of broad- and narrow-spectrum instruments would be most useful, and having a variety of reporters (parents, the child, and teachers) complete instruments would provide the most complete assessment of the presenting concerns.

Given the complexity of Jamie's case, longitudinal observation, or what is referred to as "active monitoring" over time, might be the best aid in sorting out persistent severe mood and anxiety symptoms versus transient, environmen-tally triggered states. Meeting with the child and family relatively frequently over the course of 1–2 months might be indicated prior to recommending spe-cific treatment interventions.

DSM-IV-TR DIAGNOSIS

Axis I   296.22 Major depressive disorder (MDD), moderate severity, without psychotic features

309.21 Separation anxiety disorder

Rule out adjustment disorder with mixed anxiety and depressed mood

Axis II   None

Axis III   None

Axis IV   Family relationship stresses

            Academic functioning problems

Axis V   Current Global Assessment of Functioning=55

            Highest Global Assessment of Functioning in past year=80

TREATMENT RECOMMENDATIONS

Treatment intervention recommendations would need to take into account the final diagnostic impression, evidence-based treatment principles, available mental health resources, and family preferences. Jamie does not appear to be a serious danger to herself or others, and although she is experiencing suicidal thinking, it appears to be passive rather than active, she has no well-formed plan, and she appears to have no suicidal intent and no history of previous dangerous behavior. Outpatient care would seem to be appropriate for her presentation.

If the clinician determines from the diagnostic assessment that Jamie's presentation is most compatible with an adjustment disorder, no pharmacologic treatment would be indicated. Supportive counseling that addresses reactions to change and loss or technique-specific psychotherapy addressing mood and anxiety symptoms would be indicated. Longitudinal observation for worsening of symptoms and pharmacologic intervention could be offered as a component of a treatment plan.

If the final diagnosis is a MDD and/or a specific pediatric anxiety disorder (e.g., separation anxiety disorder), the decision making regarding pharmacologic intervention is much more complex. Medication treatments can be used alone or in conjunction with psychotherapeutic approaches to help alleviate symptoms of depression and anxiety in children.

Antidepressant medications have been studied in children and adolescents with mood and anxiety disorders. Although the evidence for the superiority of antidepressants over placebo for pediatric depression in short-term randomized controlled trials is not overwhelmingly and uniformly positive, some evidence suggests that antidepressants can be an important component of a comprehensive treatment plan approach (Bridge et al. 2007). Fluoxetine is approved by the FDA for the acute treatment of major depression in children and adolescents ages 8–17. Although other agents have been studied, no other medication has approval for this indication in this age group. The research track record of antidepressants for the acute treatment of pediatric anxiety disorders is actually stronger than that for pediatric depressive disorders (Bridge et al. 2007). Additionally, fluoxetine, sertraline, and fluvoxamine carry FDA approval for the treatment of pediatric obsessive-compulsive disorder for youth ages 7–17. With the caveat that this is not the anxiety disorder being considered in this vignette, these three antidepressants are considered to have favorable risk-benefit profiles in at least one pediatric anxiety disorder and can be considered to be reasonable treatment options in this case.

Most of the available evidence and practice guidelines suggest that SSRIs, a subclass of antidepressants, are the medications of first choice for pediatric depressive and anxiety disorders. Other non-SSRI antidepressants (i.e., tricyclic antidepressants, serotonin-norepinephrine reuptake inhibitors) have been studied in youth with these disorders, but none have strong research support for their use as a first-line agent. Other antidepressants used to treat depression in adults (i.e., bupropion, monoamine oxidase inhibitors) have not been adequately studied in youth to make any kind of reasonable evidence-based recommendation, and should likely only be used in treatment-refractory cases. Likewise, alternative medication approaches to anxiety commonly used in adults (i.e., benzodiazepines, buspirone) have not been adequately studied in children and adolescents.

Providing the family with adequate information about the potential benefits and risks of SSRI therapy is important prior to initiating therapy. SSRIs are generally safe and well tolerated in adults and children. Adverse events are possible but occur relatively infrequently. Significant concern has been raised about whether SSRI therapy increases the risk of treatment-emergent suicidality specifically in younger patients. Since 2004, the FDA has required that SSRIs and all antidepressants carry a black box warning about treatment-emergent suicidality for pediatric patients, encouraging close observation of youth taking SSRIs, especially during the initial phases of treatment (Hammad et al. 2006). A full understanding of the adverse event profile of these medications may lead some families to consider SSRI therapy unacceptable either as an initial treatment intervention or at any time.

Access to and availability of evidence-based treatment approaches have to be considered in developing a final treatment plan. On the one hand, if an initial psychotherapy monotherapy approach was chosen, ideally it would be an evidence-based approach, but families may have problems accessing therapists with adequate training in evidence-based psychotherapy approaches for specific pediatric psychiatric disorders. On the other hand, most families potentially could have access to SSRI therapy through the child's primary care provider if he or she is adequately trained and has confidence in offering this treatment to families.

In Jamie's case, the family clearly will have a variety of options available in terms of reasonable treatment plans. Some but not all evidence in adolescents with depression suggests that combining SSRI therapy with an evidence-based psychotherapy may be the best and safest treatment for major depression

(Treatment for Adolescents with Depression Study Team 2004), but equivalent studies are not currently available for preadolescent patients. SSRI monotherapy has some support as being safe and effective in preadolescent youth with common anxiety disorders (Birmaher et al. 2003; Research Unit on Pediatric Psychopharmacology Anxiety Study Group 2001), but studies comparing medication monotherapy with either psychotherapy monotherapy or combination medication plus psychotherapy treatment are not currently available. An approach commonly used in clinical practice in these situations, and suggested by some treatment guidelines (Birmaher et al. 2007; National Institute for Clinical Excellence 2005), is a "sequenced" approach, such as beginning with psychotherapy treatment, observing the acute response to psychotherapy, and then adding medication for subjects who show little or no improvement or whose symptoms worsen during acute treatment. Alternatively, SSRI therapy could be the first treatment in the sequence, with psychotherapy added for treatment nonresponders, depending on patient characteristics and family preferences.

Integrative Perspective

Sharlene A. Wolchik, Ph.D.
Irwin N. Sandler, Ph.D.

DIAGNOSTIC FORMULATION

Although Jamie presents with some symptoms of MDD, including depressed/irritable mood and diminished interest in activities, as well as some symptoms of separation anxiety disorder, including excessive distress when separation from her mother occurs or is anticipated and fear of being away from her mother, she does not meet full diagnostic criteria for either disorder. Thus, a DSM-IV-TR diagnosis is not appropriate in this case. Jamie's psychological symptoms are viewed as responses to a series of divorce-related stressors that have affected multiple arenas of her life.

Researchers have repeatedly found that parental divorce can have serious negative effects on the mental health of children and adolescents and on their accomplishment of age-appropriate developmental tasks. Across age and gender, children in divorced families have more conduct, internalizing, social, and academic problems than those in nondivorced families (see Amato 2000; Amato and Keith 1991). Adolescents in divorced families are more likely than those in nondivorced families to report elevated levels of drug and alcohol use (e.g., Furstenberg and Teitler 1994; Hoffmann and Johnson 1998) and are two to three times more likely than their counterparts in nondivorced families to experience clinically significant levels of mental health problems, receive mental health services (e.g., Hetherington et al. 1992), drop out of school (McLanahan 1999), leave home early, cohabitate, and experience premarital childbearing (Goldscheider and Goldscheider 1998; Hetherington 1999).

From the perspective of the transitional-events model (e.g., Felner et al. 1983; Kurdek 1981; Sandler et al. 1988), children's postdivorce adjustment is viewed as a consequence of the multiple stressful environmental events that occur to them and their family during this transition and the interpersonal and intrapersonal protective resources available to them. Jamie's parents' divorce led to multiple changes that included moving to another house, changing schools, losing contact with friends, and spending less time with her father and possibly her paternal aunts, uncles, and grandparents. This transition also led to additional demands on her mother, including dealing with financial difficulties, developing relationships with new partners, and handling new household and work responsibilities. Dealing with these stressors and the loss of her relationship with her ex-spouse has taxed the mother's emotional and tangible resources, which has affected her relationships with her children. Research has consistently demonstrated that the quality of parenting following a divorce and the ongoing interparental conflict are two of the most significant factors affecting the mental health of children following a divorce (Amato and Keith 1991; Hetherington et al. 1992). Although neither Jamie nor her mother reports a high level of continuing conflict between Jamie's parents, evidence indicates that the quality of parenting provided by Jamie's mother decreased significantly following the divorce. Her mother has spent less time with the children, has been less emotionally available to them, and seems disorganized and inconsistent in her approach to setting and enforcing household rules.

Jamie's score on the Children's Depression Inventory (CDI; Kovacs 1992) was in the clinical range. Her mother's ratings on the Child Behavior Checklist (CBCL; Achenbach 1991) were in the clinical range on the Internalizing Behavior Problems subscale and in the nonclinical range on the Externalizing subscale. Measures assessing family functioning indicated a high number of divorce-related stressors on the Divorce Events Schedule for Children (Sandler et al. 1988) and low levels of parental warmth and high inconsistent discipline on the Child Report of Parental Behavior Inventory (Schaefer 1965). Jamie's report on the Children's Perception of Interparental Conflict Scale (Grych et al. 1992) was not elevated. Jamie reported that she sees her father about once a week and that the level of contact has been stable for the last year.

DSM-IV-TR DIAGNOSIS

Axis I   V71.09 No diagnosis or condition
           V61.20 Parent-child relational problem
Axis II   No diagnosis
Axis III   None
Axis IV   Parental divorce
Axis V   Global Assessment of Functioning=62 (current)

TREATMENT RECOMMENDATIONS

I recommend that Jamie's mother participate in an empirically validated, manualized intervention to improve parenting practices and to change other interpersonal factors that affect children's postdivorce adjustment and over which residential parents have some influence (e.g., interparental conflict, nonresidential parent visitation). The orientation of New Beginnings is cognitive-behavioral (Wolchik et al. 2000). The didactic material is presented in a conversational, interactive style, and the teaching of the skills is experiential, with exercises and role-play aimed at learning the skills accurately and applying them in interactions with one's children and ex-spouse. Each session consists of a short didactic presentation, skills demonstration and practice, home-practice assignments for using the skills with the children, and home-practice review. Parents are expected to practice the program skills with all the children who live with them.

The skills in the program build on each other. The first half of the program teaches skills to enhance the quality of the mother-child relationship and to reverse the negative cycle of interaction between mothers and children that frequently accompanies divorce. Improving mother-child communication early in the program helps reduce children's misbehaviors so that there is less need to address misbehaviors in later sessions. The first three sessions (Family Fun Time, One-on-One Time, and Catch 'em Being Good) teach relationship-building skills that mothers are to do during and after completing the program. This section is followed by a three-session segment on listening skills. The program also has three sessions that focus on effective discipline skills, including setting and communicating clear rules and use of appropriate positive and negative consequences to enforce rules. Mothers practice these skills by developing and using a plan to change one misbehavior. In addition to the strong focus on parenting, the program also includes a session to reduce children's exposure to interparental conflict and to encourage children's access to both parents after divorce. The final session includes a review of the program skills and discussion of ways to maintain the program skills.

Randomized experimental trials of this program, as presented in a group format, have shown positive short-term and long-term effects (Wolchik et al. 1993, 2000, 2002). For example, 6 years after participation, positive program effects occurred for a wide range of youth outcomes, including reductions in 1) the odds of having a diagnosis of mental disorder in the last year (odds ratio= 2.70); 2) the number of sexual partners; 3) the symptoms of mental disorder; and 4) the frequency of alcohol, marijuana, and other drug use (Wolchik et al. 2002, 2007). In addition, the program has been shown to improve multiple aspects of children's healthy functioning, including self-esteem and academic performance. Research has also shown that positive changes in parenting accounted for program-related improvements in children's mental health problems posttest and at long-term follow-up (Tein et al. 2004; Zhou et al. 2008). Evidence also indicates that children who were functioning more poorly at program entry and who experienced more stressful divorces received greater benefits from the program than those with lower levels of problems at program entry (Dawson-McClure et al. 2003; Hipke et al. 2002; Wolchik et al. 1993, 2000, 2002, 2007).

Before the first session, Jamie and her mother would have completed the CDI and CBCL, respectively. After the final session, Jamie and her mother would be interviewed to assess whether meaningful changes occurred in Jamie's moodiness and clinginess. In addition to participating in the semistructured interview, Jamie and her mother would again complete the CDI and CBCL, respectively, to assess reduction in Jamie's mental health problems. If clinically significant changes did not occur, the family would be referred to a therapist with expertise in implementing CBT with children and their parents. CBT has been shown to be an effective treatment for children with depressive and separation anxiety symptoms (Eisen and Schaefer 2005; Masi et al. 2001; Stark et al. 1987).

EDITORS' NOTE

From this case presentation, a clinician cannot determine whether Jamie does or does not meet full criteria for major depressive disorder. Life stressors in and of themselves cannot be used to rule out whether the diagnosis of depression should be made. One clinician might make the diagnosis of MDD; another might refer to depression NOS; and a third might favor a V-code diagnosis, such as adjustment disorder with depressed mood. Cognitive-behavioral methods (either a full-blown CBT, or CBT as part of a preventive intervention) may be similarly effective regardless of whether they are used in a postdivorce context to help children with depressive symptoms that do not meet full DSM-IV-TR criteria, or used with children and youth with depressive symptoms that do meet full criteria. Although no evidence is available from controlled clinical trials to support the use of medication treatments such as SSRIs for subthreshold MDD or depression NOS, should Jamie fail to respond to CBT and show significant or increasing impairment, such medication alternatives might be considered.

REFERENCES

Achenbach TM: Manual for the Child Behavioral Checklist/4–18 and 1991 Profile. Burlington, VT, University of Vermont, Department of Psychiatry, 1991

Amato PR: The consequences of divorce for adults and children. J Marriage Fam 62:1269–1287, 2000

Amato PR, Keith B: Parental divorce and the well-being of children: a meta-analysis. Psychol Bull 110:26–46, 1991

Birmaher B, Axelson DA, Monk K, et al: Fluoxetine for the treatment of childhood anxiety disorders. J Am Acad Child Adolesc Psychiatry 42:415–423, 2003

Birmaher B, Brent D; AACAP Work Group on Quality Issues, et al: Practice parameter for the assessment and treatment of children and adolescents with depressive disorders. J Am Acad Child Adolesc Psychiatry 46:1503–1526, 2007

Bridge JA, Iyengar S, Salary CB, et al: Clinical response and risk for reported suicidal ideation and suicide attempts in pediatric antidepressant treatment: a meta-analysis of randomized controlled trials. JAMA 297:1683–1696, 2007

Dawson-McClure SR, Sandler IN, Wolchik SA: Divorce, adolescents, in The Encyclopedia of Primary Prevention and Health Promotion. Edited by Gullotta TP, Bloom M. New York, Kluwer Academic/Plenum Publishers, 2003, pp 441–448

Eisen A, Schaefer C: Separation Anxiety in Children and Adolescents: An Individualized Approach to Assessment and Treatment. New York, Guilford, 2005

Felner RD, Farber SS, Primavera J: Transitions and Stressful Life Events: A Model for Primary Prevention. New York, Pergamon Press, 1983

Freud A: Adolescence. Psychoanal Study Child 13:255–278, 1958

Furstenberg FF, Teitler JO: Reconsidering the effects of marital disruption: what happens to children of divorce in early adulthood? J Fam Issues 15:173–190, 1994

Goldscheider FK, Goldscheider C: The effects of childhood family structure on leaving and returning home. J Marriage Fam 60:745–756, 1998

Grych JH, Seid M, Fincham FD: Assessing marital conflict from the child's perspective: the Children's Perception of Interparental Conflict Scale. Child Dev 63:558–572, 1992

Hammad TA, Laughren T, Racoosin J: Suicidality in pediatric patients treated with antidepressant drugs. Arch Gen Psychiatry 63:332–339, 2006

Hetherington EM: Social capital and the development of youth from nondivorced, divorced, and remarried families, in Relationships as Developmental Contexts, Vol 30: The Minnesota Symposia on Child Psychology. Edited by Laursen B, Collins WA. Mahwah, NJ, Erlbaum, 1999, pp 177–209

Hetherington EM, Clingempeel WG, Anderson ER, et al: Coping with marital transitions: a family systems perspective. Monogr Soc Res Child Dev 57:2–3, 1992

Hipke KN, Wolchik SA, Sandler IN, et al: Predictors of children's intervention-induced resilience in a parenting program for divorced mothers. Fam Relat 51:121–129, 2002

Hoffmann JP, Johnson RA: A national portrait of family structure and adolescent drug use. J Marriage Fam 60:633–645, 1998

Huurre T, Junkkari H, Aro H: Long-term psychosocial effects of parental divorce: a follow-up study from adolescence to adulthood. Eur Arch Psychiatry Clin Neurosci 256:256–263, 2006

Kelly JB: Children's adjustment in conflicted marriage and divorce: a decade review of research. J Am Acad Child Adolesc Psychiatry 39:963–973, 2000

Kestenbaum CJ: The creative process in child psychotherapy. Am J Psychother 39:479–489, 1985

Kestenbaum CJ: Memory, narrative, and the search for identity in psychoanalytic psychotherapy: a second chance. J Am Acad Psychoanal Dyn Psychiatry 31:647–661, 2003

King RA: Practice parameters for the psychiatric assessment of children and adolescents. American Academy of Child and Adolescent Psychiatry. J Am Acad Child Adolesc Psychiatry 36 (suppl 10):4–20, 1997

Kovacs M: Children's Depression Inventory: CDI Manual. North Tonawanda, NY, Multi-Health Systems, 1992

Kurdek LA: An integrative perspective on children's divorce adjustment. Am Psychol 36:856–866, 1981

Masi G, Mucci M, Millepiedi S: Separation anxiety disorder in children and adolescents: epidemiology, diagnosis, and management. CNS Drugs 15:93–104, 2001

McLanahan S: Father absence and the welfare of children, in Coping With Divorce, Single Parenting, and Remarriage. Edited by Hetherington EM. Mahwah, NJ, Erlbaum, 1999, pp 117–144

National Institute for Clinical Excellence: Depression in Children and Young People: Identification and Management in Primary, Community and Secondary Care (National Clinical Practice Guideline, No. 28). London, National Institute for Clinical Excellence, 2005

Olfson M, Marcus SC, Druss B, et al: Parental depression, child mental health problems, and health care utilization. Med Care 41:702–705, 2003

Research Unit on Pediatric Psychopharmacology Anxiety Study Group: Fluvoxamine for the treatment of anxiety disorders in children and adolescents. N Engl J Med 344:1279–1285, 2001

Sandler IN, Wolchik SA, Braver SL: The stressors of children's post divorce environments, in Children of Divorce: Empirical Perspectives on Adjustment. Edited by Wolchik SA, Karoly P. New York, Gardner Press, 1988, pp 111–143

Schaefer ES: Children's reports of parental behavior: an inventory. Child Dev 36:413–424, 1965

Stark KD, Reynolds WM, Kaslow NJ: A comparison of the relative efficacy of self-control therapy and a behavioral problem-solving therapy for depression in children. J Abnorm Child Psychol 15:91–113, 1987

Tein J-Y, Sandler IN, MacKinnon DP, et al: How did it work? Who did it work for? Mediation and mediated moderation of a preventive intervention for children of divorce. J Consult Clin Psychol 72:617–624, 2004

Treatment for Adolescents with Depression Study Team: Fluoxetine, cognitive-behavioral therapy, and their combination for adolescents with depression: Treatment for Adolescents with Depression Study (TADS). JAMA 292:807–820, 2004

Weissman MM: Juvenile-onset major depression includes childhood- and adolescent-onset depression and may be heterogeneous. Arch Gen Psychiatry 59:223–224, 2002

Wolchik SA, West S, Westover S, et al: The Children of Divorce Intervention Project: outcome evaluation of an empirically based parent training program. Am J Community Psychol 21:293–331, 1993

Wolchik SA, West SG, Sandler IN, et al: An experimental evaluation of theory-based mother and mother-child programs for children of divorce. J Consult Clin Psychol 68:843–856, 2000

Wolchik SA, Sandler IN, Millsap RE, et al: Six-year follow-up of a randomized, controlled trial of preventive interventions for children of divorce. JAMA 288:1874–1881, 2002

Wolchik S, Sandler IN, Weiss L, et al: New Beginnings: an empirically based intervention program for divorced mothers to promote resilience in their children, in Handbook of Parent Training: Helping Parents Prevent and Solve Problem Behaviors. Edited by Briesmeister JM, Schaefer CE. Hoboken, NJ, Wiley, 2007, pp 25–62

Zhou Q, Sandler IN, Millsap RE, et al: Mediation of six-year effects of the New Beginnings Program for children of divorce. J Consult Clin Psychol 76:579–594, 2008

■ CHAPTER 29 ■

It Should Have Been Me

Childhood Bereavement

Cynthia R. Pfeffer, M.D.

CASE PRESENTATION

IDENTIFYING INFORMATION

Ben is a 13-year-old male who lives with his father and is in eighth grade. Ben's mother died when he was 11 years old.

CHIEF COMPLAINT

Ben's father brought Ben to a child psychiatrist for treatment because of increasing concerns about his problems since his mother's death 2 years ago.

HISTORY OF PRESENT ILLNESS

One year after his mother's death, Ben and his father moved from Pittsburgh, Pennsylvania, to New York City so his father could take a job that did not require him to travel. Ben was fearful about moving and worried that he would be alone and would miss his school, friends, neighbors, and grandmother. He had problems adjusting to the move. His academic performance declined, and he was sad, felt as if part of him had died, had problems sleeping, intensely longed for his mother, and felt empty, lonely, and hopeless about the future. He was frequently truant from school because he preferred to stay with teenagers who refused to go

Cynthia R. Pfeffer, M.D., is Professor of Psychiatry and Director of the Childhood Bereavement Program at Weill Cornell Medical College/New York Presbyterian Hospital in White Plains, New York (for complete biographical information, see "About the Contributors," p. 613).

to school. With these peers, Ben drank alcohol and smoked marijuana, which enabled him to avoid his painful feelings about his mother's death and subsequent events of his life. He knew that substance abuse was not healthy, but he could not overcome his intense prolonged loneliness, anxiety, and sadness. Often, he wanted to die in hopes that he could be with his mother.

Past Psychiatric History

Ben was 11 years old when his mother suddenly died of complications from breast cancer. Although she had been ill for 3 years, her death was unexpected, caused by a brain hemorrhage during a course of chemotherapy to treat metastasis to the brain and lungs that developed 6 months before she died. Ben's father had been optimistic that the chemotherapy would stop the spread of cancer and that his wife would live for many years. Because Ben's father had great difficulty telling Ben that his mother's cancer had worsened, he told Ben that his mother was being treated with medications to prevent recurrence of her past cancer.

Ben visited his mother in the hospital as often as possible, but he did not see her during the week of her death because he had cold symptoms and was told that he could spread his infection to his mother. Ben's father, summoned to the hospital when his wife became comatose, did not know how to tell Ben that his mother had become fatally ill. The doctors advised that Ben come to the hospital to be with his mother and talk about her deteriorating state. Before his father could bring Ben to the hospital, his mother died. Ben was at school when his mother died.

Immediately after her death, Ben's father called the school principal to tell him what happened and to request help in telling Ben that his mother had died. That day, the school psychologist and principal sympathetically helped Ben's father in this difficult endeavor. Ben reacted intensely with crying, agitation, and repeated statements that if he had been at the hospital with her, his mother would have gotten better. His father explained that the doctors had told him that she was improving, but then she began to bleed in her brain; this caused her unexpected death. Ben repeatedly asked his father, "Who will take care of me if something happens to you? You are away a lot." His father patiently told Ben about how much he loved Ben and said that he would be with him, always.

Ben, an only child, was very close to his mother. His father was often away because of travel assignments associated with his work. During his father's absences, his maternal grandmother, who lived nearby, helped his mother care for Ben. When his mother became ill, Ben became noticeably anxious and was reluctant to go to school. The school psychologist helped him to overcome some of his fears that his mother would die.

Ben's fears of parental death began when he was 5 years old, shortly after his father was almost killed in a car accident on his way to work. Ben's father was hospitalized for 2 days for diagnostic tests because he had suffered a concussion with loss of consciousness as a result of the car accident. Four months after his father's car accident, Ben exhibited agitation, tearfulness, problems sleeping, and intense clinging to his mother. He was treated with psychotherapy by a child psychiatrist for several months to decrease his anxiety symptoms.

SUBSTANCE ABUSE HISTORY

After moving to New York City, Ben became increasingly truant from school and abused marijuana and alcohol with other teenagers who stayed away from school.

MEDICAL HISTORY

Ben had been a healthy child with normal developmental milestones as an infant and toddler. He had never been hospitalized and did not suffer from chronic illness or allergies.

DEVELOPMENTAL HISTORY

Ben had long-standing fears of separation from his parents. As a school-age child, he would choose to be with his parents rather than with schoolmates. He was fearful that something bad would happen to his parents and did not like being away from them.

SOCIAL HISTORY

One year after his mother's death, Ben and his father moved from Pittsburgh, Pennsylvania, to New York City because his father started a job that did not require him to travel.

FAMILY HISTORY

Ben's mother was the only person in her family to have had cancer, and no person in his father's family had had cancer. No maternal or paternal first- or second-degree relatives were known to have had major psychiatric disorders, including anxiety, mood, substance abuse, and psychotic disorders.

MENTAL STATUS EXAMINATION

Ben is a handsome young adolescent who showed signs of pubertal development. He responded logically to the psychiatrist's questions and spoke about his increasingly intense dysphoria and constant thoughts of his deceased mother. He appeared sad, did not consistently look at the psychiatrist, and fidgeted with his fingers. Ben acknowledged that he was anxious and fearful that if his father died, he would be left alone in the world. He thought that it would be better for him if he were dead, and he looked forward to reuniting with his mother. He denied psychotic symptoms of auditory, visual, or tactile hallucinations or delusions. He wanted to feel better and described his drug experiences as helpful in decreasing his emotional pain.

COMMENTARIES

Psychotherapeutic Perspective

Elizabeth B. Weller, M.D.
Ronald A. Weller, M.D.
Thomas A. Dixon, B.S.

DIAGNOSTIC FORMULATION

Many questions remain to be asked regarding Ben's prior history; the answers would help greatly in providing an accurate diagnosis. First, the clinician needs to know if Ben is performing at a developmentally appropriate grade level. Second, the clinician should explore the reason(s) for Ben's truancy (e.g., loss of interest, lack of concentration). Third, although no family history of psychiatric illness is reported, it should be examined in greater detail, because Ben's anxiety and depressive symptoms may be familial.

A number of stressful life events have occurred during Ben's life. When Ben was age 5, his father was in a near-fatal car accident. At this point, Ben almost lost his role model. Four months after the accident, he exhibited anxiety and depressive symptoms (tearfulness, clinginess, agitation, and problems sleeping). When he was age 8, Ben's mother became ill. Ben was very close to his mother because his father traveled often for his job. Ben was visibly anxious at this time and unwilling to go to school. His maternal grandmother cared for him when his father

Elizabeth B. Weller, M.D., is Professor of Psychiatry and Pediatrics at the University of Pennsylvania in Philadelphia, Pennsylvania.

Ronald A. Weller, M.D., is on the faculty of the Departments of Psychiatry and of Neuroscience at the University of Pennsylvania in Philadelphia, Pennsylvania.

Thomas A. Dixon, B.S., is Research Assistant in the Mood and Anxiety Disorders Center at Children's Hospital of Philadelphia in Philadelphia, Pennsylvania.

For complete biographical information, see "About the Contributors," p. 613.

was away on business. Six months before her death, Ben's mother began a course of chemotherapy to treat metastasis to the lungs and brain. However, Ben did not know that this was the reason for his mother's treatment (he was told that she was receiving preventive treatment). Ben's mother died unexpectedly when he was age 11. A year later, Ben moved from Pittsburgh to New York City, away from his maternal grandmother; his prior school, friends, and social environment; and the presumed burial site of his mother.

MAJOR DEPRESSIVE DISORDER

The main stressor (precipitating event) of Ben's present difficulties seems to be his recent move away from his familiar environment and support structure. Given his past history of traumatizing experiences and losses of support structures (potential death of father, mother's prolonged illness, and death of mother), and his long-standing concerns of being separated from his parents, he was sensitized to be more prone to depressive and anxiety symptoms. The clinician should consider whether Ben meets DSM-IV-TR criteria for major depressive disorder.

Ben is described as being sad for more than 2 weeks, actually close to a full year. He suffers feelings of worthlessness, has problems with sleeping, and is preoccupied with thoughts of death and suicide (Criterion A). The case presentation does not indicate if Ben has a loss of energy or diminished interest in activities, perhaps demonstrated by his not going to school, or if he has indecisiveness. A more detailed interview and the use of the Children's Depression Rating Scale—Revised (Poznanski et al. 1984) may help to ascertain which of these symptoms he has. He has no history of manic symptoms or mixed episodes (Criterion B) or psychotic symptoms. Ben's symptoms are causing him significant impairment academically and socially (Criterion C). His symptoms do not appear to be the result of substance use or a general medical condition (Criterion D), although his use of alcohol to heal his psychic pain is of concern because of depressogenic effects of alcohol on the central nervous system. Lastly, Ben's symptoms are not better accounted for by bereavement because his present illness far exceeds the time frame for bereavement, and he is preoccupied with thoughts of worthlessness and suicide (Criterion E).

COMPLICATED GRIEF

Immediately after his mother's unanticipated death, Ben had intense reactions when his father, the school psychologist, and the principal told him. He reacted with crying, agitation, and statements that he could have prevented the death had he been at the hospital. Ben was very worried that something might happen to his father and that no one would be present to take care of him if something did happen. Ben's father responded very optimistically by telling

Ben that he would always be there for him. During his mother's treatment, Ben's father had told Ben what Ben might have hoped to hear, namely that his mother's condition was not worsening and that she was receiving treatment to prevent the recurrence of her past cancer. Ben was unaware of his mother's worsening condition, and her sudden death made it impossible for Ben to talk with his mother before she died.

It has been 2 years since his mother's death, and Ben has been showing depressive symptoms. Of the several traumatic experiences that Ben has had, his mother's death is a necessary focus of clinical care. The possibility that bereavement is a risk factor for psychopathology has been considered for many years (Weller et al. 2002). In a study by Cerel et al. (2006), bereaved children presented with symptoms of depression that were not as severe as those of depressed children but were clinically significant when compared to those of controls. Children presenting with complicated grief are the "walking wounded," and Ben's mother's death must be addressed in his treatment.

Children who come to treatment after the death of a loved one are at increased risk for psychiatric disorders. Although much debate has occurred over what is likely to be observed in children with complex bereavement, the most likely disorders are major depressive disorder, attention-deficit disorders, disruptive behavior disorders, eating disorders, anxiety disorders, and substance-related disorders (American Psychiatric Association 2000).

ALCOHOL AND MARIJUANA ABUSE

Ben's intake of alcohol and marijuana is consistent with a diagnosis of abuse of both substances. For over a 12-month period, he has become more frequently truant from school because of the increased amount of time he has spent acquiring and using these substances with other teenagers who were not in school (Criterion A). To date, his abuse of alcohol and marijuana does not meet substance dependence criteria for either substance (Criterion B). His substance abuse should be treated promptly because it may represent a desire to self-medicate for feelings of sadness, loneliness, and anxiety. The continued abuse of these substances may cause Ben to progress to a substance dependence disorder.

SEPARATION ANXIETY

Ben had symptoms of separation anxiety disorder as a child; the onset of symptoms closely followed his father's near-fatal car accident. He became overly preoccupied with fear of separation from his parents, began to prefer the company of his parents over his peers, was overly concerned that something bad would happen to them, and strongly resisted being away from them (Criterion A). These symptoms were present for at least 4 months after his father's accident (Criterion B) and caused Ben significant distress (Criterion D) but were not simultaneous with other psychotic or anxiety disorders (Criterion E). Ben's fears and concerns may have been exacerbated by his mother's illness that began when Ben was age 8. Throughout his childhood he exhibited anxiety symptoms. He was treated with psychotherapy for a period of a few months to reduce his anxiety symptoms. The case presentation does not thoroughly cover the family's history of psychiatric disorders. A detailed psychiatric history looking into anxiety, depression, and substance abuse of three generations from both his mother's and father's families is necessary.

Ben is likely to be at increased risk of psychiatric disorders because he has several potential risk factors. These include 1) a preexisting separation anxiety disorder; 2) the unexpected sudden death of his mother, to whom he was very close, after a debilitating disease; 3) and male gender (Dowdney 2000). Other stressors include a history of his not having a close relationship with his father (due to his father's frequent travels to be the provider for the family) and a high level of discomfort with his move to a new home and school environment, leaving behind his maternal grandmother who was a caretaker for him, a school that was supportive to him, and his peers with whom he had grown up.

DIAGNOSTIC INSTRUMENTS

The Children's Depression Rating Scale—Revised (Poznanski et al. 1984) could be used to assess the severity of Ben's current depressive symptoms. This instrument has high interrater reliability and test-retest validity. The Hamilton Rating Scale for Depression, which is used to measure depressive symptomatology in adults (Hamilton 1967), could be used to determine whether Ben's father should also be a focus of treatment. The father should be assessed for clinical depression due to multiple stressors in his life, including a near-death experience in a car accident, his wife's 3-year battle with cancer and unanticipated sudden death, moving to a new job and a new city, and having to be the primary caretaker of his teenage son without supportive extended family immediately available.

DSM-IV-TR DIAGNOSIS

Axis I   V62.82 Bereavement

296.33 Major depressive disorder, recurrent, moderate, without psychotic features

Rule out dysthymic disorder

305.00 Alcohol abuse

305.20 Cannabis abuse

309.21 Separation anxiety disorder, in partial remission, early onset

Axis II   No diagnosis

Axis III   None

Axis IV   Recent move

          Death of mother

Axis V   Global Assessment of Functioning=41–50 (current)

TREATMENT RECOMMENDATIONS

INITIAL TREATMENT PLAN

Ben is a good candidate for supportive directive therapy followed by cognitive-behavioral therapy (CBT). He needs help to stop his alcohol and marijuana abuse. Involving the school with his treatment is also essential to help him acclimate to the new school and new friends. Furthermore, his father may need treatment himself, given the importance of his support for Ben and his avoidant tendencies in discussing potentially hurtful issues with Ben. The father also needs help with parenting, because the child's primary caretaker had been the mother.

A therapeutic approach that is both supportive and directive is important to motivate Ben's involvement with treatment. Because Ben's depression is at least of moderate severity, initiating fluoxetine treatment with CBT should be considered (Treatment for Adolescents with Depression Study [TADS] Team 2004).

Ben should have a complete physical examination by his pediatrician, with laboratory tests to rule out medical conditions that mimic depression. Family therapy may also be needed. The father may be underreporting the son's depressive symptoms because he simply is not aware of them or because he himself is depressed and overwhelmed with his move, his new job, and serving as primary caretaker of his son.

RATIONALE FOR CHOICE

CBT is likely to help Ben with depressive or anxiety symptoms. An extensive literature exists on the treatment of anxiety symptoms in children with CBT (for a review, see Roblek and Piacentini 2005). Because his mother has died, he must learn how to cope without her daily presence. Participation in a group for bereaved teenagers might be very helpful.

Bibliotherapy has been shown to be effective in treating mild to moderate depression in adolescents. Throughout the course of treatment, bibliotherapy, using stories with characters and experiences with which Ben can relate, may be a helpful source of information and motivation for Ben. Bibliotherapy requires the therapist to work together with Ben to help frame Ben's interpretation and exploration of available material (Ackerson et al. 1998).

CBT works well alone or when concordantly administered with fluoxetine in treating major depressive disorder (TADS Team 2004). It minimizes the cognitive aspects of depressive symptoms and the self-medicating pattern of substance abuse. Psychoeducation may also help Ben to overcome his grief. With the change in his school situation, he may be able to develop and maintain a positive, supportive social network that increases his sense of self-worth.

DESCRIPTION OF TREATMENT

CBT would include 15 one-hour sessions, over a period of 12 weeks (TADS Team 2004), and would focus on psychoeducation for depression and anxiety. In Ben's case, therapy modules should also be tailored to how he understands death, how he understands his depression, how he can monitor his mood, and how to incorporate pleasant activities into his life. Treatment would include sessions with Ben alone, with Ben and his father, and with the father alone (to provide the father with psychoeducation about depression, anxiety, and bereavement).

Although medication is discussed more extensively in the next commentary, concordantly administered fluoxetine might be considered, beginning at a dosage of 10 mg/day and increasing the dosage to 20 mg/day at week 1 and, if necessary, up to 40 mg/day thereafter (for further information, see TADS Team 2004).

OTHER TREATMENTS

If the initial treatment is not successful, other forms of psychotherapy may be useful. Multidimensional family therapy, as described by Hogue et al. (2006), includes individual, adolescent-focused treatment; parent treatment; and family treatment. Because this treatment has been shown to be effective only when used for an extensive period of time, the clinician may have more difficulty convincing the family that the treatment will be effective. Additional CBT sessions may also be considered. Regardless, a strong therapeutic alliance between Ben and his therapist is essential if the therapy is to be maximally effective.

Psychopharmacologic Perspective

Karen Dineen Wagner, M.D., Ph.D.

DIAGNOSTIC FORMULATION

Ben is a 13-year-old boy whose mother died 2 years previously. Although his mother had been ill with cancer, her death was unexpected for Ben. His initial reaction to learning of her death was age appropriate: crying, agitation, and believing he might have been able to help his mother if he had been in the hospital with her. His concern about who would take care of him if something happened to his father was also developmentally appropriate. The case history does not indicate how Ben coped with the death of his mother in the ensuing year. One year after his mother's death, Ben moved with his father out of state and experienced the loss of his friends, neighbors, and grandmother. In that ensuing year, he developed symptoms of depression, including sadness, sleeping problems, hopelessness, and emptiness. Other problems included truancy, decline in academic performance, and alcohol and marijuana use. His depression worsened during the course of the year to the point that he currently has constant thoughts about his deceased mother and a desire to reunite with her. Ben's depression is also exacerbated by his anxiety; he fears being left alone if his father should die. Fear of separation from his parents has been a long-standing problem for Ben. Although Ben's initial reaction to the death of his mother was a normal grief reaction, the development of significant depressive symptoms and continued intense longing for his mother with overall functional impairment is beyond the realm of a normal grief reaction.

Ben exhibits symptoms of major depression, including depressed mood, sleep difficulties, hopelessness, emptiness (which may reflect diminished interest or pleasure in activities), and suicidal ideation. Other symptoms such as low energy, weight loss, and psychomotor agitation/retardation were not mentioned in the vignette but may be present. To rule out a diagnosis of bipolar disorder, the clinician should also inquire whether Ben has had manic or hypomanic symptoms, which could be related to his alcohol and marijuana use. Al-

Karen Dineen Wagner, M.D., Ph.D., is Marie B. Gale Professor and Vice Chair of the Department of Psychiatry and Behavioral Sciences, and Director of the Division of Child and Adolescent Psychiatry at the University of Texas Medical Branch in Galveston, Texas (for complete biographical information, see "About the Contributors," p. 613).

though he exhibits anxiety, he does not appear to have sufficient symptoms to specify a current anxiety disorder. Administration of the Children's Depression Rating Scale—Revised (Poznanski et al. 1984, 1985) would be helpful to further elucidate the extent and severity of his depressive symptoms.

DSM-IV-TR DIAGNOSIS

Axis I   296.22 Major depressive disorder, single episode, moderate

305.00 Alcohol abuse

305.20 Cannabis abuse

History of separation anxiety disorder

Axis II   None

Axis III None

Axis IV   Death of mother

Academic problems

Problems with peer group

Axis V   Global Assessment of Functioning=50

TREATMENT RECOMMENDATIONS

The initial treatment plan should include an assessment of Ben's father to determine whether he has adequately coped with the loss of his wife so that he can deal effectively with Ben's grief. Ben would benefit from individual psychotherapy, as well as a support group for children who have lost a parent. The extent of his alcohol and substance abuse requires further assessment, and he may need substance abuse counseling. Because he has been frequently truant from school and his grades have declined, he will require academic remediation. Importantly, medication treatment is warranted given the severity of Ben's depressive symptoms, his hopelessness about the future, and his suicidality related to a desire to join his dead mother. Sood et al. (2006) recommended medication if a bereaved child develops symptoms of depression, has a significant deterioration in functioning, or develops suicidal thoughts.

Selective serotonin reuptake inhibitors (SSRIs) have the most evidence of efficacy in the treatment of depressed adolescents (Emslie et al. 2002; TADS Team 2004; Wagner et al. 2003, 2004) and would be the treatment of choice. If Ben's father prefers a medication approved by the U.S. Food and Drug Administration (FDA), the SSRI fluoxetine would be selected because it is the only medication to have FDA approval for treatment of major depression in this age group. The FDA warning about possible increased suicidality with antidepressant use in children and adolescents and the need for careful monitoring of suicidality (FDA News 2004) should be discussed with Ben and his father. The clinician may wish to inform them that a recent analysis of antidepressant trials in youth showed that the benefits for treatment of depression far outweigh potential risks of suicidal thinking or attempts (Bridge et al. 2007). Commonly occurring side effects of fluoxetine, such as headache, nausea, abdominal pain, insomnia, and increased sweating, should be discussed prior to treatment and monitored during the course of treatment. Suicidality should be assessed at every visit.

Fluoxetine treatment should be initiated at a low dosage of 10 mg/day and the dosage increased gradually based on clinical response up to 40 mg/day over the course of 8–10 weeks. The dose may need to be decreased if side effects emerge. If Ben shows no improvement in his condition when taking fluoxetine at a dosage of 40 mg/day, then treatment with fluoxetine should be discontinued. Recent guidelines recommend the use of an alternative SSRI when a patient fails to respond to one SSRI (Hughes et al. 2007). Alternative treatment with citalopram, sertraline, escitalopram, or paroxetine would be appropriate. If Ben has a partial response to alternative SSRI treatment, then augmentation with lithium, bupropion, or mirtazapine could be considered. If no improvement is seen after a trial with this alternative SSRI, then treatment with a different class of antidepressant, such as venlafaxine, bupropion, mirtazapine, or duloxetine, should be initiated. If Ben fails to respond to a different class of antidepressant, then reassessment of diagnosis, family situation, comorbid disorders, and medication adherence should be done.

When an effective medication is identified, it should be continued for at least 6–12 months after symptom remission at the full therapeutic dose that was used to achieve remission (Emslie et al. 2004).

Integrative Perspective

Cynthia R. Pfeffer, M.D.

DIAGNOSTIC FORMULATION

The psychiatrist determined that Ben suffered from major depression and complicated bereavement. Children who experience death of a parent experience severe stress associated with psychosocial and neurobiological morbidities that may increase risk for psychopathology and medical illness in the future (Pfeffer et al. 2007). Earlier vulnerabilities prior to death of a parent, such as Ben's separation fears, increase the risk for morbid outcomes of bereaved children. In the present example, Ben experienced the traumatic stress of the near death of his father from a motor vehicle accident, an event that intensified Ben's propensity to anxiety. As a result, Ben was sensitized to worrying about loss of his parents, an issue that recurred after his mother died and he moved to a distant city where he had problems adjusting to the loss of former social support from his grandmother, school, and friends. The fact that his father was often absent from the home because of work obligations intensified Ben's attachment to his mother and anticipation of her death while she was ill.

Ben's bereavement, characterized by a prolonged and unremitting pattern, was complicated and included intense longings for his deceased mother, loneliness, avoidance of painful feelings, loss of trust and security, and hopelessness about the future, and these symptoms interfered with his social and academic functioning (Prigerson and Jacobs 2001). As reported in several longitudinal studies of childhood bereavement, onset of psychopathologies involving anxiety disorders, major depressive disorder, and substance abuse also frequently occurs subsequent to parent death, whether expected or unexpected (Cerel et al. 2006; Pfeffer et al. 2007). Suicidal ideation or suicide attempts are generally rare among children with uncomplicated bereavement, but they may occur as a feature of complicated bereavement (Prigerson et al. 1999).

DSM-IV-TR DIAGNOSIS

Axis I	296.22 Major depressive disorder, single episode, moderate
	300.00 Anxiety disorder not otherwise specified
	305.00 Alcohol abuse
	292.9 Cannabis-related disorder not otherwise specified
	V62.82 Bereavement
Axis II	None
Axis III	Healthy
Axis IV	Family, social, and school problems
Axis V	Global Assessment of Functioning=70

TREATMENT RECOMMENDATIONS

The psychiatrist began treating Ben with fluoxetine and psychotherapy that would focus on relieving symptoms of the mood disorder and complicated bereavement. Within 2 months of weekly treatment, Ben felt much better. He enjoyed the conversations with the psychiatrist and felt less lonely and sad. He realized that his mother would want him to finish school and plan for his future. As he internalized these ideas, he felt more enthusiastic about attending school, stopped abusing marijuana and alcohol, and began to participate in sports activities after school. His grades improved and he was enthusiastic about learning.

Ben acknowledged that his father was very important to him and that when he grew up, Ben wanted to be a successful professional and father.

Few studies have described empirically tested treatments for children with bereavement (Cohen et al. 2004; Pfeffer et al. 2002). Treatment planning must define targets for treatment, such as symptoms of complicated bereavement versus manifestations of uncomplicated bereavement. Treatment for complicated bereavement should address features of the prolonged incapacitating distress. Intervention should address children's features of shock over the death, emotional discomfort, and acceptance of the death that make up uncomplicated bereavement. A useful approach for children with uncomplicated bereavement is group intervention with developmentally matched bereaved children. This group promotes discussion of parent death and enables bereaved children to appreciate that they are not alone in experiencing loss of a parent. Provision of consistent social support is a mainstay of intervention for bereaved children.

Treatment also should target symptoms of psychiatric disorders. Combined use of effective, empirically tested psychopharmacologic strategies and psychotherapeutic treatments, such as cognitive-behavioral or interpersonal psychotherapy, can target symptoms of anxiety and depression (American Academy of Child and Adolescent Psychiatry 2001).

REFERENCES

Ackerson J, Scogin F, McKendree-Smith N, et al: Cognitive bibliotherapy for mild and moderate adolescent depressive symptomatology. J Consult Clin Psychol 66:685–690, 1998

American Academy of Child and Adolescent Psychiatry: Practice parameter for the assessment and treatment of children and adolescents with suicidal behavior. J Am Acad Child Adolesc Psychiatry 40 (suppl 7):24–51, 2001

American Psychiatric Association: Diagnostic and Statistical Manual of Mental Disorders, 4th Edition, Text Revision. Washington, DC, American Psychiatric Association, 2000

Bridge JA, Iyengar S, Salary CB, et al: Clinical response and risk for reported suicidal ideation and suicide attempts in pediatric antidepressant treatment: a meta-analysis of randomized controlled trials. JAMA 297:1683–1696, 2007

Cerel J, Fristad MA, Verducci J, et al: Childhood bereavement: psychopathology in the 2 years postparental death. J Am Acad Child Adolesc Psychiatry 45:681–690, 2006

Cohen JA, Mannarino AP, Knudsen K: Treating childhood traumatic grief: a pilot study. J Am Acad Child Adolesc Psychiatry 43:1225–1233, 2004

Dowdney L: Childhood bereavement following parental death. J Child Psychol Psychiatry 41:819–830, 2000

Emslie GJ, Heiligenstein JH, Wagner KD, et al: Fluoxetine for acute treatment of depression in children and adolescents: a placebo-controlled, randomized clinical trial. J Am Acad Child Adolesc Psychiatry 41:1205–1215, 2002

Emslie GJ, Heiligenstein JH, Hoog SL, et al: Fluoxetine treatment for prevention of relapse of depression in children and adolescents: a double-blind, placebo-controlled study. J Am Acad Child Adolesc Psychiatry 43:1397–1405, 2004

FDA News: FDA launches a multi-pronged strategy to strengthen safeguards for children treated with antidepressant medications. October 15, 2004. Available at: http://www.fda.gov/bbs/topics/news/2004/NEW01124.html. Accessed August 2, 2008.

Hamilton M: Development of a rating scale for primary depressive illness. Br J Soc Clin Psychol 6:278–296, 1967

Hogue A, Dauber S, Samuolis J, et al: Treatment techniques and outcomes in multidimensional family therapy for adolescent behavior problems. J Fam Psychol 20:535–543, 2006

Hughes CW, Emslie GJ, Crismon ML, et al; Texas Consensus Conference Panel on Medication Treatment of Childhood Major Depressive Disorder: Texas Children's Medication Algorithm Project: update from Texas Consensus Conference Panel on Medication Treatment of Childhood Major Depressive Disorder. J Am Acad Child Adolesc Psychiatry 46:667–686, 2007

Pfeffer CR, Jiang H, Kakuma T, et al: Group intervention for children bereaved by suicide of a relative. J Am Acad Child Adolesc Psychiatry 41:505–513, 2002

Pfeffer CR, Altemus M, Heo M, et al: Salivary cortisol and psychopathology in children bereaved by the September 11, 2001 terror attacks. Biol Psychiatry 61:957–965, 2007

Poznanski EO, Grossman JA, Banegas M, et al: Preliminary studies of the reliability and validity of the Children's Depression Rating Scale. J Am Acad Child Adolesc Psychiatry 23:191–197, 1984

Poznanski EO, Freeman LN, Mokros HB: Children's Depression Rating Scale—Revised. Psychopharmacol Bull 21:979–989, 1985

Prigerson HG, Jacobs SC: Caring for bereaved patients: "all the doctors just suddenly go." JAMA 286:1369–1376, 2001

Prigerson HG, Bridge J, Maciejewski PK, et al: Influence of traumatic grief on suicidal ideation among young adults. Am J Psychiatry 156:1994–1995, 1999

Roblek T, Piacentini J: Cognitive-behavior therapy for childhood anxiety disorders. Child Adolesc Psychiatr Clin N Am 14:863–876, 2005

Sood AB, Razdan A, Weller EB, et al: Children's reactions to parental and sibling death. Curr Psychiatry Rep 8:115–120, 2006

Treatment for Adolescents with Depression Study Team: Fluoxetine, cognitive-behavioral therapy and their combination for adolescents with depression: Treatment for Adolescents with Depression Study (TADS) randomized control trial. JAMA 292:807–820, 2004

Wagner KD, Ambrosini PJ, Rynn M, et al: Efficacy of sertraline in the treatment of children and adolescents with major depressive disorder. JAMA 290:1033–1041, 2003

Wagner KD, Robb AS, Findling RL, et al: A randomized, placebo-controlled trial of citalopram for the treatment of major depression in children and adolescents. Am J Psychiatry 161:1079–1083, 2004

Weller EB, Weller RA, Benton T, et al: Grief, in Child and Adolescent Psychiatry: A Comprehensive Textbook, 3rd Edition. Edited by Lewis M. Philadelphia, PA, Lippincott Williams & Wilkins, 2002, pp 470–477

■ CHAPTER 30 ■

Won't Settle Down

Disinhibited Attachment in a Toddler

Stacy S. Drury, M.D., Ph.D.
Charles H. Zeanah, M.D.

CASE PRESENTATION

IDENTIFYING INFORMATION

Tonya was 18 months old and in foster care when she first came to clinical attention. She was living with her foster parents and several other foster children. She had been removed from her parents' custody due to neglect, and she was evaluated and treated in a comprehensive intervention program for young maltreated children.

CHIEF COMPLAINT

Tonya's foster mother reported, "She'll go off with anyone."

Stacy S. Drury, M.D., Ph.D., is Assistant Professor in the Department of Psychiatry and Neurology, Section of Child and Adolescent Psychiatry, at Tulane University Medical Center in New Orleans, Louisiana.

Charles H. Zeanah, M.D., is Sellars Polchow Professor of Psychiatry and Vice Chair and Chief of Child and Adolescent Psychiatry at the Tulane University School of Medicine in New Orleans, Louisiana.

For complete biographical information, see "About the Contributors," p. 613.

History of Present Illness

After being removed from her parents' custody due to neglect, Tonya was briefly placed with relatives. However, because the relatives allowed unsupervised visits by her parents, despite being admonished by child protective services, Tonya was removed from the "kin" foster placement and placed in a regular foster home.

Within days of her placement, Tonya began calling the foster mother "Mom." The foster mother initially took this as a good sign. However, Tonya was having some difficulties in her new home. According to her foster mother, Tonya was "moody." She would be cheerful one moment but rapidly switch to showing frustration or throwing a tantrum, especially when her foster parents tried to set limits. When unfamiliar clinicians made a home visit, Tonya readily approached them and initiated a game. Additional home visits over several weeks revealed a pattern of Tonya's readily approaching and engaging strange adults in play and, when injured, turning to the unfamiliar adults rather than attempting to engage her foster mother for comfort. Even after 6 weeks in this foster placement, Tonya did not seek comfort preferentially from her foster mother, who reported that Tonya "cannot get attached to me." Her foster mother was worried that she might "put herself in harm's way." Tonya walked up to strangers without hesitation both in and out of the home. Her foster mother was worried that Tonya was not listening to her; when Tonya was in a novel situation and began to explore the environment, she did not check back with her foster mother. In addition, when Tonya was injured or startled, she did not turn to her foster mother for comfort. Multiple observations of interactions between Tonya and her foster mother, both at home and in the clinic, did not show any attempts by Tonya to engage her foster mother in play or to share any experiences or toys with her. Tonya also was unable to effectively play with peers and became emotionally dysregulated when other children came into physical contact with her.

During supervised visits with her biological parents, Tonya was noted to be either fussy or irritable by the clinicians.

Substance Abuse History

Tonya has no known history of substance exposure prenatally.

Past Medical and Psychiatric History

Tonya has no previous history of medical or psychiatric problems.

Developmental History

Tonya's biological parents reported that Tonya "did everything early." They noted that she crawled at 3 months, walked at 5 months, and walked "good" at

8 months. Both parents reported that Tonya was "a friendly person" who approached anyone, even strangers, and asked for hugs.

When Tonya was 18 months of age, a developmental assessment was conducted as part of her involvement with child protective services. Her gross motor, fine motor, problem-solving, and personal-social skills were all within the expected limits for children her age. She was noted to have speech and language delay and had an expressive vocabulary that was limited to fewer than eight words. She continued to exhibit markedly indiscriminate behavior in a variety of settings. In addition, Tonya ate rapidly and often too much. She did not exhibit any evidence of developmental delay other than language difficulties.

SOCIAL HISTORY

Tonya was born after an unplanned but wanted pregnancy by unwed parents. Both of Tonya's biological parents spent an unspecified amount of time in foster care when they were children.

FAMILY HISTORY

Although little was known about the family's history of psychological illness, psychiatric evaluation of Tonya's biological parents revealed some important findings. Tonya's biological mother had significant disturbances of mood, consistent with mood disorder not otherwise specified and schizotypal personality disorder. A diagnosis of mild mental retardation was confirmed by the mother's scores on the Wechsler Adult Intelligence Scale—Third Edition (WAIS-III; Wechsler 1997) and the Vineland Adaptive Behavior Scales, Second Edition (Sparrow et al. 2005). Psychological evaluation of Tonya's biological father did not reveal any Axis I diagnosis, but he did report symptoms of mild depression and anxiety. He demonstrated poor cognitive and reasoning abilities and declined to reveal any details about his own past history or childhood involvement with child protection, although child protective services confirmed that he had been sexually abused.

MENTAL STATUS EXAMINATION

Generally, Tonya was an engaging and normally developing young child. Initial concerning behaviors included marked indiscriminate behavior with unfamiliar adults, unwillingness to approach or check with her parents when either injured or in an unfamiliar environment, and overeating. Her mood and affect were labile, and in the presence of her biological parents, she often became fussy and irritable and was not easily comforted by them. Although she initially had an expressive language delay, her intelligence, attention span, thought process, and play content were normal and consistent with those of other children her age. She did not exhibit any indications of developmental delays, stereotypies, or repetitive behaviors.

COMMENTARIES

Psychotherapeutic Perspective

Alicia F. Lieberman, Ph.D.

DIAGNOSTIC FORMULATION

The assessment of toddlers is guided by the principle that young children's functioning is profoundly influenced by the quality of their relationships with their parents and other caregivers and by the characteristics of the situations in which they are assessed. Observation of Tonya in interaction with the biological parents, with other primary caregivers, and with the assessor offers a multifaceted view of the child's quality of attachment, range of social skills and coping mechanisms, and attainment of age-expected cognitive and motor milestones. Tonya's developmental history and exposure to traumatic stressors and other adversities, including separation from attachment figures, allow the assessor to arrive at a differential diagnosis involving the etiology of the child's problems. Tonya's presenting problem, although a useful barometer of functioning, should not be used as the exclusive organizing focus of the assessment because the reporting adults' preconceptions and subjective experience of the child may color their report of her behavior. The parents' and caregivers' behavior toward Tonya should be carefully evaluated as part of the assessment, because young children can be very quick to adapt their behavior to match the perceived expectations from caregivers. The absence of preferential responses to the primary caregiver may reflect Tonya's experience-based expectation that the caregiver will not be responsive to her signals of need.

Tonya's presenting problem of indiscriminate sociability toward strangers is consistent with a DSM-IV-TR diagnosis of reactive attachment disorder (RAD) of infancy or early childhood, disinhibited type. She displays the key criterion for this diagnosis, namely, a pattern of indiscriminate sociability and lack of

Alicia F. Lieberman, Ph.D., is Irving B. Harris Endowed Chair of Infant Mental Health, Professor in Psychiatry, and Vice Chair for Academic Affairs at the University of California, San Francisco; Director of the Child Trauma Research Project at San Francisco General Hospital; Director of the Early Trauma Treatment Network; and President (2008) of the Board of Zero to Three: The National Center for Infants, Toddlers and Families (for complete biographical information, see "About the Contributors," p. 613).

selectivity in responding to adults. The diagnosis is supported by the criterion that she was subjected to pathogenic care, as evidenced by at least four concrete indicators: neglect by her biological parents; separation from her biological parents; separation from the relatives with whom she was placed after the first removal; and possible marginal care by her foster mother, who showed negative attributions to the child by stating, "She cannot get attached to me," in spite of the fact that the child started calling her "Mom" within days of her placement. Indeed, the foster mother may be creating a self-fulfilling prophecy by not responding to the child's signals of need. For example, the report does not indicate that the foster mother initiated care for the child when Tonya was injured or startled; instead, she seemed to wait for the child to initiate contact with her. This might be an unrealistic expectation from a toddler who was separated twice from her primary caregivers and who, as a result, has endured the disruption of emotional bonds in addition to neglect.

DIFFERENTIAL DIAGNOSIS

The diagnosis of mental retardation can be ruled out because of Tonya's overall age-appropriate developmental performance in gross motor, fine motor, problem-solving, and personal-social skills. She does not meet criteria for another frequent differential diagnosis, autistic disorder or pervasive developmental disorder. Although she is described as being unable to play effectively with peers and becoming dysregulated when other children come into physical contact with her, the diagnosis of attention-deficit/hyperactivity disorder can be ruled out because these behaviors are more parsimoniously explained as a response to repeated separation and neglect.

CO-OCCURRING DIAGNOSES

The Diagnostic Classification of Mental Health and Developmental Disorders of Infancy and Early Childhood—Revised Edition (DC:0-3R; Zero to Three 2005) offers a set of diagnostic categories specifically geared to the developmental characteristics of infants, toddlers, and preschoolers. Coexisting disorders are frequently diagnosed in young children because their limited behavioral repertoire leads them to similar manifestations for different underlying psychological processes.

The observation that Tonya shows labile affect indicates the possibility of a co-occurring disorder of affect, although more specific information is needed to make a specific diagnosis. Prolonged bereavement/grief reaction as the result of separation from her biological parents needs to be ruled out. Tonya became fussy and irritable with her biological parents and was not easily comforted by them. As elucidated by Bowlby (1973), anger, irritability, and defiance are frequent responses to prolonged separation by children during the first 3 years of life. Two of the criteria for prolonged bereavement/grief reaction in response to separation from or loss of the parent are marked disturbance in the face of reminders of the loss (e.g., visitation with the parents) and disruption in eating patterns.

DSM-IV-TR DIAGNOSIS

Axis I   313.89 Reactive attachment disorder of infancy or early childhood
          Rule out prolonged bereavement/grief reaction on DC:0-3R classification
Axis II   None
Axis III None
Axis IV   Disruption of emotional bonds with parents and relatives
          Neglect of child
          Inadequate social support in surrogate care with foster parent
Axis V   Global Assessment of Functioning=45
          Serious inability to engage in age-appropriate attachment relationships

TREATMENT RECOMMENDATIONS

The most important mental health intervention for toddlers in the foster care system is to ensure that the child is placed in a permanent home with attachment figures capable of providing adequate long-term care. In many cases, placement of a toddler in foster care is not recommended unless the child is at immediate risk and the parents are unable to profit from interventions designed to improve their parenting practices and the quality of the parent-child relationship. The disruption of attachment patterns caused by separation from the parents may have long-term negative repercussions unless the child is placed in a home where there can be continuity of developmentally appropriate care.

Tonya's parents should be offered intensive joint psychotherapy with their child, as in infant-parent psychotherapy (Fraiberg 1980; Lieberman et al. 2000) or child-parent psychotherapy (Lieberman 2004). The psychiatric profile reported for the parents does not indicate severe psychopathology incompatible with the capacity to provide adequate parenting. The parents' childhood experience in foster care suggests the possibility of a reenactment of their past in the present, as in the "ghosts in the nursery" model described by Fraiberg (1980).

Treatment should begin with a clear understanding with the child protective system that reunification is the first goal of treatment. Treatment should include the following components: 1) assessment of the parents' motivation for reunification and their ability to participate consistently in the treatment; 2) developing an empathic and supportive therapeutic relationship with the parents that provides a corrective emotional experience for their own childhood deprivation, neglect, and perhaps more severe maltreatment; 3) modeling for the parents an attitude of interest in emotional experience and investment in intersubjective attunement; 4) providing guidance to enable the parents to learn and practice developmentally appropriate parenting practices and to correct parental misunderstandings of the meaning of their child's behavior; 5) guiding the parents' ability to observe the child's behavior as a manifestation of the child's feelings, with specific attention to the age-appropriate needs to feel loved and protected and fear of separation and loss; 6) helping the parents reflect on their affective experiences taking care of Tonya, including the feelings evoked by her behavior and her responses to their ministrations, and linking these responses to the parents' emotional responses while growing up; 7) creating experiences of pleasure in the child-parent interaction through play, storytelling, reading books, singing, and other age-appropriate activities; and 8) ascertaining the presence of possible traumatic events in the parents' lives and providing treatment to alleviate the impact of these events and the transmission of traumatic patterns to their parenting of Tonya (Lieberman and Van Horn 2005, 2008).

Monitoring of Tonya's ability to relate preferentially to the parents and the parents' ability to respond appropriately to Tonya should be used as the basis for recommending increased visitation and, when appropriate, overnight visits. Monitoring of the child's safety should be coordinated with the child protection worker. Reunification should take place as soon as it is safe to do so to prevent the consolidation of preferential attachment to the foster mother and the deleterious effects of disrupting the bonds formed. Treatment should continue after reunification to monitor the ongoing stability of the parents' progress in their ability to provide appropriate parenting.

If the relationship-based treatment approach recommended above does not succeed in promoting a safe and appropriate parent-child relationship and preferential child attachment to the parents, the search for an adoptive or permanent home should be instituted as soon as possible. Preference should be given to relatives whom the child already knows. If ongoing contact with the parents can be maintained without risk to the child's safety, this should be encouraged as a way of helping the child acquire a sense of continuity and family belonging. If sufficiently protective and nurturing relatives are not available, an adoptive home is the next preferred alternative.

Psychopharmacologic Perspective

Mary Margaret Gleason, M.D.
L. Eugene Arnold, M.D., M.Ed.

DIAGNOSTIC FORMULATION

Tonya's case illustrates both vulnerability and resilience. A high-risk child with genetic loading for intellectual limitations, schizotypal traits, and mood disturbance suffers neglect and a succession of foster homes and manifests language delay, but manages to attain normal development in many domains after a few months of good nurturing. Nevertheless, she continues to show some aberrant behaviors: indiscriminate relating to strangers without preference for a mother figure, overeating, and lability/irritability, especially in the presence of biological parents. Most of these behaviors seem to be related to Tonya's early adverse experiences.

The chief complaint and most pervasive symptom described is a pattern of indiscriminate social interactions and attachment behaviors. The best diagnostic fit appears to be RAD, uninhibited type, for which the DSM-IV-TR description is "diffuse attachments as manifest by indiscriminate sociability" and "excessive familiarity with relative strangers or lack of selectivity in choice of attachment figures," with a history of "pathogenic care" (American Psychiatric Association 2000, p. 130).

In a healthy attachment relationship, a child will seek proximity to and comfort from a caregiver in times of distress or in unfamiliar settings. In RAD, children do not demonstrate this focused attachment behavior with their primary caregiver, even in new situations, with new people, or under stress. RAD can manifest with either an inhibited pattern, in which the child shows dimin-

Mary Margaret Gleason, M.D., is Assistant Professor in the Department of Psychiatry and Human Behavior at Warren Alpert Medical School, and Acting Associate Training Director for Child Psychiatry and Triple Board (Pediatrics, Psychiatry, Child Psychiatry) Training at Brown University in Providence, Rhode Island.

L. Eugene Arnold, M.D., M.Ed., is Professor Emeritus of Psychiatry; Former Director of the Division of Child and Adolescent Psychiatry; Former Vice Chair of Psychiatry; and Interim Director of the Nisonger Center of Excellence in Developmental Disabilities at The Ohio State University in Columbus, Ohio.

For complete biographical information, see "About the Contributors," p. 613.

ished attachment behaviors, limited comfort seeking, and flat or irritable affect, or an uninhibited pattern, with indiscriminate relating to strangers. Although Tonya demonstrates the irritable affect of the inhibited type, her uninhibited patterns appear to be more prominent and problematic. Assessment of young children, especially those at risk for RAD (Boris et al. 2005), includes multiple assessments over multiple sessions with multiple reporters. Tonya's presentation is not uncommon in young children in foster care; in one study, 40% of children in foster care had symptoms of RAD on a semistructured interview (Zeanah et al. 2004).

DIFFERENTIAL DIAGNOSIS

A more extensive differential diagnosis should also be considered. Tonya's history suggests adverse experiences and possibly traumatic events. Her increased distress around her biological parents and with physical contact may suggest that she is reexperiencing symptoms of posttraumatic stress disorder (PTSD), although hyperarousal and numbness symptoms are not described. Diagnosis of PTSD in very young children is challenging because it requires that the caregiver identify trauma-related triggers and recognize the child's internal state (Scheeringa 2003).

Historically, "anaclitic depression" described young children who had experienced an extreme of pathological caregiving—that is, institutionalization (Spitz 1947). The clinical presentation included social withdrawal, limited social interactions, weeping, failure to thrive, eczema, and colds. Of the characteristics of this syndrome, the mood symptoms and withdrawn patterns of social interactions persist in the DSM-IV-TR nosology, in the forms of pervasive developmental disorders, mood disorders, and RAD. Tonya presents with problems in social interactions and language impairment. However, her type of social impairment is not qualitatively the same as in pervasive developmental disorders, and her language deficits improved more quickly than would be seen in pervasive developmental disorders. DSM-IV-TR mood disorders have not been studied in children under age 36 months (Luby and Belden 2006; Luby et al. 2003) and would not explain the prominent relationship symptoms described in Tonya's vignette.

DSM-IV-TR has limitations when applied to very young children. A growing evidence base demonstrates validity of RAD, PTSD, sleep disorders, and feeding disorders in very young children (Boris et al. 2004; Chatoor et al. 1997, 2001; Goodlin-Jones et al. 2001; Scheeringa et al. 2001, 2005), but few other DSM-IV-TR disorders have been examined. In this age group, psychopathology—and mental health—may be best understood within the context of the primary caregiving relationship, rather than as isolated disorders in an individual. The caregiving relationship provides the context in which young children experience the world and learn to organize affective experiences. Further research will enhance understanding of the early presentations of psychopathology, but certainly a formulation should include attention to all five axes plus the parent-child relationship.

DSM-IV-TR DIAGNOSIS

Axis I	313.89 Reactive attachment disorder of infancy or early childhood, uninhibited type
	Rule out posttraumatic stress disorder
Axis II	Expressive language disorder
Axis III	No major physical health problems
Axis IV	Stressors: neglect, maternal deprivation, numerous caregiving disruptions
Axis V	Global Assessment of Functioning=50

TREATMENT RECOMMENDATIONS

The most important "treatment" for Tonya will be provision of consistent, loving caregiving. Psychopharmacologic intervention does not play a role in treatment of RAD in infants and toddlers. Intervention modalities for RAD are usually relationship focused and work through the foster caregiver. Quality foster care itself can be a powerful intervention. In a randomized controlled trial of institutionalized young children, quality foster care placement was associated with less impairment associated with RAD and resolution of inhibited RAD (Zeanah et al. 2005a). Uninhibited patterns of RAD persisted even in adequate caregiving relationships, as in other longitudinal studies (Chisholm 1998).

Attachment and biobehavioral catch-up is an intervention developed for U.S. foster parents and very young foster children (Dozier et al. 2006). It includes relationship-focused treatment with the foster parent to address issues that might interfere with developing a healthy relationship with a foster child and helps the foster parent to reinterpret the child's behaviors. The treatment also targets the child's behavioral and emotional regulation by allowing foster parents to practice child-led play, identify emotions, and use safe physical contact. This intervention is associated with increases in appropriate attachment-related behaviors, decreased problematic child behaviors, and normalized diurnal cortisol patterns (Dozier et al. 2006). Other attachment-focused therapies that were not specifically developed for children in foster care, such as infant-parent psychotherapy (Lieberman et al. 2000) or the circle of security (Marvin et al. 2002), may also be useful in treating this population. When reunification with biological parents is the goal, a multimodal treatment approach should address the child's needs within those relationships as well. Such an approach may include dyadic or family therapy and individual psychopharmacologic or other therapy of the parents.

PSYCHOPHARMACOLOGIC CONSIDERATIONS

There are neither theoretical reasons nor empirical data to support psychopharmacologic treatment of the core symptoms of RAD (Boris et al. 2005). Although some biological factors may be associated with RAD, this disorder is clearly etiologically linked to adverse caregiving experiences (Boris et al. 2004). Some older children with a history of RAD may present with comorbid disorders for which medications may be appropriate. However, the nosological validity of most of these disorders has not been established in infants and toddlers, and the safety and efficacy of medications to treat mental health problems in infants and toddlers are also not established. On the other hand, some data support the use of family-focused attachment-based interventions for very young children (Dozier et al. 2006). Thus, psychopharmacologic treatment in infants and toddlers with RAD is not indicated. Even in preschoolers, biological, relationship, and developmental factors warrant special considerations and caution in use of medication (as reviewed in Gleason et al. 2007).

For children in foster care, interventions must go beyond psychotherapeutic modalities and incorporate multimodal approaches. A child's emotional and physical safety during visits with the biological parents should be monitored, especially when the child becomes more distressed during or after visits, as Tonya does. The child may benefit from having the foster mother (the primary attachment figure) attend visits and serve as a secure emotional base during the potentially stressful visit. If visits cannot be done without causing distress, their schedule and role can be reevaluated. Legal advocacy is an important part of working with children in foster care. In some cases, a guardian ad litem is advisable to protect the child's interests against a variety of competing forces, including bureaucratic policies and a tendency of some courts to focus on parental rights despite the mandate to consider the child's best interests. Permanency planning for young children should be timely, as required by the Adoption and Safe Families Act (1997). Placement disruptions, for reunification with biological parents or transfer to adoptive placements, should be done only when necessary, and with attention to the child's emotional needs to avoid traumatic relationship disruptions. For this reason, initial placement with pre-adoptive foster parents may be optimal.

Integrative Perspective

Stacy S. Drury, M.D., Ph.D.
Charles H. Zeanah, M.D.

DIAGNOSTIC FORMULATION

Reactive attachment disorder arises in early childhood in some children who have been raised in aberrant caregiving environments, such as in families in which children are severely neglected or in institutions with large child/caregiver ratios (Smyke et al. 2002; Zeanah et al. 2004). Two patterns of RAD have been described: an emotionally withdrawn/inhibited pattern and an indiscriminately social/disinhibited pattern. Beyond severely depriving caregiving environments, little is known about other risk factors for the disorder, and nothing is known about why some children exhibit a withdrawn/inhibited pattern and other children exhibit an indiscriminate/disinhibited pattern (Zeanah and Smyke 2008).

According to DSM-IV-TR (American Psychiatric Association 2000), the child diagnosed with RAD fails "to initiate or respond in a developmentally appropriate fashion to most social interactions" (p. 130). Furthermore, the disinhibited type is marked by a pattern of "diffuse attachments as manifest by indiscriminate sociability with marked inability to exhibit appropriate selective attachments" (p. 130). The child exhibits indiscriminate sociability or a lack of selectivity in the choice of attachment figures. The disturbance is "not accounted for solely by developmental delay (as in mental retardation) and does not meet criteria for a pervasive developmental disorder" (p. 130). By definition, the condition is associated with grossly pathogenic care that may take the form of physical or emotional neglect or repeated changes of primary caregiver that prevent formation of stable attachments. The pathogenic care is presumed to be responsible for the disturbed social relatedness.

Tonya, who was observed initially after she had been neglected and placed in foster care, exhibited markedly disturbed interpersonal relatedness, indicated by her failure to seek comfort from her primary caregiver and her willingness to approach, engage with, and seek comfort from complete strangers instead of her primary caregiver. Based on these behaviors, and the fact that they followed severe neglect and several caregiving disruptions (i.e., pathogenic care), the clinician diagnosed Tonya with the disinhibited type of RAD. The child's behaviors exceeded the limits of high levels of sociability in typically developing children, and she had no signs of pervasive developmental disorders or developmental delay.

DSM-IV-TR DIAGNOSIS

Axis I   313.89 Reactive attachment disorder, disinhibited type

           315.31 Expressive language disorder

Axis II   None

Axis III   None

Axis IV   History of neglect

           Foster care placement

Axis V   Global Assessment of Functioning=55

TREATMENT RECOMMENDATIONS

Because of multiple concerns about the appropriateness of Tonya's first foster placement, including her failure to develop an attachment to the foster mother and the number of other children in the home, Tonya was moved to a second foster placement where she was the only child in the home. After only a week in this second placement, with an available and nurturing caregiver, several changes were noted in Tonya. She began talking more and had a significantly brighter affect. Additionally, although Tonya continued to be friendly with unfamiliar adults, she remained in close proximity to her new foster mother and referenced her before approaching others. Tonya also initiated interaction with her second foster mother by reaching up to her to be picked up, a behavior that had not been noted in her previous placement or with her biological parents. During this placement, rapid declines occurred both in Tonya's willingness to approach strangers and in her overeating.

After 3 months in her second foster placement, a semistructured interview and interaction assessment was performed with Tonya and her foster mother. Tonya's foster mother was able to describe Tonya's personality in detail and provide specific examples of her relationship with Tonya, which contrasted with her biological parents and her first foster mother, each of whom was unable to provide specific or qualitative information about Tonya's personality or relationship to him or her. The second foster mother did note that Tonya did not like to be alone and would not stay in a room by herself. The foster mother reported that Tonya's excessive eating declined after several weeks in this placement. She also reported that although initially "anybody could have taken her, now she stays with me more." In a clinic-based interactional assessment, Tonya actively engaged her foster mother during play and the two sat close together, and Tonya exhibited a significant amount of eye contact and shared positive affect with the foster mother. Upon a planned separation during this assessment, Tonya became immediately upset, but when her foster mother returned to the room, Tonya made direct eye contract with her and reached up to be picked up and comforted. She was easily soothed by her foster mother and quickly began playing again.

Thus, when placed in a nurturing environment, Tonya formed a new attachment to the foster mother. She showed some residual symptoms of disturbed attachment, such as unwillingness to be separated and somewhat excessive clinginess to her foster mother, but she developed a clear preference for the foster mother as her preferred attachment figure. Concomitantly, she had significant reductions in her indiscriminate behaviors.

Interestingly, Tonya began to demonstrate discriminated attachment behaviors within days to weeks of placement in a nurturing foster home. Once infants are 7–9 months of age, they begin to direct their bids for comfort, support, nurturance, and protection to those caregivers whom they have learned are able to provide comfort, support, and nurturance—in other words, those individuals who provide substantial amounts of care to them. When this happens, the children have developed focused or preferred attachments. The cognitive capacity needed for selective attachment appears to develop around 7–9 months of age, and if infants are raised in reasonably caregiving environments, they will develop focused or preferred attachments after this point.

Children who initially experience severe neglect, as Tonya did in her biological parents' home, may require extra effort on the part of caregiving adults to engage them; this may explain why Tonya seemed not to become attached in her first regular foster home but did so readily in her second placement. Tonya clearly demonstrated in this second home that she had the capacity to form a preferred attachment and quickly did so when placed in a nurturing environment. Although signs of disinhibited attachment diminished in Tonya as she became attached to the new foster mother, this does not always happen, particularly when children are older than age 2 years at the time of placement in an enhanced environment (Zeanah et al. 2005b). For example, a number of children who are adopted out of institutions in Romania have exhibited high levels of indiscriminate behavior even after they have developed attachments to their new caregivers (Chisholm 1998; O'Connor et al. 2003). For children living in institutions, no relationship exists between signs of indiscriminate behavior and the degree to which a child has formed a preferred attachment to a caregiver within the institution (Zeanah et al. 2005a).

The only intervention that has been shown to be effective in reducing signs of disinhibited attachments is placement of the child in an enhanced caregiving environment, but little is known about the specific aspects of enhanced caregiving that are necessary or sufficient to eliminate signs of disinhibited RAD. For example, in one recent study, the quality of care that young children received in an institutional setting was not related to signs of disinhibited attachment (Zeanah et al. 2005a). Given the lack of evidence, current clinical practice should include recommendations that parents, foster or adoptive, minimize contacts between young children who have recently come into their care and other, unfamiliar adults until the children have had an opportunity to develop attachments with them, a period believed to encompass several months (Zeanah and Smyke 2005). Parental behaviors known to be associated with fostering secure attachments in typically developing infants include sensitivity, emotional availability, and psychological and physical protection. These behaviors are appropriate treatment targets to foster in caregivers of children with RAD, given the current state of research in this field.

REFERENCES

Adoption and Safe Families Act, Pub. L. No. 10589, 42 U.S.C. 671.

American Psychiatric Association: Diagnostic and Statistical Manual of Mental Disorders, 4th Edition, Text Revision. Washington, DC, American Psychiatric Association, 2000

Boris NW, Hinshaw-Fuselier SS, Smyke AT, et al: Comparing criteria for attachment disorders: establishing reliability and validity in high-risk samples. J Am Acad Child Adolesc Psychiatry 43:568–577, 2004

Boris NW, Zeanah CH; Work Group on Quality Issues: Practice parameter for the assessment and treatment of children and adolescents with reactive attachment disorder of infancy and early childhood. J Am Acad Child Adolesc Psychiatry 44:1206–1219, 2005

Bowlby J: Attachment and Loss, Vol 2: Separation: Anxiety and Anger. New York, Basic Books, 1973

Chatoor I, Getson P, Menvielle E, et al: A feeding scale for research and clinical practice to assess mother-infant interactions in the first three years of life. Infant Ment Health J 18:76–91, 1997

Chatoor I, Ganiban J, Harrison J, et al: Observation of feeding in the diagnosis of posttraumatic feeding disorder. J Am Acad Child Adolesc Psychiatry 39:743–751, 2001

Chisholm KL: A three year follow-up of attachment and indiscriminate friendliness in children adopted from Romanian orphanages. Child Dev 69:1092–1106, 1998

Dozier M, Manni M, Gordon M: Foster children's diurnal production of cortisol: an exploratory study. Child Maltreat 11:189–197, 2006

Fraiberg S: Clinical Studies in Infant mental Fealth. New York, Basic Books, 1980

Gleason MM, Egger HL, Emslie GJ, et al: Psychopharmacological treatment for very young children: contexts and guidelines. J Am Acad Child Adolesc Psychiatry 46:1532–1572, 2007

Goodlin-Jones BL, Burhman MM, Gaylor EE: Night waking, sleep-wake organization, and self-soothing in the first year of life. J Dev Behav Pediatr 22:226–233, 2001

Lieberman AF: Child-parent psychotherapy: a relationship-based approach to the treatment of mental health disorders of infancy and early childhood, in Treating Parent-Infant Relationship Problems. Edited by Sameroff AJ, McDonough SC, Rosenblum KL. New York, Guilford, 2004, pp 97–122

Lieberman AF, Van Horn P: Don't Hit My Mommy: A Manual for Child-Parent Psychotherapy With Young Witnesses of Family Violence. Washington, DC, Zero to Three Press, 2005

Lieberman AF, Van Horn P: Psychotherapy With Infants and Young Children: Repairing the Effects of Stress and Trauma on Early Attachment. New York, Guilford, 2008

Lieberman AF, Silverman R, Pawl JH: Infant-parent psychotherapy: core concepts and current approaches, in Handbook of Infant Mental Health, 2nd Edition. Edited by Zeanah CH. New York, Guilford, 2000, pp 472–484

Luby J, Belden A: Defining and validating bipolar disorder in the preschool period. Dev Psychopathol 18:971–988, 2006

Luby JL, Mrakotsky C, Heffelfinger A, et al: Modification of DSM-IV criteria for depressed preschool children. Am J Psychiatry 160:1169–1172, 2003

Marvin R, Cooper G, Hoffman K, et al: The Circle of Security Project: attachment-based intervention with caregiver–preschool child dyads. Attach Hum Dev 4:107–124, 2002

O'Connor TG, Marvin RS, Rutter M, et al: Child-parent attachment following early institutional deprivation. Dev Psychopathol 15:19–38, 2003

Scheeringa MS, Peebles CD, Cook CA, et al: Toward establishing procedural, criterion, and discriminant validity for PTSD in early childhood. J Am Acad Child Adolesc Psychiatry 40:52–60, 2001

Scheeringa MS, Zeanah CH, Myers L, et al: Predictive validity in a prospective follow-up of PTSD in preschool children. J Am Acad Child Adolesc Psychiatry 44:899–906, 2005

Scheeringa MS, Zeanah CH, Myers L, et al: New findings on alternative criteria for posttraumatic stress disorder in preschool children. J Am Acad Child Adolesc Psychiatry 42:561–570, 2003

Smyke AT, Dumitrescu A, Zeanah CH: Disturbances of attachment in young children, I: the continuum of caretaking casualty. J Am Acad Child Adolesc Psychiatry 41:972–982, 2002

Sparrow S, Balla D, Cicchetti D: Vineland Adaptive Behavior Scales, Second Edition. Upper Saddle River, NJ, Pearson Education, 2005

Spitz RA, Wolf K: Anaclytic depression: an inquiry into the genesis of psychiatric conditions in early childhood, II. Psychoanal Study Child 2:313–342, 1947

Wechsler D: Wechsler Adult Intelligence Scale — Third Edition. San Antonio, TX, The Psychological Corporation, 1997

Zeanah CH, Smyke AT: Building attachment relationships following maltreatment and severe deprivation, in Enhancing Early Attachments. Edited by Berlin L, Ziv Y, Amaya-Jackson L, et al. New York, Guilford, 2005, pp 195–216

Zeanah CH, Smyke AT: Reactive attachment disorder in the context of deprivation, in Rutter's Child and Adolescent Psychiatry, 5th Edition. Edited by Rutter M, Bishop D, Pine D, et al. Oxford, UK, Blackwell Scientific, 2008, pp 906–915

Zeanah CH, Scheeringa M, Boris NW, et al: Reactive attachment disorder in maltreated toddlers. Child Abuse Negl 28:877–888, 2004

Zeanah CH, Smyke AT, Koga SF, et al; Bucharest Early Intervention Project Core Group: Attachment in institutionalized and community children in Romania. Child Dev 76:1015–1028, 2005a

Zeanah CH, Smyke AT, Koga SFM, et al: The Bucharest Early Intervention Project. Paper presented at the biennial meeting of the Society for Research in Child Development, Atlanta, GA, March 2005b

Zero to Three: Diagnostic Classification of Mental Health and Developmental Disorders of Infancy and Early Childhood, Revised Edition: DC:0-3R. Washington, DC, Zero to Three Press, 2005

▪ P a r t V ▪

DIAGNOSTIC AND TREATMENT DECISION MAKING

■ CHAPTER 31 ■

Diagnostic Decision Making

Cathryn A. Galanter, M.D.
Peter S. Jensen, M.D.

For this book, we brought together 90 of the field leaders in child and adolescent mental health to present cases and explain their diagnostic impressions and treatment recommendations. We chose commentators who offer a range of perspectives, in terms of how they conceptualize the cases and what types of treatment they recommend.

VARIATION AMONG CLINICIANS

A self-evident yet easily overlooked fact is that clinicians' perceptions and beliefs arising out of their experiences—personal, educational, or professional—have significant impact on how each professional practices. These varied perspectives are part of what makes the different professions rich and exciting, and children and adolescents may be treated by a team in which different professionals can offer different perspectives and treatments. However, variability can be troubling when it leads to inaccurate diagnosis and inappropriate treatment. In the current climate of evidence-based medicine, with an increasing number of evidence-based assessments and treatments available for children and adolescents, most clinicians struggle to maintain both the art and the science of medicine, seeking an approach that is both individualized *and* scientifically accurate.

Many potentially troubling examples of variability in diagnosis and treatment are documented in the literature. For example, the interrater reliability

---

Cathryn A. Galanter, M.D., is Assistant Professor of Clinical Psychiatry in the Division of Child and Adolescent Psychiatry at Columbia University/New York State Psychiatric Institute in New York, New York.

Peter S. Jensen, M.D., is President and Chief Executive Officer of the REACH Institute (Resource for Advancing Children's Health) in New York, New York.

For complete biographical information, see "About the Contributors," p. 613.

between clinicians for the assessment and diagnosis of childhood psychopathology is often poor (Piacentini et al. 1993). If two clinicians evaluate the same child and arrive at different diagnoses, one must assume that children are often misdiagnosed and consequently may receive inappropriate treatment. Research has shown that treatment may vary across settings, as illustrated by the differences in antipsychotic medications most commonly prescribed in various inpatient state hospital settings (Pappadopulos et al. 2002) or the differences in treatment for attention-deficit/hyperactivity disorder (ADHD) in specialty mental health care versus primary care practices (Zarin et al. 1998; Zito et al. 1999). When such variations in diagnosis and treatment reflect clinician rather than patient differences, significant adverse consequences for children seem likely.

One way to avoid harmful diagnostic or treatment decisions or medical errors is to think carefully about clinical decision making. A great deal of research in medicine, and some of it in mental health, focuses on how clinicians make decisions about their patients (Galanter and Patel 2005). The following section reviews some of the concepts that are particularly germane to clinical decision making and the use of this book.

CLINICAL PROBLEM SOLVING

Children and parents present to the clinician with their own concerns. The clinician then interprets their story, or narrative, into a medical framework, which can be used to arrive at a diagnosis and treatment options. During this process, clinicians are faced with the dual challenge of building an alliance while also needing to be careful diagnosticians.

The "translation" process has several steps, and clinicians are at risk for error along the way. Beginning with a patient's narrative, the clinician translates and restructures this story into a coherent medical and psychological framework. As part of this process, the clinician elicits additional information. For example, a parent may bring an adolescent daughter to treatment with concerns that she is isolating herself in her room, fighting more with her brother, and no longer keeping up her grades. Clinicians then need more information to determine how to interpret this story. Are the daughter's irritability, anhedonia, and decreased concentration associated with depression? Or is she perhaps paranoid and internally preoccupied due to an emerging psychotic disorder?

One model, the epistemological framework for medical comprehension and problem solving (Evans and Gadd 1989; Patel et al. 1989, 2001), is useful as a way to consider the diagnostic decision making of clinicians. Investigators have proposed that clinical information is represented hierarchically. (Please see Figure 31–1 for a graphic depiction of this model.) We have modified the framework so that it is especially applicable to problem solving in child and adolescent psychiatry and so that it shows decision nodes (points in the process where clinicians make decisions) as well as suggested interventions that might support clinician decision making.

The model begins with *observations* (to the left in Figure 31–1). These are units of information that are recognized as potentially useful during problem solving. In psychiatry, observations are clinical material from both the history and the mental status examination. For example, in the case of the adolescent described above, observations include the parent's report that the daughter stays in her room, the adolescent's report that hanging out with her friends "isn't as fun as it used to be," and the clinician's report that during the interview the girl never smiled and started to cry. *Findings* are observations with diagnostic implications. They are the observations that indicate a symptom or example of pathology. Negative findings are observations that indicate the absence of a symptom (e.g., if a patient denies a specific behavior). Returning to the example of the adolescent, the findings would be that she is socially withdrawn, is anhedonic, and has constricted affect in the dysphoric range. She also denied hallucinations and demonstrated a linear thought process. At the next level are *facets* — clusters of findings suggestive of diagnostic components. Examples in psychiatry include a depressive episode or a panic attack. Finally, the level of *diagnosis* subsumes all these sublevels. For the adolescent described above, the diagnosis was major depressive disorder. Investigators have used the framework of the hierarchical model to characterize clinical reasoning (Patel et al. 1994) as well as doctor-patient interaction (Patel et al. 1989).

We indicate the steps (or decision nodes) of diagnostic problem solving as part of our modifications of the framework. These decision nodes include data gathering (acquisition of observations), interpretation of observations (translating observations to findings), or data integration (combining findings to determine facets and make diagnoses (Bowen 2006; Graber 2005). Our model also includes suggested interventions that support different aspects of the decision making process. These interventions are elaborated upon in the "Recommendations" portion of the chapter.

ANALYTIC THINKING AND PATTERN RECOGNITION AND CHANGES WITH EXPERIENCE

Investigators in cognitive psychology and in medical decision making have identified different ways that clinicians diagnose patients (for reviews, see Bowen 2006; Norman 2005, 2006). Clinicians use both analytic and intuitive problem solving, while applying formal knowledge (e.g., pathophysiology) and procedural knowledge (Bowen 2006; Norman 2005, 2006).

An important aspect of problem solving is that it changes as clinicians gain experience. Not surprisingly, the process by which an intern or resident solves

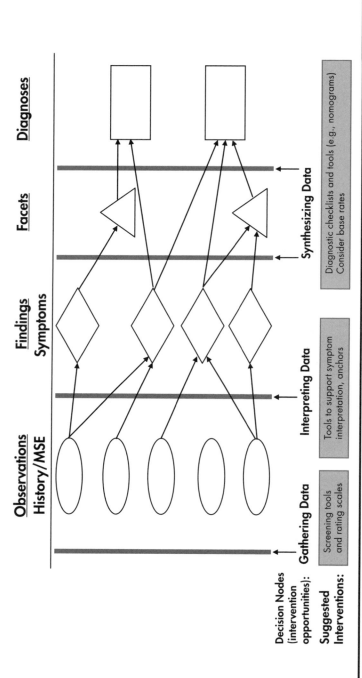

FIGURE 31–1. Modified epistemological framework with decision nodes (intervention opportunities) and suggested interventions.

MSE = mental status examination.

diagnostic problems differs from that of a clinician who has been practicing for many years. As clinicians gain experience with patients, they learn to recognize patterns more easily and also learn when symptoms do not fit the patterns (Bordage 1999; Norman et al. 2007).

Cognitive scientists who study expertise in physicians have demonstrated differences in the ways that experts and nonexperts use their knowledge and reasoning strategies. Theories of human memory indicate that humans can only manage 5–10 "chunks" of information in their short-term or working memory (Miller 1956). Studies of physicians by Patel and colleagues show that experts are better able to organize information into manageable and related chunks, they do not process irrelevant information, and they generate specific knowledge-based problem-solving inferences based on expertly recognized patterns of clinical information (Patel and Groen 1991; Patel et al. 1994). These patterns, called *schemas* or *prototypes*, allow for management of greater amounts of information (Bordage and Zacks 1984; Patel et al. 2001). Such schemas are helpful in that they allow a physician to make effective use of the limitations of working memory by decreasing the cognitive burden. In addition, they serve as a "filter" for distinguishing between relevant and irrelevant information (Patel et al. 2001).

Scientists have elaborated different cognitive and behavioral theories to describe how clinicians conceptualize illness, including exemplar models of categorization (Norman et al. 2005; Schmidt et al. 1990) or illness scripts, which are storylike narrations of a case condition (Barrows and Feltovich 1987). When a patient's symptoms do not match the exemplar model or script, clinicians may rely on more analytic processes. These are slower, and clinicians may be more aware of these more labored and conscious processes (Norman 2006). As clinicians become more experienced, they develop more coherent explanations of patients' illnesses and are more selective in their use of data (Patel and Groen 1991).

Experts are also able to conceptualize illness in a more medically or psychologically sophisticated manner. For example, in one study in internal medicine, investigators examined how novice and expert residents in internal medicine presented a case of knee pain (Bordage 1999; Chang et al. 1998). The more experienced resident described "multiple discrete episodes with abrupt onset of extremely severe pain involving a single joint, with evidence of inflammation on exam," whereas the novice explained that the pain "started last night" and "hurts a lot" and that "he's had this problem twice before." The expert resident was also able to clearly lay out the pertinent positive and negative findings, which supported the correct diagnostic conclusion of acute gout. The novice resident reported the positive findings and some of the negative findings and admitted to being unsure about the concluded (and incorrect) diagnosis. Although this is an example from medicine, one might expect to find similar examples in child and adolescent psychiatry; for example, a less experienced clinician might describe the adolescent described in our example above by stating, "She has spent several months isolated in her room and has been fighting with her brother," whereas a more advanced clinician would speak about "several months of gradually increasing depressed and irritable mood, with decreased enjoyment of activities and increasing social withdrawal from her parents and friends at school."

COGNITIVE ERRORS, HEURISTICS, AND BIASES

The concepts of cognitive errors, heuristics, and biases are important when considering problem-solving methods and decision making. Much of the earlier work in decision making began in economics (e.g., Bernoulli 1738/1954; see Baron 2000 for a review). As early as the eighteenth century, economists and scientists could calculate a probability of a given outcome based on mathematical formulas. If humans made decisions based on these equations, or if their decisions always matched the outcome of the equations (even if the decision-making process were unconscious), their decision-making process would be normative (Baron 2000) and presumed entirely "rational." One example of this type of rational decision making is to accurately use probability and base rates to estimate the likelihood of a given disease. For example, clinicians know that common disorders are more likely to occur than rare disorders. Returning to the adolescent who was isolating herself in her room, she more likely has major depressive disorder than schizophrenia because the former is a fairly common condition and the latter is very rare in early adolescents.

In the second half of the twentieth century, Nobel Prize–winning economist Daniel Kahneman, and his long-time collaborator, Amos Tversky, argued that people do not always behave rationally (e.g., do not base their decisions on all available information) as the normative model proposed (Tversky and Kahneman 1974). Instead, people tend to use heuristics, or shortcuts, in their thought processes. These cognitive strategies can result in biases under certain circumstances. Many biases have been studied and described in the literature (for reviews in the medical arena, see Bornstein and Emler 2001; Chapman and Elstein 2000; Elstein and Schwarz 2002). Medical decision-making experts have articulated the need to study biases so as to understand the cognitive processes underlying physicians' decision making and to learn where improvements may be made (Chapman and Elstein 2000). We have identified a number of these biases in Table 31–1.

One common heuristic, for example, is the *availability* heuristic. People tend to overestimate the frequency of an easily recalled (available) event and underestimate the frequency of an ordinary or difficult-to-recall (unavailable)

TABLE 31–1. Heuristics, biases, and cognitive errors useful to consider in diagnostic and treatment decision making

Heuristics, biases, and cognitive errors	Definitions
Anchoring	Overfocusing on salient aspects of patient presentation very early in diagnostic procedure, with no subsequent adjustment (Tversky and Kahneman 1982)
Availability	Overestimating probability of a diagnosis because it is especially memorable, salient, or recently encountered (Christensen-Szalanski and Bushyhead 1981; Custers et al. 1996; Poses and Anthony 1991)
Base-rate neglect	Failing to consider prevalence rates of disease, including both over- and underestimates of likelihood (Ajzen 1977; Kahneman and Tversky 1973; Yates 1990)
Clinician's illusion	Believing that people with a disorder in the population as a whole are more likely to be chronically ill because of experience with those in treatment (Cohen and Cohen 1984)
Commission bias	Tending to intervene instead of "first doing no harm" (Sharpe and Faden 1998)
Confirmation	Selectively gathering and interpreting evidence that confirms a diagnosis and ignoring evidence that contradicts it (Christensen-Szalanski and Bushyhead 1981; Eddy 1982; Elstein 1988; Joseph and Patel 1990)
Effect of description/ unpacking principle	Providing more detail of an event, which increases its judged probability (Redelmeier et al. 1995; Tversky and Koehler 1994)
Framing	Choosing riskier treatments when they are described in negative (e.g., mortality) rather than positive (e.g., survival) terms (Bornstein et al. 1999; Christensen et al. 1995; Marteau 1989; Mazur and Hickam 1990; McNeil et al. 1982; Tversky and Kahneman 1982, 1992)
Hindsight	Overestimating probability of a diagnosis when the correct diagnosis is already known (Arkes et al. 1981; Dawson et al. 1988; Fischhoff 1975)

TABLE 31–1. Heuristics, biases, and cognitive errors useful to consider in diagnostic and treatment decision making *(continued)*

Heuristics, biases, and cognitive errors	Definitions
Number of alternatives	Introducing additional options, which can increase decision difficulty and effect treatment choice (Redelmeier and Shafir 1995; Schwartz and Chapman 1999)
Omission bias	Being reluctant to intervene due to fear of causing harm (Elstein et al. 1986; Spranca et al. 1991)
Order effects	Giving more weight to information presented at the beginning and the end of the case (primacy and recency) than to information presented in the middle (Bergus et al. 1995)
Outcome bias	Fixating on a decision course with positive ends, causing the possibility of minimizing or ignoring the gravity of circumstances; based partially on hopes rather than rational decision making (Gruppen et al. 1994)
Premature closure	Committing oneself to a diagnosis without gathering all the data necessary to rule in or out other possibilities (Kassirer and Kopelman 1989; Kovacs and Croskerry 1999; Voytovich et al. 1985)
Regret	Overestimating probability of a diagnosis with a severe outcome because of anticipated regret if diagnosis were missed; the anticipated emotional response to a decision process becoming a part of the input to decision making (Dawson and Arkes 1987; Feinstein 1985; Wallsten 1981)
Representativeness	Overemphasizing pattern recognition, estimating the probability of a disease by judging how similar the case is to a diagnostic category or prototype, which can lead to base-rate neglect (Ayanian and Berwick 1991; Casscells et al. 1987; Elstein 1988; Tversky and Kahneman 1974)

event. For example, conditions of particularly hard-to-treat patients, illnesses that receive media attention, or disorders that were the subject of a recent conference are often thought to be more common than they actually are. One can easily appreciate how the availability heuristic may lead to diagnostic errors in the field of child psychiatry: in recent years, certain disorders, such as bipolar disorder or Asperger's disorder, have received widespread media coverage, including being featured on the cover of national news magazines. Although this publicity fortunately leads to increased recognition of cases that may have gone undiagnosed, it is also likely to lead to overdiagnosis. Another common error is premature closure. This bias occurs when a clinician decides on a diagnosis prematurely without gathering sufficient evidence to rule out other diagnoses. In child and adolescent psychiatry, many of the patients clinicians treat have comorbidity. Thus, even if a clinician established one diagnosis, it is important to rule out other conditions, especially those that are commonly comorbid with the first condition.

Examining biases has been formally applied in a number of medical fields, wherein authors have examined medical records to determine the cause of diagnostic errors. For example, Graber et al. (2005) reviewed 100 cases and categorized diagnostic error into three categories: no-fault errors, system-related errors, and cognitive errors (faulty knowledge, faulty data gathering, and faulty synthesis). Approaches such as Graber's are useful in determining how to best support and improve clinical decision making.

RECOMMENDATIONS

To decrease diagnostic errors, clinicians might usefully keep in mind several lessons from the decision-making literature. These "lessons" are presented below, organized according to the different steps of the diagnostic problem-solving sequence (see Figure 31–1): gathering data, interpreting data, and synthesizing data (Bowen 2006; Graber et al. 2005).

GATHERING DATA

Clinicians are at risk of making mistakes while gathering data. For example, clinicians may make the error of premature closure (Graber et al. 2002). Several recommendations may be helpful in avoiding errors in the data gathering step.

1. **Use screening tools and rating scales to support decision making.** These types of tools can be helpful for several reasons. A generalized screening tool, such as the Child Behavior Checklist (Achenbach 1991) or the Strengths and Difficulties Questionnaire (Goodman 1997), can help ensure that the clinician is not missing anything. Disorder-specific scales are helpful for gathering more specific data about a condition. Some scales also include data about

how likely it is that a child has a condition given a specific score. Additionally, for children with comorbid conditions or complicated presentations, rating scales can help structure the patients', parents', and clinicians' decision making and help sort through a great amount of data. Rating scales can also help in tracking a child's improvement over time. Clinicians can think of a score as a "lab value" to follow to see whether a child is responding to an intervention. In this book, we include a list of rating scales in the appendix.

2. **Use a psychiatric review of systems.** Conducting a brief psychiatric review of systems helps to rule in or rule out certain conditions. This review can help clinicians avoid missing comorbid conditions or misattributing symptoms to one disorder instead of attributing symptoms correctly to another. For example, in a child or adolescent with depressed mood and neurovegetative symptoms, it is important to rule out periods of mania or hypomania.

Additionally, many symptoms in childhood disorders are shared among disorders. For example, sleep disturbance, poor concentration, psychomotor agitation, and irritability can occur with anxiety disorders, mood disorders, substance abuse, and ADHD. By quickly attributing these symptoms to one condition, a clinician may miss that they are actually part of another condition. Using a brief psychiatric review of systems can help avoid such errors.

3. **Consider commonly co-occurring conditions.** Studies that compare diagnoses obtained from structured interviews to those obtained in treatment as usual (e.g., admission or discharge diagnoses from a chart) have generally found that structured interviews are more likely to identify comorbid diagnoses (Jensen and Weisz 2002; Lewczyk et al. 2003). Clinicians may be inclined to stop questioning once they have established a diagnosis. This error can be avoided by keeping epidemiology in mind to help identify comorbid conditions. Clinicians who are familiar with which conditions "travel together" are less likely to miss something. For example, oppositional defiant disorder, conduct disorder, learning disorders, and anxiety disorders are the most common comorbid conditions with ADHD. Mood disorders such as major depressive disorder or bipolar disorder may also co-occur. A careful assessment of a child with ADHD should include ruling out the most common comorbid conditions.

4. **Obtain details about specific symptoms.** When determining whether a symptom is absent or present, the clinician needs to obtain as much detail as possible and make an effort to get specific examples and find out what precipitated the symptoms.

Interpreting Data

In addition to eliciting information, clinicians need to think carefully about how to interpret it. This step is comparable to the conversion of an observation to a finding. A clinician uses judgment to determine whether information is clinically relevant, whether a symptom is pathological, and with which disease state the symptom may be associated (e.g., whether a finding of inattention is associated with ADHD, anxiety, or major depressive disorder). "Anchors" can be used to help describe symptoms and assist clinicians in discerning what is clinically significant. In research instruments, anchors often help clinicians determine what qualifies as minimal, moderate, and severe and are especially useful in helping clinicians be more reliable in interpreting symptoms. For example, investigators found increased interrater reliability when anchors were included as part of clinician rating scales (Hughes et al. 2000). The field would likely benefit from decision support tools that included anchors, especially for less common disorders for which clinicians are less likely to have accumulated an inventory through experience with patients. For instance, examples describing manic symptoms in young children, or which developmental delays are subthreshold and which are severe enough to qualify as autistic. However, we recommend that in all child and adolescent psychiatry, both in the absence and in the presence of such decision support tools, it is crucial to examine a symptom in its developmental and psychosocial context as we describe below.

5. **Think about symptoms developmentally.** When working with children, a clinician needs to think of how they present from a developmental context and to interpret their symptoms developmentally. For example, healthy toddlers have more frequent tantrums than healthy school-age children. Thus, whether tantrums and their frequency should be considered pathological or normative will vary as children age. Another example is that according to the research and the current diagnostic criteria, children (but not adults) with major depressive disorder may present with irritability (and not sadness) as their primary mood symptom. A young child may normatively exhibit pronounced anxiety in the presence of a stranger (the clinician), whereas a similar level of anxiety in youth and adults might be considered more likely pathological.

6. **Look at symptoms in a psychosocial context.** Many of the youth described in this book have experienced severe psychosocial stress, such as the death of a parent, parental divorce, or trauma. Their presentations must be considered in light of these experiences. However, clinicians must take care not to overweigh the stressor when thinking about a diagnosis. As an example, many children, such as those in the foster care system or those who have been otherwise traumatized, may in fact suffer from depression and not posttraumatic stress disorder per se. Clinicians need to take a careful psychosocial and trauma history, and be careful not to overdiagnose all traumatized children as having posttraumatic stress disorder or to assume that the symptoms that are present are necessarily caused by psychosocial stressors.

In addition to evaluating the potential impact of psychosocial contexts on symptoms, clinicians often make interpretations and inferences about how the context lends meaning and form to specific symptoms. At times, clinicians may be tempted to discount symptoms because of the context. For example, in two related studies, investigators presented clinicians with vignettes of children who had symptoms of conduct disorder, but the vignettes varied in whether they presented symptoms only, symptoms in the context of a negative environment, or symptoms caused by internal dysfunction (Kirk and Hsieh 2004; Wakefield et al. 2002). These investigators found that clinicians were less likely to diagnose conduct disorder if the child's behavior presented in the context of a negative environment. Additionally, Kirk and Hsieh (2004) found that the clinicians' professions correlated with the likelihood of diagnosing conduct disorder—social workers were less likely to diagnose conduct disorder than psychiatrists or psychologists—thus indicating that professionals' training and experiences may affect how they conceptualize diagnosis.

This concept of considering symptoms and a disorder in context is very complex (see Jensen et al. 2006). Although we believe that a phenomenological approach to diagnosis is essential at this state in the profession's knowledge, this approach must be enhanced by clinicians' understanding of psychosocial contextual factors and awareness that such factors may shape treatment decision making. For example, a child with severe and long-standing ADHD and conduct disorder expressed in the context of a disordered environment may benefit from an array of services, including a therapeutic foster care setting, intensive parent training, and medication, whereas a child with similar problems in a more benign environment may respond simply to carefully managed medication.

7. **Gather data in different settings and from multiple informants.** Often, learning about a child's behavior in multiple settings helps the clinician to better understand a child's difficulty. For some disorders, such as ADHD, data from two settings are required to make a diagnosis. For children, who spend much of their time at school, feedback from the school is incredibly useful. For example, if a child has difficulty with attention in school but not at home, the clinician might consider whether the child has a learning disability. Children with selective mutism may be talkative at home but silent at school or in the grocery store. Understanding how the child's behavior presents to different persons and across different settings provides useful information about the variability of symptoms and behaviors from the viewpoints of and in the presence of particular raters.

Differences observed and reported by raters within or across settings can be understood not merely as differences in behavior but also as a function of any or all of three other factors: variations in demands and tasks, different interpersonal relationships (e.g., mother-child vs. father-child vs. teacher-child relationship), and biases in the judgments of a rater (see next paragraph). On the other hand, consistency of reports about the child across informants and settings creates additional confidence in the clinician's determination that the behaviors should be interpreted as a symptom within the child, as opposed to an adverse psychosocial context.

8. **Be wary of biased informants.** In addition to considering the possibility that various informants can be biased, the clinician also should be careful not to attribute too much of the pathology to biased reporting alone. Investigators have demonstrated that parents with depression or anxiety (compared to parents without) may report more symptoms in their children than are reported from the child (Najman et al. 2000, 2001), the teacher (Chilcoat and Breslau 1997), the other parent (Jensen et al. 1988a, 1988b), or all of the raters (Jensen et al. 1988a, 1988b). Additionally, family characteristics (e.g., parents' marital status or gender) impact the reports of symptoms by parents, teachers, and children (Jensen et al. 1988b).

Synthesizing Data

The clinician should keep several principles in mind when integrating data. While combining information to come up with a diagnosis, the clinician risks weighing some information too heavily and forgetting other information.

9. **Keep base rates in mind when thinking about diagnosis.** As part of their training, clinicians may learn about the epidemiology of childhood mental disorders. However, they are rarely taught how to make use of these data. Research indicates that physicians are especially poor at calibration (i.e., predicting how often an event will occur over a series of cases) because they do not know the local base rates of a disease that they see in their practice (Wigton 2006). To avoid potential biases, the clinician should realize that a child or adolescent is much more likely to have a common disorder than a rare one. Rates of conditions also vary across different settings. For example, childhood schizophrenia is very rare. Thus, the young adolescent who isolates herself in her room is unlikely to be schizophrenic. Even if a child has psychotic symptoms, he or she is *still* unlikely to have schizophrenia. This inference would especially apply in school settings and outpatient community clinics. However, this calculation changes slightly at an inpatient state hospital or at a tertiary care inpatient unit specializing in psychotic disorders. In these settings, psychotic symptoms are still more likely to represent bipolar disorder or depression with psychotic features (both more common than schizo-

phrenia), yet a child presenting to one of those settings is more likely to have schizophrenia than a child presenting to an outpatient community clinic.

10. **Think of each query as a test.** In diagnosing child and adolescent mental disorders, clinicians do not yet have lab tests to guide them. As we noted above, some screening tools can be used like a lab test, by supplementing clinical decision making based on history and mental status examination. Additionally, at times clinicians can think of each query as a test from which to adjust the likelihood of a certain disorder. Thus, the pretest probability that a child has schizophrenia is very low. The probability increases given psychotic symptoms but still remains very low.

11. **Be systematic about making a diagnosis.** Experienced clinicians may be more likely to rely on pattern recognition when making diagnoses. However, less experienced clinicians and experienced clinicians working with complicated cases need to be systematic about considering symptoms to arrive at a diagnosis. In situations like this, rating scales or symptom checklists can help support decision making.

12. **Evaluate and integrate information from different informants.** In child and adolescent psychiatry, clinicians gather data from children, their parents, their teachers, and other informants. Thus, clinicians often need to integrate discrepant information. This task is often a matter of clinical judgment whereby the clinician scrutinizes the discrepant data and decides whether both data points are valid and, if not, which informant might be more reliable.

    This process of evaluation and integration takes into account many of the aspects described previously in the "Interpreting Data" section. However, several other rules of thumb may be useful. One example is using the "or" rule: if either informant endorses a symptom, the clinician might count that symptom as positive (Cohen et al. 1987). Another rule of thumb for integrating data is that parents tend to be better informants for externalizing symptoms such as oppositional defiant disorder, whereas children and adolescents are often better reporters for internalizing symptoms (Jensen and Wantanabe 1999). As another example, investigators have demonstrated that parent-rated scales are better predictors of bipolar disorder than are child- or teacher-rated scales (Youngstrom et al. 2004).

13. **Consider the need for several observation opportunities or an extended evaluation.** In some cases, a clinician may have great difficulty giving a definitive diagnosis after one meeting with a child. This problem presents for several reasons. Children and adolescents may take several sessions to be comfortable enough to share (or show) all the data pertinent to an accurate diagnosis. Additionally, for some conditions, mental

status may fluctuate. For example, diagnosing bipolar disorder would be premature if the child presents with manic symptoms during a trial of antidepressants. However, if the child has a manic episode 1 year later that is unrelated to medication, the clinician can be more confident of the bipolar disorder diagnosis.

14. **Use DSM-IV-TR as a framework to structure decision making, but use the Robins and Guze model to conceptualize diagnosis.** DSM-IV-TR is very useful as a framework to structure clinical decision making, and it serves as a bridge to communicate between clinicians and patients using a consistent and validated language. DSM-IV-TR offers clear guidelines and rules on how to consider symptoms, both cross-sectionally and when considering course. For example, it provides guidelines about the length of an episode in bipolar disorder and also for differentiating between psychosis occurring during a mood episode or distinct from a mood episode.

However, DSM-IV-TR may inadvertently lead the unwise user to assume that the causes (and treatments) of the disorder lie only within the child's biological substrate. For this reason, we recommend also considering Robins and Guze's (1970) framework, as well as the child-oriented modifications by Cantwell (1995). Robins and Guze's framework includes distinct clinical characteristics (or symptoms), distinct biological characteristics, genetics, and outcome. This broader framework was introduced to validate and distinguish overlapping disorders; therefore, these different categories are useful when considering diagnosis beyond current phenomenology. For example, for "gray" cases, such as when a child with some manic symptoms does not meet formal DSM-IV-TR criteria for bipolar I disorder but does meet all the criteria for ADHD, the presence of a strong family genetic history of bipolar disorder may help the clinician reconceptualize the problem as emergent bipolar disorder, and give earlier emphasis to selecting bipolar rather than ADHD treatment strategies.

CONCLUSION

In this casebook, the case-writer experts tended to use different methods for data collection, even though we encouraged all to draw upon common data gathering methods, including using reliable and valid rating scales. All of them used the DSM-IV-TR framework, however, and we applaud the extent to which the current DSM edition provides a common framework that, to some extent, guides data collection across clinicians. We caution, however, that whenever data collection frameworks are incomplete or incorrect (i.e., if one only collected DSM-IV-TR symptom information and failed to conduct all necessary aspects of a complete evaluation), all subsequent data synthesis and interpretation steps are likely flawed, including ultimate DSM-IV-TR diagnoses. Nonetheless, we predict that the reader will reach the same conclusion we do: available evidence across our 30 cases suggests that DSM-IV-TR, though always in need of improvement, does fairly well, if accompanied by all the other necessary aspects of a high-quality evaluation.

Even with this common ground, variations in ultimate diagnoses and treatment decisions did occur within cases, despite the fact that all three expert teams drew upon the same observations (i.e., information provided by the case writer[s]). Therefore, to the extent that the three expert teams varied, we suggest that important differences exist among clinicians—even among expert clinicians—in how they synthesize and interpret clinical data and in the extent to which they arrive at the same or different treatment decisions. We hope that this casebook begins to usefully illuminate these differences, lighting the path forward for future studies to better understand diagnostic and treatment decision-making processes. The extent to which clinicians' current differences in decision making reflect biases or incomplete understanding of patients and the success of all future attempts to improve patients' outcomes will depend on how well research studies and diagnostic systems focus and direct this light.

REFERENCES

Achenbach TM: Integrative Guide for the 1991 CBCL/4–18 YSR and TRF Profiles. Burlington, VT, University of Vermont, Department of Psychiatry, 1991

Ajzen I: Intuitive theories of events and the effects of base-rate information on prediction. J Pers Soc Psychol 35:303–314, 1977

Arkes HR, Wortmann RL, Saville PD, et al: Hindsight bias among physicians weighing the likelihood of diagnoses. J Appl Psychol 66:252–254, 1981

Ayanian JZ, Berwick DM: Do physicians have a bias toward action? A classic study revisited. Med Decis Making 11:154–158, 1991

Baron J: Thinking and Deciding, 3rd Edition. Cambridge, UK, Cambridge University Press, 2000

Barrows HS, Feltovich PJ: The clinical reasoning process. Med Educ 21:86–91, 1987

Bergus GR, Chapman GB, Gjerde C, et al: Clinical reasoning about new symptoms in the face of pre-existing disease: sources of error and order effects. Fam Med 27:314–320, 1995

Bernoulli D: Specimen theoriae novae de mensura sortis. Commentarii Academiae Scientrum Imperialis Petropolitanae 5:175–192, 1738 (English translation by Sommer L: Exposition of a new theory of the measurement of risk. Econometrica 22:23–36, 1954)

Bordage G: Why did I miss the diagnosis? Some cognitive explanations and educational implications. Acad Med 74 (suppl 10):S138–S143, 1999

Bordage G, Zacks R: The structure of medical knowledge in the memories of medical students and general practitioners: categories and prototypes. Med Educ 18:406–416, 1984

Bornstein BH, Emler AC: Rationality in medical decision making: a review of the literature on doctors' decision making biases. J Eval Clin Pract 7:97–107, 2001

Bornstein BH, Emler AC, Chapman GB: Rationality in medical treatment decisions: is there a sunk-cost effect? Soc Sci Med 49:215–222, 1999

Bowen JL: Educational strategies to promote clinical diagnostic reasoning. N Engl J Med 355:2217–2225, 2006

Cantwell DP: Child psychiatry: introduction and overview, in Comprehensive Textbook of Psychiatry, 6th Edition. Edited by Kaplan HI, Sadock BJ. Baltimore, MD, Williams & Wilkins, 1995, pp 2151–2154

Casscells W, Schoenberger A, Graboys TB: Interpretation by physicians of clinical laboratory results. N Engl J Med 299:999–1001, 1987

Chang RW, Bordage G, Connell KJ: The importance of early problem representation during case presentations. Acad Med 73 (suppl 10):S109–S111, 1998

Chapman GB, Elstein AS: Cognitive processes and biases in medical decision making, in Decision Making in Health Care: Theory, Psychology and Applications. Edited by Chapman G, Sonnenberg F. Cambridge, UK, Cambridge University Press, 2000, pp 183–210

Chilcoat HD, Breslau N: Does psychiatric history bias mothers' reports? An application of a new analytic approach. J Am Acad Child Adolesc Psychiatry 36:971–979, 1997

Christensen C, Heckerling P, Mackesy-Amiti ME, et al: Pervasiveness of framing effects among physicians and medical students. Journal of Behavioral Decision Making 8:169–180, 1995

Christensen-Szalanski JJJ, Bushyhead JB: Physicians' use of probabilistic information in a real clinical setting. J Exp Psychol Hum Percept Perform 7:928–935, 1981

Cohen P, Cohen J: The clinician's illusion. Arch Gen Psychiatry 41:1178–1182, 1984

Cohen P, Velez N, Kohn M, et al: Child psychiatric diagnosis by computer algorithm: theoretical issues and empirical tests. J Am Acad Child Adolesc Psychiatry 26:631–638, 1987

Custers E, Boshuizen H, Schmidt HG: The influence of medical expertise, case typicality, and illness script component on case processing and disease probability estimates. Mem Cognit 24:384–399, 1996

Dawson NV, Arkes HR: Systematic errors in medical decision making: judgment limitations. J Gen Intern Med 2:183–187, 1987

Dawson NV, Arkes HR, Siciliano C, et al: Hindsight bias: an impediment to accurate probability estimation in clinicopathologic conferences. Med Decis Making 8:259–264, 1988

Eddy DM: Probabilistic reasoning in clinical medicine: problems and opportunities, in Judgment Under Uncertainty: Heuristics and Biases. Edited by Kahneman D, Slovic P, Tversky A. Cambridge, UK, Cambridge University Press, 1982, pp 249–267

Elstein AS: Cognitive processes in clinical inference and decision making, in Reasoning, Inference, and Judgment in Clinical Psychology. Edited by Turk D, Salovey P. New York, Free Press, 1988, pp 17–50

Elstein AS, Schwarz A: Clinical problem solving and diagnostic decision making: selective review of the cognitive literature. BMJ 324:729–732, 2002

Elstein AS, Holzman GB, Ravitch MM, et al: Comparison of physicians' decisions regarding estrogen replacement therapy for menopausal women and decisions derived from a decision analytic model. Am J Med 80:246–258, 1986

Evans DA, Gadd CS: Managing coherence and context in medical problem-solving discourse, in Cognitive Science in Medicine: Biomedical Modeling. Edited by Evans DA, Patel VL. Cambridge, MA, MIT Press, 1989

Feinstein AR: The "chagrin factor" and qualitative decision analysis. Arch Intern Med 145:1257–1259, 1985

Fischhoff B: Hindsight ≠ foresight: the effect of outcome knowledge on judgment under uncertainty. J Exp Psychol Hum Percept Perform 1:288–299, 1975

Galanter CG, Patel VL: Medical decision making: a selective review for child psychiatrists and psychologists. J Child Psychol Psychiatry 46:675–689, 2005

Goodman R: The Strengths and Difficulties Questionnaire: a research note. J Child Psychol Psychiatry 38:581–586, 1997

Graber M, Gordon R, Franklin N: Reducing diagnostic errors in medicine: what's the goal? Acad Med 77:981–992, 2002

Graber ML, Franklin N, Gordon R: Diagnostic error in internal medicine. Arch Intern Med 165:1493–1499, 2005

Gruppen LD, Margolin J, Wisdom K, et al: Outcome bias and cognitive dissonance in evaluating treatment decisions. Acad Med 69 (suppl 10):S57–S59, 1994

Jensen AL, Weisz JR: Assessing match and mismatch between practitioner-generated and standardized interview-generated diagnoses for clinic-referred children and adolescents. J Consult Clin Psychol 70:158–168, 2002

Jensen PS, Wantanabe H: Sherlock Holmes and child psychopathology assessment approaches: the case of the false-positive. J Am Acad Child Adolesc Psychiatry 38:138–146, 1999

Jensen PS, Davis H, Xenakis SN, et al: Child psychopathology rating scales and interrater agreement, II: child and family characteristics. J Am Acad Child Adolesc Psychiatry 27:451–461, 1988a

Jensen PS, Traylor J, Xenakis SN, et al: Child psychopathology rating scales and interrater agreement, I: parents' gender and psychiatric symptoms. J Am Acad Child Adolesc Psychiatry 27:442–450, 1988b

Jensen PS, Knapp P, Mrazek DA: Toward a New Diagnostic System for Child Psychopathology: Moving Beyond the DSM. New York, Guilford, 2006, pp 11–37

Joseph G-M, Patel VL: Domain knowledge and hypothesis generation in diagnostic reasoning. Med Decis Making 10:31–46, 1990

Kahneman D, Tversky A: On the psychology of prediction. Psychol Rev 80:237–251, 1973

Kassirer JP, Kopelman RI: Cognitive errors in diagnosis: instantiation, classification, and consequences. Am J Med 86:433–441, 1989

Kirk SA, Hsieh DK: Diagnostic consistency in assessing conduct disorder: an experiment on the effect of social context. Am J Orthopsychiatry 74:43–55, 2004

Kovacs G, Croskerry P: Clinical decision making: an emergency medicine perspective. Acad Emerg Med 6:947–952, 1999

Lewczyk CM, Garland AF, Hurlburt MS, et al: Comparing DISC-IV and clinician diagnoses among youths receiving public mental health services. J Am Acad Child Adolesc Psychiatry 42:349–356, 2003

Marteau TM: Framing of information: its influence upon decisions of doctors and patients. Br J Soc Psychol 28:89–94, 1989

Mazur DJ, Hickam DH: Treatment preferences of patients and physicians: influences of summary data when framing effects are controlled. Med Decis Making 10:2–5, 1990

McNeil BJ, Pauker SG, Sox HC, et al: On the elicitation of preferences for alternative therapies. N Engl J Med 306:1259–1262, 1982

Miller GA: The magical number seven plus or minus two: some limits on our capacity for processing information. Psychol Rev 63:81–97, 1956

Najman JM, Williams GM, Nikles J, et al: Mothers' mental illness and child behavior problems: cause-effect association or observation bias? J Am Acad Child Adolesc Psychiatry 39:592–602, 2000

Najman JM, Williams GM, Nikles J, et al: Bias influencing maternal reports of child behaviour and emotional state. Soc Psychiatry Psychiatr Epidemiol 36:186–194, 2001

Norman G: Research in clinical reasoning: past history and current trends. Med Educ 39:418–427, 2005

Norman G: Building on experience: the development of clinical reasoning. N Engl J Med 355:2251–2252, 2006

Norman G, Young M, Brooks L: Non-analytical models of clinical reasoning: the role of experience. Med Educ 41:1140–1145, 2007

Pappadopulos E, Jensen PS, Schur SB, et al: "Real world" atypical antipsychotic prescribing practices in public child and adolescent inpatient settings. Schizophr Bull 28:111–121, 2002

Patel VL, Groen GJ: The general and specific nature of medical expertise: a critical look, in Towards a General Theory of Expertise: Prospects and Limits. Edited by Ericsson A, Smith J. Cambridge, UK, Cambridge University Press, 1991, pp 93–125

Patel VL, Evans DA, Kaufman DR: Cognitive framework for doctor-patient interaction, in Cognitive Science in Medicine: Biomedical Modeling. Edited by Evans DA, Patel VL. Cambridge, MA, MIT Press, 1989, pp 257–312

Patel VL, Arocha JF, Kaufman DR: Diagnostic reasoning and expertise. Psychology of Learning and Motivation: Advances in Research and Theory 31:187–252, 1994

Patel VL, Arocha JF, Kaufman DR: A primer on aspects of cognition for medical informatics. J Am Med Inform Assoc 8:324–343, 2001

Piacentini J, Shaffer D, Fisher P, et al: The Diagnostic Interview Schedule for Children—Revised Version (DISC-R), III: concurrent criterion validity. J Am Acad Child Adolesc Psychiatry 32:658–665, 1993

Poses RM, Anthony M: Availability, wishful thinking, and physicians' diagnostic judgments for patients with suspected bacteremia. Med Decis Making 11:159–168, 1991

Redelmeier DA, Shafir E: Medical decision making in situations that offer multiple alternatives. JAMA 273:302–305, 1995

Redelmeier DA, Koehler DJ, Liberman V, et al: Probability judgment in medicine: discounting unspecified possibilities. Med Decis Making 15:227–230, 1995

Robins E, Guze SB: Establishment of diagnostic validity in psychiatric illness: its applicability to schizophrenia. Am J Psychiatry 126:983–987, 1970

Schmidt HG, Norman GR, Boshuizen HPA: A cognitive perspective on medical expertise: theory and implications. Acad Med 65:611–621, 1990

Schwartz JA, Chapman GB: Are more options always better? The attraction effect in physicians' decisions about medications. Med Decis Making 19:315–323, 1999

Sharpe VA, Faden AI: Medical Harm. Cambridge, UK, Cambridge University Press, 1998

Spranca M, Minsk E, Baron J: Omission and commission in judgment and choice. J Exp Soc Psychol 27:76–105, 1991

Tversky A, Kahneman D: Judgment under uncertainty: heuristics and biases. Science 185:1124–1131, 1974

Tversky A, Kahneman D: The framing of decisions and the psychology of choice. Science 211:453–458, 1982

Tversky A, Kahneman D: Advances in prospect theory: cumulative representation of uncertainty. J Risk Uncertain 5:297–323, 1992

Tversky A, Koehler DJ: Support theory: a nonextensional representation of subjective probability. Psychol Rev 101:547–567, 1994

Voytovich AE, Rippey RM, Suffredinin A: Premature conclusions in diagnostic reasoning. J Med Educ 60:302–307, 1985

Wakefield JC, Pottick KJ, Kirk SA: Should the DSM-IV diagnostic criteria for conduct disorder consider social context? Am J Psychiatry 159:380–386, 2002

Wallsten TS: Physician and medical student bias in evaluating diagnostic information. Med Decis Making 1:145–164, 1981

Wigton RS: What do the theories of Egon Brunswik have to say to medical education? Adv Health Sci Educ Theory Pract 13:109–121, 2006

Yates JF: Judgment and Decision-Making. Englewood Cliffs, NJ, Prentice Hall, 1990

Youngstrom EA, Findling RL, Calabrese JR, et al: Comparing the diagnostic accuracy of six potential screening instruments for bipolar disorder in youths aged 5 to 17 years. J Am Acad Child Adolesc Psychiatry 43:847–858, 2004

Zarin DA, Pincus HA, West JC, et al: Practice-based research in psychiatry. Am J Psychiatry 154:1199–1208, 1998

Zito JM, Safer DJ, dosReis S, et al: Psychotherapeutic medication patterns for youths with attention-deficit/hyperactivity disorder. Arch Pediatr Adolesc Med 153:1257–1263, 1999

■ CHAPTER 32 ■

Research and Clinical Perspectives on Diagnostic and Treatment Decision Making

Whence the Future?

Peter S. Jensen, M.D.
David A. Mrazek, M.D., F.R.C.Psych.
Cathryn A. Galanter, M.D.

Since the classic contribution of Robins and Guze (1970), a commonly accepted approach to validating a given set of commonly occurring symptoms has been by demonstration—that is, by showing that the purported disorder demonstrates a number of distinguishing characteristics. More recently, this approach has been modified by Cantwell (1996), with validation of a putative disorder assumed to be accomplished if the candidate disorder can be shown to be discriminable from other disordered states (as well as normal functioning) by any or all of the following: clinical descriptors, psychosocial factors,

David A. Mrazek, M.D., F.R.C.Psych., is Chair of the Department of Psychiatry and Psychology at the Mayo Clinic and Professor of Psychiatry and of Pediatrics at the Mayo Clinic College of Medicine in Rochester, Minnesota (for complete biographical information, see "About the Contributors," p. 613).

Adapted with permission from Jensen PS, Mrazek DA: "Research and Clinical Perspectives in Defining and Assessing Mental Disorders in Children and Adolescents," in *Toward a New Diagnostic System for Child Psychopathology: Moving Beyond the DSM.* Edited by Jensen PS, Knapp P, Mrazek DA. New York, Guilford Press, 2006, pp. 11–37. Copyright 2006, Guilford Press.

demographic factors, biological factors, family genetic factors, family environmental factors, natural history, and response to treatment.

Despite the potential usefulness of this approach, most current diagnoses,
as implemented within DSM-IV (and DSM-IV-TR), fall short of this ideal validation standard. For example, at the 1998 National Institutes of Health Consensus Development Conference on attention-deficit/hyperactivity disorder
(ADHD), the conference panelists concluded that there was *some* evidence of
validity for the diagnosis of ADHD, in terms of a number of these validating
characteristics (principally family genetic factors, natural history, and response
to treatment), but evidence was lacking to support other validating characteristics (e.g., specific biological factors). Notably, Werry et al. (1987) conducted
a careful comparison of these criteria among ADHD, conduct disorder, and
anxiety disorders, finding little support for the discrimination of even these
major syndromes from one another. Despite the lack of validating evidence
concerning the major classification schemas for many of the most common
childhood mental disorders, researchers have done little to pursue this line of
reasoning in the interim, instead taking most of the major disorder categories at
face value (if only by default) or, when conducting comparisons, confining the
categories principally to either cases of disorder versus normal controls or comorbid versus noncomorbid cases (e.g., see Jensen et al. 2002). Work groups
on the upcoming DSM-V (due to be published in 2012) may be addressing
some of these issues, such as whether the symptoms of ADHD need be present
prior to age 7 years for an individual to qualify for the disorder.

This situation is not unique to childhood disorders but also bedevils most
adult conditions defined by DSM-IV-TR. Thus, if one asks whether the current
DSM "carves nature at its joints," the research literature principally answers in
the negative. For example, in a study of the diagnostic criteria for depression using a sample of monozygotic and dizygotic twins, Kendler and Gardner (1998)
examined the diagnostic criteria for number of symptoms, severity, and duration, finding that number of symptoms and severity (but not duration) predicted
increased likelihood of subsequent episodes in both the index case and the
twin. However, a natural cut point did not occur at four symptoms; even persons with fewer than five symptoms, as well as those having less severe symptoms (below diagnostic threshold), were at greater risk for subsequent episodes
of depression, both in the index case and the twin. These findings suggested
that even subthreshold depressive symptoms reveal the same underlying diathesis. In addition, no support was found for the requirement of 2 weeks' duration or some threshold of clinical severity. Thus, major depressive disorder
appeared to be a diagnostic convention imposed on a continuum of depressive
symptoms of varying severity, impairment, and duration. Similar findings have
been found in the area of genetic studies of ADHD, where heritability analyses

of full-syndrome versus subthreshold symptom states suggested that the condition likely reflected a continuum versus an all-or-none, present-absent psychopathological state (Levy et al. 1997; Rasmussen et al. 2002).

DISORDER DEFINITION VERSUS MEDICAL NECESSITY

Despite the well-specified criteria in the most recent DSM versions, different methods of determining the presence or absence of these criteria can have a profound impact on prevalence estimates. For example, Boyle et al. (1996) found that differing strategies, such as using a 3-point checklist that inquires about the presence of symptoms on a frequency scale (*0=never; 1=sometimes; 2=often*), a structured diagnostic interview, or statistical strategies that require a range of deviation from the norm, result in dramatic (120-fold) differences in prevalence (Boyle et al. 1996), as well as substantial differences in test-retest reliability, interrater reliability, and comorbidity. Thus, a range of methodological issues—including the type of measurement instrument, nature of the informant (e.g., parent, teacher, child), scoring system, chosen cutoffs for symptom levels and symptom severity—can contribute to substantial variations in mental disorder caseness determination. As a result, the general conclusion is that the presence of the diagnostic criteria alone is insufficient for determining "when a case is a case" (Boyle et al. 1996).

Even when one determines the presence or absence of symptoms using the most rigorous methods, such as face-to-face diagnostic interviews, variations in mental disorder definition are marked, based on ancillary determinations that are not necessarily part of the DSM criteria. For example, Angold et al. (1999) examined the impact of various definitions of *impairment* on rates of serious emotional disturbance, after first requiring that all children considered meet all DSM-III-R symptomatic criteria. Using five different definitions of *impairment* in their study, Angold et al. compared children with neither impairment nor a diagnosis, those with no full-blown disorder but with impairment, those with disorder but no impairment, and those with both disorder and impairment. Even among those who met both symptom and more stringent impairment criteria, only 59% reported "need for services," and fewer still (19%) of those meeting diagnostic criteria with levels of impairment as specified within the DSM-III-R criteria reported any need for services. Even with the most stringent impairment criteria, two-thirds of those with a defined serious emotional disturbance were not being served.

In an important sense, then, clinicians, researchers, and clinical policy makers wishing for precision in the determination of mental disorder have been troubled by the major differences in reported prevalence rates in state-of-the-art studies intended to address this major question, such as the dramatic (more than threefold, in some instances) differences in prevalence rates in the National Institute of Mental Health Epidemiologic Catchment Area study and the National Comorbidity Survey (Regier et al. 1998). To address this problem, particularly because the differences in prevalence rates occur principally around more commonly occurring syndromes, and to avoid future controversies that may incite suspicion or ridicule from opponents of parity for mental health care, Regier et al. (1998) recommended that only the more severe disorders with public policy implications be examined in future epidemiological studies. Recounting the differences between epidemiological survey–identified "cases" and clinically identified cases, they noted that community-defined cases are not likely to be as severe, and may in fact be transient, "nonpathologic homeostatic responses." Yet, as noted by Spitzer (1998), both the Epidemiologic Catchment Area study and the National Comorbidity Survey accounts of disorder are similarly related to external validators of psychopathology, suggesting that both measured something valid. Spitzer (1998) cautioned that researchers should not confuse the identification of valid syndromes with the need for treatment, either by avoiding such studies altogether or by requiring extraordinary levels of impairment to justify determination of mental disorder, just to appease a skeptical public, when such conditions are indeed valid disorders.

This situation may not differ much from other areas of medicine—thus, if respiratory disease specialists were to conduct surveys of the nationwide prevalence of "respiratory illness," inclusion of conditions ranging from upper respiratory illness, chronic obstructive pulmonary disease, and asthma to mild upper respiratory illnesses would likely result in nearly 100% rates of "disorder." Turning the question on its head, Spitzer (1998) asked why the field of psychiatry needs such studies when other areas of medicine do not.

Frances (1998) suggested that there are indeed clear limitations in defining clinical cases within epidemiological studies, in part because DSM fails to provide clear boundaries between normality and psychopathology, and also because the concepts of *clinical significance* and *medical necessity* are difficult to operationalize and beyond the capability of lay interviewers. In addition, given the inherent variability in rates of disorder across settings, times, and cultures, epidemiological studies may overestimate the prevalence and/or significance of milder conditions.

To avoid the conceptual muddles noted above, to answer the question "When is a case a case?" the first issue that must be addressed is "a case for what purpose?" For example, Sonuga-Barke (1998) noted that to distinguish between various definitions of disorder, one must clarify whether one wishes to define mental disorder for purposes of the clinical utility of such a definition (the "pragmatic" view) and construct validity (the ontological view). Although the ultimate goal of classification is *usefulness* (Frances 1998), as Eisenberg (1995) noted, there are many "usefulnesses." What works for researchers to define some presumably homogeneous entity (i.e., the attempt to "carve nature at its joints") may not work well for clinicians and policy makers, who often wish to know "who needs care."

Consistent with Galanter and Jensen's recommendations in Chapter 31, one potential route out of such impasses of objectives was first described by Zarin and Earls (1993), who recommended that methods of decision analysis be applied to such issues. They noted that the essential components of diagnostic decision making—choice of external validator, choice of discriminator, and choice of cutoff scores—might be implemented very differently, depending on the clinician investigator's objective: 1) to determine which children need psychiatric care, where overall assessments of disability are most relevant; 2) to determine what clinicians do in real-world practice—that is, services research, which often varies from the "ideal world" practice; or 3) to determine which children are valid cases of a specific disorder, for purposes of research into etiology, genetic factors, treatment response, and likelihood of persistence and/or recurrence.

Thus, "caseness for what purpose" is the relevant question, and one must appreciate that any cutoff or disciminator will result in some false negatives and some false positives. The choice of cutoffs will often depend on the relative costs of false negatives versus false positives, vis-à-vis the clinical or research objectives.

PROBLEMS IN DEFINING CASENESS OF MENTAL DISORDER

Inspection of the range of challenges in determining mental disorder caseness in children and adolescents suggests that many of these issues are not unique to children and adolescents per se, but are shared with the caseness challenges that are part and parcel of adult studies (as noted above), as well as with other aspects of medicine. These issues include questions concerning categorical versus dimensional distinctions, choice of cutoffs, distinguishing diagnosis from the need for treatment, cultural factors affecting diagnosis and impairment, and the role of context. With children, however, a set of somewhat unique items appear of relatively greater import in defining mental disorder within child and adolescent populations, namely, the role of children's caretaking environments vis-à-vis mental disorder, determining how to combine information from multiple informants, and special considerations that must be taken into account with young persons, principally as a function of the rapid rates of change occurring within their biological, psychological, and social capacities. We discuss these special challenges below, beginning first with those issues common to children and adults.

CATEGORIES VERSUS DIMENSIONS

A major conceptual consideration underpinning determination of mental disorder involves reflection about 1) whether the underlying construct is a true category, qualitatively different from other disordered as well as normal states, or 2) whether caseness simply reflects difficulties in functioning at the extreme end of a continuum. Although most psychiatric disorders, child and adult alike, can be shown to be quantitatively different from "normal" states, such differences do not necessarily reflect qualitative differences. Large differences between two groups on a number of markers do not necessarily make them different in kind. For example, tall persons and short persons are not said to be from two different species simply because there appears to be a "tall syndrome"—weighing a lot, having long fingers, and requiring large hat sizes. Both quantitative and qualitative distinctions are needed to make an effective argument that a "mental disorder" requires the presence of differences in kind. Finding different kinds *might* constitute a partial argument in support of a particular definition of mental disorder, yet both quantitative and qualitative differences are needed to make the case for different kinds. Although two different kinds, even when such can be identified, may have the same final common pathway, in terms of the observable phenomenology, two cases of the same kind may have very different outcomes, making the sole use of qualitative distinctions as an indicator of mental disorder problematic (Andreasen et al. 1988). To use the model of height, being short alone does not indicate whether someone is "pathologically" short or normally short. This differentiation requires knowledge of other associated factors, such as the presence of a disturbance in an endocrine system or bone metabolism (Eisenberg 1995).

At present, little evidence is available to indicate *natural* dichotomies between "cases" and "noncases" in child and adolescent psychopathology. That is, even for disorders for which a great deal of empirical evidence has been brought to bear on the selection of thresholds between normality and disorder in DSM-IV (e.g., Lahey et al. 1994), DSM-IV diagnoses are perhaps best considered to represent expert judgments more than natural dichotomies. This view has led many scholars to advocate *dimensional* approaches to the definition and assessment of child and adolescent psychopathology rather than *categorical* diagnostic approaches. Yet both clinical practice and policy making often require dichotomous decisions about the mental health of youths. Clinicians must make dichotomous decisions to treat or withhold treatment on a daily basis; researchers seek to classify the "phenotypes" of psychopathology to conduct neurobiological and genetic studies; and policy makers often engage in activities such as counting the number of youths who need but have not received mental health services. Thus, a tension exists between the need for categorical definitions of mental disorder for many important purposes and the lack of evidence to support such dichotomous categorizations.

Cutoffs and Their Determination

Because qualitative distinctions have been difficult to demonstrate and, even when demonstrable, do not appear to be a fully trustworthy guide to caseness determination, clinicians and researchers alike rely on some more or less arbitrary cutoff on a severity or impairment dimension to determine caseness. Other than severity and impairment, factors that have been considered as potential cutoffs for determination of mental disorder include the family's acknowledgment of the need for treatment, their considering the child's condition a "problem," and the degree of family burden (Angold et al. 1998). At least in part, the search for appropriate cutoffs has been spurred on by the fact that the sole application of DSM criteria has yielded implausibly high rates of disorder for those wanting to make arguments for parity of health coverage for these conditions (Regier et al. 1998; Spitzer 1998). In addition, the presence of a diagnosis does not necessarily indicate the need for treatment, any more than the presence of a mild upper respiratory infection or warts necessitates commitment of health care dollars or treatment resources—even though most would agree that such conditions are not "normal" from the perspective of actual differences in tissue structure and/or function.

The Impairment Criterion

The most common cutoff applied to determine mental disorder caseness is the construct of impairment, such that to be considered a true case of disorder, one must suffer from some degree of impairment. This is an interesting distinction, and one not necessarily applied equally to other supposed disorders. For example, persons with hypertension may have no apparent impairment at the time of diagnosis, and treatment is employed because of the statistical likelihood of future impairment as a result of the untreated condition. In fact, the treatment itself is likely to result in side effects that could be reasonably construed as impairment.

Even if one accepts that impairment is needed to establish mental disorder caseness, the problem of determining the precise cutoff for the degree of impairment is inescapable. Although a number of strategies have been employed to minimize the numbers of false positives and false negatives (Hsiao et al. 1989; Lahey et al. 1994; Piacentini et al. 1992), such strategies still must rely on some other criterion against which the determination of a "false" positive or negative is made. Critical considerations are how much impairment and as judged by whom. The requirement of impairment may seem a comfortable position at first glance, but close inspection reveals that the many definitions of *impairment* can yield dramatically different rates of disorder (Angold et al. 1999).

Similarly, it is not uncommon that a child, or adult for that matter, will be severely impaired and have many symptoms of a disorder but not meet full DSM-IV-TR criteria. For example, subthreshold major depressive disorder or symptoms of depression not meeting full DSM-IV-TR criteria for major depressive disorder are often associated with impairment. Moreover, children and adolescents who do not meet full criteria for a disorder but have many symptoms as well as impairment have a high rate of conversion to the disorder. For example, the Course and Outcome of Bipolar Youth Study purposely enrolled youth who did not meet full criteria for bipolar disorder but who were impaired. Most of these youth did not meet criteria because their episodes were too brief. Approximately 30% of them converted to bipolar I or II disorder within a 2-year follow-up period (Birmaher et al. 2006).

In part, the current requirement for impairment as embodied in DSM-IV (and DSM-IV-TR) stems from the fact that clinicians have no sure knowledge of the underlying disease processes for mental disorders, children's as well as adults'. As with hypertension, the presence of an asymptomatic malignant tumor, while not resulting in current impairment, is known to have certain consequences if left untreated; therefore, medical necessity is generally taken for granted. From a symptomatic perspective, asymptomatic hypertension and tumors might be viewed as analogues to mental disorders' "subthreshold" conditions. For example, once reliable markers have been obtained for the likelihood of future onsets of autism, mood disorders, or schizophrenia, prevention and early intervention strategies become possible. Eisenberg (1995) noted that as science progresses, so do the assumptions of what constitutes mental disorder. Over 100 years ago, knowledge of hemoglobinopathies such as thalassemia was limited to the overdescription of the clinical phenomenology of symptoms and affected bodily organs. After decades of research, precise knowledge of the point mutations in the molecular structure of the hemoglobin molecule underlying these conditions is now available, and persons totally asymptomatic can be identified and are considered "cases" from the perspective of prevention, early intervention, and genetic counseling. With time, better knowledge of the basic neural, psychological, and social processes underlying the mental disorders should allow clinicians to worry less about what should be a "case" and more about the health merits and ethical issues involved in intervening with an illness process that is reasonably well understood, at least in terms of prediction of subsequent health impairments.

CULTURAL AND CONTEXTUAL CONSIDERATIONS

As noted by many commentators on most recent versions of DSM, cultural factors play an important role in determining when a "symptom" is a symptom, what constitutes impairment, and which cases need treatment. Rogler (1993) noted that a fine-grained analysis of psychotic symptoms with highly structured diagnostic instruments is difficult to make without knowledge of the culture's social values and traditions. Even when question items are appropriately translated, the language and culture may use constructs that do not map neatly onto

DSM. For example, Manson (1995) noted that one item from the Diagnostic Interview Schedule that combined guilt, shame, and sinfulness required three different questions among Hopi, to avoid confounding different items and meanings. Rogler (1993) noted that the configuring of symptoms into disorders may require some changes from culture to culture, yet few studies have taken these issues fully into account. By way of exception, Canino et al. (1987), in implementing an epidemiological survey of Puerto Rico, not only conducted tests to ascertain the reliability and validity of the diagnostic instruments but also added new items as needed and changed algorithms for various disorders in Puerto Rico. As a consequence of these changes, they found 66% lower disorder rates of obsessive-compulsive disorder using the adjusted algorithms than using the unadjusted diagnostic algorithms. In contrast, dysthymia was 60% higher (Rogler 1993) when adjusting for cultural factors.

Within a given culture, symptoms, impairment, and mental disorder are likely to be defined in the context of what is expected and "normal" within that culture, rather than because of some underlying etiological process or biological substrate (Cantwell 1996). Therefore, current diagnostic systems such as DSM-IV-TR have a nearly impossible task of trying to accomplish a reliable description for all possible purposes, even though "purposes" are likely to vary greatly from setting to setting and culture to culture. For example, from various studies of children in Puerto Rico (Piacentini et al. 1992; Shaffer et al. 1996), although parents of Puerto Rican children rate their children as having somewhat more symptoms on the Child Behavior Checklist and similar levels of symptoms on face-to-face diagnostic interviews using the Diagnostic Interview Schedule for Children (compared to mainland U.S. samples), they attribute much lower levels of overall impairment to those same symptoms than do parents of mainland children (Shaffer et al. 1996).

Rather than reifying a "mental disorder" as a simple symptom count that crosses some relatively arbitrary threshold, Rogler (1993) suggested that within given cultures, a quick decision with substantial face validity can be accomplished for many purposes to avoid attributing symptom, case, or impairment status to conditions or situations that actually reflect some form of goal-directed, culturally situated behavior. Although this idea is eminently sensible, we are unaware of any systematic testing of such approaches to determine whether they can be reliably done and whether multiple, culturally informed raters would agree among themselves with such "face valid" decisions. This recommendation hearkens back to the etiological diagnostic formulations of previous DSMs, but such an approach, if cautiously implemented, even in Anglo-American cultures, may help avoid according mental disorder status to some conditions that many would regard instead as adaptive responses (e.g., certain forms of conduct disorder; Richters and Cicchetti 1993) and avoid criticisms that diagnostic approaches too often ignore the obvious (Jensen and Hoagwood 1997).

In an important sense, expert clinicians' judgments concerning symptom, impairment, and mental disorder status that make use of all available data over time are an irreplaceable LEAD (Spitzer 1983), if not gold standard, yet such judgments also are situated in culture and time, reflecting in part both scientific findings and cultural norms (Eisenberg 1995). As culture changes or science advances, these determinations do as well. To this extent, the judgment of what constitutes a "case" (in terms of medical necessity or need for treatment) can never be fully satisfied by statistical approaches or complex equations, and must instead take into account societal values, willingness to pay, determination of what constitutes a "problem in living" versus a disorder (e.g., the boundaries between transient sadness and major depressive disorder), and the assembled experience and norms of the expert mental health care providers within that cultural context. Without some metric that has carefully calibrated itself by taking into account these dimensions, any determination of "mental disorder" (apart from scientifically established qualitative differences in underlying disease processes) must remain more or less arbitrary.

CHILDREN'S CARETAKING ENVIRONMENTS

Important contextual considerations concerning impairment pertain to the finding that under many circumstances, persons may be impaired, yet their symptom picture is such that it does not fit full DSM criteria. For example, Angold et al. (1999) noted that a substantial subset of children evidence quite substantial impairment, yet these children often only meet criteria for various V codes. Nonetheless, along a number of important external validators, these same children can be shown to suffer substantially and can benefit from treatment. Most frequently, these difficulties are problems concerning their external surroundings, particularly their caretaking environments. Although such difficulties might also be considered "problems in living," a substantial body of evidence suggests that these difficulties are related to the onset and persistence of diagnosable conditions. To the extent that such conditions may reflect pathogenic processes that result in current suffering and may consolidate over time into an enduring pattern of problematic behavior, such situations may be on a par with other latent disease processes whose effects are only seen over time (e.g., hypertension) yet which are afforded full disorder status. To address this problem, Angold et al. (1999) recommended that greater use be made of the not otherwise specified (NOS) category, because children categorized as having an NOS disorder usually need and benefit from care at the same levels of those who meet traditional DSM disorder status. Similarly, Emde (1994) and others have suggested that alternative diagnostic schemas are required to include "relationship disorders," particularly in the early years of life. However, such schemas might also be applicable to other ages. But in young children, individual problems are so embedded in the caregiving relationships that their primary diagnostic location may need to occur at the level of the relationship, because interventions and process-based understanding are most explanatory at that level of analysis (Anders 1992). Other approaches to this problem, including the development of new axes (Global Assessment of Relational Functioning scale 1996), have been proposed, but these ideas thus far have not received widespread acceptance.

MENTAL DISORDER DEFINITIONS FOR DIFFERENT AGES, ETHNIC GROUPS, OR GENDERS

It is not clear at this point whether the most valid definitions of child and adolescent psychopathology should or should not differ according to the individual's age, gender, or ethnicity. Similarly, it is not known if different measures of distress and impairment would optimize the identification of impaired cases in youths of different ages, genders, and ethnicities, apart from the cultural factors noted above. Different symptoms, or different symptom thresholds, might identify impaired youths at different ages or with different demographic characteristics, but this possibility has not been adequately examined to date. Some evidence in this regard can be found in examining national norms that have been developed for instruments such as the Child Behavior Checklist, where youths of differing ages and genders had differing symptom profiles and actual symptom levels, yet how this information should map onto definitions of mental disorder is not clear (Achenbach 1995). Although an array of epidemiological evidence suggests that children of different ages and genders are at a greater risk for various disorders and comorbidities (Nottelmann and Jensen 1995), beyond differences in rates, it is not clear whether there are actually different syndromes in these subgroups.

Differences in psychopathology related to age, gender, and ethnicity are unlikely to be identified, however, unless professionals look for them. Future studies that allow comparisons among representative samples of youths of different ages, genders, and ethnicities should include diagnostic criteria for which differences might be expected. For example, in the study of gender differences in psychopathology, the inclusion of items describing "relational aggression" (Crick et al. 1997) may reveal gender differences in conduct disorder that would not be identified if these items were not included. In the case of ethnic differences, the inclusion of the few symptoms of *ataque de nervios* that are not included in other DSM-IV-TR syndromes would allow clinicians to determine if this potential culturally specific syndrome is found in Hispanic adolescents but not in adolescents from other ethnic groups. The inclusion of a small number of such additional items in future population-based studies would be of great importance to the understanding of potential age, gender, and ethnic differences in psychopathology.

A final important consideration that must be addressed in considering issues of caseness in children and adolescents is the issue of children's actual trajectories of functioning. Given the rapidly evolving nature of the child's burgeoning capacities, important information can be gleaned from the *rate* of the child's growth and development, and evidence of delays (e.g., failure to thrive, mental or growth retardation) might constitute grounds for consideration of caseness. A major impediment to such issues in the case of children and adolescents is the fact that as currently written, diagnostic criteria are static across ages and, as a general rule, symptoms presenting at most ages are taken at face value without consideration of the extent to which a given symptom (e.g., motor activity, inattention, fears of specific objects, separation fears, aggression to others) may actually be normative at given ages. Although no good evidence to date indicates that such considerations make any difference (e.g., Ryan et al. 1987), these issues have been insufficiently explored, and studies that have examined these questions have likely been greatly underpowered, particularly when examining these issues in nonclinical settings.

WHAT THE SENSIBLE CLINICIAN SHOULD DO

In our view, the experienced clinician takes into account the above-mentioned issues—that is, not placing too much emphasis on categorical versus dimensional distinctions, distinguishing diagnosis from the need for treatment, examining the impact of cultural factors on diagnosis and impairment, evaluating the role of context and caretaking factors, evaluating and when appropriate combining information from multiple informants, and carefully considering developmental factors. In an attempt to characterize this process, we suggest that a reasonable clinician consider doing the following, though not necessarily in this order:

1. Determine the nature of the presenting problems/chief complaints, considering who needs help and why.
2. Evaluate the developmental nature of symptoms.
3. Examine cultural and contextual factors affecting presentations.
4. Ascertain levels of impairment.
5. Understand key aspects of the syndrome.
6. Determine the presence of comorbidity and other factors that may affect choice and/or ordering of treatments.

In contrast to using research-based approaches that often focus principally on assessing symptoms primarily conceptualized as "within the child," working with these additional considerations requires a "Meyerian" (Adolf) approach to historical diagnosis (Lief 1948). "An accurate diagnosis much more akin to detective work or archeology—a quasijudicial procedure," according to Meehl (1973). Figure 32–1 shows how a sensible clinician might approach the complex mass of information presented by a patient and family, and how this clinician can organize his or her approach to intervention. Notably, such an approach to intervention does not necessarily presume the same approach or prioritization of etiological factors.

As suggested by Figure 32–1, a number of moderating factors may affect the clinician's decision making or recommendations in the ordering, timing, and/or combining of treatments. Such factors include 1) the child's degree of impairment (with more impairment, most clinicians will increase the range, type, and amount of treatments); 2) interference with developmental lines (with presumed interference, the clinician may be more likely to make or suggest environmental modifications that serve to increase the child's developmental opportunities, with the assumption that normal developmental processes will take hold if not otherwise thwarted); 3) the responsiveness of the child's problem to intervention type(s) (all things being equal, the clinician is likely to recommend or choose specific treatments known to impact the disorder, symptom, or type of impairment); and 4) setting specificity of the problem and the intervention (if problems are setting specific, the clinician is likely to target the intervention to that setting).

In addition to these considerations, however, several other principles are likely to operate to guide clinicians' decision making: individualizing the clinical approach and working with families in the therapeutic process described.

INDIVIDUALIZED CLINICAL APPROACH

Given the enormous complexity of the range of factors shaping the child's clinical presentation, treatment approaches must embed and tailor the intervention within the child's specific developmental stage/status and ecological niche. Such considerations mean that the clinician must of necessity take into careful account whether an intervention will be implemented in a single setting or must cross multiple settings (e.g., home, school), whether it should focus on one or multiple domains of functioning (e.g., self-concept, parent-child behavior management, peer relationships), and how it should incorporate a family's values and inputs into the treatment design and selection.

Almost no areas of medicine use a "one size fits all" approach to treating pathology: medication dosages are adjusted to a patient's body size or surface area, the pace and order of cancer chemotherapies are changed to address each patient's type and severity of side effects, and even surgical procedures are modified to be better tolerated by frail or compromised patients. Likewise, a good clinician

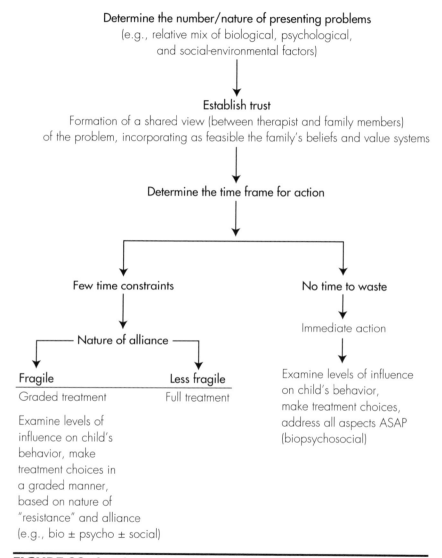

FIGURE 32–1. Sensible clinician's approach to intervention.

worth his or her salt does not continue with a tightly focused didactic approach with parents if significant dissension between parents threatens to scuttle the entire therapeutic enterprise. Nor does a skilled therapist continue trying to "unload" his or her therapeutic goods on a family if overarching issues of trust/distrust or like/dislike seem to be undermining the family's confidence in the therapist's abilities. Yet too many of the modern-day managed care–driven treatments seem to forget that these issues are paramount to the integrity of the treatment.

PARENTS AND FAMILIES AS PARTNERS IN THE THERAPEUTIC PROCESS

To address concerns about the palatability of therapies to families, an effective clinician is usually very attentive to relating to children and families as partners in the therapeutic process. Therapies that fail to build this principle into the approach to families are likely to miss a critical component of treatment effectiveness. Unlike more traditional biomedical procedures that are presumably active once the intervention has been delivered or ingested (e.g., medications), the psychotherapies are inextricably intertwined with the psychopathological conditions, to the extent that both are embedded in behavioral patterns of human social exchange. Without the full enlistment of all critical family members in using their behaviors to change the child's behaviors, success is much less certain. This recruitment of family effort is possible only to the extent that the therapy itself represents a *partnership* between therapist and family participants, and to the degree that the therapist communicates this principle effectively and convincingly to these would-be therapeutic partners. Such partnerships, both in the course of pharmacotherapy and/or psychotherapy, are key to long-term success.

PUTTING IT ALL TOGETHER: UNDERSTANDING AND APPLYING PRINCIPLES OF BEHAVIOR CHANGE

Clinicians should proceed with treatment only if 1) they possess a clear theory and/or understanding of the principles of treatment (e.g., what are the *necessary though not sufficient* elements of change in this treatment paradigm); 2) given these therapeutic principles, they know what types of person- or family-specific obstacles may hamper the delivery and effectiveness of the treatment (including the family's commitment to *the therapeutic partnership*); and 3) they know which modifications in pacing, ordering, and timing of treatments must be accommodated to minimize the effects of these potential obstacles on the active components of treatment. For example, an overarching hierarchy of therapeutic principles (based on the clinicians' best "wisdom") might be constructed that supersedes (or must precede) the implementation of an effective psychosocial intervention. Such principles might include the family's/parents' need for control and autonomy in directing family affairs, the apparent consistency of an intervention with the family's values, sufficient marital harmony so that both parents can actively support the intervention, trust and/or liking for the therapist, the apparent sensibility and credibility of the intervention to the family, the "fairness" of the intervention to family members affected by it, the family partners' ability to "attend to" and learn the intervention, and the presence of appropriate and sufficient emotional reserves and equilibrium in those who must deliver and receive the intervention.

Together, the presence of these therapeutic principles coupled with elements or principles of change might constitute the *necessary and sufficient* ingredients to deliver a reasonably effective psychosocial intervention with an active treatment component. However, in a *therapeutic partnership*, some autonomy is likely to be surrendered to the partner/therapist (if change is to occur), but this best occurs in the presence of trust, liking, and confidence in the therapist. If the intervention is inconsistent with family values, seems unfair, or "just doesn't make sense" from the family's perspective, a very high degree of trust is needed before such an intervention can proceed (if at all), or the differences between the therapist's and family's values and treatment rationales must be fully adjudicated. Likewise, the presence of marital difficulties, preoccupation with other problems, or severe emotional distress (sadness, anger, anxiety) in any of the therapeutic partners must be monitored. Just as the cancer chemotherapist delays the delivery of more antitumor agents when the platelets drop too low, the psychotherapist monitors these core emotional levels within the family therapeutic partners and at critical junctures addresses these issues directly, in the service of providing the most effective psychotherapy for the child's identified difficulties.

We close this chapter by noting the enormity of the decision-making challenges that face a clinician who attempts to deal with a troubled child and concerned family. Although DSM-IV-TR provides much guidance, diagnostic categories often fail to capture the critical issues of context, a child's development, and the nature of the child's fit within his or her particular setting. However, keeping so many issues and clinical principles in view is difficult for the clinician when facing diagnostic and treatment decision–making challenges. We suggest that there are indeed models and theories that are simultaneously developmental, contextual, and adaptational, and that accord with much of the basic research that guides modern-day biology (e.g., see Jensen et al. 2006). Sustained dialogues among clinicians, researchers, and DSM developers are essential to continuing the improvement in mapping DSM approaches to patients. We hope that this casebook will constitute a useful stimulus to these dialogues.

REFERENCES

Achenbach TM: Empirically based assessment and taxonomy: applications to clinical research. Psychol Assess 7:261–274, 1995

Anders TF: Clinical syndromes, relationship disturbances, and their assessment, in Relationship Disturbances in Early Childhood: A Developmental Approach. Edited by Sameroff AJ, Emde RN. New York, Basic Books, 1992, pp 125–144

Andreasen NC, Shore D, Burke JD, et al: Clinical phenomenology. Schizophr Bull 14:345–363, 1988

Angold A, Messer SC, Stangl D, et al: Perceived parental burden and service use for child and adolescent psychiatric disorders. Am J Public Health 88:75–80, 1998

Angold A, Costello EJ, Farmer EM, et al: Impaired but undiagnosed. J Am Acad Child Adolesc Psychiatry 38:129–137, 1999

Birmaher B, Axelson D, Strober M, et al: Clinical course of children and adolescents with bipolar spectrum disorders. Arch Gen Psychiatry 63:175–183, 2006

Boyle MH, Offord DR, Racine Y, et al: Identifying thresholds for classifying childhood psychiatric disorder: issues and prospects. J Am Acad Child Adolesc Psychiatry 35:1440–1448, 1996

Canino GJ, Bird HR, Shrout PE, et al: The prevalence of specific psychiatric disorders in Puerto Rico. Arch Gen Psychiatry 44:727–735, 1987

Cantwell DP: Classification of child and adolescent psychopathology. J Child Psychol Psychiatry 37:3–12, 1996

Crick NR, Casa JF, Mosher M: Relational and overt aggression in preschool. Dev Psychol 33:579–588, 1997

Eisenberg L: Doing away with the illusion of homogeneity: medical progress through disease identification. First Leo Kanner Lecture, Division of Child and Adolescent Psychiatry, Johns Hopkins Hospital, Baltimore, MD, June 9, 1995

Emde R: Individuality, context, and the search for meaning. Child Dev 65:719–737, 1994

Frances A: Problems in defining clinical significance in epidemiological studies. Arch Gen Psychiatry 55:119, 1998

Global Assessment of Relational Functioning scale (GARF), I: background and rationale. Group for the Advancement of Psychiatry Committee on the Family. Fam Process 35:155–172, 1996

Hsiao JK, Bartko JJ, Potter WZ: Diagnosing diagnoses: receiver operating characteristic methods and psychiatry. Arch Gen Psychiatry 46:664–667, 1989

Jensen PS, Hoagwood K: The book of names: DSM-IV in context. Dev Psychopathol 9:231–249, 1997

Jensen PS, and members of the MTA Cooperative Group: ADHD comorbidity findings from the MTA Study: new diagnostic subtypes and their optimal treatments, in Defining Psychopathology in the 21st Century: DSM-V and Beyond. Edited by Helzer JE, Hudziak JJ. Washington, DC, American Psychiatric Publishing, 2002, pp 169–192

Jensen PS, Knapp P, Mrazek DA (eds): Toward a New Diagnostic System for Child Psychopathology: Moving Beyond the DSM. New York, Guilford, 2006

Kendler KS, Gardner CO: Boundaries of major depression: an evaluation of DSM-IV criteria. Am J Psychiatry 55:172–177, 1998

Lahey BB, Applegate B, McBurnett K, et al: DSM-IV trials for attention deficit hyperactivity disorder in children and adolescents. Am J Psychiatry 151:1673–1685, 1994

Levy F, Hay DA, McStephen M, et al: Attention-deficit hyperactivity disorder: a category or continuum? Genetic analysis of a large-scale twin study. J Am Acad Child Adolesc Psychiatry 36:737–744, 1997

Lief A (ed): The Commonsense Psychiatry of Dr Adolf Meyer. New York, McGraw-Hill, 1948

Manson SM: Culture and major depression: current challenges in the diagnosis of mood disorders. Psychiatr Clin North Am 18:487–501, 1995

Meehl PE: When shall we use our heads instead of a formula? in Psychodiagnosis: Selected Papers. Edited by Meehl. New York, WW Norton, 1973, pp 81–89

Nottelmann ED, Jensen PS: Bipolar affective disorder in children and adolescents. J Am Acad Child Adolesc Psychiatry 34:705–708, 1995

Piacentini JC, Cohen P, Cohen J: Combining discrepant diagnostic information from multiple sources: are complex algorithms better than simple ones? J Abnorm Child Psychol 20:51–63, 1992

Rasmussen ER, Neuman RJ, Heath AC, et al: Replication of the latent class structure of attention-deficit/hyperactivity disorder (ADHD) subtypes in a sample of Australian twins. J Child Psychol Psychiatry 43:1018–1028, 2002

Regier DA, Kaelber CT, Rae DS, et al: Limitations of diagnostic criteria and assessment instruments for mental disorders: implications for research and policy. Arch Gen Psychiatry 55:109–115, 1998

Richters JE, Cicchetti D: Mark Twain meets DSM-III-R: conduct disorder, development, and the concept of harmful dysfunction. Dev Psychopathol 5:5–29, 1993

Robins E, Guze SB: Establishment of diagnostic validity in psychiatric illness: its application to schizophrenia. Am J Psychiatry 126:983–987, 1970

Rogler LH: Culture in psychiatric diagnosis: an issue of scientific accuracy. Psychiatry 56:324–327, 1993

Ryan ND, Puig-Antich J, Ambrosini P, et al: The clinical picture of major depression in children and adolescents. Arch Gen Psychiatry 44:854–861, 1987

Shaffer D, Fisher P, Dulcan MK, et al: The NIMH Diagnostic Interview Schedule for Children Version 2.3 (DISC-2.3): description, acceptability, prevalence rates, and performance in the MECA Study (Methods for the Epidemiology of Child and Adolescent Mental Disorders Study). J Am Acad Child Adolesc Psychiatry 35:865–877, 1996

Sonuga-Barke EJ: Categorical models of childhood disorder: a conceptual and empirical analysis. J Child Psychol Psychiatry 39:115–133, 1998

Spitzer RL: Psychiatric diagnosis: are clinicians still necessary? Compr Psychiatry 24:399–411, 1983

Spitzer RL: Diagnosis and need for treatment are not the same. Arch Gen Psychiatry 55:119, 1998

Werry JS, Reeves JC, Elkind GS: Attention deficit, conduct, oppositional, and anxiety disorders in children, I: a review of research on differentiating characteristics. J Am Acad Child Adolesc Psychiatry 26:133–143, 1987

Zarin DA, Earls F: Diagnostic decision making in psychiatry. Am J Psychiatry 50:197–206, 1993

Screening Tools and Rating Scales Useful in the Screening, Assessment, and Monitoring of Children and Adolescents

Screening tools and rating scales (C = Clinician; P = Parent; T = Teacher; Y = Youth)

Screening tool or rating scale	Rater[a]	Age (years)	Reference[b]	Publisher and location	Public domain[c]
GENERAL SCREENING TOOLS					
Behavior Assessment System for Children— Second Edition (BASC-2)	Y, P, T	2–21	Reynolds and Kamphaus 2004	Pearson Assessments* http://ags.pearsonassessments.com/group.asp?nGroupInfoID=a30000	N
Brief Psychiatric Rating Scale for Children (BPRS-C)	C, P	3–18	Overall and Pfefferbaum 1982	Carroll W. Hughes, Ph.D.*	Y
Caregiver-Teacher Report Form (C-TRF)	T	1.5–5 and 6–18	Achenbach and Rescorla 2000	Thomas M. Achenbach, Ph.D.* http://www.aseba.org/products/c-trf1-5.html	N
Child Behavior Checklist/ 1½–5/LDS (CBCL)	P	1.5–5	Achenbach and Rescorla 2000	Thomas M. Achenbach, Ph.D.* http://www.aseba.org/products/cbcl1-5.html	N
Child Behavior Checklist/ 6–18 (CBCL)	P	6–18	Achenbach and Rescorla 2001	Thomas M. Achenbach, Ph.D.* http://www.aseba.org/products/cbcl6-18.html	N
Children's Impairment Rating Scale	P, T	≥4	Fabiano et al. 2006	Center for Children and Families at the University at Buffalo http://ccf.buffalo.edu/pdf/Impairment_scale.pdf	Y
Conners' Parent Rating Scale—Revised (CPRS-R)	P	3–17	Conners 1997	Pearson Assessments* http://www.pearsonassessments.com/tests/crs-r.htm	N

Screening tools and rating scales (C = Clinician; P = Parent; T = Teacher; Y = Youth) (continued)

Screening tool or rating scale	Rater[a]	Age (years)	Reference[b]	Publisher and location	Public domain[c]
GENERAL SCREENING TOOLS (continued)					
Conners' Teacher Rating Scale—Revised (CTRS-R)	T	3–17	Conners et al. 1998	Pearson Assessments* http://www.pearsonassessments.com/tests/crs-r.htm	N
Early Childhood Inventory–4: Parent Checklist (ECI-P)	P	3–5	Gadow and Sprafkin 1997	Checkmate Plus* http://www.checkmateplus.com/products/eci-4.html	N
Early Childhood Inventory–4: Teacher Checklist (ECI-T)	T	3–5	Sprafkin and Gadow 1996	Checkmate Plus* http://www.checkmateplus.com/products/eci-4.html	N
Eyberg Child Behavior Inventory (ECBI)	P	2–16	Eyberg and Pincus 1999	Psychological Assessment Resources* http://www3.parinc.com/products/product.aspx?Productid=ECBI	N
Millon Adolescent Clinical Inventory (MACI)	Y	13–19	Millon et al. 1993	Pearson Assessments* http://www.pearsonassessments.com/tests/maci.htm	N
Parent General Behavior Inventory (P-GBI)	P	5–17	Youngstrom and Duax 2005	Eric A. Youngstrom, Ph.D.*	Y

Screening tools and rating scales (C = Clinician; P = Parent; T = Teacher; Y = Youth) *(continued)*

Screening tool or rating scale	Rater[a]	Age (years)	Reference[b]	Publisher and location	Public domain[c]
GENERAL SCREENING TOOLS *(continued)*					
Teacher Report Form/ 6–18 (TRF)	T	6–18	Achenbach and Rescorla 2001	Thomas M. Achenbach, Ph.D.* http://www.aseba.org/products/trf.html	N
Temperament and Atypical Behavior Scale (TABS)	P	11–71 months	Neisworth et al. 1999	Brookes Publishing* http://www.brookespublishing.com/store/books/ bagnato-tabs/index.htm	N
Youth Self-Report (YSR)	Y	11–18	Achenbach and Rescorla 2001	Thomas M. Achenbach, Ph.D.* http://www.aseba.org/products/ysr.html	N
FUNCTIONING					
Children's Global Assessment Scale (CGAS)	C	4–16	Shaffer et al. 1983	David Shaffer, M.D.*	Y
Reasons for Living Inventory for Adolescents (RFL-A)	Y	Adolescent	Osman et al. 1998	Marsha Linehan, Ph.D.*	Y
Social Skills Rating System (SSRS)	Y	3–18	Gresham and Elliott 1990	Pearson Assessments* http://ags.pearsonassessments.com/ Group.asp?nGroupInfoID=a3400	N
Symptom Checklist–90– Revised (SCL-90-R)	Y	≥13	Derogatis 1983	Pearson Assessments* http://www.pearsonassessments.com/tests/ scl90r.htm	N

Screening tools and rating scales (C = Clinician; P = Parent; T = Teacher; Y = Youth) *(continued)*

Screening tool or rating scale	Rater[a]	Age (years)	Reference[b]	Publisher and location	Public domain[c]
PARENT AND FAMILY FUNCTIONING AND PSYCHOSOCIAL STRESSORS					
Children's Perception of Interparental Conflict Scale (CPIC)	Y	9–12	Grych et al. 1992	Frank Fincham, Ph.D.* http://www.chs.fsu.edu/~ffincham/measures/ CPIC.htm	Y
Children's Report of Parental Behavior Inventory (CRPBI)	Y	12–18	Schaefer 1965	National Auxiliary Publications*	N
Divorce Events Schedule for Children (DESC)	Y, P	8–18	Sandler et al. 1988	Prevention Research Center* http://www.asu.edu/clas/asuprc	Y
Parenting Stress Index: Short Form (PSI-SF)	P	Infant– adolescent	Abidin 1995	Psychological Assessment Resources* http://www3.parinc.com/products/ product.aspx?Productid=PSI-SF	N
ANXIETY DISORDERS					
Anxiety Disorders Interview Schedule for DSM-IV, Child and Parent Versions (ADIS-IV))	Y, P	6–17	Silverman and Albano 1996	Oxford University Press* http://www.us.oup.com/us/catalog/general/subject/ Psychology/PractitionerClientGuides/ ?view=usa&ci=9780195183870	N
Beck Anxiety Inventory (BAI)	C	≥17	Beck 1993; Beck and Steer 1988	Harcourt Assessment* http://harcourtassessment.com/HAIWEB/Cultures/ en-us/Productdetail.htm?Pid=015-8018- 400&Mode=summary	N

Screening tools and rating scales (C = Clinician; P = Parent; T = Teacher; Y = Youth) *(continued)*

Screening tool or rating scale	Rater[a]	Age (years)	Reference[b]	Publisher and location	Public domain[c]
ANXIETY DISORDERS *(continued)*					
Multidimensional Anxiety Scale for Children (MASC)	Y	8–19	March 1997	Harcourt Assessment* http://harcourtassessment.com/HAIWEB/Cultures/en-us/Productdetail.htm?Pid=015-8036-905&Mode=summary	N
Revised Child Anxiety and Depression Scales (RCADS)	Y	6–18	Chorpita et al. 2000	Bruce F. Chorpita, Ph.D.* http://www2.hawaii.edu/~chorpita/	N
Selective Mutism Supplement Questionnaires	P, T	4–10	Black 2001a, 2001b	Comprehensive Psychiatric Associates Questionnaire for Parents (SM Supplement): http://wellpsych.com/SM_parent_qstnr.pdf School Questionnaire (SM Supplement): http://www.wellpsych.com/SM_school_qstnr.pdf	N
Screen for Child Anxiety Related Disorders (Child and Parent Versions) (SCARED)	Y, P	8–18	Birmaher et al. 1997	http://www.wpic.pitt.edu/research/carenet/CARE-NETPROVIDERS/PDFForms/ScaredChild-final.pdf http://www.wpic.pitt.edu/research/carenet/CARE-NETPROVIDERS/PDFForms/ScaredParent-final.pdf	Y

Screening tools and rating scales (C = Clinician; P = Parent; T = Teacher; Y = Youth) *(continued)*

Screening tool or rating scale	Rater[a]	Age (years)	Reference[b]	Publisher and location	Public domain[c]
ATTENTION-DEFICIT/HYPERACTIVITY DISORDER					
ADHD Rating Scale–IV	C, Y, P, T	6–12	DuPaul et al. 1998	ADD WareHouse* http://www.addwarehouse.com/shopsite_sc/store/html/adhd-rating-scale-iv.html	N
Conners' Rating Scales—Revised (CRS-R)	Y, P, T	3–17	Conners 1997	Pearson Assessments* http://www.pearsonassessments.com/tests/crs-r.htm	N
Swanson, Nolan and Pelham Rating Scale, Fourth Edition (SNAP-IV) Teacher and Parent Rating Scale	P, T	6–18	Swanson 1992	James M. Swanson, M.D.*	Y
DEVELOPMENTAL DISORDERS					
Autism Diagnostic Interview—Revised (ADI-R)	C	≥18 months	Lord et al. 2003	Western Psychological Services* http://portal.wpspublish.com/portal/page?_pageid=53,70436&_dad=portal&_schema=PORTAL	N
Autism Screening Questionnaire (ASQ)			*Now called Social Communication Questionnaire (see below)*		

Screening tools and rating scales (C = Clinician; P = Parent; T = Teacher; Y = Youth) *(continued)*

Screening tool or rating scale	Rater[a]	Age (years)	Reference[b]	Publisher and location	Public domain[c]
DEVELOPMENTAL DISORDERS *(continued)*					
Autism Spectrum Screening Questionnaire (ASSQ)	Y	7–16	Ehlers and Gillberg 1993	Available in referenced article	Y
Childhood Autism Rating Scale (CARS)	C, T	≥2	Schopler et al. 1988	Pearson Assessments* http://ags.pearsonassessments.com/Group.asp?nGroupInfoID=aCARS	N
Social Communication Questionnaire (SCQ, previously ASQ)	P	≥4	Rutter et al. 2003	Western Psychological Services* http://portal.wpspublish.com/portal/page?_pageid=53,70432&_dad=portal&_schema=PORTAL	N
DISRUPTIVE DISORDERS					
Aberrant Behavior Checklist (ABC)	Y	6–54	Aman et al. 1985	Stoelting* http://www.stoeltingco.com/tests/store/ViewLevel3.asp?keyword3=1164	N
Modified Overt Aggression Scale (MOAS)	C	Adult	Kay et al. 1988	Available in referenced article	Y
Nisonger Child Behavior Rating Form (NCBRF)	P, T	3–16	Aman et al. 1996	Michael Aman, Ph.D.* http://psychmed.osu.edu/ncbrf.htm	Y
Nisonger Child Behavior Rating Form, Typical IQ Version (NCBRF-IQ)	P	5–15	Aman et al. 2008	Michael Aman, Ph.D.* http://psychmed.osu.edu/ncbrf.htm	Y

Screening tools and rating scales (C = Clinician; P = Parent; T = Teacher; Y = Youth) *(continued)*

Screening tool or rating scale	Rater[a]	Age (years)	Reference[b]	Publisher and location	Public domain[c]
EATING DISORDERS					
Eating Attitudes Test (EAT)	Y	6–18	Garner et al. 1982	River Centre Clinic http://www.river-centre.org/selftest.html	Y
Eating Disorder Examination (EDE)	C	8–15 (Child Version) and ≥16	Fairburn and Cooper 1993	Oxford University, Department of Psychiatry, Centre for Research on Eating Disorders at Oxford* http://www.psychiatry.ox.ac.uk/research/researchunits/credo/assessment-measures	N
INTELLIGENCE AND LANGUAGE					
Clinical Evaluation of Language Fundamentals—3rd Edition (CELF)	Y	6–11	Wiig et al. 2006	Harcourt Assessment* http://harcourtassessment.com/HAIWEB/Cultures/en-us/Productdetail.htm?Pid=015-8035-305&Mode=summary	N
Peabody Picture Vocabulary Test—4th Edition (PPVT-IV)	Y	≥2 years, 6 months	Dunn and Dunn 2006	Pearson Assessments* http://ags.pearsonassessments.com/Group.asp?nGroupInfoID=a30700	N
Test of Language Development—Intermediate, 4th Edition (TOLD-I:4)	C	8–12	Hammill and Newcomer 2008	PRO-ED* http://www.proedinc.com/customer/productLists.aspx?brandid=2	N

Screening tools and rating scales (C = Clinician; P = Parent; T = Teacher; Y = Youth) *(continued)*

Screening tool or rating scale	Rater[a]	Age (years)	Reference[b]	Publisher and location	Public domain[c]
INTELLIGENCE AND LANGUAGE *(continued)*					
Test of Language Development—Primary, 4th Edition (TOLD-P:4)	C	4–8	Newcomer and Hammill 2008	PRO-ED* http://www.proedinc.com/customer/productLists.aspx?brandid=2	N
Wechsler Intelligence Scale for Children—4th Edition (WISC-IV)	Y	6–16	Wechsler 2003	Harcourt Assessment* http://harcourtassessment.com/HAIWEB/Cultures/en-us/Productdetail.htm?Pid=015-8979-044&Mode=summary	N
MOOD DISORDERS (DEPRESSION AND BIPOLAR)					
Beck Depression Inventory–II (BDI-II)	Y	≥13	Beck et al. 1996	Harcourt Assessment* http://harcourtassessment.com/HAIWEB/Cultures/en-us/Productdetail.htm?Pid=015-8018-370&Mode=summary	N
Center for Epidemiological Studies Depression Scale for Children (CES-DC)	Y	6–17	Weissman et al. 1980	Bright Futures http://www.brightfutures.org/mentalhealth/pdf/professionals/bridges/ces_dc.pdf	Y
Child Mania Rating Scale—Parent Version (CMRS-P)	P	5–17	Pavuluri et al. 2006	Depression and Bipolar Support Alliance http://www.dbsalliance.org/pdfs/ChildManiaSurvey.pdf	Y

Screening tools and rating scales (C = Clinician; P = Parent; T = Teacher; Y = Youth) *(continued)*

Screening tool or rating scale	Rater[a]	Age (years)	Reference[b]	Publisher and location	Public domain[c]
MOOD DISORDERS (DEPRESSION AND BIPOLAR) *(continued)*					
Children's Depression Inventory (CDI)	Y, P, T	7–17	Kovacs 1992	Multi-Health Systems* https://www.mhs.com/ecom/ (nmehbjmxfyt3zo2xu1olh545)/ product.aspx?RptGrpID=CDI	N
Children's Depression Rating Scale–Revised (CDRS-R)	C	6–12 and adolescent	Poznanski and Mokros 1996	Western Psychological Services* http://portal.wpspublish.com/portal/ page?_pageid=53,69676&_dad=portal&_schema =PORTAL	N
Hamilton Rating Scale for Depression (Ham-D)	C	Adult	Hamilton 1960	http://library.umassmed.edu/ementalhealth/ clinical/ham_depression.pdf	Y
Parent Version of the Young Mania Rating Scale (P-YMRS)	P, T	5–17	Gracious et al. 2002	Child and Adolescent Bipolar Foundation http://www.bpkids.org/site/PageServer? pagename=lrn_08_20_03	Y
Quick Inventory of Depressive Symptomatology (QIDS)	C, Y	Adult	Rush et al. 2003	University of Pittsburgh, Epidemiology Data Center IDS/QIDS: http://www.ids-qids.org Clinician-Rated Version: http://www.ids-qids.org/ translations/english/QIDS-C%20English.pdf Self-Report Version: http://www.ids-qids.org/ translations/english/QIDS-SREnglish2page.pdf	Y

Screening tools and rating scales (C = Clinician; P = Parent; T = Teacher; Y = Youth) (continued)

Screening tool or rating scale	Rater[a]	Age (years)	Reference[b]	Publisher and location	Public domain[c]
OBSESSIVE-COMPULSIVE DISORDER					
Children's Yale-Brown Obsessive Compulsive Scale (CY-BOCS)	C	6–17	Scahill et al. 1997	Wayne Goodman, M.D.*	Y
Leyton Obsessional Inventory, Child Version (LOI-CV)	Y	12–16	Berg et al. 1986	Available in referenced article	Y
POSTTRAUMATIC STRESS DISORDER AND TRAUMA					
Child and Adolescent Trauma Survey (CATS)	Y, T	10–16	March et al. 1997	Not publicly available at time of publication; in development by Multi-Health Systems	N
Child PTSD Symptom Scale (CPSS)	Y	8–18	Foa et al. 2001	Edna Foa, Ph.D.*	Y
Extended Grief Inventory (EGI)	Y	8–18	Layne et al. 2001	Christopher M. Layne, Ph.D.*	Y
Traumatic Events Screening Inventory for Children (TESI-C)	Y	≥8	Ford et al. 1999	National Center for Posttraumatic Stress Disorder http://www.ncptsd.va.gov/ncmain/ncdocs/assmnts/TESI-C.pdf	Y
UCLA PTSD Reaction Index for DSM-IV (Revision 1) (UCLA-PTSD-R1)	P, Y	Child–adolescent	Rodriguez et al. 1999	UCLA Trauma Psychiatry Service*	N

Screening tools and rating scales (C = Clinician; P = Parent; T = Teacher; Y = Youth) *(continued)*

Screening tool or rating scale	Rater[a]	Age (years)	Reference[b]	Publisher and location	Public domain[c]
PSYCHOTIC DISORDERS					
Bunney-Hamburg Psychosis Rating Scale	C	Adult	Bunney and Hamburg 1963	Available in referenced article	Y
Scale for the Assessment of Negative Symptoms (SANS)	C	Adult	Andreasen 1982	Nancy P. Andreasen, M.D., Ph.D.*	N
Scale for the Assessment of Positive Symptoms (SAPS)	C	Adult	Andreasen 1984	Nancy P. Andreasen, M.D., Ph.D.*	N
Structured Interview for Prodromal Syndromes and Scale of Prodromal Symptoms (SIPS)	C	≥12	Miller et al. 2003	Barbara Walsh, Ph.D.*	N
SUBSTANCE ABUSE DISORDERS					
Problem Recognition Questionnaire (PRQ)	Y	≥16	Cady et al. 1996	Ken Winters, Ph.D.*	Y
Teen Addiction Severity Index (T-ASI)	Y	Adolescent	Kaminer et al. 1991	Yifrah Kaminer, M.D.*	Y

Screening tools and rating scales (C = Clinician; P = Parent; T = Teacher; Y = Youth) *(continued)*

Screening tool or rating scale	Rater[a]	Age (years)	Reference[b]	Publisher and location	Public domain[c]
SUICIDE RISK					
Beck Suicide Intent Scale (SIS)	C	Adult	Beck et al. 1974	Available in referenced book	N
Columbia Suicide-Severity Rating Scale (C-SSRS)	C, Y	6–17	Posner et al. 2007	Kelly Posner, Ph.D.*	Y
Suicidal Ideation Questionnaire (SIQ)	Y	Grades 7–9 and 10–12	Reynolds 1987	Psychological Assessment Resources* http://www3.parinc.com/products/product.aspx?Productid=SIQ	N
TIC DISORDERS					
Premonitory Urge for Tics Scale (PUTS)	Y	8–17	Woods et al. 2005	Available in referenced book	Y
Yale Global Tic Severity Scale (Y-GTSS)	C	Child, adolescent, adult	Leckman et al. 1989	James Leckman, M.D.*	Y

[a]C=Clinician; P=Parent; T = Teacher; Y=Youth.
[b]See section "References" at end of appendix.
[c]N=No; Y=Yes.
*More information about source is provided in the Publishers list that follows the table.

PUBLISHERS

Thomas M. Achenbach, Ph.D., Department of Psychiatry, University of Vermont College of Medicine, 1 South Prospect Street, Burlington, VT 05401; Phone: 802-656-2629; Fax: 802-656-9965; E-mail: Thomas.Achenbach@uvm.edu; http://www.aseba.org

ADD WareHouse, 300 Northwest 70th Avenue, Suite 102, Plantation, FL 33317; Phone: 800-233-9273; Fax: 954-792-8545; http://www.addwarehouse.com

Michael Aman, Ph.D., Research Unit on Pediatric Psychopharmacology, Ohio State University, Columbus, OH; Phone: 614-688-4196; E-mail: aman.1@osu.edu; http://psychmed.osu.edu/ncbrf.htm

Nancy P. Andreasen, M.D., Ph.D., University of Iowa, 200 Hawkins Drive, Room 2911 JPP, Iowa City, IA 52242; Phone: 319-356-1553; E-mail: nancy-andreasen@uiowa.edu

Brookes Publishing, Customer Service Department, P.O. Box 10624, Baltimore, MD 21285-0624; Phone: 800-638-3775; Fax: 410-337-8539; E-mail: custserv@brookespublishing.com; http://www.brookespublishing.com

Checkmate Plus, P.O. Box 696, Dept. D, Stony Brook, NY 11790-0696; Phone: 800-779-4292; Fax: 631-360-3432

Bruce F. Chorpita, Ph.D.; Phone: 601-984-5805; E-mail: chorpita@hawaii.edu; http://www2.hawaii.edu/~chorpita

Frank Fincham, Ph.D., Family Institute, Sandels Building, Florida State University, Tallahassee, FL 32306-1491; Phone: 850-644-4914; http://www.chs.fsu.edu/~ffincham/measures/CPIC.htm

Edna Foa, Ph.D., Center for the Treatment and Study of Anxiety, Department of Psychiatry, University of Pennsylvania School of Medicine, 3535 Market Street, 6th Floor, Philadelphia, PA 19104; Phone: 215-746-3327; E-mail: foa@mail.med.upenn.edu

Wayne Goodman, M.D., Department of Psychiatry, University of Florida, P.O. Box 100256, Gainesville, FL 32610

Harcourt Assessment, Customer Service, P.O. Box 599700, San Antonio, TX 78259; Phone: 800-872-1726; Fax 800-232-1223; http://harcourtassessment.com

Carroll W. Hughes, Ph.D., Department of Psychiatry, University of Texas Medical Center–Dallas, 5323 Harry Hines Boulevard, Dallas, TX 75390-8589; Phone: 214-648-4325; E-mail: carroll.hughes@utsouthwestern.edu

Yifrah Kaminer, M.D., Division of Child and Adolescent Psychiatry, University of Connecticut Health Center, 263 Farmington Avenue, Farmington, CT 06030-2103; Phone: 860-679-4344; Fax: 860-679-4077; E-mail: Kaminer@psychiatry.uchc.edu

Christopher M. Layne, Ph.D., National Center for Child Traumatic Stress, University of California, Los Angeles, 11150 West Olympic Boulevard, Suite 650, Los Angeles, CA 90064; Phone: 310-235-2633 Ext 223; Fax: 310-235-2612; E-mail: CMLayne@mednet.ucla.edu

James Leckman, M.D., Yale University Child Study Center, 230 South Frontage Road, P.O. Box 207900, New Haven, CT 06520; Phone: 203-785-7971; E-mail: James.Leckman@yale.edu

Marsha Linehan, Ph.D., Department of Psychology, University of Washington, Box 351525, Seattle, WA 98195-1525; Phone: 206-685-2037; Fax: 206-616-1513; E-mail: linehan@u.washington.edu

Multi-Health Systems, P.O. Box 950, North Tonawanda, NY 14120-0950; Phone: 800-456-3003; Fax: 888-540-4484; E-mail: customerservice@mhs.com; http://www.mhs.com/mhs/

National Auxiliary Publications, c/o Microfiche Publications, P.O. Box 3513, Grand Central Station, New York, NY 10163-3513; Phone: 516-481-2300

Oxford University, Department of Psychiatry, Centre for Research on Eating Disorders at Oxford; E-mail: credo@medsci.ox.ac.uk; http://www.psychiatry.ox.ac.uk/research/researchunits/credo/assessment-measures

Oxford University Press, Customer Service; Phone: 800-451-7556; custserv.us@oup.com; http://www.us.oup.com/us/catalog

Pearson Assessments Order Department, P.O. Box 1416, Minneapolis, MN 55440; Phone: 800-627-7271; Fax: 800-632-9011; agsinfo@pearson.com; http://ags.pearsonassessments.com

Kelly Posner, Ph.D., New York State Psychiatric Institute, 1051 Riverside Drive, New York, NY 10032; E-mail: posnerk@childpsych.columbia.edu

Prevention Research Center, Arizona State University, 900 South McAllister Avenue (Room 205), Tempe, AZ 85281-2001; Phone: 480-965-7420; Fax: 480-965-5430; http://www.asu.edu/clas/asuprc/publications.html

PRO-ED, 8700 Shoal Creek Boulevard, Austin, TX 78757-6897; Phone: 800-897-3202; Fax: 800-397-7633; http://www.proedinc.com

Psychological Assessment Resources, 16204 North Florida Avenue, Lutz, FL 33549; Phone: 800-331-8378; Fax: 800-727-9329; http://www3.parinc.com

David Shaffer, M.D., Department of Psychiatry, College of Physicians and Surgeons, Columbia University, 1051 Riverside Drive, New York, NY 10032; Phone: 212-543-5948; Fax: 212-543-5966; E-mail: shafferd@childpsych.columbia.edu

Stoelting, 620 Wheat Lane, Wood Dale, IL 60191; Phone: 630-860-9700; Fax: 630-860-9775; E-mail: Info@StoeltingCo.com; http://www.stoeltingco.com

James M. Swanson, Ph.D., UCI Child Development Center, 19722 MacArthur Boulevard, Irvine, CA 92612; Phone: 949-824-1824; Fax: 949-824-1811; E-mail: jmswanso@uci.edu

UCLA Trauma Psychiatry Service, 300 UCLA Medical Plaza, Suite 2232, Los Angeles, CA 90095-6968; Phone: 310-206-8973; E-mail: Asteinberg@mednet.ucla.edu; rpynoos@mednet.ucla.edu

Barbara Walsh, Ph.D., Department of Psychiatry, Yale University, 34 Park Street, New Haven, CT 06519-1187; Phone: 203-974-7052; Barbara.Walsh@yale.edu

Western Psychological Services, 12031 Wilshire Boulevard, Los Angeles, CA 90025-1251; Phone: 800-648-8857; Fax: 310-478-7838; http://portal.wpspublish.com

Ken Winters, Ph.D., Department of Psychiatry, University of Minnesota, F282/2A West 8393, 2450 Riverside Avenue, Minneapolis, MN 55454; Phone: 612-273-9815, 612-273-9800; Fax: 612-273-9779; E-mail: winte001@umn.edu

Eric A. Youngstrom, Ph.D., 248 Davie Hall, Department of Psychology, University of North Carolina–Chapel Hill, Chapel Hill, NC 27599-3270; Phone: 919-962-3997; E-mail: eay@unc.edu

REFERENCES

Abidin RR: Parenting Stress Index: Professional Manual, 3rd Edition. Odessa, FL, Psychological Assessment Resources, 1995

Achenbach TM, Rescorla LA: Manual for the ASEBA Preschool Forms and Profiles. Burlington, University of Vermont, Department of Psychiatry, 2000

Achenbach TM, Rescorla LA: Manual for the ASEBA School-Age Forms and Profiles. Burlington, VT, University of Vermont, Research Center for Children, Youth, and Families, 2001

Aman MG, Singh NN, Stewart AW, et al: The Aberrant Behavior Checklist: a behavior rating scale for the assessment of treatment effects. Am J Ment Defic 89:485–491, 1985

Aman MG, Tassé MJ, Rojahn J, et al: The Nisonger CBRF: a child behavior rating form for children with developmental disabilities. Res Dev Disabil 17:41–57, 1996

Aman MG, Leone S, Lecavalier L, et al: The Nisonger Child Behavior Rating Form— Typical IQ Version, for children with typical IQ. Int Clin Psychopharmacol 23:232–242, 2008

Andreasen NC: Negative symptoms in schizophrenia. Arch Gen Psychiatry 39:784–788, 1982

Andreasen NC: Scale for the Assessment of Positive Symptoms. Iowa City, University of Iowa, 1984

Beck AT: Beck Anxiety Inventory. San Antonio, TX, Harcourt Assessment, 1993

Beck AT, Steer RA: An inventory for measuring clinical anxiety: psychometric properties. J Consult Clin Psychol 56:893–897, 1988

Beck A, Schuyler D, Herman I: Development of suicidal intent scales, in The Prediction of Suicide. Edited by Beck A, Resnik H, Lettieri D. Bowie, MD, Charles Press, 1974, pp 45–56

Beck AT, Steer RA, Brown GK: Beck Depression Inventory–II. San Antonio, TX, Harcourt Assessment, 1996

Berg CJ, Rapoport JL, Flament M: The Leyton Obsessional Inventory — Child Version. J Am Acad Child Psychiatry 25:84–91, 1986

Birmaher B, Khetarpal S, Brent D, et al: The Screen for Child Anxiety Related Emotional Disorders (SCARED): scale construction and psychometric properties. J Am Acad Child Adolesc Psychiatry 36:545–553, 1997

Black B: Questionnaire for Parents (SM Supplement). 2001a. Available at: http://wellpsych.com/SM_parent_qstnr.pdf. Accessed July 19, 2008.

Black B: School Questionnaire (SM Supplement). 2001b. Available at: http://www.wellpsych.com/SM_school_qstnr.pdf. Accessed July 19, 2008.

Bunney WE Jr, Hamburg DA: Methods for reliable longitudinal observation of behavior. Arch Gen Psychiatry 9:280–294, 1963

Cady M, Winters KC, Jordan DA, et al: Measuring treatment readiness for adolescent drug abusers. J Child Adolesc Subst Abuse 5:73–91, 1996

Chorpita BF, Yim LM, Moffitt CE, et al: Assessment of symptoms of DSM-IV anxiety and depression in children: a revised child anxiety and depression scale. Behav Res Ther 38:835–855, 2000

Conners CK: Conners' Rating Scales — Revised: Technical Manual. North Tonawanda, New York, Multi-Health Systems, 1997

Conners CK, Sitarenios G, Parker JD, et al: Revision and restandardization of the Conners' Teacher Rating Scale (CTRS-R): factor structure, reliability, and criterion validity. J Abnorm Child Psychol 26:279–291, 1998

Derogatis LR: SCL-90-R: Administration, Scoring and Procedures Manual–II. Towson, MD, Clinical Psychometric Research, 1983

Dunn LM, Dunn DM: Peabody Picture Vocabulary Test, 4th Edition. Minneapolis, MN, AGS/Pearson Assessments, 2006

DuPaul GJ, Power TJ, Anastopoulos AD, et al: ADHD Rating Scale — IV: Checklists, Norms, and Clinical Interpretation. New York, Guilford, 1998

Ehlers S, Gillberg C: The epidemiology of Asperger syndrome: a total population study. J Child Psychol Psychiatry 34:1327–1350, 1993

Eyberg SM, Pincus D: Eyberg Child Behavior Inventory and Sutter-Eyberg Student Behavior Inventory: Professional Manual. Odessa, FL, Psychological Assessment Resources, 1999

Fabiano GA, Pelham WE Jr, Waschbusch DA, et al: A practical measure of impairment: psychometric properties of the Impairment Rating Scale in samples of children with attention deficit hyperactivity disorder and two school-based samples. J Clin Child Adolesc Psychol 35:369–385, 2006

Fairburn CG, Cooper Z: The Eating Disorder Examination, 12th Edition, in Binge Eating: Nature, Assessment, and Treatment. New York, Guilford, 1993, pp 317–360

Foa EB, Treadwell K, Johnson K, et al: The Child PTSD Symptom Scale: a preliminary examination of its psychometric properties. J Clin Child Psychol 30:376–384, 2001

Ford JD, Racusin R, Daviss WB, et al: Trauma exposure among children with oppositional defiant disorder and attention deficit-hyperactivity disorder. J Consult Clin Psychol 67:786–789, 1999

Gadow KD, Sprafkin J: Early Childhood Symptom Inventory–4 Norms Manual. Stony Brook, NY, Checkmate Plus, 1997

Garner DM, Olmsted MP, Bohr Y, et al: The Eating Attitudes Test: psychometric features and clinical correlates. Psychol Med 12:871–878, 1982

Gracious BL, Youngstrom EA, Findling RL, et al: Discriminative validity of a parent version of the Young Mania Rating Scale. J Am Acad Child Adolesc Psychiatry 41:1350–1359, 2002

Gresham FM, Elliott SN: Social Skills Rating System Manual. Circle Pines, MN, American Guidance Service, 1990

Grych JH, Seid M, Fincham FD: Assessing marital conflict from the child's perspective: the Children's Perception of Interparental Conflict Scale. Child Dev 63:558–572, 1992

Hamilton M: A rating scale for depression. J Neurol Neurosurg Psychiatry 23:56–62, 1960

Hammill DD, Newcomer PL: Test of Language Development, Intermediate, 4th Edition. Austin, TX, PRO-ED, 2008

Kaminer Y, Bukstein O, Tarter RE: The Teen-Addiction Severity Index: rationale and reliability. Int J Addict 26:219–226, 1991

Kay SR, Wolkenfeld F, Murrill LM: Profiles of aggression among psychiatric patients, I: nature and prevalence. J Nerv Ment Dis 176:539–546, 1988

Kovacs M: The Children's Depression Inventory (CDI). Psychopharmacol Bull 21:995–998, 1985

Kovacs M: Children's Depression Inventory. North Tonawanda, NY, Multi-Health Systems, 1992

Layne CM, Savjak N, Saltzman WR: Extended Grief Inventory. Los Angeles, University of California at Los Angeles and Brigham Young University, 2001

Leckman JF, Riddle MA, Hardin MT, et al: Yale Global Tic Severity Scale: initial testing of a clinician-rated scale of tic severity. J Am Acad Child Adolesc Psychiatry 28:566–573, 1989

Lord M, Le Couteur A, Lord C: Autism Diagnostic Interview—Revised. Los Angeles, CA, Western Psychological Services, 2003

March JS: Manual for the Multidimensional Anxiety Scale for Children (MASC). North Tonawanda, NY, Multi-Health Systems, 1997

March J, Amaya-Jackson L, Terry R, et al: Post-traumatic stress in children and adolescents after an industrial fire. J Am Acad Child Adolesc Psychiatry 36:1080–1108, 1997

Miller TJ, McGlashan TH, Rosen JL, et al: Prodromal assessment with the Structured Interview for Prodromal Syndromes and the Scale of Prodromal Symptoms: predictive validity, interrater reliability, and training to reliability. Schizophr Bull 29:703–715, 2003

Millon T, Millon C, Davis R, et al: The Millon Adolescent Clinical Inventory. Minneapolis, MN, National Computer Systems, 1993

Neisworth JT, Bagnato SJ, Salvia JJ, et al: Temperament and Atypical Behavior Scale (TABS): Early Childhood Indicators of Developmental Dysfunction. Baltimore, MD, Paul H Brookes, 1999

Newcomer PL, Hammill DD: Test of Language Development, Primary, 4th Edition. Austin, TX, PRO-ED, 2008

Osman A, Downs WR, Kopper BA, et al: The Reasons for Living Inventory for Adolescents (RFL-A): development and psychometric properties. J Clin Psychol 54:1063–1078, 1998

Overall JE, Pfefferbaum B: The Brief Psychiatric Rating Scale for Children. Psychopharmacol Bull 18:10–16, 1982

Pavuluri MN, Henry D, Devineni B, et al: Child Mania Rating Scale: development, reliability, and validity. J Am Acad Child Adolesc Psychiatry 45:550–560, 2006

Posner K, Melvin GA, Stanley B, et al: Factors in the assessment of suicidality in youth. CNS Spectr 12:156–162, 2007

Poznanski E, Mokros HB: Children's Depression Rating Scale, Revised. Los Angeles, CA, Western Psychological Services, 1996

Reynolds CR, Kamphaus RW: Behavior Assessment System for Children, 2nd Edition. Bloomington, MN, Pearson Assessments, 2004

Reynolds WM: Suicidal Ideation Questionnaire. Odessa, FL, Psychological Assessment Resources, 1987

Rodriguez N, Steinberg A, Pynoos RS: ULCA PTSD Reaction Index for DSM-IV Instrument Information: Child Version, Parent Version, Adolescent Version. Los Angeles, CA, UCLA Trauma Psychiatry Service, 1999

Rush AJ, Trivedi MH, Ibrahim HM, et al: The 16-Item Quick Inventory of Depressive Symptomatology (QIDS), Clinician Rating (QIDS-C), and Self-Report (QIDS-SR): a psychometric evaluation in patients with chronic major depression. Biol Psychiatry 54:573–583, 2003

Rutter M, Bailey A, Lord C, et al: Social Communication Questionnaire. Los Angeles, CA, Western Psychological Services, 2003

Sandler IN, Wolchik SA, Braver SL: The stressors of children's post divorce environments, in Children of Divorce: Empirical Perspectives on Adjustment. Edited by Wolchik SA, Karoly P. New York, Gardner Press, 1988, pp 111–143

Scahill L, Riddle MA, McSwiggin-Hardin M, et al: Children's Yale-Brown Obsessive Compulsive Scale: reliability and validity. J Am Acad Child Adolesc Psychiatry 36:844–852, 1997

Schaefer ES: Children's Report of Parental Behavior: an inventory. Child Dev 36:413–424, 1965

Schopler E, Reichler RJ, Renner BR: The Childhood Autism Rating Scale. Los Angeles, CA, Western Psychological Services, 1988

Shaffer D, Gould MS, Brasic J, et al: A Children's Global Assessment Scale (CGAS). Arch Gen Psychiatry 40:1228–1231, 1983

Silverman WK, Albano AM: The Anxiety Disorders Interview Schedule for DSM-IV—Child and Parent Versions. San Antonio, TX, Graywind/Psychological Corporation, 1996

Sprafkin J, Gadow KD: Early Childhood Inventories. Stony Brook, NY, Checkmate Plus, 1996

Swanson JM: School-Based Assessments and Interventions for ADD Students. Irvine, CA, KC Press, 1992

Wechsler, D: The Wechsler Intelligence Scale for Children, 4th Edition. San Antonio, TX, Harcourt Assessment, 2003

Weissman MM, Orvaschel H, Padian N: Children's symptom and social functioning self report scales: comparison of mothers' and children's reports. J Nerv Ment Dis 168:736–740, 1980

Wiig EH, Secord WA, Semel E: Clinical Evaluation of Language Fundamentals, 3rd Edition, Spanish Edition. San Antonio, TX, Harcourt Assessment, 2006

Woods DW, Piacentini J, Himle MB, et al: Premonitory Urge for Tics Scale (PUTS): initial psychometric results and examination of the premonitory urge phenomenon in youths with tic disorders. J Dev Behav Pediatr 26:397–403, 2005

Youngstrom EA, Duax J: Evidence-based assessment of pediatric bipolar disorder, part I: base rate and family history. J Am Acad Child Adolesc Psychiatry 44:712–717, 2005

About the Contributors

J. Stuart Ablon, Ph.D., is associate director and cofounder of the Collaborative Problem Solving Institute in the Department of Psychiatry at Massachusetts General Hospital and an associate clinical professor of psychiatry at Harvard Medical School, Boston, Massachusetts. Dr. Ablon received his doctorate in clinical psychology from the University of California at Berkeley and completed his predoctoral and postdoctoral training at Massachusetts General Hospital and Harvard Medical School. He specializes in the treatment of explosive, inflexible, easily frustrated children and adolescents and is coauthor of *Treating Explosive Kids: The Collaborative Problem-Solving Approach.* In addition to his work with families with children with social, emotional, and behavioral challenges, Dr. Ablon consults extensively to schools and therapeutic facilities.

Jean Addington, Ph.D., is a professor of psychiatry at the University of Toronto and a research scientist at the Centre for Addiction and Mental Health (CAMH) in Toronto, Ontario, Canada. She is director of psychosocial treatments in the First Episode Psychosis Program at CAMH and director of the PRIME Research Clinic for the investigation and treatment of young people at high risk of developing psychosis. She played a major role in developing the First Episode Psychosis Program in Calgary, Alberta. In Toronto, she has been responsible for developing research on the prodromal phase of schizophrenia. She has been awarded a major National Institutes of Health grant dedicated to developing models of prediction of conversion to psychosis and a major grant from the Ontario Mental Health Foundation to develop a research program investigating psychological intervention for those at ultrahigh risk of developing psychosis. She is currently president of the International Early Psychosis Association.

Anne Marie Albano, Ph.D., A.B.P.P., is an associate professor of clinical psychology in the Division of Child and Adolescent Psychiatry at Columbia University and director of the Columbia University Clinic for Anxiety and Related

Disorders. She is a principal investigator for the National Institute of Mental Health (NIMH) multisite Child/Adolescent Anxiety Multimodal Treatment Study and was a principal investigator for the NIMH Treatment for Adolescents with Depression Study. Dr. Albano has authored over 80 articles and chapters, conducts clinical research, supervises the research and clinical development of interns and postdoctoral fellows in psychology and psychiatry, and is involved in advanced training of senior clinicians in cognitive-behavioral therapy.

L. Eugene Arnold, M.D., M.Ed., is a board-certified child and adolescent psychiatrist. He is professor emeritus of psychiatry at the Ohio State University (OSU), where he was formerly director of the Division of Child and Adolescent Psychiatry and vice-chair of psychiatry, and is currently interim director of the Nisonger Center of Excellence in Developmental Disabilities, Columbus, Ohio. He graduated from the OSU College of Medicine; interned at the University of Oregon; took residencies at Johns Hopkins, where he earned his M.Ed.; and served in the U.S. Public Health Service. He is a coinvestigator in the OSU Research Unit on Pediatric Psychopharmacology. He has more than 38 years of experience in child psychiatric treatment research, including the National Institute of Mental Health's multisite Multimodal Treatment Study of Children with ADHD (MTA), for which he continues as executive secretary and current chair of the steering committee. For his work on the MTA, he received the National Institutes of Health Director's Award. He has a particular interest in alternative and complementary treatments for ADHD. His publications include 9 books, over 55 chapters, and more than 160 articles.

Andrea Auther, Ph.D., received her doctoral degree in clinical psychology from St. John's University in Queens, New York. Since 2000, she has been working with the Recognition and Prevention (RAP) program, an early intervention research center and clinic for adolescents and young adults experiencing prodromal symptoms of psychosis located at the Zucker Hillside Hospital in Glen Oaks, New York. She is currently assistant director of the RAP program and supervises clinical diagnostic interviews, provides individual and group psychotherapy, and collaborates on a wide variety of research endeavors. Dr. Auther was a recipient of a Young Investigator Award from the National Alliance for Research on Schizophrenia and Depression to study the role of substance use in the development of psychosis, her main research interest.

Susan Bacalman, M.S.W., is a licensed clinical social worker and is a member of the research core at the M.I.N.D. Institute (Medical Investigation of Neurodevelopmental Disorders Institute), University of California, Davis Medical

Center, Sacramento, California. She administers diagnostic measures to research participants in a range of studies being conducted at the M.I.N.D. She works with Dr. Robert L. Hendren on the child psychiatry clinic team, evaluating children and adolescents with neurodevelopmental and psychiatric symptoms. She also established and continues to facilitate an Asperger's disorder support group for adolescents and young adults. Prior to coming to U.C. Davis, she worked under Drs. Helen Tager-Flusberg and Susan Folstein at the Shriver Center in Waltham, Massachusetts, doing research focusing on language and communication impairments in children with autism. She has co-authored articles on neurodevelopmental disorders, including autism and fragile X syndrome.

Gail A. Bernstein, M.D., is head of the Program in Child and Adolescent Anxiety and Mood Disorders and holds the endowed professorship in child and adolescent anxiety disorders in the Division of Child and Adolescent Psychiatry at the University of Minnesota Medical School, Minneapolis. She is an internationally recognized expert in pediatric anxiety disorders. Dr. Bernstein is board certified in pediatrics, general psychiatry, and child and adolescent psychiatry. She was director of the Division of Child and Adolescent Psychiatry at the University of Minnesota from 1996 to 2000. Dr. Bernstein has served on several editorial boards and on the American Academy of Child and Adolescent Psychiatry (AACAP) Work Group on Quality Issues. She was a principal author of each of the three AACAP Practice Parameters for Assessment and Treatment of Anxiety Disorders. She has been principal investigator on grants from the National Institute of Mental Health titled "Imipramine in the Treatment of School Refusal" and "Early Interventions for Anxious Children." Dr. Bernstein won the 2000 AACAP Children's Mental Health Alliance Psychotherapy Award and the 2006 AACAP Norbert and Charlotte Rieger Award for Scientific Achievement.

Boris Birmaher, M.D., is the endowed chair in early-onset bipolar disease and a professor of psychiatry at the University of Pittsburgh School of Medicine. He has board certifications in both general psychiatry and child psychiatry. He received his medical degree from Valle University in Cali, Colombia, and completed his training in general psychiatry at the Hebrew University, Hadassah Medical Center in Jerusalem, Israel. He received training in biological psychiatry at the Albert Einstein College of Medicine in New York and training in child psychiatry at Columbia University/New York Psychiatric Institute, in New York, New York. Dr. Birmaher is also the director of the Child and Adolescent Anxiety Program and codirector of the Child and Adolescent Bipolar Services program at Western Psychiatric Institute and Clinic, Pittsburgh, Pennsylvania. Dr. Birmaher is a well-known researcher in pharmacologic and biological studies of children and adolescents with mood and anxiety disorders. Dr. Birmaher has published over 185 papers in peer-reviewed journals and also recently published *New Hope for Children and Teens With Bipolar Disorder.* The American Psychiatric Association recently named Dr. Birmaher a distinguished fellow in recognition of his academic, research, and service work. In addition, Dr. Birmaher is the recipient of an endowment from the University of Pittsburgh School of Medicine to study early-onset bipolar disease.

Bruce Black, M.D., is founder and director of Comprehensive Psychiatric Associates, a multidisciplinary mental health group practice in Wellesley, Massachusetts. He has previously served as director of the Pediatric Psychopharmacology Program at the University of Maryland School of Medicine in Baltimore, Maryland; as staff psychiatrist in the Biological Psychiatry Branch at the National Institute of Mental Health in Bethesda, Maryland; and as director of Outpatient Psychiatry and of the Mood and Anxiety Disorders Program at New England Medical Center in Boston, Massachusetts. He is currently an assistant professor of psychiatry at Tufts University School of Medicine, Boston, Massachusetts. Dr. Black is the author of over 35 scholarly papers and chapters in major medical textbooks.

Caroline Lewczyk Boxmeyer, Ph.D., is a research scientist in the Center for the Prevention of Youth Behavior Problems at the University of Alabama, Tuscaloosa. Her work focuses on identifying the effective elements of prevention and intervention programs for children with disruptive behavior problems and training community clinicians to implement cognitive-behavioral interventions. Dr. Boxmeyer is also a supervising psychologist in the psychology clinic at the University of Alabama.

David A. Brent, M.D., is academic chief of child and adolescent psychiatry at Western Psychiatric Institute and Clinic, and is a professor of child psychiatry, pediatrics, and epidemiology and endowed chair of suicide studies at the University of Pittsburgh School of Medicine, Pittsburgh, Pennsylvania. Dr. Brent received his undergraduate education at Pennsylvania State University and graduated from Jefferson Medical College of Thomas Jefferson University. He trained in pediatrics at the University of Colorado, trained in general and child psychiatry at Western Psychiatric Institute and Clinic, and completed a master's degree in psychiatric epidemiology at the University of Pittsburgh School of Public Health. He cofounded and now directs Services for Teens at Risk, a Commonwealth of Pennsylvania–funded program for suicide prevention, education of professionals, and treatment of at-risk youth and their families. His work has helped to shape clinical guidelines on the assessment of suicidal risk, prevention of adolescent suicide, and treatment of adolescent depression.

Oscar G. Bukstein, M.D., M.P.H., is an associate professor of psychiatry at the University of Pittsburgh School of Medicine, Pittsburgh, Pennsylvania. He is board certified in psychiatry, child and adolescent psychiatry, and addiction psychiatry. His master's and doctoral degrees are from the University of Texas, Austin. Dr. Bukstein received his specialty training in psychiatry at the University of Pittsburgh and Western Psychiatric Institute and Clinic, where he continues as a faculty member. In addition to his experience in the treatment of adolescents with comorbid substance use disorders and psychiatric disorders, Dr. Bukstein has published extensively on the topic of adolescent substance use disorders. He was primary author of the American Academy of Child and Adolescent Psychiatry's "Practice Parameter for the Assessment and Treatment of Children and Adolescents With Substance Use Disorders." He was director of the clinical core of the Pittsburgh Adolescent Alcohol Research Center. He is currently conducting several pharmacologic trials for children and adolescents with substance use disorders, depression, and attention-deficit/hyperactivity disorder. He is also principal investigator on a National Institute on Drug Abuse–funded study to develop a home-based treatment for younger adolescents with early substance use problems. He is the principal investigator at the Pittsburgh site of the National Institute of Mental Health's Treatment of Adolescent Suicidal Attempters Study and was a coinvestigator at the Pittsburgh site of the National Institute of Mental Health's Multimodal Treatment Study of Children With ADHD. He also has organized controlled clinical trials involving youth with conduct disorder and the use of pharmacotherapies and behavioral interventions.

John V. Campo, M.D., is chief of the Division of Child and Adolescent Psychiatry, medical director of Pediatric Behavioral Health, and a professor of clinical psychiatry at the Ohio State University and Nationwide Children's Hospital in Columbus, Ohio. He is board certified in pediatrics, psychiatry, and child and adolescent psychiatry, and has focused much of his career at the interface between pediatrics and psychiatry. Dr. Campo's clinical and research interests include the development and implementation of effective treatments for common pediatric mental disorders in real-world settings; novel models of service delivery that integrate evidence-based mental health services into general medical settings, particularly primary care; and the relationship between medically unexplained physical symptoms, anxiety, and depression in youth. He is the recipient of funding from the National Institute of Mental Health.

Gabrielle A. Carlson, M.D., has been a professor of psychiatry and pediatrics and director of the Division of Child and Adolescent Psychiatry at State University of New York at Stony Brook since 1985. She was educated at Wellesley College and Cornell University Medical College. She did her adult psychiatry training at Washington University in St. Louis and at the National Institute of Mental Health. She completed a fellowship and research fellowship in child and adolescent psychiatry at the University of California, Los Angeles, where she subsequently taught on the faculty. Dr. Carlson specializes in childhood psychopathology and psychopharmacology in general, and specifically in the subjects of childhood and adolescent depression and bipolar disorder. Her first publications on bipolar disorder in the 1970s redirected the field toward accurately diagnosing this disorder in youth. She has written over 200 papers and chapters and 2 books on the phenomenology of bipolar disorder, the long-term follow-up and treatment of young people with bipolar disorder, and the relationship of bipolar disorder to behavior disorders such as attention-deficit/hyperactivity disorder, developmental disorders, and mood disorders.

Bruce F. Chorpita, Ph.D., is a professor of psychology at the University of California, Los Angeles. He received his doctorate in psychology from the University at Albany, State University of New York, and held a faculty position with the Department of Psychology at the University of Hawaii from 1997 to 2008. From 2001 to 2003, Dr. Chorpita served as clinical director of the Hawaii Department of Health's Child and Adolescent Mental Health Division. With roughly 100 publications on children's mental health, he has been the recipient of multiple awards and honors for his work. Dr. Chorpita has held grants from the National Institute of Mental Health, the Hawaii Departments of Education and Health, and the John D. and Catherine T. MacArthur Foundation, and he recently published *Modular Cognitive Behavior Therapy*.

Greg Clarke, Ph.D., has been conducting mental health research for 20 years. He received his doctorate in clinical psychology from the University of Oregon in 1985. From 1985 to 1996, he was an assistant and associate professor in the Child Psychiatry Division of Oregon Health and Science University in Portland, Oregon. In 1996, he joined the Kaiser Permanente Center for Health Research in Portland, where he currently conducts research. Dr. Clarke's areas of interest include depression treatment and prevention, child and adolescent mental health and treatments, and treatment of substance abuse comorbid with mental disorders. Dr. Clarke has been the principal investigator and co-investigator of several grants funded by the National Institute of Mental Health, conducting controlled outcomes trials of depression treatment and prevention in at-risk populations. Some of his most recent controlled trials examine the costs and clinical outcomes of preventing and treating depression in adolescent offspring of depressed parents enrolled in a health maintenance organization; the medication and psychotherapy treatment of depression in adolescents who have failed to respond to an initial course of selective serotonin reuptake inhibitor medication; treatment of depression in adults also receiving outpatient treatment for alcohol addiction; simultaneous psychotherapy and medication for depressed adolescents treated in primary care; and Internet self-care programs for depressed adults and adolescents.

Barbara J. Coffey, M.D., M.S., is director of the Institute for Tourette and Tic Disorders at the New York University Child Study Center, and an associate professor in the Department of Child and Adolescent Psychiatry at New York University School of Medicine, New York, New York. Dr. Coffey received her B.A. in biology and psychology from the University of Rochester, her M.D. from Tufts University School of Medicine, and her M.S. in epidemiology from the Harvard School of Public Health. She completed a residency in general psychiatry at Boston University Hospital and a residency in child and adolescent psychiatry at Tufts University School of Medicine. Dr. Coffey is the former director of pediatric psychopharmacology at McLean Hospital and director of the Tourette's Clinics at McLean and Massachusetts General Hospitals in Boston. She remained on the faculty of Harvard Medical School as a clinical associate at Massachusetts General Hospital until January 2007. A past member of the Medical Advisory Board of the Tourette Syndrome Association, Dr. Coffey is the author of numerous manuscripts in peer-reviewed journals, abstracts, and book chapters, and is a featured speaker at conferences all over the world. Her research has focused on the clinical course, comorbidity, phenomenology, and treatment of Tourette's disorder.

Judith A. Cohen, M.D., is a board-certified child and adolescent psychiatrist and medical director of the Center for Traumatic Stress in Children and Adolescents at Allegheny General Hospital in Pittsburgh, Pennsylvania. With her colleagues, Dr. Cohen has developed and tested trauma-focused cognitive behavioral therapy (TF-CBT) for traumatized children, as described in the book *Treating Trauma and Traumatic Grief in Children and Adolescents.* Dr. Cohen has served on the board of directors for the American Professional Society on the Abuse of Children and for the International Society for Traumatic Stress Studies (ISTSS), and is associate editor of ISTSS's *Journal of Traumatic Stress* and coeditor of its forthcoming published guidelines for treating posttraumatic stress disorder. Dr. Cohen is principal author of the "Practice Parameters on Posttraumatic Stress Disorder," published by the American Academy of Child and Adolescent Psychiatry, which awarded her its 2004 Rieger Award for Scientific Achievement. Dr. Cohen publishes, trains, consults, teaches extensively, and sees clinical cases related to the assessment and treatment of childhood trauma. She and her colleagues have recently revised TF-CBT for childhood traumatic grief and have conducted three pilot studies supporting the efficacy of this treatment approach for traumatically bereaved children and their parents.

Christine A. Conelea, M.S., is a graduate student in the clinical psychology doctoral program at the University of Wisconsin–Milwaukee. Her current work focuses on understanding the behavioral processes involved in Tourette's syndrome, habit disorders, and associated comorbid conditions, as well as the functional impact and treatment of these disorders.

Cheryl M. Corcoran, M.D., is the Florence Irving Assistant Professor of Clinical Psychiatry at Columbia University/New York State Psychiatric Institute, New York, New York. Dr. Corcoran is director of the Center of Prevention and Evaluation, a clinical research program for young people identified as at increased risk for nonaffective psychosis. Dr. Corcoran has studied the psychosis prodrome for more than a decade. Dr. Corcoran specializes in the phenomenology of the psychosis prodrome and the trajectory to a first episode of psychosis in young people. Dr. Corcoran also examines the role of stress and drug use in symptom fluctuations in prodromal patients. She has published widely on the psychosis prodrome, including ethics and family perspectives.

Barbara A. Cornblatt, Ph.D., M.B.A., is currently a professor of psychiatry at the Albert Einstein College of Medicine, an investigator at the Feinstein Institute for Medical Research, and director of the Recognition and Prevention (RAP) program at the Zucker Hillside Hospital, Glen Oaks, New York. Her early research focused on identifying neurocognitive, social, and behavioral predictors of later illness in the young offspring and siblings of patients with schizophrenia. In 1998, she founded the RAP program, one of the first research and treatment programs dedicated to the prevention of psychosis. Since the program's inception, close to 250 adolescents and young adults (ages 13–22) have participated in the RAP clinic and research program. The RAP program is supported by grants from the National Institute of Mental Health and recently was one of five centers nationally to receive an award from the Robert Wood Johnson Foundation to evaluate the preventive benefits of a newly introduced psychosocial intervention. Dr. Cornblatt also developed the Continuous Performance Test—Identical Pairs (CPT-IP), a measure of attention and working memory that has been used in a large number of studies both nationally and internationally. The CPT-IP has become a principal component of the MATRICS battery, the current standard for measuring neuropsychological change in clinical trials. Dr. Cornblatt is on the board of directors for the International Early Psychosis Association and is on the editorial board of the journal *Early Intervention in Psychiatry*.

Christoph U. Correll, M.D., is medical director at the Zucker Hillside Hospital's Recognition and Prevention (RAP) program, a National Institute of Mental Health–funded research program for the identification and treatment of adolescents and young adults at risk for psychosis and bipolar disorder. He is also an assistant professor of psychiatry and behavioral sciences at the Albert Einstein College of Medicine, Bronx, New York. Having completed his medical studies at the Free University of Berlin, Germany, and Dundee University Medical School, Scotland, Dr. Correll finished his general psychiatry residency and child and adolescent psychiatry fellowship at the Zucker Hillside Hospital, Glen Oaks, New York. He served as a member of the Consensus Development Conference on Antipsychotic Drugs and Obesity and Diabetes, Expert Consensus Panel on Atypical Antipsychotic Related Adverse Effects in Children and Adolescents, and Roadmap Expert Consensus Survey on the Pharmacology and Use of Antipsychotics. He currently serves as a member of the American Psychiatric Association Work Group on Diabetes and Second-Generation Antipsychotic Agents and as a member of the German Bipolar Disorder Treatment Guideline Project. Dr. Correll's research focuses on the identification and treatment of individuals with established mood and psychotic disorders, as well as individuals who are considered at high risk for the development of schizophrenia and bipolar disorder. In addition, his work focuses on psychopharmacologic treatment options, especially the risk/benefit ratio of psychotropic medications used in children and adolescents and adults with severe psychiatric disorders.

Sarah A. Crawley, M.A., is a doctoral student in clinical psychology at Temple University, Philadelphia, Pennsylvania, where she does research on anxiety disorders in children and adolescents. Her current work focuses on the role of somatic symptoms in childhood anxiety disorders.

Kathryn R. Cullen, M.D., is an assistant professor in the child psychiatry division in the department of psychiatry at the University of Minnesota Medical School. Her research interests have been focused on understanding the developmental underpinnings of mental disorders such as schizophrenia and depression, and how treatment may harness the neuroplasticity that is inherent to developing periods in order to positively alter trajectories. After her clinical training in child and adolescent psychiatry, she completed a National Institutes of Health T32 postdoctoral research fellowship at the Center for Neurobehavioral Development at the University of Minnesota, during which she examined neural circuitry and stress reactivity in adolescents with major depressive disorder. Dr. Cullen uses integrative methodology to study developmental mechanisms that underlie pediatric depression. Her current work involves neuroimaging and measurement of stress reactivity in adolescents with depression.

Lisa M. Cullins, M.D., is the corporate medical director at EMQ Children and Family Services, which is a nonprofit organization headquartered in Campbell, California, with three regional sites throughout California that provide comprehensive mental health care to children and adolescents predominantly in the child welfare system. Dr. Cullins also is an adjunct assistant clinical professor of psychiatry at the University of California, San Francisco. Prior to joining EMQ Children and Family Services, Dr. Cullins was medical director of the District of Columbia Kids Integrated Delivery System (DC KIDS) in the Department of Psychiatry at Children's National Medical Center and assistant professor of psychiatry in behavioral sciences and pediatrics at George Washington University School of Medicine in Washington, D.C. In addition to providing leadership to the DC KIDS program, Dr. Cullins was also associate training director for the Child Psychiatry Fellowship Program in the Department of Psychiatry. Dr. Cullins has worked extensively with youth and families in the foster care system and has been an avid advocate for policy and system of care reform.

Ronald E. Dahl, M.D., is the Staunton Professor of Psychiatry and Pediatrics, and professor of psychology at the University of Pittsburgh in Pittsburgh, Pennsylvania. He is a pediatrician with research interests in sleep/arousal and affect regulation and their relevance to the development of behavioral and emotional disorders in youth. His work focuses on early adolescence and pubertal development as a neurodevelopmental period with unique opportunities for early intervention. He codirects a large program of research on child and adolescent anxiety and depression with more than 20 years of continuous funding from the National Institute of Mental Health, and he has received grants focusing on questions of neurobehavioral development and adolescent health outcomes from the National Institute on Alcohol Abuse and Alcoholism, National Institute on Drug Abuse, and National Institute of Child Health and Human Development. His research is interdisciplinary and bridges from basic work in affective neuroscience and development to clinical work focusing on early intervention for behavioral and emotional health problems. Dr. Dahl has participated in several interdisciplinary research groups, including the MacArthur Foundation Research Network on Psychopathology and Development and the Robert Wood Johnson Foundation Research Network on Tobacco Dependence. He has published extensively on adolescent development, sleep disorders, and behavioral and emotional health in children and adolescents.

Tara L. Deliberto, B.S., is the laboratory manager for the Laboratory for Clinical and Developmental Research in the Department of Psychology at Harvard University, Cambridge, Massachusetts. Ms. Deliberto received her bachelor's degree in rehabilitation counseling from Boston University. Her current research interests are focused on the etiology, assessment, and treatment of self-injurious behaviors.

David R. DeMaso, M.D., is a professor of psychiatry and pediatrics at Harvard Medical School and psychiatrist-in-chief at Children's Hospital Boston. As a child and adolescent psychiatrist, the underlying essence of his work has been to understand what facilitates or hinders an individual's ability to cope with physical illnesses. In 2002, he received the Simon Wile Leadership in Consultation Award from the American Academy of Child and Adolescent Psychiatry (AACAP) for his work in the field of pediatric psychosomatic medicine. In 2006, he received the AACAP Klingenstein Third Generation Foundation Award for Research in Depression or Suicide for the best paper on depression and/or suicide published in the *Journal of the American Academy of Child and Adolescent Psychiatry*, and coauthored the *Clinical Manual of Pediatric Psychosomatic Medicine: Mental Health Consultation With Physically Ill Children and Adolescents.*

Thomas A. Dixon, B.S., graduated from Ursinus College in 2007 after serving as a research assistant in the fields of child development and cognitive neuroscience. During this time he presented findings at both local and national conferences. He has also worked in clinical practices associated with the University of Pennsylvania: The Center for Cognitive Therapy and the Children's Hospital of Philadelphia Mood and Anxiety Disorders Center. At the latter, he serves as a research assistant to Elizabeth B. Weller, M.D., and to Ronald A. Weller, M.D., studying bereavement, bipolar disorders, mania, and the depressive disorders, in a study coordinator capacity.

Stacy S. Drury, M.D., Ph.D., is an assistant professor in the Department of Psychiatry and Neurology, Section of Child and Adolescent Psychiatry, at Tulane University Medical Center in New Orleans, Louisiana. She completed her M.D. and her Ph.D. in genetics from Louisiana State University and her psychiatry and child and adolescent psychiatry training at Tulane University.

Her current clinical work and research focus on medical traumatic stress in pediatric cancer and transplant patients and on gene × environment interactions in early negative life events.

Helen Egger, M.D., is an assistant professor at the Center for Developmental Epidemiology in the Department of Psychiatry and Behavioral Sciences at Duke University Medical Center, and clinical director at the Duke Preschool Psychiatric Clinic, Durham, North Carolina. Dr. Egger is a child psychiatrist and epidemiologist who graduated from Yale Medical School and completed adult and child psychiatry residencies and postdoctoral research training at Duke University Medical Center. Dr. Egger has been a leader in the development of measures for assessing psychiatric symptoms and disorders in young children, such as the Preschool Age Psychiatric Assessment (PAPA) and the ePAPA, the computerized version. Her current research program focuses on anxiety disorders in preschool children. She is a collaborator on the Bucharest Early Intervention Project, a longitudinal study of the effects of early deprivation with children living in orphanages in Romania. Her work is funded by the National Institute for Mental Health, the National Institute on Drug Abuse, the National Alliance for Research in Schizophrenia and Depression (NARSAD), a Pfizer Faculty Scholar's Grant in Clinical Epidemiology, and the National Alliance for Autism Research/Autism Speaks. She has been the recipient of many awards, including the Gerald L. Klerman Award for outstanding clinical research by a NARSAD Young Investigator. Dr. Egger currently serves in leadership positions for the American Academy of Child and Adolescent Psychiatry and serves as a board member for Zero to Three.

Graham J. Emslie, M.D., a professor with tenure, is chief of the Child and Adolescent Psychiatry Division at the University of Texas Southwestern Medical Center at Dallas (UTSW) and Children's Medical Center of Dallas. He holds the Charles E. and Sarah M. Seay Chair in Child Psychiatry at UTSW. Dr. Emslie completed his medical training at Aberdeen University in Scotland; his general psychiatry training and research fellowship at the University of Rochester, New York; and child psychiatry training at Stanford University. He has published extensively on the psychopharmacologic treatments of early-onset psychiatric disorders, including depression, anxiety disorders, and attention-deficit/hyperactivity disorder, and is currently involved in research projects integrating psychopharmacology and psychosocial interventions.

Jeffery N. Epstein, Ph.D., is an associate professor of pediatrics in the Division of Behavioral Medicine and Clinical Psychology at Cincinnati Children's Hospital Medical Center with a joint appointment in the University of Cincinnati's Department of Psychology. He is also director of the Cincinnati Children's Center for Attention Deficit Hyperactivity Disorder. He earned his doctorate in clinical psychology from State University of New York at Stony Brook and completed a clinical internship at the Medical University of South Carolina. Dr. Epstein is a licensed psychologist whose research and clinical work focus on the diagnosis and treatment of attention-deficit/hyperactivity disorder and other psychological disorders originating in childhood. He is a coinvestigator on the Multimodal Treatment Study of Children with ADHD. He has published numerous empirical papers on a variety of ADHD-related topics, including ADHD-related cognitive deficits and the promotion of evidence-based guidelines among community physicians.

Christianne Esposito-Smythers, Ph.D., is an assistant professor (research) in the Department of Psychiatry and Human Behavior at Brown University and on the training faculty at the Brown University Center for Alcohol and Addiction Studies, Providence, Rhode Island. She is also a licensed clinical psychologist. Her primary area of research interest is the development of cognitive-behavioral interventions for adolescents with co-occurring mental health and substance use disorders. She is the principal investigator on a research study, funded by the National Institute on Alcohol Abuse and Alcoholism, which compares an integrated cognitive-behavioral treatment for adolescents with co-occurring suicidality and substance use disorder to enhanced community care. She is also a coinvestigator on a research study jointly funded by the Adolescent Medicine Trials Network for HIV/AIDS and the National Institute of Child Health and Human Development to develop a substance abuse treatment program tailored for adolescents with HIV.

Sheila M. Eyberg, Ph.D., A.B.P.P., is a distinguished professor in the Department of Clinical and Health Psychology at the University of Florida, Gainesville. She obtained her doctorate in clinical psychology at the University of Oregon and completed a 2-year postdoctoral fellowship in clinical child psychology at Oregon Health and Science University, where she developed parent-child interaction therapy (PCIT) and its related assessment measures, including the Dyadic Parent-Child Interaction Coding System, the Eyberg Child Behavior Inventory, and the Therapy Attitude Inventory. Dr. Eyberg has published over 130 research articles and papers related to PCIT and has been an associate editor of *Behavior Therapy* and the *Journal of Clinical Child and Adolescent Psychology*. She has served on the Child Psychopathology and Treatment Review Committee of the National Institute of Mental Health and is a diplomate in clinical psychology and in clinical child and adolescent psychology of the American Board of Professional Psychology. Dr. Eyberg is a fellow of the American Psychological Association and is past president of the Society for Child and Family Policy and Practice, the Society of Clinical Child and Adolescent Psychology, the Society of Pediatric Psychology, and the Southeastern Psychological Association. She received the Distinguished Contributions to Education and Training Award from the American Psychological Association in 2007. Currently she is conducting a 5-year National Institute of Mental Health study comparing individual versus group PCIT for preschoolers with attention-deficit/hyperactivity disorder.

Robert L. Findling, M.D., is the Rocco L. Motto, M.D., Chair of Child and Adolescent Psychiatry at Case Western Reserve University School of Medicine, Cleveland, Ohio. Dr. Findling is also director of the Division of Child and Adolescent Psychiatry at University Hospitals Case Medical Center. Dr. Findling earned his undergraduate degree at Johns Hopkins University and went to medical school at the Medical College of Virginia. Dr. Findling then completed a triple board joint residency-training program in pediatrics, psychiatry, and child and adolescent psychiatry at Mt. Sinai Hospital in New York City. Dr. Findling's research endeavors have focused on pediatric psychopharmacology and serious psychiatric disorders in the young. Dr. Findling has been honored with numerous awards and has received both national and international recognition as a clinical investigator. Dr. Findling's research is supported in part by the National Institutes of Health, the Stanley Medical Research Institute, the American Foundation for Suicide Prevention, and the pharmaceutical industry. In addition, Dr. Findling is a fellow of the American Academy of Pediatrics.

E. Blake Finkelson, B.A., is a doctoral student in clinical psychology and a graduate research assistant in the Children, Families and Cultures (CFC) Laboratory at the Catholic University of America, Washington, D.C. Prior to graduate school, she worked as a research assistant for the Eating Disorders Research Unit at the Columbia University Medical Center and as a project coordinator for the Metro Region New York State Comprehensive Care Center for Eating Disorders (NYCCCED). Ms. Finkelson completed her bachelor's degree in psychology at the University of Pennsylvania in 2003.

Mary A. Fristad, Ph.D., A.B.P.P., is a professor of psychiatry and psychology and director of research and psychological services in the Division of Child and Adolescent Psychiatry at the Ohio State University in Columbus, Ohio, where she has been on the faculty since 1986. Dr. Fristad has published over 125 articles and book chapters addressing the assessment and treatment of childhood-onset depression, suicidality, and bipolar disorder. She coauthored

Childhood Mental Health Disorders: Evidence Base and Contextual Factors for Psychosocial, Psychopharmacological, and Combined Intervention and a book for families titled *Raising a Moody Child: How to Cope With Depression and Bipolar Disorder*. Dr. Fristad has served on and chaired many National Institute of Mental Health review committees. She has been a member and now serves as president of the executive board for the Society of Clinical Child and Adolescent Psychology, has chaired the Serious Emotional Disturbance Committee of the American Psychological Association (APA) Task Force for Serious Mental Illness/Serious Emotional Disturbance, and served on the APA Task Force on Psychotropic Medications and Children. She serves on the boards of directors for five web-based education and support groups for children and families with mood disorders. Dr. Fristad has been the principal or co-principal investigator on over two dozen federal, state, and local grants focusing on the assessment and biopsychosocial treatment of mood disorders in youth.

Jami M. Furr, M.A., is an upper-level doctoral student in clinical psychology and a student research assistant in the Child and Adolescent Anxiety Disorders Clinic at Temple University, Philadelphia, Pennsylvania. She investigates anxiety disorders in youth and the use of cognitive-behavioral therapy with children and adolescents. Her current work focuses on trauma in youth and, more specifically, the effects of disasters on posttrauma symptoms in youth. Ms. Furr also is interested in the mindfulness and awareness of inner emotional states in youth with anxiety disorders and their parents.

Cathryn A. Galanter, M.D., is an assistant professor of clinical psychiatry in the Division of Child and Adolescent Psychiatry at Columbia University. Her research interests include understanding and improving the diagnostic and treatment decision making of clinicians, educating physicians using theory-based interventions, and understanding bipolar disorder and its overlap with attention-deficit/hyperactivity disorder. Her research is currently funded by the National Institute of Mental Health. She also teaches trainees; treats children, adolescents, and adults; and is active in the American Academy of Child and Adolescent Psychiatry and the American Psychiatric Association. She has received many awards and authored numerous chapters and peer-reviewed publications.

Mary Kay Gill, R.N., M.S.N., J.D., is program coordinator of Course and Outcome for Bipolar Youth (MH 59929) and Longitudinal Assessment of Manic Symptoms (MH 73953), Western Psychiatric Institute and Clinic, University of Pittsburgh Medical Center, Pittsburgh, Pennsylvania. Ms. Gill received her master's degree in psychiatric mental health nursing and her juris doctorate from the University of Pittsburgh. She has more than 25 years of clinical psychiatric nursing experience, including 10 years working in various research projects with bipolar children and adolescents.

Mary Margaret Gleason, M.D., is an assistant professor in the Department of Psychiatry and Human Behavior, Warren Alpert Medical School of Brown University, Providence, Rhode Island. She is a pediatrician and child psychiatrist with specialty training in early childhood mental health. She is currently the acting associate training director for child psychiatry and triple board (pediatrics, psychiatry, child psychiatry) training at Brown University and a fellow in Zero to Three's Leaders for the 21st Century program, which promotes early childhood research and advocacy. She co-led the Preschool Psychopharmacology Working Group, which recently published treatment guidelines focused on rational, evidence-based psychiatric treatment for young children. Her clinical work focuses on assessment and treatment of high-risk children under age 6 in Louisiana's Early Childhood Supports and Services program, and she has a specific interest in maltreated children.

Daniel A. Gorman, M.D., F.R.C.P.C., is a staff psychiatrist in the neuropsychiatry program at the Hospital for Sick Children and an assistant professor in the Department of Psychiatry at the University of Toronto, Ontario, Canada. His clinical and research interests include Tourette's disorder, attention-deficit/hyperactivity disorder, obsessive-compulsive disorder, and child psychopharmacology. Dr. Gorman completed his postgraduate clinical training at New York-Presbyterian Hospital/Weill Cornell Medical Center and Children's Hospital Boston. He then completed a National Institute of Mental Health postdoctoral research fellowship in child psychiatry at Columbia University and New York State Psychiatric Institute, focusing on Tourette's disorder and neuroimaging techniques. His current work investigates psychosocial outcomes in young adults with Tourette's disorder and obsessive-compulsive disorder.

Ross W. Greene, Ph.D., is an associate clinical professor in the Department of Psychiatry at Harvard Medical School; cofounder of the Collaborative Problem Solving Institute in the Department of Psychiatry at Massachusetts General Hospital, Boston; and originator of a model of psychosocial treatment for challenging kids called Collaborative Problem Solving. He is the author of three books—*The Explosive Child*; *Treating Explosive Kids*; and *Lost at School: Why Our Behaviorally Challenging Kids Are Falling Through the Cracks and How We Can Help Them*—along with numerous articles, chapters, and scientific papers on the effectiveness of the Collaborative Problem Solving approach, the classification of and outcomes in youth with oppositional defiant disorder and severe social impairment, and teacher stress. Dr. Greene's research has been funded by, among others, the Stanley Research Institute, the National Institute on Drug Abuse/National Institute of Mental Health, the U.S. Department of Education, and the Maine Juvenile Justice Advisory Group. He consults extensively to general and special education schools, inpatient and residential facilities, and systems of juvenile detention, and lectures widely throughout the world.

Laurence L. Greenhill, M.D., is Ruane Professor of Psychiatry and Pediatric Psychopharmacology at Columbia University, director of the New York State Research Unit of Pediatric Psychopharmacology at the New York State Psychiatric Institute (NYSPI), and attending and consultant physician at the Disruptive Behavior Disorders Clinic at Columbia Presbyterian Medical Center, New York, New York. He obtained his medical degree at the Albert Einstein College of Medicine. He interned in pediatrics at Jacobi Medical Center and then trained at the National Institute of Mental Health (NIMH) and was later awarded an NIMH Research Career Development Award in the psychopharmacology of child disorders, specializing in ADHD. He has completed several NIMH grants and pharmaceutical company contracts to study ADHD medications and currently serves as a principal investigator of three NIMH multisite grants: the Multimodal Treatment Study of Attention Deficit Hyperactivity Disorder Follow-up Study, the Preschool ADHD Treatment Study of methylphenidate safety and efficacy in preschool children with ADHD, and the Treatment Study of Adolescent Suicide Attempters. He is president of the American Academy of Child and Adolescent Psychiatry (AACAP) and past chair of AACAP's Workgroup on Research and the Pediatric Psychopharmacology Initiative. He is the senior editor of ADHD articles for the *Journal of Child and Adolescent Psychopharmacology*. He serves as senior investigator in the NYSPI's Center for Study of Suicidal Behavior and is a member of the Principal Research Core of the NIMH Advanced Center for Intervention Services Research at the NYSPI Intervention Research Center. He is the author of over 95 published articles and has edited 3 books, including a monograph on methylphenidate.

Angela S. Guarda, M.D., is an associate professor of psychiatry and behavioral sciences at Johns Hopkins School of Medicine, Baltimore, Maryland, and has been director of the Johns Hopkins Eating Disorders Program since 1997. Dr. Guarda is nationally recognized as an expert in the inpatient and partial hospital treatment of eating disorders. Her clinical research interests include perceived coercion and ambivalence toward treatment among patients with anorexia nervosa and bulimia. Dr. Guarda is also involved in translational research on the biological basis of eating disorders in the areas of receptor neuroimaging and endocrine responses to feeding.

Allison G. Harvey, Ph.D., is an associate professor of clinical psychology and director of the Sleep and Psychological Disorders Laboratory at the University of California, Berkeley. She completed her clinical training and doctorate in Sydney, Australia, and then served on the faculty at Oxford University in the United Kingdom before moving to Berkeley in 2004. Her research seeks to improve treatments for chronic insomnia and for insomnia that is comorbid with psychiatric disorders, particularly transdiagnostic approaches. The editorial boards on which she serves include the journal *SLEEP* and *Behavioral Sleep Medicine*. She has been the recipient of numerous awards, most recently from NARSAD (National Alliance for Research in Schizophrenia and Depression) and the American Association for Behavior Therapy, and has received research funding from the Wellcome Trust, the Jules Thorn Charitable Trust, the Economic and Social Research Council in the United Kingdom, and the National Institute of Mental Health.

Robert L. Hendren, D.O., is a professor of psychiatry, executive director and Tsakopoulos-Vismara Chair of the M.I.N.D. Institute (Medical Investigation of Neurodevelopmental Disorders Institute), and chief of child and adolescent psychiatry at the University of California, Davis. He is president of the American Academy of Child and Adolescent Psychiatry for 2007–2009. His primary areas of research and publication are translational clinical pharmacology and nutritional trials using biomarkers (magnetic resonance imaging, measures of inflammation, oxidative stress, immune function, and pharmacogenomics) in neurodevelopmental disorders such as pervasive developmental disorder, bipolar disorder, schizophrenia spectrum disorders, and impulse control disorders.

Scott W. Henggeler, Ph.D., is a professor of psychiatry and behavioral sciences and director of the Family Services Research Center (FSRC) at the Medical University of South Carolina, Charleston. He received his doctorate in clinical psychology from the University of Virginia in 1977. The FSRC has received the Annie E. Casey Families Count Award, the GAINS Center National Achievement Award, and the Points of Light Foundation President's Award in recognition of excellence in community service directed at solving community problems. Dr. Henggeler has published more than 225 journal articles, book chapters, and books; is on the editorial boards of 9 journals; and has received grants from the National Institute of Mental Health, National Institute on Drug Abuse, National Institute on Alcohol Abuse and Alcoholism, Office of Juvenile Justice and Delinquency Prevention, Center for Substance Abuse Treatment, Annie E. Casey Foundation, and others.

Stephen P. Hinshaw, Ph.D., is a professor of psychology and chair of the Department of Psychology at the University of California, Berkeley. After receiving his bachelor's degree from Harvard in 1974, he directed day school and residential programs for children with developmental disabilities before obtaining his doctorate in clinical psychology from the University of California, Los Angeles in 1983. Following a postdoctoral fellowship at the Langley Porter Psychiatric Institute of the University of California, San Francisco, he joined the Berkeley faculty in 1990. His work focuses on developmental psychopathology, with particular emphasis on peer and family relationships, neuropsychological risk factors, psychosocial and pharmacologic treatment strategies for youth with attention-deficit/hyperactivity disorder, conceptual and definitional issues related to mental disorder, and stigma. Internationally recognized as an expert in developmental psychopathology, Dr. Hinshaw has authored over 200 articles, chapters, and reviews on child psychopathology, plus 6 books. He has received numerous research grants from the National Institute of Mental Health and is editor of the journal *Psychological Bulletin* and associate editor of *Development and Psychopathology*. He is past president of the International Society for Research in Child and Adolescent Psychopathology and of the Society for Clinical Child and Adolescent Psychology. A fellow of the American Psychological Association, the Association for Psychological Science, and the American Association for the Advancement of Science, he received the Distinguished Teaching Award, College of Letters and Sciences, University of California, Berkeley, in 2001.

Brian L. Isakson, Ph.D., is a clinical psychology postdoctoral fellow at the Center for Rural and Community Behavioral Health in the department of psychiatry at the University of New Mexico Health Science Center, Albuquerque. As a graduate student at Georgia State University, Dr. Isakson's work included program development and supervision of refugee adolescent mentoring programs, as well as conducting therapy and assessments with adult refugee torture survivors. Dr. Isakson conducted research on the effects of war trauma on Bosnian adolescents, and his dissertation examined adult refugee torture survivors' understanding of the healing process. As a postdoctoral fellow, Dr. Isakson coordinates a research study examining the impact of a community-based refugee wellness program, the African Refugee Well-Being Project, which pairs refugees with undergraduate students to engage in cultural exchanges, one-on-one learning, and advocacy. In addition, Dr. Isakson conducts research on behavioral health services and health disparities.

Peter S. Jensen, M.D., is president and chief executive officer of the REACH Institute (Resource for Advancing Children's Health Institute), New York, New York. He has been studying ADHD for over 20 years. He first served as chief of the Child and Adolescent Research Disorders branch of the National Institute of Mental Health (NIMH) and later as associate director for child and adolescent research for NIMH. While there, he served as the lead NIMH investigator on the multisite Multimodal Treatment Study of Children with ADHD. In 1999, he moved to Columbia University as the Ruane Professor of Child and Adolescent Psychiatry to start the Center for Advancement of Children's Mental Health. His current work emphasizes the implementation of evidence-based approaches via the development of field-consensus guidelines and toolkits, and application of basic science–driven behavior change approaches as applied to clinicians. He led the development of the Treatment Recommendations for Atypical Antipsychotics in Youth and Guidelines for Adolescent Depression—Primary Care. In his role at the REACH Institute, he continues to spearhead other national consensus and dissemination efforts for children in the child welfare, juvenile justice, education, and primary care systems.

Paramjit T. Joshi, M.D., is the endowed professor and chair of the Department of Psychiatry and Behavioral Sciences at Children's National Medical Center and professor in the Departments of Psychiatry and Behavioral Sciences and Pediatrics at the George Washington University School of Medicine in Washington, D.C. She first trained as a pediatrician and then proceeded to complete her training in general and child and adolescent psychiatry at Johns Hopkins University School of Medicine, where she remained on the faculty until 1999. She is a distinguished fellow of the American Psychiatric Association (APA) and the American Academy of Child and Adolescent Psychiatry and is president of the Society of Professors of Child and Adolescent Psychiatry (2006–2008). Dr. Joshi is an internationally recognized expert in the area of pediatric disaster psychiatry and the psychosocial effects of war and trauma on children. She is a recipient of the APA's Bruno Lima Award for outstanding contributions in the care and understanding of disaster psychiatry. Dr. Joshi has also been studying mood disorders for over two decades and is currently conducting a multisite study on the treatment of early-age mania. She has taught and published extensively on the issues of depression, bipolar disorder, and childhood trauma.

Yifrah Kaminer, M.D., M.B.A., is a professor of psychiatry in the Department of Psychiatry and Alcohol Research Center and codirector of research in the Division of Child and Adolescent Psychiatry at the University of Connecticut

Health Center, Farmington. His main interest has focused on clinical research of assessment and treatment of high-risk behaviors, particularly substance abuse, gambling behavior, and suicidal behavior in youth with comorbid psychiatric disorders. He has received funding for research from the National Institute on Alcohol Abuse and Alcoholism, National Institute on Drug Abuse, Center for Substance Abuse Treatment, and Donaghue Foundation. Dr. Kaminer has been teaching about addictive disorders in youth at the Yale Child Study Center since 2003. Dr. Kaminer is a member on the board of the International Society for Addiction Medicine and is on the editorial board of several peer-reviewed journals. Dr. Kaminer has developed rating scales, including the Teen Addiction Severity Index and the Teen Treatment Services Review, and treatment manuals. He has authored or coauthored more than 120 publications, including articles and book chapters. Dr. Kaminer authored *Adolescent Substance Abuse: A Comprehensive Guide to Theory and Practice,* coedited *Adolescent Substance Abuse: Psychiatric Comorbidity and High-Risk Behaviors,* and authored the forthcoming *Aftercare Phone Therapy* for adolescent substance abusers.

Sandra J. Kaplan, M.D., is director of the Division of Trauma Psychiatry, North Shore University Hospital–Zucker Hillside Hospital, Long Island Jewish Medical Center, in Manhasset, New York; a professor of psychiatry at New York University School of Medicine; and director of the Adolescent Trauma Treatment Development Center of the National Child Traumatic Stress Network and of the Florence and Robert A. Rosen Center for Law Enforcement and Military Personnel and Their Families. She is a diplomat of the American Board of Pediatrics and of the American Board of Psychiatry and Neurology in general psychiatry, child and adolescent psychiatry, and with special expertise in forensic psychiatry. Dr. Kaplan's leadership of research and clinical efforts, which have focused on enhancing the mental health of children, adolescents, and families exposed to traumatic events, has made the North Shore–Long Island Jewish Health System a national authority in this area. She has received numerous research and service grants, including funding from the National Institute of Mental Health for the ongoing "Follow-Up: Young Adults Physically Abused as Adolescents" and a New York State Temporary Aid to Needy Families Grant to support a Foster Care Prevention program. Dr. Kaplan was the project director of the North Shore–Long Island Jewish Health System site of the Child and Adolescent Trauma Treatment Services program to provide and evaluate interventions for children impacted by the September 11, 2001, attacks, and recipient of the American Psychiatric Association's (APA's) McGavin Award for Research Contributions to Primary Prevention in Child Psychiatry. Her work has included membership on the Steering Committee of the American Medical Association's National Advisory Council on Violence and Abuse, the U.S.

Department of States Civilian Psychiatric Response Team, the Steering Committee of the Interdisciplinary Forum on Mental Health and Family Law of the Bar Association of the City of New York, and the APA's Council on Children and Families. She served as chair of the APA's Committee on Family Violence and Sexual Abuse and the Corresponding Committee on Childhood Trauma. Dr. Kaplan is also the author of numerous publications in medical journals and editor of *Family Violence: A Clinical and Legal Guide.*

Niranjan S. Karnik, M.D., Ph.D., is an assistant adjunct professor in the Department of Psychiatry and the Department of Anthropology, History, and Social Medicine at the University of California School of Medicine in San Francisco. He also serves as a staff psychiatrist at the Palo Alto Medical Foundation in Fremont, California. He has interests in the mental health needs of underserved and vulnerable youth, cultural psychiatry, delinquency, and childhood trauma.

Courtney Pierce Keeton, Ph.D., is an instructor of psychiatry and behavioral sciences in the Division of Child and Adolescent Psychiatry, Johns Hopkins Medical Institutions, in Baltimore, Maryland. She completed her psychology doctoral training at the University of Massachusetts Amherst. She continued her training in cognitive-behavioral therapy in a predoctoral internship at the Duke University Medical Center and a postdoctoral fellowship at Johns Hopkins. Currently, Dr. Keeton is developing a project focused on young child anxiety, including selective mutism.

Philip C. Kendall, Ph.D., A.B.P.P., is the Laura H. Carnell Professor of Psychology and director of the Child and Adolescent Anxiety Disorders Clinic at Temple University in Philadelphia, Pennsylvania. Dr. Kendall develops and evaluates treatments for emotional and behavioral disorders in youth, specifically cognitive-behavioral therapy (CBT) for anxiety disorders. He has twice been a fellow at the Center for Advanced Study in Behavioral Sciences, Stanford, California, and is a fellow of both the American Association for the Advancement of Science and the American Psychological Association (APA). As author/coauthor of over 400 publications, he is an internationally recognized expert on clinical child and adolescent psychology. Coping Cat, the treatment he developed for anxious youth, has been reported to be effective in over a dozen randomized clinical trials, and the treatment materials have been translated into over a dozen languages. Dr. Kendall has received several National Institute of Mental Health (NIMH) research grants. He is currently completing a multisite NIMH-sponsored project evaluating CBT and medications for the treatment of childhood anxiety disorders and an NIMH-sponsored study of the features of the therapy process that predict differential improvement. Dr. Kendall is editor of *Clinical Psychology: Science and Practice*, and past president of Division 53 (Clinical Child Psychology) of the APA and the American Board of Clinical Child and Adolescent Psychology of the American Board of Professional Psychology. He has been recognized with the State of Pennsylvania Distinguished Contribution to the Science and Profession of Psychology Award and, in 1996, was presented with the Great Teacher Award by Temple University. He received the Anxiety Disorders Association of America's Research Recognition Award in 2005 and the Award for Distinguished Scientific Contributions in 2006 from the Society of Clinical Psychology (the APA's Division 12). Based on a quantitative study of scientific citations, he was identified as one of the most "highly cited" researchers.

Clarice J. Kestenbaum, M.D., is a professor of clinical psychiatry and director of training emerita in the Division of Child and Adolescent Psychiatry at Columbia University College of Physicians and Surgeons, New York, New York. Dr. Kestenbaum completed her general and child and adolescent psychiatry residency training at Columbia University and graduated from the Columbia Psychoanalytic Center for Training and Research in both adult and child psychoanalysis. Dr. Kestenbaum is a past president of the American Academy of Child and Adolescent Psychiatry and of the American Academy of Psychoanalysis and Dynamic Psychiatry. Her extensive hospital-based and outpatient clinical experience includes many years of working with children at risk for affective disorders, with an emphasis on children with bipolar disorder. For almost 30 years, Dr. Kestenbaum has been studying the children of parents with schizophrenia in her role as consultant to the New York Longitudinal Study of Children at Risk for Schizophrenia. She has maintained expertise in the application of both psychotherapy and medication in her clinical work with children and adolescents. Currently, she is a consultant to the Prodromal Schizophrenia Program (Center for Prevention and Evaluation) of Columbia University. Dr. Kestenbaum is a cofounder of CARING at Columbia, an organization that helps inner-city at-risk children. The program is a model for prevention and intervention that brings together artists, poets, and musicians to work with mental health professionals in school and hospital settings.

Dena A. Klein, Ph.D., is a staff psychologist and director of the child and adolescent psychological assessment service in the Child Outpatinet Psychiatry Department and Adolescent Depression and Suicide Program at Montefiore Medical Center in Bronx, New York. Her current research and clinical work involves the assessment and treatment of suicidal and nonsuicidal self-injurious adolescents using dialectical behavior therapy. She received her doctoral degree in clinical psychology from Rutgers, The State University of New Jersey, where her research and clinical training focused on empirically supported prevention and intervention for children and adolescents.

Rachel G. Klein, Ph.D., is the Fascitelli Family Professor of Child and Adolescent Psychiatry and director of the Institute for Anxiety and Mood Disorders at the Child Study Center, New York University (NYU) Langone Medical Center, New York, New York. She has conducted multiple National Institute of Mental Health–funded studies of medical and psychosocial treatments in children and adolescents with anxiety disorders, depression, or learning disorders, and multiple treatment studies of ADHD. To identify early precursors of anxiety and depression, Dr. Klein has studied children at high risk for anxiety and mood disorders. She has undertaken follow-up studies of large cohorts of several childhood disorders (anxiety disorders, ADHD, and learning disorders), with systematic focus on multiple aspects of function, including educational and occupational attainment, social development, and the evolution of substance use and abuse. At this time, Dr. Klein and colleagues are following a cohort of nearly 200 children with ADHD, and matched controls, now in their early 40s. Dr. Klein has been a member of the DSM-III, DSM-III-R, and DSM-IV committees on the nomenclature for children, and is a member of the DSM-V work groups. In recognition of her contribution to psychiatry, she was elected honorary fellow of the American Psychiatric Association. Prior to joining the NYU Child Study Center in 1999, she was a professor of psychiatry at Columbia University and director of clinical psychology at the New York State Psychiatric Institute and the New York–Presbyterian Hospital.

Penelope Knapp, M.D., is a professor emerita of psychiatry and pediatrics at the University of California, Davis, where she served as chief of the Division of Child, Adolescent and Family Psychiatry. She is currently the medical director of the California Department of Mental Health. She has been the project director of the CA First 5–funded Infant Preschool Family Mental Health Initiative and codirector of the California BEST PCP project as part of ABCD II. She is currently cochair of CalMEND: California Mental Health Care Management Program, a quality improvement initiative led by the Department of Health Care Services and Department of Mental Health. Dr. Knapp is a member or fellow of several national organizations, including the American Academy of Child and Adolescent Psychiatry and the American Academy of Pediatrics, serving on the Bright Futures Infancy Panel, the Mental Health Task Force, and the Developmental Psychosocial Toolkit task force. Her principal current interests are prevention and early intervention for high-risk parents, infants, and toddlers; evidence-based practices for mental health services; and screening and intervention in primary care settings for social-emotional, behavioral, and relationship problems.

Robert A. Kowatch, M.D., Ph.D., is a professor of psychiatry and pediatrics and director of psychiatry research at Cincinnati Children's Hospital Medical Center, Cincinnati, Ohio. He completed his internship in internal medicine at the Graduate Hospital under the auspices of the University of Pennsylvania, and his residency in general psychiatry at the Hospital of the University of Pennsylvania. In 2006, he completed a doctorate in cognition and neuroscience at the University of Texas at Dallas. Dr. Kowatch has authored or coauthored more than 60 articles, 14 book chapters, and a book. He has published in the areas of the diagnosis and treatment of children and adolescents with bipolar disorders, sleep disorders, and depression. His articles have been published in the *Journal of the American Academy of Child and Adolescent Psychiatry, Neuropsychopharmacology, Archives of General Psychiatry*, and the *Journal of Child Neurology*, among others. He is a member of the American Academy of Child and Adolescent Psychiatry, the Society of Biological Psychiatry, and the American College of Neuropharmacology. His research interests are in the diagnosis, treatment, and neurobiology of child and adolescent mood disorders.

Harvey N. Kranzler, M.D., is a professor of clinical psychiatry, director of the Division of Child and Adolescent Psychiatry at the Albert Einstein College of Medicine, and clinical director of Bronx Children's Psychiatric Center, Bronx, New York. Dr. Kranzler's expertise is in the psychopharmacologic management of treatment-resistant patients who have not responded to the usual medications. He teaches the advanced psychopharmacology course in the Albert Einstein College of Medicine Child Psychiatry Fellowship and has been a coinvestigator in a National Institute of Mental Health–funded research protocol for treatment-refractory schizophrenia in children and adolescents.

Christopher J. Kratochvil, M.D., is a professor in the department of psychiatry and a member of the graduate faculty at the University of Nebraska Medical Center (UNMC) in Omaha. He is also assistant director of the Psychopharmacology Research Consortium at UNMC. Board certified in psychiatry as well as child and adolescent psychiatry, Dr. Kratochvil received both his bachelor's and medical degrees from Creighton University in Omaha, Nebraska. He completed a residency in psychiatry at the Creighton–Nebraska Joint Residency Program. He went to the Duke University Medical Center, where he completed a residency in child and adolescent psychiatry and served as chief resident from 1996 to 1997. He is currently a member of the American Academy of Child and Adolescent Psychiatry, the American Psychiatric Association, the American Medical Association, the Nebraska Regional Council of Child and Adolescent Psychiatry, and the Nebraska Psychiatric Association. He was recently elected to the board of directors of the American Academy of

Child and Adolescent Psychiatry. Dr. Kratochvil's research interests include pediatric psychopharmacology, with an emphasis on the treatment of attention-deficit/hyperactivity disorder and pediatric depression. He is the UNMC principal investigator in the Treatment for Adolescents with Depression Study (TADS), funded by the National Institute of Mental Health.

Sanjiv Kumra, M.D., M.S., is an associate professor of psychiatry and division chief of the Department of Child and Adolescent Psychiatry at the University of Minnesota, Minneapolis. After completing a postdoctoral fellowship at the National Institute of Mental Health (NIMH) with Dr. Judith L. Rapoport, he became the lead investigator for the Treating Refractory Childhood Schizophrenia study at the Zucker Hillside Hospital. Currently, he is funded by NIMH to apply diffusion tensor imaging to understand the impact of recurrent exposure to cannabis on white matter development in adolescents with schizophrenia.

Joshua M. Langberg, Ph.D., is an assistant professor in the Cincinnati Children's Hospital Medical Center (CCHMC) Center for ADHD. He received his doctorate in clinical psychology from the University of South Carolina. He completed a clinical internship at the Duke University Medical Center and a postdoctoral fellowship at CCHMC. His research and professional interests include the assessment and treatment of children and adolescents with ADHD. His current work has focused on developing interventions to improve the academic functioning of young adolescents and college students with ADHD.

Christopher M. Layne, Ph.D., is director of treatment and intervention development for the University of California, Los Angeles/Duke National Center for Child Traumatic Stress, Los Angeles, California. With Robert Pynoos, he developed a pioneering group treatment protocol in 1993 for high school students exposed to community violence–related trauma and traumatic bereavement. Dr. Layne then served as field director of the UNICEF School-Based Program for War-Exposed Adolescents in postwar Bosnia between 1997 and 2001. He has taught research methods and psychometrics for over 10 years and has consulted with schools following school shootings. Following the September 11, 2001, terrorist attacks, he provided extensive methodological support, training, and consultation to clinicians in adopting a trauma and grief–focused intervention that he codeveloped to treat adolescents exposed to severe trauma and the traumatic death of close life figures. Dr. Layne's research and clinical interests include mental health interventions for adolescents exposed to trauma and loss; traumatic bereavement and grief; and research methodology, test construction, and developmental psychopathology approaches to understanding resilience and vulnerability in high-risk settings, including war, terrorism, community violence, and natural disasters.

Patricia K. Leebens, M.D., a board-certified adult, child, and adolescent psychiatrist, is currently consulting child and adolescent psychiatrist at Family and Children's Aid in Danbury, Connecticut. She is an assistant clinical professor of child psychiatry at the Yale Child Study Center in New Haven, Connecticut, and the University of Connecticut School of Medicine in Farmington. After completing medical school at the University of Colorado and adult and child psychiatry and research training at Yale University School of Medicine, Dr. Leebens served as a unit chief in charge of an adolescent inpatient psychiatric unit at Riverview Hospital for Children and Youth, a state psychiatric hospital in Connecticut. She later became the director of psychiatry for the Department of Children and Families in Connecticut, where she developed policies and procedures within the agency to oversee the use of psychotropic medications with the 6,000+ children in the care of the state. Prior to her medical career, Dr. Leebens worked as a junior high school teacher and school counselor for 6 years. Given her background in education and extensive work with children in state psychiatric facilities, Dr. Leebens has a particular interest in learning disabilities, autistic spectrum disorders, trauma in children, and early-onset psychosis.

Daniel le Grange, Ph.D., is an associate professor of psychiatry in the Department of Psychiatry, Section for Child and Adolescent Psychiatry, and director of the Eating Disorders Program at the University of Chicago, Chicago, Illinois. He trained in family-based treatment for adolescent anorexia nervosa at the Maudsley Hospital in London, where he was a member of the team that developed the Maudsley Approach as a treatment for early-onset anorexia nervosa. Most of Dr. le Grange's scholarly work is in the area of family-based treatment for adolescent eating disorders, including the first study of two outpatient family-based treatments for adolescents with anorexia nervosa. He is coauthor of two family-based treatment manuals based on the Maudsley Approach, one for anorexia nervosa and one for bulimia nervosa. He is also coauthor of a parent handbook for eating disorders in children and adolescents. Dr. le Grange's clinical and research work focus on psychosocial treatments, and he has been the recipient of several federal and nonfederal grants to evaluate the efficacy of these treatments for adolescents with anorexia or bulimia nervosa. Dr. le Grange was elected fellow of the Academy for Eating Disorders (AED) in 2002 and over the past few years has held several leadership positions at AED. He is also a member of the Eating Disorders Research Society and serves on the clinical and scientific advisory council of the National Eating Disorders Association.

Alicia F. Lieberman, Ph.D., is the Irving B. Harris Endowed Chair of Infant Mental Health and professor in psychiatry and vice-chair for academic affairs at the University of California, San Francisco, and director of the Child Trauma Research Project, San Francisco General Hospital. She directs the Early Trauma Treatment Network, a center of the National Child Traumatic Stress Network. She is currently president of the board of Zero to Three: The National Center for Infants, Toddlers and Families. She is the author or senior author of several books for parents and clinicians, including *The Emotional Life of the Toddler*; *Losing a Parent to Death in the Early Years: Treating Traumatic Bereavement in Infancy and Early Childhood*; *Don't Hit My Mommy: A Manual for Child-Parent Psychotherapy With Young Witnesses of Domestic Violence*; and *Psychotherapy With Infants and Young Children: Repairing the Effect of Stress and Trauma on Early Attachment*. She is senior editor of *DC:0–3 Casebook: A Guide to the Use of Zero to Three's Diagnostic Classification of Mental Health and Developmental Disorders of Infancy and Early Childhood*. Dr. Lieberman served on the National Research Council and Institute of Medicine Committee on Integrating the Science of Early Childhood Development, whose work resulted in the publication of the influential *From Neurons to Neighborhoods: The Science of Early Childhood*, and has been a member of National Institute of Mental Health grant review committees. She is the author of over 50 articles and chapters about infancy and therapeutic interventions in the early years. She lectures extensively on four continents and is a consultant to government agencies and private foundations nationally and abroad.

John E. Lochman, Ph.D., A.B.P.P., is professor and Doddridge Saxon Chairholder in Clinical Psychology at the University of Alabama, Tuscaloosa, where he also directs the Center for Prevention of Youth Behavior Problems (CPYBP). A major focus of the CPYBP is to investigate how evidence-based programs can be effectively disseminated into real-world settings. Dr. Lochman is also an adjunct professor in the Department of Psychiatry and Behavioral Sciences at the Duke University Medical Center, and he is a special visiting professor in interdisciplinary behavioral research (Department of Social Sciences), and in the Rudolf Magnus Institute of Neuroscience at the University of Utrecht from 2007 to 2009. He has received the Blackmon-Moody Outstanding Professor and the Burnum Distinguished Faculty Awards at the University of Alabama, and was awarded an honorary doctorate by the University of Utrecht in the Netherlands in 2004 for his prevention research. Dr.

Lochman has over 250 publications on risk factors, social cognition, and intervention and prevention research with aggressive children. His research has been funded with federal research grants for the past 22 years, including 14 grants as principal investigator and 9 grants as coinvestigator. Dr. Lochman is editor-in-chief of the *Journal of Abnormal Child Psychology*; serves on the National Institutes of Health study section on Psychosocial Development, Risk and Prevention; is a fellow in the American Psychological Association and in the Academy for Cognitive Therapy; is a member of the board of directors of the Society for Prevention Research; and is president-elect of the American Board for Clinical Child and Adolescent Psychology.

Joan L. Luby, M.D., is an associate professor of psychiatry (child) at Washington University School of Medicine in St. Louis, Missouri, and is founder and director of the Washington University School of Medicine Early Emotional Development Program, a clinical research program that focuses on the study and treatment of affective disorders in preschool-age children. Dr. Luby's clinical work and research (funded by the National Institute of Mental Health and NARSAD [National Alliance for Research in Schizophrenia and Depression]) focuses more broadly on infant/preschool psychopathology and nosology and the social/emotional development of young children. Her contributions include the first large-scale empirical studies that have established the criteria for identification, validation, and clinical characteristics of depressive syndromes in the preschool age group. Dr. Luby was awarded the Joseph Fischoff, M.D., Honorary Lectureship in Child and Adolescent Psychiatry in 2002 and the Gerald Klearman award for outstanding research from NARSAD in 2004. She chairs the infancy committee of the American Academy of Child and Adolescent Psychiatry. Dr. Luby has published extensively in numerous general and child psychiatric journals on the issue of preschool mood disorders and young child psychopathology.

Richard P. Malone, M.D., is a professor of psychiatry at Drexel University College of Medicine, Philadelphia. Pennsylvania. He received his medical degree from Hahnemann University, completed his general and child adolescent psychiatry residency at Medical College of Pennsylvania/Eastern Pennsylvania Psychiatric Institute in Philadelphia, and completed a 2-year fellowship in research training in child psychopharmacology at New York University Medical Center. He has been the recipient of National Institute of Mental Health grants to investigate the treatment of aggression in conduct disorder and grants from the U.S. Food and Drug Administration (FDA) and the National Institute of Mental Health (NIMH) to investigate treatment in autism. Dr. Malone is the author of a number of papers in the areas of aggression in conduct disorder and in autism, and he has presented his work both nationally and internationally. In addition, Dr. Malone has served on a number of national committees, including for the American Academy of Child and Adolescent Psychiatry, NIMH, and the FDA.

Anthony P. Mannarino, Ph.D., is director of the Center for Traumatic Stress in Children and Adolescents and vice president of the Department of Psychiatry, Allegheny General Hospital, Pittsburgh, Pennsylvania. He is also professor of psychiatry at Drexel University College of Medicine. Dr. Mannarino has been a leader in the field of child traumatic stress for the past 25 years. He has been awarded numerous federal grants from the National Center on Child Abuse and Neglect and the National Institute of Mental Health to investigate the clinical course of traumatic stress symptoms in children and to develop effective treatment approaches for traumatized children and their families. Dr. Mannarino has received many honors for his work, including the Betty Elmer Outstanding Professional Award, the Most Outstanding Article Award for papers published in the journal *Child Maltreatment* given by the American Professional Society on the Abuse of Children (APSAC), the Model Program Award from the Substance Abuse and Mental Health Services Administration for "Cognitive Behavioral Therapy for Child Traumatic Stress," and the Legacy Award from the Greater Pittsburgh Psychological Association. Dr. Mannarino recently completed a 2-year term as president of APSAC and is now president of the Section on Child Maltreatment, Division of Child and Family Policy and Practice, American Psychological Association.

John S. March, M.D., M.P.H., is a professor of psychiatry and chief of child and adolescent psychiatry at the Duke University Medical Center, Durham, North Carolina. Dr. March also holds faculty appointments at the Duke Clinical Research Institute and in the Department of Psychology and Neuroscience. He has extensive experience developing and testing the efficacy and effectiveness of cognitive-behavioral and pharmacologic treatments for pediatric mental disorders. He holds a career development award from the National Institute of Mental Health (NIMH) devoted to clinical trials methods and is principal or co-principal investigator on several National Institute of Mental Health–funded treatment outcome studies: the Multimodal Treatment of Children with ADHD Study, the Pediatric OCD Treatment Study, the Child/Adolescent Anxiety Multimodal Study, and the Treatment for Adolescents with Depression Study. His most recent undertaking is the creation of a practical clinical trials network in pediatric psychiatry, the Child and Adolescent Psychiatry Trials Network (http://www.captn.org). CAPTN is beginning a large study of the safety and effectiveness of antidepressants (selective serotonin reuptake inhibitors and serotonin-norepinephrine reuptake inhibitors) in youth with mental illness. Dr. March, with funding from NARSD (National Alliance for Research in Schizophrenia and Depression), will conduct a substudy looking for risk genes associated with adverse response to antidepressant treatment. Dr. March is deputy editor of *Biological Psychiatry* and is an active member of the NIMH Advisory Mental Health Council, American College of Neuropsychopharmacology, Collegium Internationale Neuro-psychopharmacologicum (International College of Neuropsychopharmacology), and the American Academy of Child and Adolescent Psychiatry.

Carla E. Marin, M.S., is a doctoral candidate in life span developmental science at Florida International University in Miami, Florida. Ms. Marin is presently involved in research at the Child Anxiety and Phobia Program at Florida International University. Ms. Marin is working toward a career in academia, where she can continue her research on Latino youth and families, focusing on internalizing problems in this population. Ms. Marin also served as editorial assistant of the American Psychological Association's Division 53 flagship journal, *Journal of Clinical Child and Adolescent Psychology.*

Jon McClellan, M.D., is a professor in the Department of Psychiatry and Behavioral Sciences at the University of Washington in Seattle, and medical director of the Child Study and Treatment Center, Division of Mental Health, Washington State. His research focuses primarily on the diagnosis and treatment of early-onset schizophrenia and bipolar disorder, and the genetics of neuropsychiatric disorders. Dr. McClellan is the primary author of the American Academy of Child and Adolescent Psychiatry's practice parameters for schizophrenia and bipolar disorder.

Alec L. Miller, Psy.D., is professor of clinical psychiatry and behavioral sciences, chief of child and adolescent psychology, director of the Adolescent Depression and Suicide Program, and associate director of the Psychology Internship Training Program at Montefiore Medical Center/Albert Einstein College of Medicine, Bronx, New York. He is also cofounder of Cognitive and Behavioral Consultants of Westchester, a private group practice in White Plains, New York. Dr. Miller is a fellow of the American Psychological Association (Divisions 12 and 53), past president of Division 12's Section on Clinical Emergencies and Crises, 2007 Division 12 program chair, past chair of the International Society for the Improvement and Training of Dialectical Behavior Therapy (ISITDBT), and recipient of the Service Award from ISITDBT in 2002. He is past associate editor of *Cognitive and Behavioral Practice*, a consultant on the U.S. Food and Drug Administration's Suicide Classification Project, and a member of the International Academy of Suicide Research. He has received federal, state, and private funding for his research. He has authored numerous scientific articles, book chapters, and books, including *Dialectical Behavior Therapy With Suicidal Adolescents*. Also, upon invitation by the American Psychological Association, Dr. Miller developed a psychotherapy training video, *DBT for Multi-Problem Adolescents*. Also, he is highly sought after as a lecturer on topics including adolescent suicide, nonsuicidal self-injury, and dialectical behavior therapy (DBT). He has given more than 250 invited lectures and workshops to both lay and professional audiences and has trained thousands of mental health professionals around the world in DBT.

Jodi A. Mindell, Ph.D., C.B.S.M., is a professor of psychology at Saint Joseph's University and of pediatrics at the University of Pennsylvania School of Medicine in Philadelphia. She is also associate director of the Sleep Center at the Children's Hospital of Philadelphia. Dr. Mindell has published extensively on pediatric sleep disorders. She is the author of *Sleeping Through the Night: How Infants, Toddlers, and Their Parents Can Get a Good Night's Sleep* and *Sleep Deprived No More: From Pregnancy to Early Motherhood*, as well as coauthor of *A Clinical Guide to Pediatric Sleep: Diagnosis and Management of Sleep Problems* and *Take Charge of Your Child's Sleep: The All-in-One Resource for Solving Sleep Problems in Kids and Teens*. Dr. Mindell is on the board of directors of the National Sleep Foundation, a foundation established to educate the public about sleep and sleep disorders, and has been on the board of directors of the Sleep Research Society. Dr. Mindell is also the cofounder and cochair of the Pediatric Sleep Medicine annual meeting.

Robert Miranda, Jr., Ph.D., is an assistant professor (research) in the Department of Psychiatry and Human Behavior at Brown University, Providence, Rhode Island. His research centers on delineating mechanisms that link disruptive behavior and substance use disorders in adolescents and on identifying promising medications to improve treatment for these youth. He is the principal or coinvestigator on several federally funded research projects in this area. Dr. Miranda is also a licensed clinical psychologist who specializes in the assessment and treatment of adolescents and has worked extensively in school settings. He holds a faculty appointment at the Brown University Center for Alcohol and Addiction Studies, where he supervises postdoctoral fellows in the area of adolescent alcohol intervention and treatment outcome research.

David A. Mrazek, M.D., F.R.C.Psych., is chair of the Department of Psychiatry and Psychology at the Mayo Clinic and a professor of psychiatry and pediatrics at the Mayo Clinic College of Medicine, Rochester, Minnesota. Dr. Mrazek previously held the position of professor and chair of the Department of Psychiatry at George Washington University Medical Center and was the Leon Yochelson Professor of Psychiatry. At Mayo, Dr. Mrazek has initiated a psychiatric pharmacogenomic research program and implemented clinical psychiatric pharmacogenomic services. Dr. Mrazek is the principal investigator of the SSRI Pharmacogenomic Project within the National Institutes of Health–funded Pharmacogenetics Research Network. He currently serves as the vice-chair of the Psychiatry Residency Review Committee and is a member of the Executive Committee of the American Board of Psychiatry and Neurology.

Matthew K. Nock, Ph.D., is the John L. Loeb Associate Professor of the Social Sciences and director of the Laboratory for Clinical and Developmental Research in the Department of Psychology at Harvard University, Cambridge, Massachusetts. Dr. Nock received his doctorate in psychology from Yale University and completed his clinical internship at the New York University Child Study Center–Bellevue Hospital Center. His research focuses primarily on the etiology, assessment, and treatment of self-injurious and aggressive behaviors. Dr. Nock has authored more than 70 scientific papers on these topics, and his research is currently funded by the National Institute of Mental Health and the Talley and Clark Funds at Harvard University. In addition to his research and clinical work, Dr. Nock teaches courses at Harvard on self-destructive behaviors, statistics, research methodology, developmental psychopathology, and cultural diversity.

Judith A. Owens, M.D., M.P.H., D'A.B.S.M., is an internationally recognized authority on pediatric sleep. She is an associate professor of pediatrics at Brown Medical School and the director of the Pediatric Sleep Disorders Clinic at Hasbro Children's Hospital and the Learning, Attention, and Behavior Program at Rhode Island Hospital, Providence, Rhode Island. She received her undergraduate and medical degrees from Brown and a master's in maternal and child health from the University of Minnesota. She completed training in pediatrics at Children's Hospital of Philadelphia and fellowships in behavioral pediatrics at Minneapolis Children's Medical Center and in child psychiatry at Brown. She is board certified in developmental/behavioral pediatrics and sleep medicine. Dr. Owens's research interests are in the neurobehavioral and health consequences of sleep problems in children, pharmacologic treatment of pediatric sleep disorders, sleep health education, and cultural and psychosocial issues impacting sleep. As a recipient of a 5-year National Institutes of Health grant in sleep education, she has developed educational materials for Brown Medical School and the American Academy of Sleep Medicine (AASM). She received the AASM Excellence in Education Award and recently completed a 4-year term as chair of the AASM Section on Childhood Sleep Disorders and Development. Dr. Owens is the author of over 100 original research and review articles in peer-reviewed journals and book chapters. She recently coauthored a book for physicians on pediatric sleep disorders, *A Clinical Guide to Pediatric Sleep: Diagnosis and Management of Sleep Problems,* and a parent book on sleep, *Take Charge of Your Child's Sleep: The All-in-One Resource for Solving Sleep Problems in Kids and Teens*. She has been interviewed about her work by numerous national news outlets.

Mani Pavuluri, M.D., Ph.D., is the founding director of the nationally recognized pediatric mood program that includes the Pediatric Translational Research in Affective and Cognitive Neurocircuitry and Treatment (P-TRACT) lab at the Center for Cognitive Medicine, University of Illinois, Chicago. After obtaining her basic medical degree, Dr. Pavuluri was trained in psychiatry in New Zealand, Australia, and the United States. She obtained her doctorate in developmental psychopathology. She has published in several peer-reviewed journals on topics such as neurocognition and the biological causes of bipolar disorder. She reviews several international journals. Dr. Pavuluri has obtained several grants, one of which is a K23 award from the National Institutes of Health for study of functional magnetic resonance imaging (fMRI) outcome pre- and post-clinical trial in pediatric bipolar disorder. Her main area of interest is the interaction between affect dysregulation and cognitive function in pediatric bipolar disorder. She and her team of scientists are actively working on translational research, developing and testing cutting-edge neuroscience and imaging methodology crucial for conducting rigorous fMRI studies. Her focus is determining the neurobiological predictors of medication response. Dr. Pavuluri is a site principal investigator for the National Institute of Child Health and Human Development and National Institute of Mental Health's multisite Collaborative Lithium Trials (COLT), in which she is taking a lead on studying the effects of lithium on neurocognitive function.

William E. Pelham, Jr., Ph.D., A.B.P.P., is a graduate of Dartmouth College and earned his doctorate in clinical psychology from the State University of New York at Stony Brook in 1976. He is currently a distinguished professor of psychology, pediatrics, and psychiatry and director of the Center for Children and Families at the State University of New York at Buffalo. His summer treatment program for children with ADHD has been recognized by the American Psychological Association, Substance Abuse and Mental Health Services Administration, and CHADD as a model program and is widely recognized as the state of the art in treatment for ADHD. Dr. Pelham has authored or coauthored more than 275 professional papers dealing with ADHD and its assessment and treatment (psychosocial, pharmacologic, and combined). Dr. Pelham is a fellow of the American Psychological Association and the American Psychological Society, and past president of the Society of Child Clinical and Adolescent Psychology and the International Society for Research in Child and Adolescent Psychopathology. He has held more than 40 research grants from federal agencies (e.g., National Institute of Mental Health, National Institute on Alcohol

Abuse and Alcoholism, National Institute on Drug Abuse), foundations, and pharmaceutical companies, and he has served as a consultant/advisor on ADHD and related topics to numerous agencies and organizations.

Bradley S. Peterson, M.D., is the Suzanne Crosby Murphy Professor in Pediatric Neuropsychiatry and director of magnetic resonance imaging research in the Department of Psychiatry at Columbia University/New York State Psychiatric Institute, New York, New York. He trained in general psychiatry at Massachusetts General Hospital and Harvard University, in child psychiatry at the Child Study Center of Yale University, and in psychoanalysis at the Western New England Institute for Psychoanalysis. His research interests concern primarily the applications of neuroimaging to the study of serious childhood neuropsychiatric disorders, including Tourette's disorder, ADHD, obsessive-compulsive disorder, autism, bipolar disorder, depression, prenatal toxin exposure, and premature birth. His imaging studies integrate measures of brain structure and function with genetic, neurochemical, behavioral, neuropsychological, and clinical measures to define disease processes and therapeutic responses in large samples of children and adults.

Cynthia R. Pfeffer, M.D., is a professor of psychiatry and director of the Childhood Bereavement Program at Weill Cornell Medical College, New York–Presbyterian Hospital, White Plains, New York. She is internationally known for her clinical and research work with suicidal children and adolescents and childhood bereavement. She has been awarded grants to study the development of children who lost a loved one on September 11, 2001, from the National Institute of Mental Health and to study the coping of children and their parents who suffered the suicide death of a loved one from the American Foundation for Suicide Prevention. Dr. Pfeffer was awarded a Distinguished Investigator Award from the National Alliance for Research in Schizophrenia and Depression to study the likelihood of developing mood or anxiety disorders related to the effects of severe stress of bereavement on children who have a specific profile of the serotonin transporter gene. She was also the recipient of the Charlotte and Norbert Rieger Award for Scientific Achievement from the American Academy of Child and Adolescent Psychiatry. After September 11th, Dr. Pfeffer was a consultant for numerous schools, corporations, and academic centers and was invited to be an expert witness at the Senate Committee Hearing on Psychological Issues of Terrorism. She has also served as a consultant on the U.S. Food and Drug Administration advisory committee to evaluate the safety of antidepressants and other drugs used to treat children and adolescents. She is the author of over 130 scientific papers, author of the book *The Suicidal Child*, and coauthor of "Practice Guideline for the Assessment and Treatment of Patients With Suicidal Behavior." She has also edited several books, including *Severe Stress and Mental Disturbances in Children* and two books on pediatric neurology, and is coeditor of the *Bulletin for the International Association for Child and Adolescent Psychiatry and Allied Professionals.*

John Piacentini, Ph.D., A.B.P.P., is a professor of psychiatry and biobehavioral sciences in the David Geffen School of Medicine and director of the Child OCD, Anxiety, and Tic Disorders Program at the Semel Institute for Neuroscience and Human Behavior at the University of California, Los Angeles. He received his doctorate in clinical psychology from the University of Georgia and completed postdoctoral training and was a faculty member at Columbia University/New York State Psychiatric Institute. Dr. Piacentini has authored over 140 papers, chapters, and books and has received numerous National Institutes of Health and other grants addressing the etiology, assessment, and treatment of childhood anxiety, obsessive-compulsive disorder, tic disorders, and adolescent suicide. He is chair of the Tourette Syndrome Association Behavioral Sciences Consortium, founding fellow of the Academy of Cognitive Therapy, president-elect of the American Board of Clinical Child and Adolescent Psychology, and a member of the Scientific Advisory Board for the Trichotillomania Learning Center. Dr. Piacentini is also deputy editor for the *Journal of the American Academy of Child and Adolescent Psychiatry* and an editorial board member for several leading psychology journals. He is a frequent lecturer and actively involved in training mental health practitioners on how to treat youngsters with obsessive-compulsive disorder, anxiety, and similar problems.

Daniel Pine, M.D., is chief of the Section on Development and Affective Neuroscience, chief of the Emotion and Development Branch, and chief of Child and Adolescent Research in the Mood and Anxiety Disorders Program of the National Institute of Mental Health (NIMH) Intramural Research Program, Bethesda, Maryland. He moved to this position in 2000, after 10 years of training, teaching, and research at the New York State Psychiatric Institute and Columbia University. Since graduating from medical school at the University of Chicago, he has been engaged in research focusing on the epidemiology, biology, and treatment of psychiatric disorders in children and adolescents. His areas of expertise include biological and pharmacologic aspects of mood, anxiety, and behavioral disorders in children, as well as classification of psychopathology across the life span. This expertise is reflected in more than 180 peer-reviewed papers on these topics. Currently, his group at NIMH is examining the degree to which mood and anxiety disorders in children and adolescents are associated with underlying abnormalities in the amygdala, prefrontal cortex, and other brain regions that modulate activity in these structures. He also serves as chair of the Psychopharmacologic Drug Advisory Committee for the U.S. Food and Drug

Administration and of the Developmental Working Group for the DSM-V Task Force. He has received a number of awards, including Career Development and R01 extramural grant support from NIMH, a National Alliance for Research in Schizophrenia and Depression Independent Investigator Award, and the Blanche Ittelson Award from the American Psychiatric Association for outstanding research contributions to the field of child psychiatry.

Nicole Powell, Ph.D., M.P.H., received her doctoral degree in clinical psychology from the University of Alabama in 2000 and completed a clinical internship at Children's Memorial Hospital in Chicago. After spending 3 years as a staff psychologist at an inpatient treatment and evaluation center for children, she now holds the position of research psychologist at the Center for the Prevention of Youth Behavior Problems at the University of Alabama, Tuscaloosa. Her interests include the effects of parental psychopathology on children's adjustment and the implementation and evaluation of manualized interventions for disruptive children and their parents.

Frank W. Putnam, M.D., is a child and adolescent psychiatrist, professor of pediatrics and psychiatry, and director of the Mayerson Center for Safe and Healthy Children, Cincinnati Children's Hospital Medical Center, Cincinnati, Ohio. Formerly chief of developmental traumatology at the National Institute of Mental Health, Dr. Putnam has received numerous awards for his research and clinical contributions to understanding the psychosocial and biological impacts of child maltreatment. His current research focuses on developing strategies for the implementation of evidence-based child trauma treatments in community-based mental health settings.

Judith L. Rapoport, M.D., is chief of the Child Psychiatry Branch at the National Institute of Mental Health in Bethesda, Maryland. The branch studies the neurobiology and treatment of severe childhood-onset neuropsychiatric disorders. For the past 20 years, she has been studying the phenomenology, treatment, neurobiology, and genetics of very early-onset psychoses. This work has been influential in the field of schizophrenia, supporting the continuity of very early-onset and later-onset schizophrenia and the progressive nature of anatomical brain abnormalities.

M. Jamila Reid, Ph.D., has worked at the Parenting Clinic at the University of Washington, Seattle, for the past 11 years. She is affiliate assistant professor in the Department of Psychology. Her work at the clinic involves delivering treatment to families of children with ADHD, oppositional defiant disorder, and other childhood behavior disorders. She is extensively involved in training and research for The Incredible Years, an evidence-based practice for children with conduct problems.

Mark A. Riddle, M.D., is a professor of psychiatry and pediatrics and director of the Division of Child and Adolescent Psychiatry at Johns Hopkins University School of Medicine, Baltimore, Maryland. He also serves as vice president for psychiatric sciences of the Kennedy Krieger Institute, a Johns Hopkins–affiliated organization for individuals with developmental disabilities. Dr. Riddle's research, teaching, and clinical practice focus on children with obsessive-compulsive and anxiety disorders, and on pediatric psychopharmacology.

Paula Riggs, M.D., is an associate professor of psychiatry at the University of Colorado School of Medicine, Denver. She and her research group have conducted the first controlled studies of combined pharmacotherapy and behavioral treatment in dually diagnosed adolescents, including a randomized controlled trial of fluoxetine with cognitive-behavioral therapy (CBT) in depressed, substance-abusing youths. She is also the principal investigator of a large multisite study in the National Institute on Drug Abuse (NIDA) Clinical Trials Network, evaluating the safety and effectiveness of psychostimulant medication for ADHD in adolescents concurrently receiving CBT for substance abuse in 11 "real-world" adolescent drug treatment programs. Based on this research, Dr. Riggs and her clinical research team have developed the first empirically supported integrated treatment model, Encompass: Integrated Treatment for Adolescents and Young Adults. Dr. Riggs has also had a career-long commitment to training and mentoring junior investigators, and is currently the principal investigator of an NIDA/American Academy of Child and Adolescent Psychiatry K12 Physician Scientist Career Development Award, the aim of which is to address the critical shortage of child and adolescent psychiatrist investigators in addiction research.

Irwin N. Sandler, Ph.D., is a Regents' Professor in the Department of Psychology and director of the Prevention Research Center for Families in Stress at Arizona State University in Tempe. He completed his psychology doctoral training at the University of Rochester. He has been the director of a National Institute of Mental Health (NIMH)–supported Preventive Research Center, and the recipient of multiple grants from NIMH to study resilience for children in stress and to develop and evaluate preventive interventions for these children and their families. His research has focused mainly on children who experience parental divorce or the death of a parent and has emphasized linking theory and research about sources of resilience with the design and evaluation of preventive interventions. He has received numerous awards for his work, including the Stanley Cohen Distinguished Research Award from the Association of Family and Conciliation Courts, the Award for Distinguished Contribution to Theory and Research in Community Psychology, and the Presidential Citation from the American Psychological Association.

Lawrence Scahill, M.S.N., Ph.D., is a professor of nursing and child psychiatry and director of the Research Unit on Pediatric Psychopharmacology (RUPP) at the Child Study Center, Yale University School of Nursing, New Haven, Connecticut. The Yale RUPP is part of a multisite consortium focused on developing and testing new treatments for children with autism and related disorders. Dr. Scahill is also actively involved in treatment research in Tourette's syndrome as part of the Behavioral Sciences Consortium and the Clinical Trials Consortium. Dr. Scahill received his master's degree in psychiatric nursing and his doctorate in epidemiology at Yale University. He joined the faculty of the Child Study Center in 1989 and was appointed assistant professor in 1997, associate professor in 2000, and professor in 2006. Dr. Scahill serves on the Medical Advisory Board of the Tourette Syndrome Association, is on the editorial board of several journals, and is the author of over 150 articles on autism, Tourette's syndrome, ADHD, and obsessive-compulsive disorder.

Laura Schreibman, Ph.D., is a distinguished professor of psychology at the University of California, San Diego, in La Jolla, where she has been on the faculty since 1984. She earned her doctorate at the University of California, Los Angeles, where she focused on the field of behavior analysis and treatment of children with autism. Her research since her degree has continued in the same vein, and she currently directs a federally funded research program focusing on the experimental analysis and treatment of autism. Her general research interests have included the analysis of speech and attentional deficits, generalization of behavior change, parent training, self-management, peer training, and issues of assessment. Her current lines of funded research involve evaluation of pictorial versus verbal communication teaching strategies for very young children with autism (funded by the National Institute of Mental Health), development of classroom Pivotal Response Training strategies (funded by the Department of Education), and the development of individualized treatments for children with autism and their families. She also heads a new research program to assess brain correlates to treatment outcome for infants with autism (a Core of an Autism Center of Excellence Award funded by the National Institutes of Health). She is the author of over 120 research articles and book chapters, as well as 3 books. Her latest book is *The Science and Fiction of Autism.*

Wendy K. Silverman, Ph.D., A.B.P.P., is professor of psychology at Florida International University in Miami. She is the recipient of several grants from the National Institute of Mental Health aimed at developing and evaluating psychosocial treatments for anxiety disorders in children. She has published 4 books on the topic of children and anxiety disorders and more than 150 scientific articles and book chapters. Dr. Silverman is the former editor of the

Journal of Clinical Child and Adolescent Psychology, current associate editor of the *Journal of Consulting and Clinical Psychology*, and past president of the American Psychological Association's Division 53, Society of Clinical Child and Adolescent Psychology. She also serves as chair of the child intervention National Institute of Mental Health review panel.

Lacramioara Spetie, M.D., is an assistant professor of psychiatry at the Ohio State University, Columbus, where she previously completed her residency and fellowship in child and adolescent psychiatry. She has been practicing psychiatry for over 10 years, with an interest in the areas of ADHD and mood disorders in children and adolescents. She has coauthored several papers reviewing the clinical presentation and treatment of ADHD.

Kevin D. Stark, Ph.D., is a professor at the University of Texas, Austin, and a licensed psychologist in the state of Texas. He earned a doctorate in school psychology from the University of Wisconsin in 1985. He has been a member of the scientific advisory boards to a number of National Institute of Mental Health (NIMH)–sponsored clinical trials of interventions for childhood disorders. He has trained mental health workers across the nation and in Western Europe in evidence-based treatments for depressed and anxious youth. He conducts research that is designed to evaluate and build models of depressive disorders in children. In addition, he conducts research into the assessment and treatment of depressive disorders in children. He is currently analyzing the results from a 5-year NIMH-funded study evaluating the relative efficacy of cognitive-behavioral therapy with and without parent training relative to a minimal contact control condition for depressed 9- to 13-year-old girls. He has published a book, written 68 articles and chapters, presented 83 papers at professional conferences, conducted many workshops for professional organizations, and received approximately $3 million in grant funding to date. He received the Lightner-Witmer Young Scholar Award in 1990 from the American Psychological Association and is a Beck Institute Scholar.

Hans Steiner, Dr. med. univ., F.A.P.A., F.A.A.C.A.P., F.A.P.M., is a professor in psychiatry and behavioral sciences, child and adolescent psychiatry, and human development at Stanford University School of Medicine, Palo Alto, California. He is one of the leading advocates of the developmental psychopathology model within psychiatry. He is an internationally known expert in the subfields of maladaptive aggression, disruptive behavior disorders and juvenile delinquency, personality development, and the overlap between primary care and psychiatry. He has led and has served on several task forces advising and consulting with the state of California and local governments on issues of health care for youth in juvenile justice systems. He is the principal author of the current practice parameters for the diagnosis and treatment of conduct disorders and oppositional defiant disorders of the American Academy of Child and Adolescent Psychiatry.

Susan E. Swedo, M.D., received her medical degree from Southern Illinois University School of Medicine and completed a pediatrics residency at Children's Memorial Hospital in Chicago. Dr. Swedo served as chief of adolescent medicine for Northwestern University until 1986, when she joined Dr. Judith L. Rapoport's laboratory at the National Institute of Mental Health (NIMH), Bethesda, Maryland. Dr. Swedo is a tenured investigator in the NIMH Intramural Research Program and serves as chief of the Pediatrics and Developmental Neuropsychiatry Branch, which conducts research on the causes and treatment of pediatric neuropsychiatric disorders, including obsessive-compulsive disorder (OCD), anxiety disorders, and autistic spectrum disorders. Dr. Swedo and her colleagues were the first to identify a postinfectious subtype of OCD, known as PANDAS (pediatric autoimmune neuropsychiatric disorders associated with streptococcal infection). This line of research has resulted in several novel treatment and prevention strategies for childhood-onset OCD, as well as a patent for a biological marker that can be used to identify at-risk children. The recipient of numerous awards, including the American Academy of Child and Adolescent Psychiatry Award for Scientific Achievement and the American College of Neuropsychopharmacology International Award for Clinical Research, Dr. Swedo is the author of more than 100 professional books and articles. She is also the coauthor of two trade books: *It's Not All in Your Head* and *Is It Just a Phase?* (a parent's guide to childhood behavior problems).

Eva M. Szigethy, M.D., Ph.D., is an assistant professor of psychiatry and pediatrics at the University of Pittsburgh School of Medicine and is the director of the Medical Coping Clinic in the Department of Gastroenterology at Children's Hospital of Pittsburgh, Pittsburgh, Pennsylvania. Since completing her child psychiatry fellowship at Harvard University/Boston Children's Hospital, she has specialized in the treatment of emotional and behavioral challenges in children and adolescents with gastrointestinal diseases. She has developed a cognitive-behavioral intervention for depressed youth with chronic physical illness and is currently testing the efficacy of this intervention in youth with inflammatory bowel disease. Her work is funded by the Crohn's and Colitis Foundation of America, a National Institute of Mental Health–funded R01 grant, and a prestigious National Institutes of Health Director's Innovator Award.

Julia W. Tossell, M.D., is a staff clinician with the Child Psychiatry Branch, National Institute of Mental Health, Bethesda, Maryland. Dr. Tossell is responsible for the clinical care of the subjects enrolled in inpatient research protocols. These protocols focus on the diagnosis, treatment, and longitudinal follow-up of childhood-onset schizophrenia. She is also involved in ongoing outpatient studies of children with attention-deficit/hyperactivity disorder, obsessive-compulsive disorder, and sex chromosome variations.

Andrea M. Victor, Ph.D., is a licensed psychologist and an assistant professor in the Child and Adolescent Anxiety and Mood Disorders Clinic at the University of Minnesota Medical School in Minneapolis. She specializes in providing cognitive-behavioral therapy (CBT) to treat children and adolescents diagnosed with anxiety and mood disorders. In addition, she teaches and supervises clinical psychology interns and child and adolescent psychiatry fellows in the practice of CBT. Dr. Victor's primary research interests include the assessment and treatment of childhood anxiety disorders. Her publications include peer-reviewed journal articles and textbook chapters pertaining to the description and treatment of children with anxiety disorders.

Karen Dineen Wagner, M.D., Ph.D., is the Marie B. Gale Professor and Vice-Chair of the Department of Psychiatry and Behavioral Sciences and director of the Division of Child and Adolescent Psychiatry at the University of Texas Medical Branch in Galveston. Dr. Wagner is an internationally recognized expert in the pharmacologic treatment of childhood mood disorders. Her work has led to the development of evidence-based treatments for children and adolescents with major depression and bipolar disorder. Dr. Wagner is the recipient of numerous honors, including an honorary doctorate from State University of New York; Distinguished Alumna, State University of New York School of Medicine at Stony Brook; Psychiatric Excellence Award from the Texas Society of Psychiatric Physicians; and the Blanche F. Ittleson Award for Research in Child and Adolescent Psychiatry from the American Psychiatric Association. Dr. Wagner has served in leadership positions in professional organizations and has been a member of the National Advisory Mental Health Council of the National Institutes of Health. She receives research support from the National Institute of Mental Health and serves as consultant to or on the advisory board of various pharmaceutical companies.

John T. Walkup, M.D., is an associate professor of psychiatry and behavioral sciences in the Division of Child and Adolescent Psychiatry at Johns Hopkins Medical Institutions in Baltimore, Maryland. He currently serves as deputy director of the Division of Child and Adolescent Psychiatry and medical director of the National Institute of Mental Health–funded Research Unit of Pediatric Psychopharmacology. Dr. Walkup is the author of a number of articles and book chapters on psychopharmacology, Tourette's syndrome, obsessive-compulsive disorder, and other anxiety disorders.

B. Timothy Walsh, M.D., is the Ruane Professor of Pediatric Psychopharmacology in the Department of Psychiatry at the College of Physicians and Surgeons, Columbia University, and Director of the Division of Clinical Therapeutics at the New York State Psychiatric Institute in New York, New York. Dr. Walsh is a member of the DSM-V Task Force and chairs the Eating Disorders Workgroup for DSM-V. He is a past president of the Academy for Eating Disorders, president of the Eating Disorders Research Society, and an associate editor of the *International Journal of Eating Disorders*.

Bruce Waslick, M.D., is a staff child psychiatrist in the Division of Child Behavioral Health at Baystate Medical Center in Springfield, Massachusetts, and an associate professor of psychiatry at Tufts University School of Medicine in Boston, Massachusetts. Dr. Waslick has had extensive research experience in understanding the etiology and treatment of pediatric mood, anxiety, and behavioral disorders, and he was a site principal investigator for the National Institute of Mental Health (NIMH)–funded Treatment for Adolescents with Depression Study. Dr. Waslick has been the principal investigator on federally funded (NIMH), industry-funded (Eli Lilly, Johnson & Johnson, Somerset), and foundation-funded research grants and contracts.

James Waxmonsky, M.D., is a board-certified child psychiatrist who is on the faculty of psychiatry at the State University of New York at Buffalo (UB) as well as the staff at the Women and Children's Hospital of Buffalo. He completed his child psychiatry training at Massachusetts General Hospital, where he worked on multiple clinical trials for pediatric and adult ADHD. Currently, he collaborates with Dr. William Pelham at the UB Center for Children and Families on the integration of behavioral and pharmacologic treatments for children with ADHD and serves as an investigator on several federally funded grants in this area. Additional research interests include the treatment of children with ADHD and comorbid affective illness and the long-term safety of stimulant medications.

Carolyn Webster-Stratton, Ph.D., is professor and director of the Parenting Clinic at the University of Washington in Seattle. She is also the developer and author of The Incredible Years programs for parents, teachers, and children, and has been researching these interventions for the past 28 years. She and her coinvestigator Dr. M. Jamila Reid have recently completed a 5-year study evaluating the effectiveness of a classroom-based social and emotional curriculum delivered by trained teachers combined with a school-based parent program. Her current National Institutes of Health–funded research involves testing the Incredible Years programs for parents and teachers with children who have been diagnosed with ADHD, as well as studying the dissemination of The Incredible Years parent program with high-risk families in California.

Lynn M. Wegner, M.D., F.A.A.P., is associate clinical professor and director for the Developmental/Behavioral Pediatrics Division of the Pediatrics Department at the University of North Carolina at Chapel Hill School of Medicine. She is immediate past-chair of the American Academy of Pediatrics (AAP) Section on Developmental and Behavioral Pediatrics and is a consultant to the AAP Task Force on Mental Health. As part of her subspecialty practice, she routinely has to identify the interplay between children's language, attention, and memory abilities as they impact daily functioning and mood regulation. She has given numerous talks before national groups and has written peer-reviewed articles about identifying developmental differences and accompanying affective disorders and functional impact in daily life.

Elizabeth B. Weller, M.D., is professor of psychiatry and pediatrics at the University of Pennsylvania in Philadelphia. She established the Child and Adolescent Psychiatry Mood and Anxiety Disorders Center at the Children's Hospital of Philadelphia in the Department of Child and Adolescent Psychiatry and is involved in multiple multicenter studies sponsored by the National Institute of Mental Health and pharmaceutical industries. Dr. Weller's research interests include grief in prepubertal children and adolescents, disorders in families of depressed hospitalized prepubertal children, suicide in depressed prepubertal children, clinical characteristics and treatment of bipolar children and adolescents, and velocardiofacial syndrome. She has conducted mood disorder research with her spouse, Dr. Ronald A. Weller, since residency training. Since 1983, they have been studying bereavement in children and adolescents and their surviving parents. They have received National Institute of Mental Health funding to study prepubertal children and adolescents and to follow up on these subjects 5 years after loss. Dr. Weller has published extensively on mood disorders and bereavement in children and adolescents, and has been principal investigator for several clinical research studies examining depression and early-onset bipolar disorder in children and adolescents. She has edited several books, including *Current Perspectives on Major Depressive Disorders in Children* and *Psychiatric Disorders in Children and Adolescents*, and is the principal author of the *Children's Interview for Psychiatric Syndromes*, a diagnostic tool that explores 21 psychiatric syndromes found in children and adolescents.

Ronald A. Weller, M.D., is on the faculty of psychiatry and neuroscience at the University of Pennsylvania in Philadelphia. He has served as president of the American Academy of Clinical Psychiatrists and as a consultant to the American Psychiatric Association on major depression. Dr. Weller has published extensively on issues of children's mental health, including on the topics of bereavement, depression, and mania, among others. Dr. Weller's research interests include grief in prepubertal children and adolescents, disorders in families of depressed hospitalized prepubertal children, suicide in depressed prepubertal children, clinical characteristics and treatment of bipolar children and adolescents, and velocardiofacial syndrome. He and his spouse, Dr. Elizabeth B. Weller, have had National Institute of Mental Health funding to study the treatment of depressed children, as well as funding from the pharmaceutical industry to test new pharmacologic agents. Dr. Weller has been principal investigator for several clinical research studies, among them examinations of bereavement and bipolar disorder in children and adolescents. Dr. Weller is a coauthor of the *Children's Interview for Psychiatric Syndromes.*

Karen C. Wells, Ph.D., is associate professor of medical psychology in the Department of Psychiatry at Duke University Medical Center in Durham, North Carolina, where she is also director of the Family Studies Program and Clinic and director of psychology internship. Prior to her tenure at Duke, she was on the psychiatry department faculties of the George Washington University School of Medicine and the University of Pittsburgh School of Medicine. Her research has focused on the development, evaluation, and dissemination of psychosocial treatments for child and adolescent psychiatric disorders, including attention-deficit/hyperactivity disorder. She has focused especially on parent- and family-based approaches to these disorders. She has been the lead investigator of the Duke site for the Multi-Modal Treatment of ADHD study and has participated as an investigator in several of the large National Institute of Mental Health–funded multisite clinical trials focusing on treatment of child and adolescent psychopathology.

Helen Nelson Willard, M.Ed., CCC-SLP, is a speech-language pathologist with 35 years of experience: 30 years in the public school setting and 5 years as a private practitioner. She is licensed to practice in the state of North Carolina and holds the Certificate of Clinical Competence in speech-language pathology from the American Speech-Language-Hearing Association. She received her bachelor's degree in education from the University of Miami in Coral Gables, Florida; completed graduate work at the University of North Carolina at Chapel Hill; and received her master's degree in speech pathology from North Carolina Central University in Durham. Mrs. Willard's 30 years of experience in the public school setting provided her with the opportunity to develop and implement program guidelines, to supervise county-wide projects, to mentor colleagues, and to provide numerous workshops on phoneme awareness and literacy interventions. She is the owner and sole practitioner of Speech-Language Professional Services, a private practice committed to making a positive difference in the lives of children and adults. Located in Cary, North Carolina, her practice provides a full range of diagnostic and therapeutic services, with unique and specialized services in the area of language-based reading deficits.

Jeffrey J. Wilson, M.D., is assistant professor of clinical psychiatry at Columbia University and the New York State Psychiatric Institute in New York, New York, and he is in private practice in Hackensack, New Jersey. Dr. Wilson is a graduate of Rutgers University and the University of Medicine and Dentistry of New Jersey. He completed a psychiatry residency at the Albert Einstein College of Medicine, child and adolescent psychiatry residency at Stanford University, and addiction psychiatry residency at Columbia University. Dr. Wilson was a recipient of the National Institute on Drug Abuse K23 Mentored Career Development Award. He has published several articles and chapters related to child and adolescent conduct disorder, ADHD, and substance abuse.

Nancy C. Winters, M.D., is an associate professor in the Department of Psychiatry, Division of Public Psychiatry, at Oregon Health and Science University (OHSU), Portland, where she also practices child/adolescent psychiatry and adult psychiatry. She is also the chief psychiatrist for Children's Mental Health and Addictions for the state of Oregon. Dr. Winters has been a leader in national efforts to develop organized systems of care for children and adolescents with serious mental and emotional disorders, including membership on the American Academy of Child and Adolescent Psychiatry Work Group on Community-Based System of Care since 1994. Dr. Winters has been active in resident education and served as child psychiatry residency training director at OHSU from 1998 to 2007. She has contributed to the child psychiatric literature in the areas of community systems of care, child psychiatric rating scales, childhood depression, case formulation, and infant and toddler feeding disorders. She was involved in development of widely used level of care assessment scales for children and adolescents. She has a long-standing interest in psychotherapy and is currently a candidate at the Oregon Psychoanalytic Institute.

Sharlene A. Wolchik, Ph.D., is a professor in the Department of Psychology at Arizona State University, Tempe. She completed her psychology doctoral training at Rutgers University. Dr. Wolchik has been a leader in the area of children's responses to parental divorce for the past 20 years. She has been awarded numerous grants from the National Institute of Mental Health and the National Institute of Child Development. Her research has examined factors that affect resilience in children who face the family transitions of parental divorce or parental bereavement. In addition, she has developed and evaluated preventive interventions for children from divorced families and parentally bereaved youth. She recently received the Stanley Cohen Distinguished Research Award from the Association of Family and Conciliation Courts for her work in divorce.

Douglas W. Woods, Ph.D., received his doctorate in clinical psychology from Western Michigan University in 1999. He is a recognized expert in the assessment and treatment of tic disorders and trichotillomania and is currently an associate professor and director of clinical training at the University of Wisconsin–Milwaukee. Dr. Woods has authored or coauthored over 100 papers and chapters. He has edited two books describing behavioral interventions for tic disorders and trichotillomania and another book on contemporary behavior analytic models of psychiatric disorders. He has presented his work nationally and internationally in over 170 conference presentations and invited talks, is on the editorial boards of 7 different journals, and has served as an ad hoc reviewer for over 28 different journals across the disciplines of psychiatry, psychology, pharmacology, and neurology. Dr. Woods is the first psychologist ever to serve as a member of the Tourette Syndrome Association's (TSA) Medical Advisory Board, and serves on the Scientific Advisory Board of the Trichotillomania Learning Center (TLC). He has been funded by the TSA Grants program, and TLC Grants program, and is currently funded by the National Institutes of Health as part of two separate multisite research projects investigating the efficacy of behavior therapy for children and adults with Tourette's syndrome.

Charles H. Zeanah, M.D., is the Sellars Polchow Professor of Psychiatry and vice-chair and chief of child and adolescent psychiatry at Tulane University School of Medicine, New Orleans, Louisiana. Dr. Zeanah has a long-standing interest in infant mental health, and his research and clinical interests concern the effects of abuse and serious deprivation on young children, parent-child attachment, psychopathology in early childhood, and infant-parent relationships. He has directed an ongoing community-based intervention for maltreated infants and toddlers in the New Orleans area for the past 14 years. He is also co-principal investigator of the Bucharest Early Intervention Project, designed to evaluate foster care as an intervention for institutionalized young children. In each of these settings, he has studied and treated young children with serious disturbances of attachment.

Alison Zisser, M.S., is a graduate student in the Department of Clinical and Health Psychology at the University of Florida, Gainesville. Her research focuses on family-based behavioral interventions for young children with ADHD and the impact of parental ADHD in their treatment. She is a graduate research assistant in the University of Florida Child Study Laboratory, where she serves as a parent child interaction therapy (PCIT) therapist on a National Institute of Mental Health–funded study of group versus individual PCIT for young children with ADHD and disruptive behavior.

DISCLOSURE OF COMPETING INTERESTS

The following contributors to this book have indicated a financial interest in or other affiliation with a commercial supporter, a manufacturer of a commercial product, a provider of a commercial service, a nongovernmental organization, and/or a government agency, as listed below:

J. Stuart Ablon, Ph.D. — Dr. Ablon receives royalties for publications from Guilford Press.

Anne Marie Albano, Ph.D., A.B.P.P. — Dr. Albano receives grant support from the National Institute of Mental Health. She receives royalties for publications from Oxford University Press and Guilford Press.

L. Eugene Arnold, M.D., M.Ed. — Dr. Arnold receives research funding from Neuropharm, Eli Lilly, and Shire; is consultant for Novartis, Organon, Targacept, Neuropharm, Abbott, and Shire; and is on the Speakers Bureau for McNeil, Novartis, and Shire.

Boris Birmaher, M.D. — Dr. Birmaher's research is funded by the National Institute of Mental Health. He has given invited lectures sponsored by the following pharmaceutical companies: JAZZ Pharmaceuticals, Solvay Pharmaceuticals, and Abcomm. He has received royalties for publications from Random House.

Bruce Black, M.D. — Dr. Black has received speaker's fees from Eli Lilly.

Oscar G. Bukstein, M.D., M.P.H. — Dr. Bukstein serves as a consultant to McNeil Pediatrics and Shire Pharmaceuticals. He is on the Speakers Bureau for McNeil Pediatrics and Novartis. Other disclosures include CME: CMP Media, Haymarket Media, i3 CME, Medscape, Information Television Network, and SciMedica Group.

Gabrielle A. Carlson, M.D. — Dr. Carlson has research grants from the National Institute of Mental Health, Eli Lilly, BMS, and Otsuka. She is on advisory boards for those companies as well.

Barbara J. Coffey, M.D., M.S. — Dr. Coffey has had research support from Bristol-Myers Squibb, Boehringer Ingelheim, the National Institute of Mental Health, and the Tourette Syndrome Association. She has served on advisory boards for Eli Lilly and JAZZ Pharmaceuticals.

Judith A. Cohen, M.D. — Dr. Cohen receives funds from the National Institute of Mental Health, Substance Abuse and Mental Health Services Administration. She also receives royalties from Guilford Press.

Christoph U. Correll, M.D. — Dr. Correll has received speaker and/or consultancy honoraria from AstraZeneca, Bristol-Myers Squibb, Eli Lilly, Organon, Otsuka, Pfizer, Supernus, and Vanda.

Helen Egger, M.D. — Dr. Egger has received funding from the National Institute of Mental Health, National Institute on Drug Abuse, Autism Speaks, and NARSAD. She does not receive any money or other support from industry.

Graham J. Emslie, M.D.—Dr. Emslie receives research support from the National Institute of Mental Health, Eli Lilly, Organon, Shire, Somerset, Forest Laboratories, and Biobehavioral Diagnostics. He is a consultant for Eli Lilly, GlaxoSmithKline, Wyeth-Ayerst, Shire, and Biobehavioral Diagnostics, and is on the Speakers Bureau for McNeil.

Sheila M. Eyberg, Ph.D., A.B.P.P.—Dr. Eyberg mentions the Eyberg Child Behavior Inventory in her contribution to this volume. She receives royalties on the sale of this instrument from Psychological Assessment Resources.

Robert L. Findling, M.D.—Dr. Findling receives or has received research support from, acted as a consultant to, and/or served on a speaker's bureau for Abbott, Addrenex, AstraZeneca, Bristol-Myers Squibb, Forest, GlaxoSmith-Kline, Johnson & Johnson, Lilly, Neuropharm, Novartis, Organon, Otsuka, Pfizer, Sanofi-Aventis, Sepracore, Shire, Solvay, Supernus Pharmaceuticals, and Wyeth.

Cathryn A. Galanter, M.D.—Dr. Galanter receives grant support from the National Institute of Mental Health and is a member of the REACH Institute Primary Pediatric Psychopharmacology Steering Committee.

Ross W. Greene, Ph.D.—Dr. Greene has relationships with publishers of his three books: *The Explosive Child* (Harper Collins), *Treating Explosive Kids* (Guilford Press), and *Lost at School* (Scribner).

Laurence L. Greenhill, M.D.—Dr. Greenhill has received research funding to study risperidone from Johnson & Johnson Pharmaceuticals and has an investigator-initiated grant to study aripiprazole by Otsuka. He has a consultant arrangement with Pfizer Pharmaceuticals to serve as chair of their Ziprasidone Pediatric Clinical Trials Data and Safety Monitoring Board.

Allison G. Harvey, Ph.D.—Dr. Harvey has served on the Speakers Bureau for Sleep Medicine Education Initiative and has served as a consultant to Actelion.

Scott W. Henggeler, Ph.D.—Dr. Henggeler is a shareholder in MST Services, which has an exclusive licensing agreement through the Medical University of South Carolina for the transport of MST technology and intellectual property.

Peter S. Jensen, M.D.—Dr. Jensen receives grant support from McNeil Consumer and Specialty Pharmaceuticals and Novartis. He is a consultant and/or advisor to Cephalon, Janssen Pharmaceutica Products, Janssen-Ortho, and UCB Pharma. He serves on the Speakers Bureau for Cephalon, Cmed, Janssen Pharmaceutica Products, Janssen-Ortho, and UCB Pharma. He is also a stockholder in Eli Lilly.

Paramjit T. Joshi, M.D.—Dr. Joshi has grant support from the National Institute of Mental Health.

Yifrah Kaminer, M.D. M.B.A. — Dr. Kaminer receives grant support from the National Institute on Alcohol Abuse and Alcoholism.

Philip C. Kendall, Ph.D., A.B.P.P. — Dr. Kendall has no conflicts of interest in connection with his contribution to this volume, but he does receive royalties from publications of books on the topic.

Robert A. Kowatch, M.D., Ph.D. — Dr. Kowatch receives research support from Bristol-Myers Squibb, the Stanley Research Foundation, the National Institute of Mental Health, and the National Institute of Child Health and Human Development. He serves on the Speakers Bureau for Astra-Zeneca and Abbott and is a consultant and/or on the advisory board for Creative Educational Concepts, CABF, Abbott, Sanofi-Aventis, GS&K, and Medscape. He is also editor of *Current Psychiatry*.

Christopher J. Kratochvil, M.D. — Dr. Kratochvil receives grant support from Eli Lilly, McNeil, Shire, Abbott, Pfizer, Somerset, and Cephalon, and also receives study drug for a National Institute of Mental Health–funded study from Eli Lilly. He is a consultant for Eli Lilly, AstraZeneca, Abbott, and Pfizer. He is also editor of the *Brown University Child and Adolescent Psychopharmacology Update*, member of the REACH Institute Primary Pediatric Psychopharmacology Steering Committee, member of the American Professional Society for ADHD and Related Disorders Board of Directors, and member of the CME Outfitters Professional Advisory Board. Dr. Kratochvil is assistant editor of the *Journal of the American Academy of Child and Adolescent Psychiatry*, chair of the American Academy of Child and Adolescent Psychiatry Pediatric Psychopharmacology Initiative, and member of the American Academy of Child and Adolescent Psychiatry Council.

Daniel le Grange, Ph.D. — Dr. le Grange receives royalties from Guilford Press.

Richard P. Malone, M.D. — No funding was provided for the preparation of his contribution to this volume. Dr. Malone has received funds to conduct studies on antipsychotic medications in autism from Bristol-Myers Squibb, Johnson & Johnson, Pfizer, and Lilly. He has also received funding from the U.S. Food and Drug Administration's Orphan Product Division and the National Institute of Mental Health to conduct research in autism.

John S. March, M.D., M.P.H. — Dr. March receives research support (PI/Invest) from Eli Lilly and has drug supplied for a National Institutes of Health study from Pfizer and Lilly. He receives consulting fees from Pfizer, Wyeth, Lilly, and GlaxoSmithKline; serves as a scientific advisor for Pfizer and Lilly; and serves on the data safety monitoring boards of Astra-Zeneca and Johnson & Johnson. His National Institute of Mental Health–funded federal disclosures include Treatment for Adolescents with Depression Study (TADS), Child/Adolescent Multimodal Study (CAMS), Pediatric OCD Treatment Study

(POTS I, II and Jr), Research Unit on Pediatric Psychopharmacology—Psychosocial Intervention (RUPP-PI), Child and Adolescent Psychiatry Trials Network (CAPTN), and K24. Dr. March also has stock in MedAvante. An additional possible competing interest is his Multidimensional Anxiety Scale for Children (Multi-Health Systems).

David A. Mrazek, M.D., F.R.C.Psych. — Dr. Mrazek has developed intellectual property at the Mayo Clinic that has been exclusively licensed by AssureRx.

Mani Pavuluri, M.D., Ph.D. — Dr. Pavuluri has no conflict of interest to declare in relation to the written material published in this book. Her research work is funded by NIH/NCRR K23 RR018638-01, NIMH MH077852, NIMH P50 HD055751, the NARSAD Foundation, the National Institute of Child Health and Human Development, the Colbeth Foundation, the Dana Foundation, and GlaxoSmithKline-NeuroHealth. She receives study medications from Abbott Pharmaceuticals and Janssen Research Foundation.

John Piacentini, Ph.D., A.B.P.P. — Dr. Piacentini receives book royalties from Oxford University Press for a child obsessive-compulsive disorder treatment manual, which is referenced in the manuscript.

Lawrence Scahill, M.S.N., Ph.D. — Dr. Scahill serves as a consultant to Janssen, Bristol-Myers Squibb, Supernus, and Neuropharm.

Wendy K. Silverman, Ph.D., A.B.P.P. — Dr. Silverman's work for this project was supported by grants from the National Institute of Mental Health (R01MH63997 and K24MH073696). She receives royalties from Oxford University Press, publisher of the Anxiety Disorders Interview Schedule for DSM-IV: Child and Parent Versions.

Hans Steiner, Dr. med. univ., F.A.P.A., F.A.A.C.A.P., F.A.P.M. — Dr. Steiner's pharmaceutical relationships are as follows: speaker for Abbott, AstraZeneca, Janssen, and Eli Lilly; advisor/consultant for Abbott, Janssen, and Otsuka; unrestricted educational grant from Abbott, Janssen, Wyeth-Ayerst, Solvay, GlaxoSmithKline, McNeil-Alza, Novartis, Forest, and Pfizer; and research grant from Pfizer, Abbott, and Janssen.

Karen Dineen Wagner, M.D., Ph.D. — Dr. Wagner receives research support from the National Institute of Mental Health. She serves as a consultant and/or on the advisory board for Abbott Laboratories, AstraZeneca, Bristol-Myers Squibb, Eli Lilly, Forest Laboratories, Johnson & Johnson, Otsuka, Solvay, and Wyeth.

John T. Walkup, M.D. — Dr. Walkup receives grant support from Pfizer, Lilly, and Abbott. He serves as a consultant for GlaxoSmithKline.

B. Timothy Walsh, M.D. — Dr. Walsh received funding from Abbott Laboratories to conduct a literature review for the peer-reviewed article "Placebo Response in Acute Mania" in the *Journal of Clinical Psychiatry.*

Bruce Waslick, M.D. — Dr. Waslick receives research support from Eli Lilly, Johnson & Johnson, and Somerset Pharmaceuticals.

James Waxmonsky, M.D. — Dr. Waxmonsky has received research support from Eli Lilly. He has served on the Speakers Board for Novartis.

Carolyn Webster-Stratton, Ph.D. — Dr. Webster-Stratton has a potential financial conflict of interest in the dissemination of the Incredible Years programs, as she stands to gain from a favorable report. Therefore, she has voluntarily agreed to distance herself from critical research activities (primary data handling and analyses), and the University of Washington has approved these arrangements.

Douglas W. Woods, Ph.D. — Dr. Woods has been a co-primary investigator on two separate National Institutes of Health–funded grants investigating the efficacy of behavior therapy in children and adults. He is a member of the Tourette Syndrome Association Medical Advisory Board and the Trichotillomania Learning Center's Scientific Advisory Board.

The following contributors have no competing interests to disclose:

Jean Addington, Ph.D.
Andrea Auther, Ph.D.
Susan Bacalman, M.S.W.
Gail A. Bernstein, M.D.
Caroline Lewczyk Boxmeyer, Ph.D.
David A. Brent, M.D.
John V. Campo, M.D.
Bruce F. Chorpita, Ph.D.
Greg Clarke, Ph.D.
Christine A. Conelea, M.S.
Cheryl M. Corcoran, M.D.
Barbara A. Cornblatt, Ph.D., M.B.A.
Sarah A. Crawley, M.A.
Kathryn R. Cullen, M.D.
Lisa M. Cullins, M.D.
Ronald E. Dahl, M.D.
Tara L. Deliberto, B.S.
David R. DeMaso, M.D.
Thomas A. Dixon, B.S.
Stacy S. Drury, M.D., Ph.D.
Jeffery N. Epstein, Ph.D.
Christianne Esposito-Smythers, Ph.D.
E. Blake Finkelson, B.A.

Mary A. Fristad, Ph.D., A.B.P.P.
Jami M. Furr, M.A.
Mary Kay Gill, R.N., M.S.N., J.D.
Mary Margaret Gleason, M.D.
Daniel A. Gorman, M.D., F.R.C.P.C.
Angela S. Guarda, M.D.
Robert L Hendren, D.O.
Stephen P. Hinshaw, Ph.D.
Brian L. Isakson, Ph.D.
Sandra J. Kaplan, M.D.
Niranjan S. Karnik, M.D., Ph.D.
Courtney Pierce Keeton, Ph.D.
Clarice J. Kestenbaum, M.D.
Dena A. Klein, Ph.D.
Rachel G. Klein, Ph.D.
Penelope Knapp, M.D.
Harvey N. Kranzler, M.D.
Sanjiv Kumra, M.D., M.S.
Joshua M. Langberg, Ph.D.
Christopher M. Layne, Ph.D.
Patricia K. Leebens, M.D.
Alicia F. Lieberman, Ph.D.
John E. Lochman, Ph.D., A.B.P.P.
Joan L. Luby, M.D.
Anthony P. Mannarino, Ph.D.
Carla E. Marin, M.S.
Jon McClellan, M.D.
Alec L. Miller, Psy.D.
Jodi A. Mindell, Ph.D., C.B.S.M.
Robert Miranda, Jr., Ph.D.
Matthew K. Nock, Ph.D.
Judith A. Owens, M.D., M.P.H., D'A.B.S.M.
William E. Pelham, Jr., Ph.D., A.B.P.P.
Bradley S. Peterson, M.D.
Cynthia R. Pfeffer, M.D.
Daniel Pine, M.D.
Nicole Powell, Ph.D., M.P.H.
Frank W. Putnam, M.D.
Judith L. Rapoport, M.D.
M. Jamila Reid, Ph.D.
Mark A. Riddle, M.D.

Paula Riggs, M.D.
Irwin N. Sandler, Ph.D.
Laura Schreibman, Ph.D.
Lacramioara Spetie, M.D.
Kevin D. Stark, Ph.D.
Susan E. Swedo, M.D.
Eva M. Szigethy, M.D., Ph.D.
Julia W. Tossell, M.D.
Andrea M. Victor, Ph.D.
Lynn M. Wegner, M.D., F.A.A.P.
Elizabeth B. Weller, M.D.
Ronald A. Weller, M.D.
Karen C. Wells, Ph.D.
Helen Nelson Willard, M.Ed., CCC-SLP
Jeffrey J. Wilson, M.D.
Nancy C. Winters, M.D.
Sharlene A. Wolchik, Ph.D.
Charles H. Zeanah, M.D.
Alison Zisser, M.S.

Subject Index

Page numbers printed in **boldface** type refer to tables or figures.

Index of Cases
by Diagnosis